Morphological and Functional Aspects of Immunity

ADVANCES IN EXPERIMENTAL MEDICINE AND BIOLOGY

Morphological and Functional Aspects of Immunity

Proceedings of the Third International Conference
on Lymphatic Tissue and Germinal Centers held in
Uppsala, Sweden, September 1–4, 1970

Edited by

Kerstin Lindahl-Kiessling

Institute for Medical Genetics
University of Uppsala
Uppsala, Sweden

G. Alm

Department of Histology
Institute of Human Anatomy
University of Uppsala
Uppsala, Sweden

and

M. G. Hanna, Jr.

Biology Division
Oak Ridge National Laboratories
Oak Ridge, Tennessee

ℚ PLENUM PRESS · NEW YORK-LONDON · 1971

Library of Congress Catalog Card Number 75-148822

SBN 306-39012-4

© 1971 Plenum Press, New York
A Division of Plenum Publishing Corporation
227 West 17th Street, New York, N.Y. 10011

United Kingdom edition published by Plenum Press, London
A Division of Plenum Publishing Company, Ltd.
Davis House (4th Floor), 8 Scrubs Lane, Harlesden, NW10 6SE, England

Printed in the United States of America

PREFACE

The Third International Conference on Lymphatic Tissue and Germinal Centers in Immune Reactions was held at the University of Uppsala in Sweden, September 1-4, 1970. The conference is obliged to Professor K. E. Fichtelius for his initiative in establishing the meeting, as well as for the assistance of his staff at the Department of Histology in organizing the meetings.

At the University of Uppsala inquiries into the lymphatic system go back to the 17th century and are marked by milestones, such as Olof Rudbeck's discovery of the thoracic duct in 1651 and August Hammar's fundamental work on the thymus in the beginning of this century. So one is justified to say that the conference gathered on historical ground. The organizing committee, naturally, hopes that the achievements presented at the conference will contribute to and provide significant advances in the history of lymphatic research.

The material presented in this volume displays a great diversity of methods and the ingenuity of different investigators in their experimental designs. It is also apparent that contemporary research on lymphatic tissues or cells no longer recognizes the artificial borderline of morphologic *versus* functional. It has become a multi-disciplinary affair in which an increasing number of different specialists are working closely together. Apparently this is one reason why so many new and important discoveries have been made recently.

Primarily, the proceedings – as should be – reflect the communications between and the achievements of a representative sample of investigators who are using different tools in their research on the lymphatic system. Also, the ascertainment value of this sample is probably very high. Nevertheless, several sections, such as those dealing with phylogeny and ontogeny of immune response, regulation of lymphoid function, cancer immunology and immunosuppression, should be of interest to a broader audience of biologists, physicians and clinical research workers.

The comprehensive invited lectures given by Drs. J. J. Trentin, J. Thorbecke and J. F. A. P. Miller were highlights during the conference and are gratefully acknowledged. Thanks are also due to Drs. C. C Congdon, O. Mäkelä, R. Peterson and L. Fiore-Donati, who acted as mediators during the discussions.

In particular, the organizing committee wishes to acknowledge the assistance of T. Brenning, O. Bäck, R. Bäck and A. S. Coulson.

The conference was supported by grants from the Swedish Medical Research Council and the Swedish Ministry of Education. At the start of the conference the participants had the pleasure of being the guests of Pharmacia Ltd., Uppsala, at a cocktail party.

The editors

K. Lindahl-Kiessling
G. Alm
M. G. Hanna, Jr.

LIST OF CHAIRMEN, SPEAKERS, AND CO-AUTHORS

ADA, G. L., Department of Microbiology, John Curtin School of Medical Research, Canberra, A.C.T., Australia.

AGAROSSI, G., CNEN-Euratom Immunogenetics Group, Animal Radiobiology Laboratory, C.S.N. Casaccia, Rome, Italy.

ALBRIGHT, J. F., Department of Pharmacology, Smith, Kline & French Laboratories, Philadelphia, Pa., U.S.A.

ALEXANDER, P., Chester Beatty Research Institute, Institute of Cancer Research, Belmont, Sutton, Surrey, England.

ALM, G., Department of Histology, Institute of Human Anatomy, University of Uppsala, Uppsala, Sweden.

ALZER, G., Medizinische Universitätsklinik, Köln, W. Germany.

ASFI, C., Immunobiology Unit, Department of Zoology, University of Edinburgh, Edinburgh, Scotland.

BÄCK, R., Department of Histology, Institute of Human Anatomy, University of Uppsala, Uppsala, Sweden.

BACULI, B. S., Department of Anatomy, School of Medicine, University of California, Los Angeles, Calif. 90024, U.S.A.

BALFOUR, B. M., Division of Immunology, National Institute for Medical Research, Mill Hill, London N.W.7, England.

BARTH, R. F., Department of Pathology and Oncology, University of Kansas Medical Center, Kansas City, Kan., U.S.A.

BAŠIĆ, I., Institute "R. Bošković" and Institute of Immunology, Zagreb, Yugoslavia.

BIANCO, C., Department of Pathology, New York University School of Medicine, New York, N. Y. 10016, U.S.A.

BIASI, G., Division of Experimental Oncology, University of Padova, Padova, Italy.

BOCKMAN, D. E., Department of Anatomy, Medical College of Ohio at Toledo, Ohio, U.S.A.

BROWN, B. A., Department of Anatomy, School of Medicine, University of California, Los Angeles, Calif. 90024, U.S.A.

BRYANT, B. J., Department of Medical Microbiology, University of California, Davis, Calif. 95616, U.S.A.

BYSTRYN, J.-C., Department of Medicine, New York University School of Medicine, New York, N. Y., U.S.A.

CEGLOWSKI, W. S., Temple University School of Medicine, Philadelphia, Pa., U.S.A.

CELADA, F., Department of Tumor Biology, Karolinska Institutet, Stockholm, Sweden.

CERNY, J., Department of Microbiology, Albert Einstein Medical Center, Philadelphia, Pa., U.S.A.

CHAN, P. L., Cancer Research Laboratory, The University of Western Ontario, London, Ontario, Canada.

CHANANA, A. D., Medical Department, Brookhaven National Laboratory, Upton, N. Y. 11973, U.S.A.

CHIECO-BIANCHI, L., Division of Experimental Oncology, University of Padova, Italy.

CHILLER, J. M., Department of Experimental Pathology, Scripps Clinic and Research Foundation, La Jolla, Calif., U.S.A.

COCKETT, A. T. K., Division of Urology, University of Rochester, Rochester, N. Y., U.S.A.

COHEN, I. R., Department of Cell Biology, The Weizmann Institute of Science, Rehovot, Israel.

COHEN, S., Department of Pathology, State University of New York at Buffalo, Buffalo, N. Y., U.S.A.

COLE, L. J., Immunobiology Program, Life Sciences Division, Stanford Research Institute, Menlo Park, Calif., U.S.A.

COLLAVO, D., Division of Experimental Oncology, University of Padova, Padova, Italy.

CONGDON, C. C, Biology Division, Oak Ridge National Laboratory, Oak Ridge, Tenn. 37830, U.S.A.

COOPER, E. L., Department of Anatomy, School of Medicine, University of California, Los Angeles, Calif. 90024, U.S.A.

COOPER, M. D., Departments of Pediatrics and Microbiology, Spain Research Laboratories, University of Alabama in Birmingham, Birmingham, Ala., U.S.A.

COTTIER, H., Department of Pathology, University of Bern, Bern, Switzerland.

CREVON, M. D., Hopital Necker Enfants Malades, Paris, France.

CRONKITE, E. P., Medical Department, Brookhaven National Laboratory, Upton, L. I., N. Y., U.S.A.

CRUCHAUD, A., Laboratory of Immunology, Department of Medicine, Hopital Cantonal, Geneva, Switzerland.

DAVIES, A. J. S., Chester Beatty Research Institute, Institute of Cancer Research, Royal Cancer Hospital, London S.W.3, England.

DEKARIS, D., INSTITUTE "R. Boskovic" and Institute of Immunology, Zagreb, Yugoslavia.

DE MACARIO, E. CONWAY, Department of Tumor Biology, Karolinska Institutet, Stockholm, Sweden.

DE SOUSA, M., Department of Bacteriology & Immunology, Glasgow University, Glasgow, Scotland.

DI PIETRO, S., CNEN-Euratom Immunogenetics Group, Animal Radiobiology Laboratory, C.S.N. Casaccia, Rome, Italy.

DORIA, G., CNEN-Euratom Immunogenetics Group, Animal Radiobiology Laboratory, C.S.N. Casaccia, Rome, Italy.

DORMONT, J., Hopital Necker Enfants Malades, University of Paris, Paris, France.

DUKOR, P., Department of Pathology, New York University School of Medicine, New York, N. Y. 10016, U.S.A.

DUQUESNOY, R. J., Department of Microbiology, Marquette School of Medicine, Milwaukee, Wisc., U.S.A.

DURKIN, H. G., Department of Pathology, New York University School of Medicine, New York, N. Y., U.S.A.

DWYER, J. M., The Walter and Eliza Hall Institute of Medical
    Research, Melbourne, Australia.

ELEKES, E., "Frédéric Joliot-Curie" National Research Institute for
    Radiobiology and Radiohygiene, Budapest, Hungary.

EVERETT, N. B., Department of Biological Structure, University of
    Washington, Seattle, Wash., U.S.A.

FAGRAEUS, A., State Bacteriological Laboratory, Stockholm, Sweden.

FELDMAN, M., Department of Cell Biology, The Weizmann Institute of
    Science, Rehovot, Israel.

FIORE-DONATI, L., Division of Experimental Oncology, University of
    Padova, Italy.

FITCH, F. W., Department of Pathology, University of Chicago,
    Chicago, Ill., U.S.A.

FORD, W. L., Institute f. Exp. Immunology, Nørre allé 71,
    Copenhagen, Denmark.

FRANCHESCHI, C., Department of Tumor Biology, Karolinska Institutet,
    Stockholm, Sweden.

FRENCH, V. I., Department of Experimental Pathology, University of
    Birmingham, Birmingham 15, England.

FRIEDMAN, H., Department of Microbiology, Albert Einstein Medical
    Center, Philadelphia, Pa., U.S.A.

GALLAGHER, M. T., Baylor University College of Medicine, Houston,
    Texas 77025, U.S.A.

GALLILY, R., Department of Immunology, The Hebrew University-
    Hadassah Medical School, Jerusalem, Israel.

GARVEY, J. S., Division of Chemistry and Chemical Engineering,
    California Institute of Technology, Pasadena, Calif., U.S.A.

GLOBERSON, A., Department of Cell Biology, The Weizmann Institute
    of Science, Rehovot, Israel.

GOOD, R. A., Pediatric Research Laboratories, University of
    Minnesota Hospital, Minneapolis, Minn., U.S.A.

GRAF, M. W., Department of Medicine, New York University School of
    Medicine, New York, N. Y., U.S.A.

GRISCELLI, C., Laboratoire d'Immunopathologie infantile, Faculté
    Necker Enfants Malades, Paris, France.

GROSS, R., Medizinische Universitätsklinik, Köln, W. Germany.

GUTMAN, G., Department of Pathology, Stanford University Medical
    School, Stanford, Calif., U.S.A.

GUY-GRAND, D., Laboratoire d'Immunopathologie infantile, Faculté
    Necker Enfants Malades, Paris, France.

HALL, J. G., Chester Beatty Research Institute, Institute of
    Cancer Research, Belmont, Sutton, Surrey, England.

HANNA, M. G., JR., Biology Division, Oak Ridge National Laboratory,
    Oak Ridge, Tenn. 37830, U.S.A.

HARD, R. C., Department of Histology, Institute of Human Anatomy,
    University of Uppsala, Uppsala, Sweden.

HEMMINGSSON, E., Department of Histology, Institute of Human
    Anatomy, University of Uppsala, Uppsala, Sweden.

HESS, M. W., Department of Pathology, University of Bern,
    Bern, Switzerland.

HILDEMANN, W. H., Department of Medical Microbiology, University
    of California, Los Angeles, Calif., U.S.A.

HIRSCHMANN, W. D., Medizinische Universitätsklinik, Köln,
    W. Germany.

HRŠAK, I., Department of Biology, Institute "R. Bošković"
    Zagreb, Yugoslavia.

HUMPHREY, J. H., Division of Immunology, National Institute for
    Medical Research, Mill Hill, London N.W.7, England.

HUNTER, R. L., Department of Pathology, University of Chicago,
    Chicago, Ill., U.S.A.

ISAKOVIČ, K., Immunology Unit, Institute for Biological Research,
    Belgrade, Yugoslavia.

JAGARLAMOODY, S. M., Department of Surgery, University of Minnesota,
    Minneapolis, Minn., 55455, U.S.A.

JANKOVIČ, B. D., Immunology Unit, Institute for Biological Research,
    Belgrade, Yugoslavia.

JENKINS, V. K., Department of Radiology, University of Texas
    Medical Branch, Galveston, Texas, U.S.A.

JÍLEK, M., Department of Immunology, Institute of Microbiology,
    Czechoslovak Academy of Sciences, Prague 4, Czechoslovakia.

JOEL, D. D., Medical Department, Brookhaven National Laboratory,
    Upton, L. I., N. Y., U.S.A.

KIM, Y. B., Department of Microbiology, University of Minnesota,
    School of Medicine, Minneapolis, Minn., U.S.A.

KINCADE, P. W., Departments of Pediatrics and Microbiology, Spain
    Research Laboratories, University of Alabama in Birmingham,
    Birmingham, Alabama, U.S.A.

KOCSÁR, L., "Frédéric Joliot-Curie" National Research Institute for
    Radiobiology and Radiohygiene, Budapest, Hungary.

KOO, G., Temple University School of Medicine, Philadelphia, Pa.,
    U.S.A.

KUNIN, S., Department of Cell Biology and Chemical Immunology,
    The Weizmann Institute of Science, Rehovot, Israel.

LAISSUE, J., Institute of Pathology, University of Bern,
    Bern, Switzerland.

LAWTON, A. R., III, Departments of Pediatrics and Microbiology,
    Spain Research Laboratories, University of Alabama in Birmingham,
    Birmingham, Alabama, U.S.A.

LEENE, W., Laboratorium v. Elektronen-Mikroscopie, Amsterdam,
    The Netherlands.

LEVINE, B. B., Department of Medicine, New York University School
    of Medicine, New York, N. Y., U.S.A.

LINNA, T. J., Department of Histology, Institute of Human Anatomy,
    University of Uppsala, Uppsala, Sweden.

MACARIO, A. J. L., Department of Tumor Biology, Karolinska
    Institutet, Stockholm, Sweden.

MÄKELÄ, O., Serobakteriologi, Hartmanink. 3, Helsinki 29, Finland.

MANSON, L. A., The Wistar Institute, Philadelphia, Pa., U.S.A.

MARIANI, T., Pediatric Research Laboratories, University of
    Minnesota Hospital, Minneapolis, Minn., U.S.A.

MATOSIĆ, M., Institute "R. Bošković" and Institute of Immunology,
  Zagreb, Yugoslavia.

MCALACK, R. F., Department of Microbiology, Albert Einstein Medical
  Center, Philadelphia, Pa., U.S.A.

MCARTHUR, W. P., Division of Immunology, Sloan Kettering Institute,
  New York, N. Y., U.S.A.

MCCLUSKEY, R. T., Department of Pathology, State University of
  New York at Buffalo, Buffalo, N. Y., U.S.A.

MCGARRY, M. P., Baylor University College of Medicine, Houston,
  Texas, U.S.A.

MCKHANN, C. F., Department of Surgery, University of Minnesota,
  Minneapolis, Minn., U.S.A.

MERÉTEY, K., "Frédéric Joliot-Curie" National Research Institute
  for Radiobiology and Radiohygiene, Budapest, Hungary.

MICHALEK, S., The Variety Club Research Center of the La Rabida
  University of Chicago Institute, University of Chicago,
  Chicago, Ill., U.S.A.

MICKLEM, H. S., Immunobiology Unit, Department of Zoology,
  University of Edinburgh, Scotland.

MILLER, J. F. A. P., Walter and Eliza Hall Institute of Medical
  Research, Royal Melbourne Hospital, Melbourne, Australia.

MÖLLER, G., Department of Bacteriology, Karolinska Institutet,
  Stockholm SW, Sweden.

MÜLLER-HERMELINK, H. K., Departments of Pathology and Hygiene,
  University of Kiel, W. Germany.

MÜLLER-RUCHHOLTZ, W., Departments of Pathology and Hygiene,
  University of Kiel, W. Germany.

NACHTIGAL, D., Department of Cell Biology, The Weizmann Institute
  of Science, Rehovot, Israel.

NIEUWENHUIS, P., Department of Histology, State University of
  Groningen, Groningen, Holland.

NUSSENZWEIG, V., Department of Pathology, New York University School
  of Medicine, New York, N. Y. 10016, U.S.A.

ODARTCHENKO, N., Department of Cell Biology, Swiss Institute for
    Experimental Cancer Research, Bugnon 21, Lausanne, Switzerland.

OERKERMANN, H., Medizinische Universitätsklinik, Köln, W. Germany.

OWEN, J. J. T., Department of Human Anatomy, University of Oxford,
    Oxford, England.

OZER, H., Department of Microbiology, Yale University, New Haven,
    Conn., U.S.A.

PARISH, C. R., Department of Microbiology, John Curtin School of
    Medical Research, Canberra, A.C.T., Australia.

PARROTT, D. M. V., Department of Bacteriology & Immunology,
    Western Infirmary, Glasgow, Scotland.

PENNELLI, N., Division of Experimental Oncology, University of Padova,
    Padova, Italy.

PETERSON, R. D. A., The Variety Club Research Center of the La Rabida
    University of Chicago, Chicago, Ill., U.S.A.

PETROVIĆ, S., Microbiological Institute, Faculty of Pharmacy,
    University of Belgrade, Belgrade, Yugoslavia.

PHILLIPS-QUAGLIATA, J. M., Department of Pathology, New York
    University School of Medicine, New York, N. Y., U.S.A.

PRENDERGAST, R. A., Wilmer Institute, Johns Hopkins University,
    School of Medicine, Baltimore, Md., U.S.A.

QUAGLIATA, F., Department of Pathology, New York University School
    of Medicine, New York, N. Y., U.S.A.

RAFF, M. C., National Institute for Medical Research, Mill Hill,
    London, N.W.7, England.

ROMBALL, C. G., Department of Experimental Pathology, Scripps Clinic
    and Research Foundation, La Jolla, Calif., U.S.A.

ROSSE, C., Department of Biological Structure, University of
    Washington, Seattle, Wash., U.S.A.

RUBIN, A. D., Department of Medicine (Hematology), The Mount Sinai
    School of Medicine, New York, N. Y., U.S.A.

SAKAI, A., Division of Urology, University of Rochester,
    Rochester, N. Y., U.S.A.

SANTOS, G. W., Johns Hopkins University School of Medicine, Baltimore, Md., U.S.A.

SCHUMACHER, K., Medizinische Universitätsklinik, Köln, W. Germany.

SEGAL, S., Department of Cell Biology, The Weizmann Institute of Science, Rehovot, Israel.

SHEAGREN, J. N., Laboratory of Clinical Investigation, National Institute of Allergy and Infectious Diseases, Bethesda, Md., U.S.A.

SILOBRČIĆ, V., Institute of Immunology, Zagreb, Yugoslavia.

SILVERSTEIN, A. M., Wilmer Institute, Johns Hopkins University School of Medicine, Baltimore, Md., U.S.A.

SIMMONS, T., The Wistar Institute, Philadelphia, Pa., U.S.A.

SINCLAIR, N. R. StC., Cancer Research Laboratory, The University of Western Ontario, London, Ontario, Canada.

SJÖBERG, O., Department of Bacteriology, Karolinska Institutet, Medical School, S-10401 Stockholm 60, Sweden.

SMITH, M. E., Chester Beatty Research Institute, Institute of Cancer Research, Belmont, Sutton, Surrey, England.

SMITH, R. T., Department of Pathology, University of Florida, Gainesville, Fla., U.S.A.

SONSINO, M., Division of Urology, University of Rochester, Rochester, N. Y., U.S.A.

SORDAT, B., Department of Pathology, University of Bern, Bern, Switzerland.

SPEIRS, R. S., Baylor College of Medicine, Houston, Texas, U.S.A.

STARK, J. M., Department of Experimental Pathology, University of Birmingham, Birmingham 15, England.

ŠTERZL, J., Department of Immunology, Institute of Microbiology, Czechoslovak Academy of Sciences, Prague 4, Czechoslovakia.

STJERNSWÄRD, J., Department of Tumor Biology, Karolinska Institutet, Radiumhemmet, Stockholm 60, Sweden.

STONER, R. D., Medical Research Center, Brookhaven National Laboratory, Upton, L. I., N. Y., U.S.A.

STUTMAN, O., Department of Laboratory Medicine, University of
    Minnesota, Minneapolis, Minn., U.S.A.

TAKAHASHI, T., Department of Pathology, New York University School
    of Medicine, New York, N. Y., U.S.A.

THEIS, G. A., Department of Pathology, New York University School
    of Medicine, New York, N. Y., U.S.A.

THORBECKE, G. J., Department of Pathology, New York University
    School of Medicine, New York, N. Y., U.S.A.

TOMAŽIČ, V., Institute "R. Bošković" Laboratory for Tumor and
    Transplantation Immunology, Zagreb, Yugoslavia.

TRENTIN, J. J., Baylor University College of Medicine, Houston,
    Texas, U.S.A.

TRIDENTE, G., Division of Experimental Oncology, University of
    Padova, Italy.

TYLER, R., Department of Biological Structure, University of
    Washington, Seattle, Wash., U.S.A.

UHLENBRUCK, G., Medizinische Universitätsklinik, Köln, W. Germany.

UHR, J. W., Irvington House Institute for Rheumatic Fever, New York
    University Medical Center, New York, N. Y., U.S.A.

UNANUE, E. R., Department of Pathology, Harvard Medical School,
    Boston, Mass., U.S.A.

VAN DEN BROEK, A. A., Department of Histology, State University of
    Groningen, Groningen, Holland.

VÀNKY, F., The Orthopaedic Clinic, Karolinska Sjukhuset,
    Stockholm 60, Sweden.

VÁRTERÉSZ, V., "Frédéric Joliot-Curie" National Research Institute
    for Radiobiology and Radiohygiene, Budapest, Hungary.

VASSALLI, P., Hopital Necker Enfants Malades, Paris, France, and
    Department of Pathology, State University of New York at Buffalo,
    Buffalo, N. Y., U.S.A.

VITALE, B., Institute "R. Bošković" Laboratory for Tumor and
    Transplantation Immunology, Zagreb, Yugoslavia.

WAKSMAN, B. H., Department of Microbiology, Yale University,
    New Haven, Conn., U.S.A.

WARNER, N. L., The Walter and Eliza Hall Institute of Medical
    Research, Melbourne, Australia.

WATSON, D. W., Department of Microbiology, University of Minnesota,
    School of Medicine, Minneapolis, Minn., U.S.A.

WEIGLE, W. O., Scripps Clinic and Research Foundation, La Jolla,
    Calif., U.S.A.

WEISSMAN, I. L., Department of Pathology, Stanford University
    Medical School, Palo Alto, Calif., U.S.A.

WEKSLER, B. B., Department of Medicine, The New York Hospital-
    Cornell Medical Center, New York, N. Y., U.S.A.

WEKSLER, M. E., Department of Medicine, The New York Hospital-
    Cornell Medical Center, New York, N. Y., U.S.A.

WHITE, R. G., Department of Experimental Pathology, University of
    Birmingham, Birmingham 15, England.

WILLIAMS, R. M., Department of Microbiology, Yale University,
    New Haven, Conn., U.S.A.

WINTZER, G., Medizinische Universitätsklinik, Köln, W. Germany.

WOLF, N. S., Department of Experimental Animal Medicine,
    University of Washington, Seattle, Wash., U.S.A.

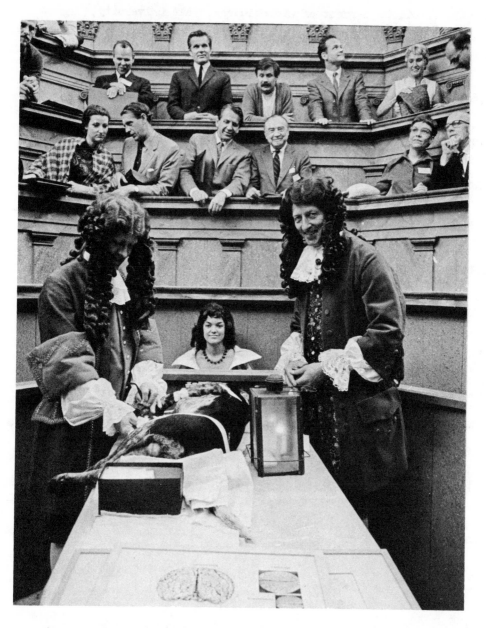

  As a pleasant historical interlude, during the closing ceremony, the Royal Lymphatic Society of Uppsala arranged a reenactment of Olof Rudbeck's demonstration in 1652 of his discovery of the lymphatic system before the Swedish sovereign of the time, Queen Kristina. The demonstration took place in the historic Rudbeckian Anatomical Theater.

CONTENTS

SESSION 2

Origin and Interaction of Immunologically Active Cells

Chairman: A. J. Davies
Co-chairman: F. W. Fitch

SESSION 3

Lymphoid Cell Migration

Chairman: J. Linna
Co-chairman: W. L. Ford

SEPTEMBER 2
Chairman for discussions: O. Mäkelä

SESSION 4

Lymphatic Tissue and Germinal Centers
in Relation to Antibody Production

Chairman: H. Cottier
Co-chairman: A. Fagraeus

SESSION 5

Localization of Antigen and Immune Complexes in Lymphatic
Tissue with Special Reference to Germinal Centers

Chairman: M. G. Hanna, Jr.
Co-chairman: R. L. Hunter

SESSION 6

Immunologically Active Cell Kinetics (Models)

Chairman: J. Šterzl
Co-chairman: J. F. Albright

SEPTEMBER 3

Chairman for the discussions: R. Peterson

SESSION 7

Regulation of Lymphatic Tissue Function

Chairman: J. W. Uhr
Co-chairman: G. Möller

SESSION 8

Modification of Immune Response by External Agents with
Special Reference to Germinal Centers

Chairman: M. Hess
Co-chairman: G. W. Santos

SESSION 9

Tolerance and Autosensitization

Chairman: W. O. Weigle
Co-chairman: N. Odartchenko

SEPTEMBER 4

Chairman for the discussion: L. Fiore-Donati

SESSION 10

Neoplastic Disease and the Immune System

Chairman: P. Alexander
Co-chairman: R. T. Smith

SESSION 11

Free Session

Chairman: R. C. Hard

CONTENTS

NEW OBSERVATIONS ON LYMPH GLAND (LM1) AND THYMUS ACTIVITY IN LARVAL BULLFROGS, RANA CATESBEIANA[1]

Edwin L. Cooper[2], Bruce A. Brown and Buena S. Baculi[3]

Department of Anatomy, School of Medicine, University of

California, Los Angeles, California 90024

INTRODUCTION

The lymphoid and myeloid (chiefly, bone marrow) systems are concerned principally with the immune response capacity in most vertebrates. With the exception of birds and certain mammals, the thymus acts alone as a major organ and is necessary for the maturation and maintenance of immune competence. I shall restrict my presentation to a review of new information on the role of lymph gland and thymus in larval bullfrogs. I will not consider the thymus or other organs of the lymphomyeloid complex in other larval anurans (1,2,3,4).

We presented evidence that the thymus of bullfrog larvae (Rana catesbeiana) is necessary for the development of cellular reactions like tissue graft destruction (5). I also reported that the thymus was, in addition, important in humoral responses thus giving it a role more analogous to the thymus of most mammals except rabbits (6,7). Recently I found that another organ, the lymph gland (LM1) appears essential for antibody synthesis (8). To resolve this conclict, past experiments done on both organs were reviewed with new insight. At this time it appears that these organs serve very different functions, with the major common feature being their possible embryologic origin from the same germ layer. The results of these reviews and new observations follow.

---

1) Supported by: American Cancer Society Research Grants E492 and IN34 and National Science Foundation Grants GB7607 and GB17767 to ELC.
2) Guggenheim Fellow, Honorary Fulbright Scholar 1970-71.

OBSERVATIONS

The Thymus and LM2

At a first glance, an inexperienced worker could equate the thymus and lymph gland owing to their anatomical positioning in the branchial cavity, as well as their dense closely packed lymphocyte population. When the tissues are not arterially perfused during fixation, the characteristic sinusoids of the lymph gland collapse, making the histological determination even more difficult. The histologic similarity is striking at low magnification (Figs. 1 and 2) and only closer observations, fixation perfusion and 1μ sectioning techniques make the distinction quite clear (Fig. 3,4,5,6). Upon careful dissection, it also becomes obvious that each element of the lymphomyeloid complex occupies a distinct anatomical position. The lymph gland is located superficially and the thymus quite deep and attached to the head cartilage (Fig.7). A thorough analysis of early laboratory notes discloses that the extirpated organs, thought to be thymus, were indeed lymph gland as revealed by notations like "extreme bleeding". According to the drawing such bleeding was probably due to severing some element of the gill apparatus, for a thymectomy can be carried out almost bloodlessly. A recent thorough search into the literature reveals that Speidel (9) may have described the same structure in Rana climitans and thought it to be thymus.

Vasculature of LM1

The vascular pattern of the lymph gland is prima facie evidence that it functions as a blood-filtering organ. We found a rete mirabile, particularly a venous portal system, of afferent and efferent vessels. Interposed between the blood vessels is a labyrinth of sinusoids. Lymphatic vessels are not present, thus they cannot be classified as true nodes, but seem to be more related to mammalian hemal nodes (10).

Stroma of LM1

The bilateral lymph gland is surrounded by a capsule composed of fibroblasts with collagenous and reticular fibers. Lymph glands do not possess trabeculae but the walls of the sinusoids and parenchymal cords are supported by the same fibers of the capsule which do not divide it into lobules. Stromal cells in close association with the meshwork of stromal fibers consist of littoral cells which line the sinusoids, primitive reticular cells, fibroblasts along collagenous fiber bundles and two morphophysiologic types of fixed

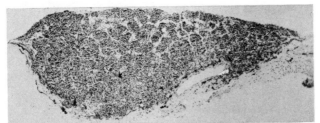

Fig. 1.   Larval lymph gland (LM1), 5μ section hematoxylin and eosin x 50.

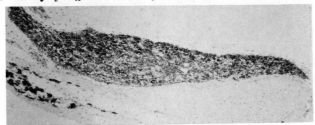

Fig. 2.   Larval thymus, same as 1.

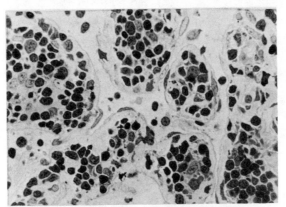

Fig. 3.   LM1, 0.5μ, perfused x 450.

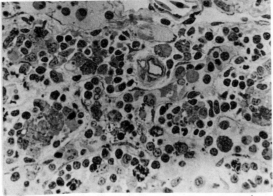

Fig. 4.   LM1, 0.5μ, non-perfused x 450.

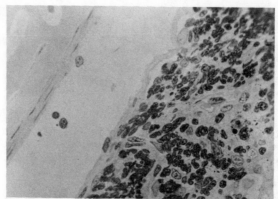

Fig. 5.   Thymus 0.5 μ non-perfused x 450.

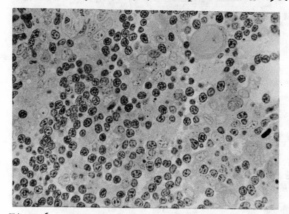

Fig. 6.   Thymus 0.5 μ perfused x 450.

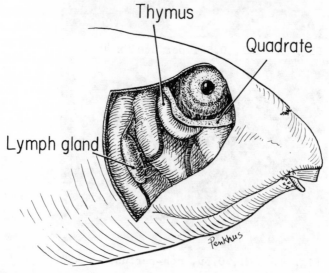

Fig. 7.   Tadpoles showing branchial region and location of lymph gland and thymus.

macrophages. Macrophages (M1 and M2) are present and distinguishable on
the basis of size and phagocytic properties. M1 is larger, 8-10μ, strongly
PAS positive with a cytoplasm that contains numerous pyknotic nuclei of
phagocytosed cells. M1 did not phagocytose India ink. M2 is smaller,
6-10μ, takes up India ink and shows lighter staining properties.

Parenchyma of LM1

The parenchyma is composed of large numbers of lymphoid cells, along with
fewer neutrophils, eosinophils and plasma cells. The greatest percentage
of lymphocytes are small, constituting about 70% of the lymphoid cell population. Often lymphoid cells were seen undergoing diapedesis to or from
the sinusoids. Stem or blast cells constituted 6-13% and were the most actively mitotic. The granulocyte population made up no more than 6% of the
total. Plasma cells, though present, were not prominent in normal unstimulated organs, but were found in increased numbers in glands of larvae after
antigenic challenge (11). In 1μ sections, it appears that the parenchymal
cords contain a centrally located blast cell with peripheral lymphocytes of
varying degrees of differentiation as well as plasma cells. These "nest-
like" structures may then represent the amphibian germinal center. Work is
currently in progress to examine the effect of antigenic challenge on these
germinal centers.

Electron Microscopy of LM1

At the ultrastructural level, lymph glands possess large lymphocytes, with
dense chromatin, accumulated around the nuclear periphery; the cytoplasm
is granular and homogeneous. The lymphocytes are found in clusters around
a larger blast cell with a more diffuse nuclear pattern and prominant nucleoli. The cytoplasm contains free and rosette ribosomes as well as varying
amounts of endoplasmic reticulum. Numerous mitochondria and a golgi complex are evident (Fig. 8). The sinusoids are lined by endothelial cells with
elongate nuclei; the cytoplasm is homogeneous, with mitochondria, and
various vesicles. Macrophages possess lysosomes and ingested carbon particles after experimental injection. Cellular debris is present in cytoplasmic
vesicles. Plasma cells show clumped chromatin in the nuclear periphery.
Their cytoplasm contains mitochondria, a golgi complex and distended endoplasmic reticulum, presumably active in antibody synthesis. The outer capsule is made up of collagen, with numerous fibroblasts and reticular fibers.
The sinusoids usually contain typical nucleated amphibian erythrocytes,
and numerous small lymphocytes. Many macrophages line the sinusoids and
show phagocytic vesicles and numerous pseudopods. These cells remain in

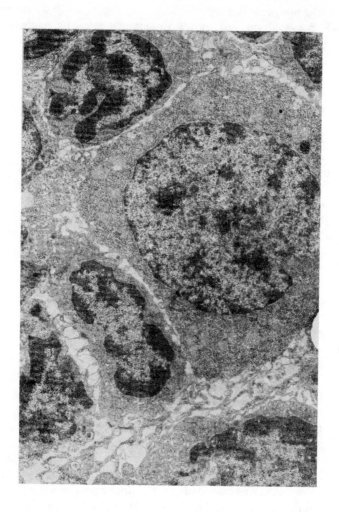

Fig. 8. LM1 electron microscopic view x 13,000 showing central blast cell and surrounding lymphocytes forming germinal center.

the sinusoids, presumably by adherence mechanism from the pseudopods, in contrast to the red blood cells which are washed out to a large extent during the perfusion process. The granulocyte population has not yet been investigated, but their presence has been recorded.

Morphology of Thymus

The thymus consists of a well developed outer connective tissue capsule with septa that pierce the underlying cortical region and form the meshwork of the medulla. A few blood vessels and thymocytes are present in close proximity to the capsule, but the thymus is not punctuated heavily with blood sinuses as is the lymph gland in Rana catesbeiana or the thymus (?), described by Speidel in Rana climitans. What he may have observed quite by mistake as in our observation, was a lymph gland and not the thymus. In bullfrog tadpoles, the cortex is composed of numerous closely-packed thymocytes and a lesser number of reticular cells. In the medulla, the stroma is more developed containing, in addition, eosinophils and reticular cells.

Function of LM1 in Larvae of Unknown Age

In 1963, Cooper et al. first reported the effects of thymectomy in amphibian larvae (6). In older bullfrog larvae at standard stages 25-29, complete or bilateral thymectomy usually failed to impair the isoimmune response to skin homografts. Statistical analysis revealed no difference in sham-operated and experimental animals. Runting was obvious in these groups and only 5 larvae showed prolonged survival. We suggested then a qualitative difference in thymectomized and sham-operated larvae at approximately 90-180 days posthatching at stages 25-29.

The thymus, according to Cooper et al. (7), is essential for antibody synthesis in larvae approximately 60-200 days post-hatching at stages 25-29. After immunization $25° + 0.5$ C with goldfish serum protein antigens, specific precipitating antibodies were found in the majority of sham-operated controls. In contrast, nearly all of the thymectomized group showed a markedly weakened response to goldfish serum antigens (Table 1). Based on new morphological observations we conclude that these results were mediated by LM-1 which was removed rather than the thymus. Removal of lymph glands failed to prevent skin allograft rejection, but inhibited antibody synthesis.

Table 1. Summary of survival times of skin allografts and antibody titers in bullfrog larvae without lymph glands at 25.5 ± 0.5°C.

Approximate age and stages of development at lymph gland removal	Group and type of operation	No. of tadpoles given skin allografts at stages 25-29	Interval between lymph gland removal and allografting (days)	Median survival time (days) ± std. error with std. deviation in parenthesis	Range of graft survival time (days)	No. of larvae with allografts showing signif. prolonged survival[2]	No. of tadpoles immunized with	Standard stage at testing	Precipitin test	Highest antibody titer detectable with passive hemagglutination
3-6 months 25-26	Lymphadenectomy	45	0-28	10.9+1.4 (4.5)	5 to >70	5	1) goldfish serum 13	25-27	1 positive, 7 slightly positive, 5	---
3-6 months 25-26	Sham lymphadenectomy	42	0-28	9.6+0.9 (3.3)	5 to 19	none	18	25-29	negative 10, positive 5, slightly positive 3	---
6-9 months 25-30	Lymphadenectomy	none	--	--	--	--	2) 1% BSA 100	25,29	negative	0
"	Unilateral lymphadenectomy						6	29		1:32
"	Sham lymphadenectomy	none					47	25-30		1:20; 1:32-1:64
"	Lymphadenectomy	8			up to 21 days	none	--			---
"	Sham lymphadenectomy	8			up to 21 days	none	--			---

1) Summary of original data taken from (Refs. 5, 6, 7, 8).
2) There was no apparent difference in survival times depending on the interval between lymphadenectomy and allografting.
3) These survival times greatly exceeded the 95% confidence limits (> 2 std. dev.) as determined by the nomographic methods of Litchfield.
   These recipients were at standard stages 25 and 26 at the time of lymph gland removal.

Function of Thymus in Larvae of Known Age

From re-examination of the material presented by Cooper and Hildemann (1965), it appears that at stage 25, 18–64 days post-thymectomy, the thymus regularly curtails the capacity to reject skin allografts.

Reconciliation of Thymus-Lymph Gland Function in Larvae of Unknown Ages.

Removal of lymph glands in tadpoles, stage 25, at similar ages to those which received goldfish serum did not interfere with their capacity to destroy skin allografts. By contrast, larvae with both glands removed were incapable of synthesizing antibodies to BSA. Those with only one lymph gland removed still showed detectable antibody titers. From this data it appears that the lymph gland in tadpoles, not the thymus, is responsible for antibody synthesis. Lymph gland removal does not affect skin allograft survival in older larvae.

SUMMARY AND CONCLUSIONS

The thymus in most amphibians is important during the early stages of development in preparing juveniles for mounting cellular immune reactions. If removed during early life, animals show a weakened capacity for rejecting skin allografts. The thymus in some anuran amphibians may play a negative feedback role in humoral reactions as evidenced by heightened serum proteins and antibodies after extirpation. In the bullfrog tadpole, two lymphoid structures, the thymus and lymph gland are present. The thymus controls the capacity to destroy skin allografts during approximately the first month of the life cycle, but not during later stages. The lymph gland contributes to the capacity to synthesize serum antibodies during later stages; we do not know its role in early life. Careful distinctions must be made between the development, anatomy and frunction of the thymus and other branchial lymphoid organs in amphibians in order to complete our understanding of the LM complex activity in immune phenomena. Absence of bone marrow during early stages of frog development provides us with an excellent model for future comparisons with emerging mammalian and avian concepts.

REFERENCES

1.   J.D. Horton. J. Exp. Zool. 170:449, 1969.
2.   R.J. Turner, J. Exp. Zool. 170:461, 1969.

3.   M.J. Manning and J.D. Horton. J. Embryol. Exp. Morph. 22:265, 1969.
4.   L. Du Pasquier. Ann. Inst. Past. 114:490, 1968.
5.   E.L. Cooper and W.H. Hildemann. Transplantation 3:446, 1965.
6.   E.L. Cooper, W.H. Hildemann and W. Pinkerton. Immunogenetics letter 3:62, 1963.
7.   E.L. Cooper, W. Pinkerton and W.H. Hildemann. Biol. Bull. 127: 232, 1964.
8.   E.L. Cooper. Anat. Rec. 162:453, 1968.
9.   C.C. Speidel. Am. J. Anat. 37:141, 1926.
10. B.S. Baculi and E.L. Cooper. J. Morph. 123:463, 1967.
11. B.S. Baculi and E.L. Cooper. J. Morph. 126:463, 1968.

THE USE OF SURFACE ALLOANTIGENIC MARKERS TO STUDY THE DIFFERENTIATION OF THYMUS-DERIVED LYMPHOCYTES IN MICE[1]

Martin C. Raff[1] and J.J.T. Owen[2]

National Institute for Medical Research, Mill Hill,

London, N.W.7, and Department of Human Anatomy,

University of Oxford, Oxford

The studies to be described involve the use of antisera directed against two alloantigens found on the surface of mouse lymphoid cells. Theta (θ) is found in brain as well as on thymocytes (1) and has recently been shown to be present on thymus-derived peripheral lymphocytes (2, 3, 4, 5). It can thus serve as a marker to distinguish thymus-derived lymphocytes from thymus-independent lymphocytes in peripheral lymphoid tissues. The thymus-leukemia antigen (TL) is normally found only on thymocytes in TL-positive strains of mice (6). We have used θ and TL as markers to study the development of thymocytes from embryonic stem cells, the differentiation of thymocytes to thymus-derived lymphocytes, and the emigration of thymus-derived lymphocytes to peripheral lymphoid tissues. ^{51}Chromium and dye-exclusion cytotoxic testing has been used to detect these alloantigens.

It is well established that in the embryo, stem cells from yolk sac and liver migrate to thymus and there proliferate and differentiate into thymocytes (7, 8). These stem cells, which

---

[1] This work was supported in part by a Post-doctoral Fellowship from the National Multiple Sclerosis Society of the United States.

[2] Work carried out while on leave of absence at the National Institute for Medical Research, Mill Hill.

are probably large, basophilic cells, first appear in thymus around
day 11 of embryonic life and do not express θ or TL on their surfaces (9). By day 15 or 16, some stem cells have differentiated to
typical lymphocytes, and it is at this time that θ and TL can first
be detected (9). By day 18, the great majority of thymus cells
express both antigens. We can exclude the possibility that the
appearance of θ and TL in thymus from day 15 onwards is the result
of immigration of cells carrying these antigens. Thus, when we
isolated 14-day thymic rudiments in Millipore diffusion chambers
on the chorioallantois of chick embryos we found that after 4 days
in culture, the majority of cells, which were initially all TL and
θ negative, expressed both antigens (9). In the adult, stem cells
migrate to thymus from bone marrow (10) but less is known about
their morphology and whether or not they express θ and TL.

Although an unknown number of thymocytes appear to die within
the thymus (11), it is now generally accepted that a significant
number migrate to peripheral lymphoid tissues where they make up
the majority, if not all, of the thymus-dependent population of
lymphocytes (12, 13, 14) and are thus appropriately called "thymus-
derived". However, there is clearly another differentiation step
whereby a thymocyte becomes an immunologically competent thymus-
derived lymphocyte, since peripheral thymus-derived lymphocytes do
not express TL (6) and have far less θ on their surface than do
thymocytes (6). This antigenic change has allowed us to demonstrate a population of cells within the thymus with the surface
antigenic characteristics of peripheral thymus-derived lymphocytes.
This suggests that at least part of the second differentiation step
occurs within the thymus, prior to emigration. We have demonstrated
these "mature lymphocytes" within the thymus in a number of ways.

Firstly, when ^{51}Cr-labelled thymocytes were injected intravenously into irradiated syngeneic hosts, the labelled cells that
were harvested from spleen as early as 3 hours after injection
looked exactly like peripheral thymus-derived lymphocytes rather
than thymocytes in terms of their behaviour in cytotoxic testing
(15). That is, they were TL negative and required much higher
concentrations of anti-θ to kill them than is required with thymocytes. The finding of cells with these surface antigenic properties
within 3 hours of injection suggests that a population of peripheral-
like lymphocytes already exists in thymus and these are the cells
that migrate to spleen. The fact that a significant percentage of
thymocytes in two TL positive strains of mice (CBA and A) are TL
negative (15) is also consistent with this view. We then found
that by pretreating ^{51}Cr-labelled thymocytes with anti-TL serum and
complement that the percentage of thymocytes that migrate to lymph
nodes is increased (15), which establishes that, as suspected, the
cells that migrate to peripheral lymphoid tissues are already TL
negative.

In a second set of experiments, we treated ^{51}Cr-labelled CBA thymocytes with a concentration of anti-θ (final dilution of 1/120) and hamster complement (final dilution of 1/7) which will kill the great majority of thymocytes but will not kill any peripheral θ-bearing cells. The remaining viable cells (less than 5% of the original number) were found to be TL negative and behaved in cyto-toxic testing with anti-θ like peripheral θ-bearing lymphocytes (Table I). In another experiment, we treated CBA mice with hydrocortisone acetate (2.5 mg intraperitoneally) and 48 hours later we tested their thymocytes with anti-θ and anti-TL sera. They behaved like peripheral thymus-derived lymphocytes (Table I). In a final experiment along these lines, we kept A strain thymocytes in suspension in Eagles medium in Millipore diffusion chambers and after 7 days in culture we tested the residual cells with anti-TL serum. All the cells were TL negative.

When these data are put together with the findings of others that thymocytes are capable of eliciting a graft-versus-host reaction, and that thymocytes treated with anti-TL (16) or taken from hydrocortisone-treated mice (17) are enriched for cells with this capacity, it is clear that there is a small but significant population of cells present in the thymus which is indistinguishable from peripheral thymus-derived lymphocytes. Although it seems very likely that these "mature" lymphocytes have differentiated within the thymus from less mature thymocytes, it has not as yet been excluded that these cells have returned to the thymus as part of the recirculating pool of lymphocytes.

Perhaps the last stage of development of the thymus-derived lymphocyte before it is ready to encounter its particular antigen, is its migration to the peripheral lymphoid tissues. This process of thymus cell migration to the periphery apparently begins before birth, at least in CBA and Balb/c mice, as there is a small but significant number of θ-bearing cells in the blood and mesenteric lymph node on the first day of life (18), which probably accounts for the failure of neonatal thymectomy to completely eliminate cell-mediated immune responses. The percentage of θ-bearing cells in the periphery rapidly increases in the first week of life, in parallel with the rapid increase in absolute numbers of lymphocytes in peripheral lymphoid tissues, suggesting that the development of these tissues is largely dependent on thymus-derived cells. The rapid rate of development in the first days of life provides an explanation for why thymectomy must be carried out at an early stage to be effective.

Adult Peyer's patches contain a significant population of θ-positive lymphocytes (18) and their development in the first days of life depend to a large extent on thymus-derived cells (18). They are, therefore, to this extent at least, a peripheral rather than a central lymphoid tissue. In mice, it remains to be established that Peyer's patches have any primary role.

The usefulness of the θ alloantigen in studying the origin, distribution and function of thymus-derived lymphocytes has served to emphasize the need for a marker for thymus-independent lymphocytes, about which relatively little is known.   In collaboration with N.A. Mitchison and S. Nase, we have raised an anti-lymphocytic serum by immunizing rabbits with lymph node cells from mice which had been thymectomized,lethally irradiated and reconstituted with syngeneic foetal liver cells.   Following absorption with mouse RBC and liver, and exhaustive absorption with thymocytes, the antiserum was no longer cytotoxic for thymocytes but killed approximately 55% of spleen cells, 30% of lymph node cells and 40% of bone marrow cells.   By using the antiserum together with anti-θ in additive and sequential cytotoxic tests we could show that it was selectively killing thymus-independent lymphocytes, and we are very optimistic about its potential usefulness as a marker for these lymphocytes.

Table I.   Cytotoxic titres* of anti-θ and anti-TL sera for CBA thymocytes, lymph node lymphocytes, residual thymocytes after treatment with anti-θ (1/120 + hamster complement, and thymocytes from hydrocortisone-treated mice**

	Anti-θ	Anti-TL
Normal thymocytes	512-1024	64-128
Normal lymph node lymphocytes	8-16	No cytotoxic activity
Residual thymocytes after treatment with anti-θ (1/120) + hamster complement	8-16	No cytotoxic activity
Thymocytes from hydrocortisone- treated mice	8-16	No cytotoxic activity

*Cytoxic titre = reciprocal of dilution of first
tube off the cytotoxic plateau

**Five-week old CBA mice received 2.5 mg of hydrocortisone
acetate intraperitoneally 48 hours prior to being killed

ACKNOWLEDGMENTS

We thank Miss P. Chivers and Miss F. Rose for excellent technical assistance, and Dr. L. J. Old for providing the anti-TL serum used in these studies.

REFERENCES

1. A. E. Reif and J. M. V. Allen, J. Exp. Med., 120:413, 1964.

2. M. C. Raff, Nature (London), 224:378, 1969.

3. M. Schlesinger and I. Yron, Science, 164:1412, 1969.

4. M. C. Raff and H. H. Wortis, Immunology, 18:929, 1970.

5. M. Schlesinger and I. Yron, J. Immunol., 104:798, 1970.

6. T. Aoki, U. Hämmerling, E. de Harven, E. A. Boyse, and
    L. J. Old, J. Exp. Med., 130:979, 1969.

7. M. A. S. Moore and J. J. T. Owen, J. Exp. Med., 126:715, 1967.

8. J. J. T. Owen and M. A. Ritter, J. Exp. Med., 129:431, 1969.

9. J. J. T. Owen and M. C. Raff (submitted to J. Exp. Med.)

10. C. E. Ford, in: Ciba Found. Symp. Thymus: Experimental and
    Clinical Studies, G. E. W. Wolstenholme, Ed., p. 131.
    London: J. A. Churchill, Ltd., 1966.

11. M. Matsuyama, M. Wiadrowski, and D. Metcalf, J. Exp. Med.,
    123:559, 1966.

12. J. F. A. P. Miller, Proc. Roy. Soc., B, 156:415, 1962.

13. I. Weissman, J. Exp. Med., 126:291, 1967.

14. A. J. S. Davies, Transplant. Rev., 1:43, 1969.

15. M. C. Raff, Nature (London) (in press).

16. E. Leckband, Fed. Proc., 29:621 (Abs.), 1970.

17. H. Blomgren and B. Anderson, Exp. Cell Res., 57:185, 1969.

18. M. C. Raff and J. J. T. Owen (submitted to Europ. J. Immunol.)

A NEW THEORETICAL MODEL OF PLASMA CELL DIFFERENTIATION[1]

M. D. Cooper, P. W. Kincade, D. E. Bockman and

A. R. Lawton, III

Departments of Pediatrics and Microbiology, Spain
Research Laboratories, University of Alabama in
Birmingham, Birmingham, Alabama, and Department of
Anatomy, Medical College of Ohio at Toledo, Ohio

Over the last several years, investigations in our laboratories
have centered around the problem of differentiation and development
of the plasma cell line. The chicken has been the primary animal
model used because this cell line can be easily manipulated by bursectomy in this species (1). Stem cells, originally located in the
yolk sac, begin migration into the bursa of Fabricius around the
13th day of incubation and assume lymphoid features in that environment (2). Removal of the bursa on or before the 17th day of incubation can prevent seeding of its lymphoid cells to extra-bursal sites.
As a consequence, subsequent germinal center and plasma cell development is prevented and agammaglobulinemia ensues (3). Chemical
bursectomy, produced by testosterone administration early in embryonic life, can similarly abort development of the plasma cell line
(4). Consistent with this and other evidence indicating that the
bursa is the site of induction for the immunoglobulin-producing
line of cells (5-7), immunoglobulin synthesis occurs in the bursa
several days prior to its appearance in other lymphoid organs (8).

The principal end products of the bursal line of cells in
chickens are two classes of immunoglobulins, commonly termed IgM
and IgG. During development, IgM synthesis precedes IgG synthesis
and the ontogeny of circulating levels reflects this production
sequence (8, 9). The following evidence indicates that this developmental sequence is controlled by the bursa: (i) Embryonic bursectomy at 19 days of incubation allows the peripheral development
of IgM producing cells but prevents or severely stunts development

[1]Research currently supported by USPHS grants No. AI08345, AI42973,
GM43118, FR00463 and AM13535, and by The American Cancer Society.

17

of IgG producers; (ii) later removal of the bursa usually does not abort development of either IgM or IgG producers (3).

The investigations summarized in this report provide insight into the mechanisms responsible for the development of immunoglobulin class heterogeneity. Our results indicate that IgG producing cells arise within the bursa as the progeny of cells which formerly were IgM producers.

The first requirement for these investigations was a sensitive and highly specific detection system for the subunits of chicken immunoglobulins. Toward this end, purified solutions of goat antibodies specific for chicken μ, γ and light chains were isolated using solid immunoadsorbent columns made with (i) IgM; (ii) IgG; and (iii) agammaglobulinemic serum (10). After appropriate testing for specificity, the antibodies were tagged with either fluorescein or rhodamine.

Using these reagents, the ontogeny of immunoglobulin-containing cells was investigated. Cells staining for μ-chain were first observed in the bursa on the 14th day of incubation; these cells also contained light chains (10). Cells containing IgG were also found within bursal follicles prior to their appearance in extra-bursal sites but they were not detected until the 21st day of incubation, around the time of hatching. Few IgM-containing cells were seen in extra-bursal sites during embryonic life; the earliest IgM-containing cell observed in an extra-bursal site was found in the tonsilla-caecalis of a 17 day embryo. IgG-containing cells were not observed in extra-bursal sites until 4 days after hatching. Rapid peripheral expansion of IgM-containing cells began around the 3rd day after hatching and rapid expansion of IgG-containing cells was initiated around the 8th post-hatching day in chicks raised in conventional environments. It was also determined that neither artificial antigenic stimulation nor sheltering from exogenous antigens alters the ontogeny of immunoglobulins within the bursa, whereas antigenic exposure causes a rapid increase in numbers of immunoglobulin-containing cells in peripheral tissues. These observations suggest that stem cells are influenced to make IgM shortly after their arrival within the bursa and to begin IgG synthesis around a week later in the same location; these seem to be normal events in differentiation of this cell line which occur independently of exogenous antigenic exposure.

Two simple models of plasma cell development consistent with these observations were constructed. One model assumes that the first yolk sac stem cells arriving in the bursa are activated for IgM synthesis and later seeded as cells committed to synthesis of antibodies of this immunoglobulin class. Later, other stem cells arriving in the bursa would be influenced to synthesize IgG antibodies. The second model proposes that all stem cells are initially activated to produce IgM; in subsequent generations the progeny of these cells switch from IgM to IgG synthesis. It seemed likely that an experimental means for selective destruction or suppression of cells containing IgM, followed by bursectomy to prevent subsequent recovery, might provide incisive evidence in favor of one of the two hypotheses. The demonstration of antibody-mediated suppression of immunoglobulin allotype synthesis in rabbits (11) coupled with the observations on the ontogeny of immunoglobulins in chickens suggested that selective antibody-mediated suppression of immunoglobulin class synthesis might be achieved by giving anti-μ antibodies during embryonic life.

Serum immunoglobulin levels were serially determined in chickens given varying amounts of anti-μ antibodies intravenously on the 13th day of incubation and in controls given similar amounts of bovine serum albumin; both groups were subjected to bursectomy at hatching. IgM synthesis was suppressed by anti-μ antibodies in a dose-dependent manner; if sufficient anti-μ were given, IgM-producing cells could be completely abolished (Fig. 1a) as confirmed by fluorescent analysis of tissues when the experiment was terminated 9 weeks after hatching. Further, IgG synthesis was suppressed at least as efficiently as IgM synthesis (Fig. 1b). Fluorescent analysis of the tissues demonstrated that deficiency of IgG-containing cells was responsible for the deficit of IgG in the circulation.

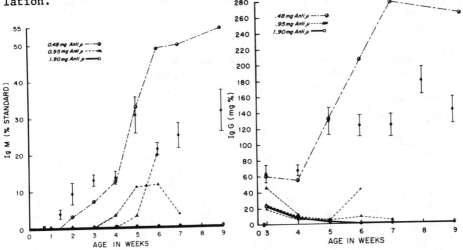

Fig. 1. Suppression of circulating IgM (a) and IgG (b) in bursectomized chickens given an embryonic injection of antibodies to IgM. Ī = Bursectomy controls, mean ± S.E.

Bursal tissues obtained in this experiment at 16, 19 and 21 days of incubation were examined grossly and by routine histology, electron microscopy, and fluorescent analysis for immunoglobulin deposition. The bursas of anti-µ treated embryos were smaller than those of controls. Within these bursas, some follicles were selectively depleted of lymphoid cells. Furthermore, healthy appearing lymphoid cells, and even dividing cells, were observed next to neighboring degenerating cells, demonstrating the selective destruction of bursal lymphocytes. Since IgM-containing cells were rarely observed in the bursas of anti-µ treated embryos, it was concluded that the effect of anti-µ on bursal cells was selective for cells which contained IgM.

Table I. Effect of embryonic injection of goat anti-µ antibodies on immunoglobulin levels in chickens.[+]

Experimental Group	Number in Group	IgM (mg%) Mean Level ± S.E.	IgG (mg%) Mean Level ± S.E.
Anti-µ Treatment	8	4 ± 2.1	12 ± 5.6
Normal γ Globulin Treatment	10	84 ± 12.4	182 ± 42.8

[+]Each experimental bird received 2 mg of purified goat antibodies specific for chicken µ-chain intravenously on the 13th day of incubation. Controls received 2 mg of normal goat gamma globulin. Both groups were bursectomized at hatching. Serum IgM and IgG levels were measured by single diffusion-in-gel when the birds were 10 weeks old.

The results of this and another similar experiment summarized in Table I strongly favor the hypothesis that IgG producing cells arise from cells which were formerly IgM producers. Results of an earlier experiment had suggested that IgM producers do not convert to IgG producers outside of the bursa. Chickens subjected to bursectomy at an appropriate age may produce IgM in supernormal amounts but make little or no IgG (3). Such birds have been observed for as long as 8 months; they did not correct their deficit in circulating IgG as would be expected if IgM producers could convert outside of the bursa (12). In order to further explore this possibility, the effect of anti-µ antibodies on cells in extra-bursal sites was evaluated. In the first experiment, chicks were subjected to bursectomy at hatching and then given injections of anti-µ antibodies; uninjected bursectomized birds served as controls.

Again, IgM suppression was observed in the group given anti-µ antibodies (Fig. 2a) but their IgG levels were not significantly different from those of bursectomy controls (Fig. 2b). These results have been confirmed in another experiment in which bursectomized controls received normal goat globulin (Table II). The observations indicate that administration of anti-µ antibodies does not affect IgG producing cells in extra-bursal sites, and therefore

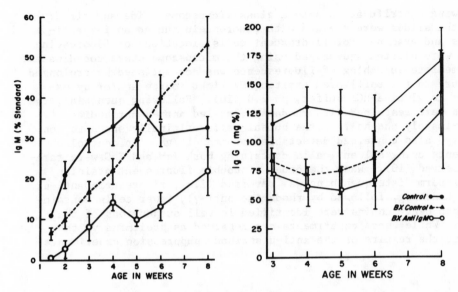

Fig. 2. Circulating IgM (a) and IgG (b) levels in bursectomized chickens given injections of antiserum to IgM after hatching.

suggests that cells outside of the bursa do not switch from IgM to IgG synthesis.

Table II. Immunoglobulin levels in chickens given anti-μ antibodies or normal IgG following bursectomy after hatching*

Experimental Group	Number in Group	IgM (mg%) Mean Level ± S.E.	IgG (mg%) Mean Level ± S.E.
Anti-μ Treatment	6	18.7 ± 6.9	176.0 ± 46.5
Normal γ Globulin Treatment	8	90.8 ± 11.7	140.5 ± 39.4

*Following bursectomy at the age of 1 day, experimental birds received 4 mg of purified goat antibodies to chicken μ-chain intravenously and controls received 4 mg of normal goat gamma globulin. Serum IgM and IgG levels were measured at age 7 weeks.

The results of these experiments and immunofluorescent studies of bursal tissue sections (10) suggested that cells containing both μ and γ chains might be found within the bursa. Therefore, cell suspensions were prepared from bursal and spleen tissues of 10 week old chickens to analyze the immunoglobulin content of single cells.

Following centrifugation onto a glass microscope slide and air dry-
ing, the slides were stained with fluorescein tagged anti-γ antibodies and examined for fluorescent cells; locations of fluorescing
cells were plotted and mapped using the microscope stage coordinates.
Intermediate quenching of fluorescence was accomplished by prolonged
exposure to the unfiltered exciting UV light source and/or by exposure to glycine-HCl buffer, pH 2.0 (10). Following quenching, the
slides were restained with rhodamine labeled anti-μ antibodies.
Approximately one-half of the bursal cells originally shown to contain IgG also contained detectable amounts of IgM. In control experiments using spleen, cells containing both IgM and IgG were rarely observed (10). When the order of double fluorescent staining
with intermediate quenching was reversed (i.e., fluorescein anti-μ,
then quenching, followed by rhodamine anti-γ), fewer cells containing both heavy chains were identified in cell suspensions of the
bursa. While these experiments are regarded as preliminary, they
support the results of the anti-μ antibody suppression experiments.

Fig. 3.

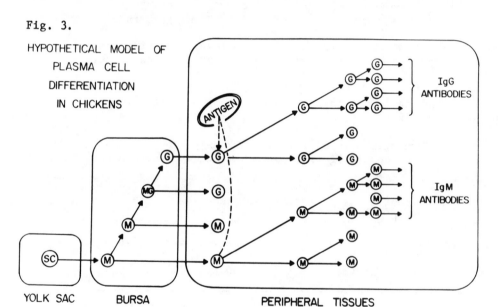

In accordance with these findings, we have constructed a hypothetical model of plasma cell differentiation in chickens (Fig. 3).
The basic premise of this hypothesis (13) is that antibody heterogeneity is generated in a stepwise pattern among the progeny of
yolk sac stem cells during their residence within the bursa. Shortly after arrival in the bursa, stem cells are influenced to begin
IgM synthesis. At some point, progeny of these cells switch from
IgM to IgG synthesis. Primarily for reasons of simplicity, we are
proposing that antibody heterogeneity is generated prior to the

conversion to IgG synthetic capability. During this process of
replication, cells migrate out of the bursa at various stages of
differentiation. Having left the bursa, these cells and their progeny are irrevocably committed to synthesis of antibodies of a
single class, sub-class and specificity. The events occurring within the bursa seem to be normal events of differentiation of the cell
line; antigen influence is exerted outside of the bursa and after
the cells are committed to synthesis of a particular kind of antibody, a view that is consistent with the clonal selection theory of
Burnet. Implicit in this model is the notion that antigen would
independently influence cells of the different immunoglobulin
classes having the same antibody specificity.

A number of observations suggest that generation of immunoglobulin class and antibody heterogeneity in mammals may follow the
same general pattern (Reviewed in ref. 13): (i) The phylogenetic
order of appearance of the three major classes of immunoglobulins
is IgM, IgG, IgA; (ii) This sequence is repeated in the ontogeny of
immunoglobulin production in mammalian species; (iii) Under certain
conditions, human lymphoid cells can produce more than one class of
immunoglobulin (14-16). The combinations of immunoglobulins produced by a single cell appear to be restricted to IgM and IgG, or
IgG and IgA; single cells synthesizing IgM and IgA have not been
observed; (iv) Recent studies on two myeloma proteins (IgM and IgG)
produced in the same patient have suggested that both immunoglobulins may be expressing the same set of variable region genes (17),
thus lending support to our hypothesis that a switch from IgM to
IgG synthesis may occur within a single clone of cells. We have
also suggested that IgA producing cells arise from cells which
formerly produced IgG within the mammalian bursa-equivalent (13).
The hypothesis can be tested in mammals; experimental efforts
directed toward this end are in progress.

REFERENCES

1. B. Glick, T. S. Chang, and R. G. Jaap, Poultry Sci., 35:224,
   1956.

2. M. A. S. Moore and J. J. T. Owen, Dev. Biol., 14:40, 1966.

3. M. D. Cooper, W. A. Cain, P. Van Alten, and R. A. Good,
   Int. Arch. Allergy, 35:242, 1969.

4. N. L. Warner, J. W. Uhr, G. J. Thorbecke, and Z. Ovary,
   J. Immun., 103:1319, 1969.

5. M. D. Cooper, R. D. A. Peterson, M. A. South, and R. A. Good,
   J. Exp. Med., 123:75, 1966.

24

M. D. COOPER ET AL.

6. M. D. Cooper, M. L. Schwartz, and R. A. Good, Science, 151:471, 1966.

7. C. C. Clawson, M. D. Cooper, and R. A. Good, Lab. Invest., 16:407, 1967.

8. G. J. Thorbecke, N. L. Warner, G. M. Hochwald, and S. H. Ohanian, Immunology, 15:123, 1968.

9. R. Van Meter, R. A. Good, and M. D. Cooper, J. Immun., 102:370, 1969.

10. P. W. Kincade and M. D. Cooper, Submitted for publication.

11. S. Dray, Nature, 195:677, 1962.

12. M. D. Cooper and K. S. Self, Unpublished observations.

13. M. D. Cooper, P. W. Kincade, and A. R. Lawton, in: B. M. Kagan and E. R. Stiehm, Eds., Immunologic Incompetence. Chicago: Year Book Medical Publishers, in press.

14. N. Costea, V. J. Yakulis, J. A. Libnoch, C. G. Pilz, and P. Heller, Am. J. Med., 42:630, 1967.

15. J. L. Fahey and I. Finegold, Cold Spring Harbor Symp. Quant. Biol., 32:283, 1967.

16. M. Takahashi, N. Tanigaki, Y. Yagi, G. E. Moore, and D. Pressman, J. Immun., 100:1176, 1968.

17. J. E. Hopper, S. K. Wilson, A. Nisonoff, A. C. Wang, and H. H. Fudenberg, Fed. Proc. 29:258, 1970.

The Rabbit Appendix: A Central or Peripheral Lymphoid Organ?

P. Nieuwenhuis

Department of Histology, State University of Groningen

Groningen, Holland

Recent experiments (Miller) (1) indicate the antibody-forming-cell-precursor (AFCP) in mice to be BM derived. On the other hand Good and coworkers demonstrated that in the chicken the Bursa of Fabricius is essential in the development of the antibody forming capacity. In the rabbit the gut-associated lymphoid tissue like Peyer's patches etc. should represent the Bursa-aequivalent (2). Fichtelius (3) claims the intimate relationship between epithelium and lymphoid tissue to be essential for its functioning as a first level lymphoid organ.

The present paper will deal with the next two problems: (i) the nature of lympho-epithelial relations in the rabbit appendix and their role - if any - in the postulated central lymphoid function of this organ, and (ii) the production of antibody-forming-cell-precursors by the rabbit appendix.

LYMPHOEPITHELIAL RELATIONS IN THE RABBIT APPENDIX

In the rabbit appendix a regular pattern of follicular structures can be readily observed. Like follicular structures in the spleen and lymph nodes they contain an outer marginal zone (sub-epithelial zone), a lymphocyte corona and a follicular center with high mitotic activity (germinal center) (fig. 1).

Heavy infiltration of the epithelial lining over these follicular structures with small lymphoid cells is evident (4,5,6). Methylgreen-pyronin staining reveals clusters of small or medium sized lymphoid cells engulfed in the highly basophilic cytoplasm of supporting epithelial cells which we have - noncommittally - called "nurse" cells (fig. 2).

From the base of the crypts upwards the number of cells/cluster

25

increases suggesting proliferation in situ. Three points, however, argue against this: (i) mitotic figures among cluster cells are extremely rare; (ii) following the injection of colcemid no metaphasic arrest was observed among cluster cells; (iii) following the i.v. injection of 0.1 μc/gr.b.w. ^{3}H-Thymidine (Amersham) only a minor fraction (< 5%) of the cluster cells were found to be labelled. However, after two or three days the number of labelled cells found within clusters had increased up to 50-70%, suggesting an immigration of labelled cells.

At about 1/3 from the top of the protruding follicle no more clusters are found within the epithelium. Above this level empty nurse cells can be found, suggesting the extrusion of the lymphoid cells into the cryptal space.

With the *electron microscope* (fig. 3) cluster cells are best characterized as medium sized lymphoid cells. A whole cluster is completely surrounded by the cell membrane of the nurse cell. Between the cluster and the nucleus of the nurse cell – which is of the open face type, containing a nucleolus and numerous pores in the nuclear membrane – a narrow electron lucent band is always present filled with some fibrillar material. The nucleus of the nurse cell itself is surrounded by a densely-packed rough surfaced endoplasmic reticulum. More to the top empty nurse cells can be observed, their surface area still disturbed by the recent extrusion of cluster cells. Migration of lymphoid cells from clusters backwards through the basement membrane to the subepithelial zone was never noticed.

Electron microscopical observations of the prenatal and neonatal appendix disclosed the following: until the time of birth no lymphoid cells occur within the epithelium covering the areas where follicular structures will develop within the first week after birth. However, nurse-cell-precursors may be observed characterized by the presence of numerous electron dense bodies (lysosomes?) intermingled with mitochondria situated between the nucleus of these cells and the still intact basement membrane. Twelve hours after birth for the first time small lesions in the basement membrane were noticed. At 24 hours the first lymphoid cells are found to migrate through the basement membrane lesions to reach a position beneath the nucleus of the nurse cell, the cytoplasm of which starting to surround the intruder. The nucleus of the nurse cell then moves to a lateral position (fig. 4) to slide down underneath the invading lymphocyte. By two or three days as a result of continuous immigration the number of cells/cluster had increased and by 6 days in principle the adult situation had been reached.

Figure 1: Normal rabbit appendix
Figure 2: Lympho-epithelial relations in normal rabbit appendix
Figure 3: Electron micrograph of cluster + nurse cell
Figure 4: Rabbit appendix 24 hours after birth.

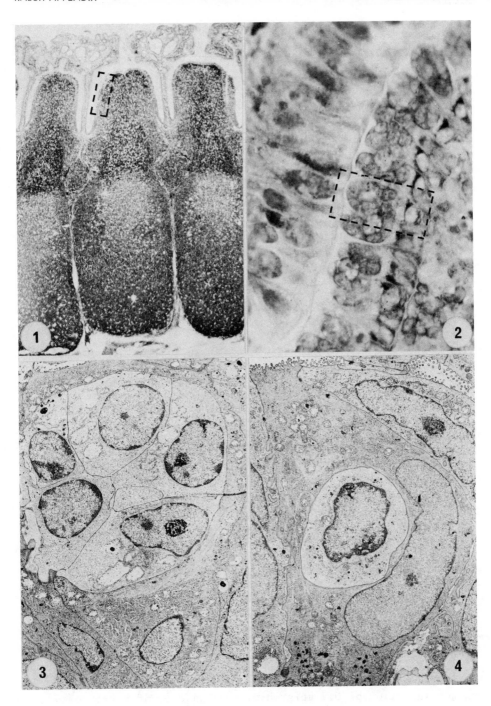

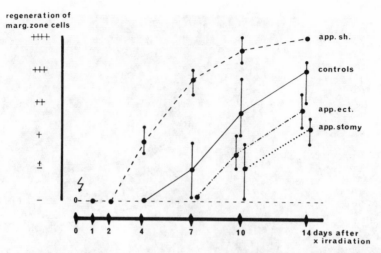

Figure 5: Regeneration of marginal zone cells in the spleen following 450 rads whole body X-irradiation.

PRODUCTION OF AFCP's BY THE RABBIT APPENDIX

Following 450 rads whole body irradiation follicular structures
are severely damaged; regeneration – at least in the spleen – does
not occur until 7-10 days later. This regeneration at first consists
of small groups of medium sized lymphoid cells, marginal zone cells,
from which in later stages regular follicular structures develop.
At the same time primary antibody forming potential – which had been
abolished as a result of the irradiation – is restored. Regeneration
of follicular structures along the digestive tract was much faster;
active germinal centers already being present around day seven post-
irradiation.

To check whether this gut-associated lymphoid tissue contributes to the regeneration of follicular structures elsewhere *appendectomized* animals or animals subjected to *appendicostomy* with cecal ligation "sterilized" through the intraluminal application of
a mixture of neomycine/phtallylsulfathazol received 450 rads. As
shown in fig.5 regeneration of follicular structures in the spleen
in both instances is delayed for about 3-4 days. In the wall of the
"sterilized" appendices no regeneration of germinal centers was observed, suggesting (i) that regeneration of germinal center activity in the appendix is antigen dependent and (ii) that appendix germinal centers contribute to the regeneration of follicular structures elsewhere through cell delivery. In the reverse experiment
(whole body X-irradiation with the *appendix shielded* regeneration
of follicular structures in the spleen was enhanced (fig.5). Following the injection of 0.2 μc/gr.b.w. ^{3}H-Thymidine 18 hours post

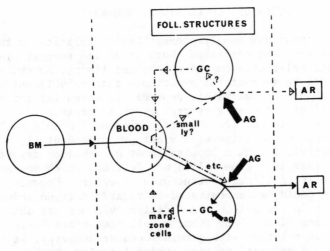

Figure 6: Hypothesis: origin of antibody-forming-cell-precursors.
         (Ag: antigen, GC: germinal center, AR: antibody response).

irradiation (appendix shielded) labelled lymphoid cells were detected 4 days post irradiation among the regenerating follicular structures.

Next appendectomized or sham-operated animals were exposed to
450 rads whole body irradiation and after 10 days injected i.v.
with a standard dose of paratyphoid vaccine. In the appendectomized
animals antibody-forming-potential of the spleen measured as 6th
day peak titer was reduced to appr. 10% of control animals. These
experiments suggest that as a result of the appendectomy less antibody-forming-cell-precursors had reached the spleen, these precursor cells presumably being the appendix-germinal-center-derived
marginal zone cells.

However, when artificially (by the i.v. injection of an antigen) induced germinal centers in the *spleen* were selectively labelled by means of local labelling of the spleen (7), the *in situ* development of marginal zone cells from these labelled germinal centers could be observed by the substantial increase in the number of
labelled cells within the marginal zone. Moreover labelled cells
were found to migrate to and home preferentially in follicular
structures elsewhere (popliteal lymph nodes, appendix). When 24
hours after the labelling of spleen germinal centers a booster injection was given labelled plasmablasts were found 24 hours later,
suggesting the production of memory cells within these germinal
centers. If, however, a non cross reacting antigen was injected
again although less numerous labelled plasmablasts were noticed.

DISCUSSION, CONCLUSIONS, SUMMARY

An as yet almost unknown lympho-epithelial relation in the
rabbit appendix has been described. Data presented suggest migration of lymphoid cells through the epithelial lining. No evidence
could be obtained to support the hypothesis that this lympho-epithelial relationship in the rabbit appendix is essential for its
functioning – if at all – as a central lymphoid organ.

Evidence was obtained for the production of lymphoid cells by
the rabbit appendix associated with – antigen dependent (?) – germinal center activity. Thus a population of germinal-center-derived
lymphoid cells (marginal zone cells) was defined, which was demonstrated to populate follicular structures elsewhere. However, the
same phenomenon could be demonstrated as regards antigen induced
germinal centers in the spleen. In addition evidence was obtained
for the generation of antibody forming cell precursors – virginal
or committed – in relation with germinal center activity. It is
suggested that all germinal centers (and follicular structures)
throughout the lymphoid tissue in principle are identical structures giving rise to a population of circulating lymphoid cells capable of homing in follicular structures elsewhere and mounting primary or secondary antibody response.

The above mentioned observations in relation with the proven
non-thymus dependency (8) of follicular structures and the observation that AFCP's are bone marrow derived (1) suggest (Fig.6) that
bone marrow precursor cells, upon reaching peripheral lymphoid
tissues may become involved in germinal center activity, the germinal center being an – antigen dependent – amplification (and perhaps selecting) mechanism for antibody forming cell precursors.

ACKNOWLEDGEMENTS

Thanks are due to the Foundation for Basic Medical Research
(FunGO) for financial support and to miss W. Kleiwerd, miss W.K.
Polman and mr. E.H. Blaauw for skilled technical assistence.

REFERENCES

1. Mitchell, G.F. and Miller, J.F.A.P., J.Exp.Med. 1968, 128, 821.
2. Perey, D.Y.E. and Good, R.A., Lab.Invest. 1968, 18, 15.
3. Fichtelius, K.E., Finstad, J. and Good, R.A., Int.Arch.Allergy
   1969, 35, 119.
4. Jolly, J., Compt.Rend. de l'Ass. des Anat. (Suppl.) 1911, 164.
5. Watzka, M., Anat.Anz.Erg.hft. 1932, 75, 150.
6. Ackerman, G.A., Anat.Rec. 1966, 154, 21.
7. Nieuwenhuis, P., Adv. in Exp.Med. and Biol. 1969, 5, 113.
8. Veldman, J.E., Acad.Thesis, Groningen – The Netherlands, 1970.

IMMUNOGLOBULIN GENE EXPRESSION IN
IMMUNOCYTE DIFFERENTIATION *

Noel L. Warner and John M. Dwyer

The Walter and Eliza Hall Institute of

Medical Research, Melbourne, Australia

Immunocompetent cells appear to exist in at least two distinct subpopulations on the basis of several different observations. (i) In chickens, a sharp dichotomy between lymphoid cells involved in cellular or humoral immune responses is associated with a separate developmental control by thymus or the bursa of Fabricius (1); (ii) in the initiation of certain antibody responses, thymic derived cells, "T" cells (2), collaborate with non-thymic derived cells, "B" cells, to induce the latter into active antibody secretion (3) ; and (iii) in peripheral lymphoid tissues, varying proportions of lymphoid cells carry thymic specific cell surface isoantigens such as theta (4). Whether these three classifications are all describing the same two cell types is not completely resolved, however it does appear that "T" and "B" cells are distinct in both their ontogenic development and functional capacity. In this article we wish to discuss the development of these two lines in terms of the type of immunoglobulin synthesised by these cells, and therefore responsible for their ability to react with antigen.

In the normal ontogeny of immunoglobulin formation in chickens, the bursa of Fabricius is the first site of immunoglobulin synthesis (5) with IgM being detected at least at embryo day 18, and in another study (6), at embryo day 14. No significant immunoglobulin synthesis was detected in the embryonic or neonatal chicken thymus. The existence however, of a population of cells capable of initiating antigen specific delayed hypersensitivity reactions in agammaglobulinemic bursaless

---
* This work was supported by USPHS grant No. AM 11234-03.

chickens, strongly suggests that the "T" cell population does carry some
form of immunoglobulin as its surface bound antigen recognition unit.
It has been shown that hemopoietic stem cells enter the avian bursa (7)
and thymus (8) only a day or so before the earliest appearance of
recognisable lymphoid cells. This indicates that the actual differentiation
of immunocompetent cells from hemopoietic stem cells may involve a
quite rapid activation (derepression) of certain immunoglobulin genes,
which is sufficient to yield surface bound immunoglobulin molecules, if
not actual secretion.

In order to determine the exact nature of the surface immunoglobulin
on lymphoid cells, two separate questions must be answered: (i) does the
immunoglobulin contain an antigen binding site?; and (ii) what is the light
and heavy chain type of the molecule? The first question has been
approached by the use of a technique of uptake of ^{125}I labelled soluble
antigens by lymphoid cell suspensions from various tissues of normal
unimmunised animals. Antigen binding cells have been found with this
technique (9 - 11)to occur inadult mouse and human peripheral lymphoid
tissues, and in fetal mammalian thymus (12) and embryonic chicken
bursa (13). Determination of the possible heavy chain type of this antigen
receptor has then been made by the attempted blocking of antigen uptake
by preincubation of the cells with the various anti-immunoglobulin sera.
Using this method, the antigen binding receptor on adult mouse lymphoid
cells was shown to be IgM (14).

Before considering these results in detail, it is important to consider
the possible ways in which these lymphoid cells may have bound antigen.
At least three different explanations exist : (i) a non-specific binding
which does not involve an immunoglobulin molecule; (ii) cytophilic
antibody bound to the surface of a cell with its antibody site still exposed;
and (iii) the lymphoid cell has itself synthesised the immunoglobulin
receptor, which may either be an intact molecule of a presently recognised
serum class, be of a new class (the hypothetical IgX) made only in these
specialised cells, or be an incomplete molecule in the sense of lacking
one of the polypeptide chains or a portion thereof. Examples of all three
possibilities have now been found, and must therefore be considered in
any new antigen binding system.

The results in Table 1. show the number of labelled lymphocytes
per million lymphocytes, in cell suspensions prepared from different
lymphoid tissues of chicken, mouse and man. In each case, a sample of
the cell suspension was first incubated with either normal rabbit serum
or Eisens balanced salt solution (control), or with a polyvalent rabbit
antiserum containing antibodies against both L chains and μ and γ chains
of the appropriate species. Human fetal bone marrow and liver, which

Table 1. Antigen uptake by different cells after pretreatment with
polyvalent anti-immunoglobulin serum.

Cell suspension	Labelled lymphocytes / 10^6 after serum treatment		Percent control uptake
	Control	Anti-Ig.	
Adult mouse spleen	856*	<40*	<5
Adult mouse spleen	116	<9	<8
Adult mouse P. E. C.	77000*	18000*	23
Adult mouse P. E. C.	5200	1600	29
1 day mouse spleen	1520*	440	29
Fetal mouse spleen	120	60	50
Fetal mouse thymus	500	120	24
Adult human P. B. L.	8200	700	8
Fetal human liver	1200	850	72
Fetal human thymus	1900	0	0
Fetal human B. M.	2300	2400	100
Chick embryo thymus	80	0	<1
Chick embryo bursa (HL)	5200	70	1
Chick embryo bursa (LL)	2790	1360	49

* Labelled antigen was hemocyanin. In all other cases antigen was
monomeric flagellin.   P. E. C. = peritoneal exudate cells. P. B. L. =
peripheral blood lymphocytes. B. M. = bone marrow. HL = grain counts
>50 per cell (heavily labelled). LL = grain counts 5-50 per cell .

are true hemopoietic organs, contain large numbers of antigen binding
cells, virtually all of which fall into the nonspecific category, as no
blocking was observed with the antiserum. Approximately one quarter of
the antigen binding cells in adult peritoneal exudate are also of this type.
With neonatal and fetal mouse tissues, a considerable proportion of non-
specific cells were found, which in the case of the chick embryo bursa,
were almost exclusively of the lightly labelled type. Most of the adult
mouse spleen lymphocytes and human blood lymphocytes were blocked by
the antiserum. This was also true for the human fetal thymus and the
heavily labelled chick embryo bursal cells.

These results with the chick embryo bursa (13) are of particular
interest in that they may indicate that the "B" line of cells, which is
known to synthesise IgM in embryo, may express an antibody specificity
region . Furthermore, as the emergence of antigen binding cells in the

chick embryo is in the bursa but not the thymus, whereas in mammals the fetal thymus is involved, a possible presence of "B" line cells in the early mammalian thymus must be considered. A degree of caution regarding this interpretation must however be added. Recent studies have shown two examples in which antigen binding cells were produced by passive antibody treatment. Basten, Miller, and Warner (unpublished) have shown that an IgG containing G-200 Sephadex fraction of a mouse anti-chicken γ-globulin serum, will confer on a proportion of mouse thoracic duct cells the ability to behave as antigen binding cells with respect to labelled chicken γ-globulin. This property could be removed by repeated washing, indicating lability of the binding of antibody to the cell. We have also recently found that pretreatment of 17 day embryonic bursal cells with a chicken anti-flagellin serum, will lead to the development of 18% of antigen binding cells to flagellin. Further studies on the nature of this passive cytophilic binding to lymphocytes are in progress, and at present can only indicate that considerable caution should be taken in interpreting results based solely on assays which only measure the presence of immunoglobulin on cells, rather than determining intra-cellular content, secretion or synthesis of immunoglobulin. These results also indicate the possibility that the antigen binding cells found in normal embryonic bursa may represent small amounts of cytophilic antibody derived from the mother via the yolk. Blocking tests with anti-μ and anti-γ are now in progress.

Our current data on the immunoglobulin class of the antigen receptor is summarised in Table 2. With both human and mouse unimmunised lymphoid cell suspensions, almost complete blocking of antigen uptake was achieved by preincubation of the cells with either anti-L or anti-μ chain antibodies, but not with any other anti-heavy chain sera. As indicated previously, the cytophilic immunoglobulin for mouse thoracic duct cells was an IgG. Unfortunately we do not yet have data on anti-L or -μ chain treatment of mammalian fetal thymus. However in one experiment with specific anti-γ chain sera and a three week newborn human thymus, no blocking at all was observed ($62/10^5$ control and $67/10^5$ in anti-γ treated), suggesting that placentally transferred maternal IgG may not be involved in coating the newborn thymus cells. In contrast to these studies, blocking of cell mediated immune reactions such as graft versus host reactions with mouse spleen cells (15), the transfer of delayed hyper-sensitivity with sensitised peritoneal exudate cells (15), and the in vitro reactions of human lymphocytes to tuberculin or HLA antigens (16), has only been achieved with anti-L chain sera, and not with any anti-H chain sera.

In view of the fact that most lymphoid cell suspensions are mixtures of "T" and "B" cells, we have also examined malignant lymphoid cells for

Table 2.   Immunoglobulin class of antigen receptors.

Cell suspension	Assay system	Ig. class
Adult mouse spleen	A. B. C*	IgM (L, μ)
Adult human blood lymphocytes	A. B. C.	IgM (L, μ)
Newborn human thymus	A. B. C.	Not IgG.
Embryonic chick bursa	Synthesis**	IgM
Embryonic chick bursa	A. B. C.	?
Adult mouse thoracic duct cells and passive antibody	A. B. C.	IgG
Adult mouse spleen	Graft versus host	L chain
Sensitised adult mouse P. E. C.	Transfer of del. hypersensitivity	L chain.

* Antigen binding cells.   ** Incorporation of ^{14}C amino acids. (5)

possible immunoglobulin synthesis. Just as plasma cell tumors represent a pure clone of their normal counterpart, and are usually synthesising a normal product, so malignant lymphoid cells which are readily obtained in quite pure form might represent their normal counterpart. Previous studies with human leukemias (chronic lymphocytic) (18) and Burkitt s lymphoma (17) have indicated low levels of synthesis of IgM.

Samples of 12 different mouse lymphoid tumors maintained by serial transplantation in vivo, were cultured in vitro with ^{14}C labelled amino acids for 24 hours. The cultures were frozen and thawed repeatedly, and the supernatant fluid was then examined in radioimmunoelectrophoresis for mouse immunoglobulin synthesis (method as in 5). Of four lymphomas which arose in peripheral sites, two showed free light chain synthesis (confirmed by sucrose gradient centrifugation), one gave complete IgM synthesis, and the other free light chains and a trace of IgM. Of 8 lines established from radiation induced thymomas, only two showed a faint trace of immunoglobulin synthesis, which in both cases was free light chains. These studies support the concept of two types of lymphocytes, one making intact IgM and the other only free light chains. However it will also be essential to apply a "T" cell surface isoantigenic marker to these cells, to ascertain whether the light chain producers, but not the IgM producers, are of "T" type.

There are still many questions to be answered about the nature of

the immunoglobulin receptors on lymphoid cells, particularly in relation
to the question of specificity in B cells, and the possibility of hidden H
chains in "T" cells. At present we feel that the data is most consistent
with the interpretation that, just as differentiation in any other system
is essentially a turning on and off of various genes carried in the genome,
so immunocompetent cell differentiation involves the induced activation of
immunoglobulin genes in progeny of hemopoietic stem cells. The thymic
environment (? hormone) appears to activate only a light chain gene
(? only the variable part of the light chain), whereas the bursa or bursal
equivalent activates light and mμ chain synthesis.

REFERENCES

1. N. L. Warner, Folia Biol., 13: 1, 1967.
2. I. M. Roitt, M. F. Greaves, G. Torrigiani, J. Brostoff, and
    J. H. L. Playfair, Lancet, ii: 367, 1969.
3. J. F. A. P. Miller and G. F. Mitchell, Transpl. Rev., 1: 3, 1969.
4. M. C. Raff, Nature, 224: 378, 1969.
5. G. J. Thorbecke, N. L. Warner, G. M. Hochwald, and S. H.
    Ohanian, Immunology, 15: 123, 1968.
6. M. D. Cooper, P. W. Kincade, and A. R. Lawton, in Immunologic
    Incompetence, edited by B. M. Kagan and E. R. Stiehm. Year book
    Med. Publishers, Chicago in press 1970.
7. M. A. S. Moore and J. J. T. Owen, Nature, 208: 956, 1965.
8. M. A. S. Moore and J. J. T. Owen, J. Exp. Med., 126: 715, 1967.
9. D. Naor and D. Sulitzeanu, Nature, 214: 687, 1967.
10. P. Byrt and G. L. Ada, Immunology, 17: 503, 1969.
11. J. M. Dwyer and I. R. Mackay, Lancet, i: 164, 1970.
12. J. M. Dwyer and I. R. Mackay, Lancet, i: 1119, 1970.
13. J. M. Dwyer and N. L. Warner, submitted for publication.
14. N. L. Warner, P. Byrt, and G. L. Ada, Nature, 226: 942, 1970.
15. S. Mason and N. L. Warner, J. Immunol., 104: 762, 1970.
16. M. F. Greaves, Transpl. Rev., 5: in press 1970.
17. E. Klein, G. Klein, J. S. Nadkarni, J. J. Nadkarni, H. Wigzell,
    and P. Clifford, Lancet, ii: 1068, 1967.
18. B. Johansson and E. Klein, Clin. Exp. Immunol., 6: 421, 1970.

CHAIRMAN'S INTRODUCTION TO DISCUSSION

THE MATURATION OF LYMPHOID TISSUE STRUCTURE AND FUNCTION

IN ONTOGENY

A. M. Silverstein and R. A. Prendergast

Wilmer Institute, Johns Hopkins University

School of Medicine, Baltimore, Maryland 21205

A number of structural organizations have been identified in
the peripheral lymphoid tissues of man and animals. In encapsulated
lymph nodes, these include a more-or-less distinct division between
cortex and medulla, the presence of primary lymphoid follicles and
subsequently mature germinal centers, and a discrete interfollicular
zone in the lymph node cortex. On a more functional basis, the lymph
node has been divided geographically into "thymus-dependent regions",
concerned primarily with cellular immunologic events, and "bursa-
dependent regions", devoted presumably to the production of humoral
antibody (1). The spleen is similarly, although less precisely,
characterized by a white pulp and a red pulp, with germinal centers
and their characteristic lymphocytic mantles prominent in the
periarterial Malpighian bodies. Intense infiltrates of lymphocytes
and plasma cells with or without germinal centers also characterize
the wall of the intestinal tract, and here a special relationship
has been postulated between the lymphoid germinal center and its
superjacent epithelium (2). As was pointed out elsewhere in this
symposium, however, all of the structural organizations and all of
the functions normally attributed to organized lymphoid tissue may
be duplicated at almost any other location within the body (3).

It appears to be a generally shared belief that these lymphoid
structures and especially the germinal center are important if not
absolutely necessary prerequisites for the mature immunologic
response to antigenic stimulus. This conclusion seems to be based
upon the almost invariable use of mature animals in studying lymphoid
function in the immune response, and on 1) the ubiquitous presence
of these structures in mature lymphoid tissue; 2) an almost invariant
lymphofollicular hyperplastic response to antigenic stimulus; and 3) a
hypoplasia or absence of some of these structures in association

37

with specific immunologic defects in certain natural or experimental immunologic deficiency diseases. The germinal center has received special attention in this respect, being variously charged with such critical roles as that of antigen trapping, focusing, and long-term antigen retention (4,5), or as the source of immunologic memory cells (6,7).

In this paper we will reexamine the relationship between lymphoid structure and immunologic function by comparing these developments in the normal fetus with those in the fetus exposed to immunogenic stimulus. It will become evident that none of the lymphoid organizations referred to above constitute a sine qua non of the immune response, and that in fact they seem more to follow than to prepare for the active immunologic response of the stimulated host.

                    *   *   *

The context for the present discussion arises from observations on the maturation of immunologic capability and of lymphoid tissues in the normal fetal lamb in utero, although evidence is rapidly accumulating that the conclusions to be drawn from this species are applicable also, with but minor variation, to the fetus and neonate of other mammalian species (8). The upper portion of Figure 1 brings out the most important aspect of the development of immunologic competence in the fetal and neonatal lamb, i.e., that at discrete times during its normal 150-day gestation period and even after birth, the ability to respond to different antigenic stimuli arises as a series of seemingly independent events. Thus, prior to about 75-days gestation in the case of allografts, or about 120-days gestation in the case of ovalbumin, the fetus does not "see" the antigen in an immunologic sense, and evinces no sign of response to stimulus. After the critical age is attained for each of these antigens, however, not only does the fetus respond actively to the antigenic stimulus, but both qualitatively and quantitatively its response equals that of the adult animal (9-11).

The significance of these findings is pointed up by a consideration of the status of the lymphoid tissues of the developing fetus. The lower portions of Figure 1 summarize the principal elements of the maturation of the lymphoid tissues of the fetal lamb. The line for each lymphoid tissue starts at the earliest gestation age at which lymphoid cells can be found in the respective locations. Thus, lymphocytes are not seen in the anlage of peripheral lymph nodes until about the 45th day of gestation, when they begin to populate the cervical nodes, nor are they seen in the developing spleen until about 58 to 65-days gestation, nor in the lamina propria of the intestinal tract until sometime between 75 and 85-days gestation. Following the first arrival of lymphoid cells in each of these tissues, there commences a slow and continuous maturation of these tissues until birth, in terms of

LYMPHOID MATURATION

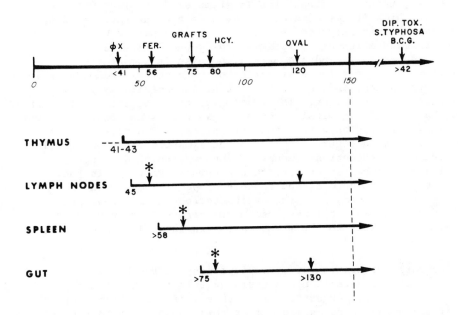

Fig. 1. Comparison of immunologic and lymphoid maturation in the fetal lamb. Numbers represent gestation ages up to normal 150-day term, and neonatal age thereafter. ϕX = bacteriophage, FER = horse ferritin, HCY = snail hemocyanin, OVAL = hen albumin. (See text for additional discussion.)

increasing numbers of lymphoid cells and their organization into geographically defined formations. But even at birth, the amount of white pulp in the spleen of the normal animal is minimal and germinal centers are absent, while the population of lymphocytes in most of the regional nodes is sparse. There is little distinction as yet between cortex and medulla, with no germinal centers evident, but only the occasional primary follicle. Only in the Peyer's patch region of the intestinal tract and in the mesenteric lymph nodes immediately draining this area is any appreciable maturity of lymphoid tissue observed (the simple arrows in Figure 1). Here increased numbers of lymphocytes can be found with more-or-less mature germinal centers, although plasma cell differentiation is almost completely lacking.

Only after birth, presumably in response to the sudden incursion of a variety of different antigenic stimuli, does one find a rapid maturation of all lymphoid tissues within the developing

host, and this in direct proportion to the proximity of the lymphoid
tissue in question to the likely routes of entry of the stimuli.
If, however, the developing fetus is stimulated in utero with an
antigen to which it has developed immunologic competence, then the
active immunologic response is found to be accompanied by a
precocious maturation of the stimulated lymphoid tissues. This
response generally includes a marked increase in lymphocyte
population, an increasing distinction between cortex and medulla in
the regional nodes, and may or may not be accompanied by frank
germinal center formation. Interestingly, this maturation of lymphoid
tissue can be induced within a given organ very soon after the first
arrival of lymphocytes within that organ, as is indicated by the
asterisk-arrows in Figure 1. Should the lymphoid organ in question
not be ready to support an immune response, then it does not
participate and some other structure becomes involved. In the
absence of any lymphoid tissue capable of participating in the
response, such as occurs in the antibacteriophage response prior
to 45-days gestation, the response occurs presumably in non-lymphoid
tissues, most likely in the liver, although this has not been
formally demonstrated.

        The early maturation of lymphoid tissue in the Peyer's patch
region and the mesenteric nodes draining this area is of some
interest in view of suggestions that this tissue may constitute a
central lymphoid control organ. That this is unlikely in the ovine
species is suggested by observations that complete removal of the
intestinal tract of the fetal lamb prior to first appearance of
lymphocytes within it is without effect on subsequent maturation of
immunologic capabilities by the fetal lamb. Furthermore, the
peripheral lymphoid nature of the Peyer's patches in this species
is attested to by demonstration that reduction of stimulus from the
empty gut lumen distal to an ileal atresia results in a marked
diminution in the development of Peyer's patch germinal centers.
Conversely, introduction of additional antigenic stimuli into the
intestinal tract of the fetus via an indwelling gastric catheter
results in marked and precocious enhancement of lymphoid maturation
both in the lamina propria of the gut and in the dependent
mesenteric lymph nodes (12).

                    *   *   *

        From the data briefly reviewed above we may make several
deductions about the relationship between immunologic reactivity
and lymphoid tissue organization in the stimulated host. First, it
becomes clear that there is no presently identifiable morphologic
hallmark to be found in lymphoid tissues which might signal the
development of immunologic competence (i.e., the potential to
respond to a given antigenic stimulus). Second, it would appear
that the fetal host can engage in any form of immunologic response
in the absence of, or at least prior to the maturation of, such

structural entities as the lymph node cortex with primary follicles or the white pulp of the spleen, or of germinal centers in any lymphoid tissue location. This is supported by the lack of direct correlation observed between plasma cell formation and lymphoid organization in human fetuses exposed to the highly antigenic Treponema pallidum in congenital syphilis (13). Third, studies of the response to antigenic stimulus in such immunologic virgin animals as the mammalian fetus in utero strongly suggest that the maturation of lymphoid tissues is not a necessary preparation for the immune response, but in fact only accompanies or even follows it as a component of the more general response to the same antigenic stimuli. Data from germ-free animals (14), representing somewhat of an extension of the protected intrauterine environment, lend further support for this view.

ACKNOWLEDGMENTS

These studies were supported in part by the U.S. Army Research and Development Command, Contract No. DA-49-193-MD-2640; an unrestricted gift from the Alcon Laboratories, Inc.; and an Independent Order of Odd Fellows Research Professorship.

REFERENCES

1. M. D. Cooper, R. D. A. Peterson, M. A. South, and R. A. Good, J. Exp. Med., 123:75, 1966.

2. K. E. Fichtelius, in: L. Fiore-Donati and M. G. Hanna, Jr., Eds., Lymphatic Tissue and Germinal Centers in Immune Response, p. 9. New York: Plenum Press, 1969.

3. A. M. Silverstein and R. A. Prendergast, this volume, p. 583.

4. G. J. V. Nossal, G. L. Ada, and C. M. Austin, Aust. J. Exp. Biol. Med. Sci., 42:311, 1964.

5. M. G. Hanna, Jr., A. K. Szakal, and H. E. Walburg, Jr., in: L. Fiore-Donati and M. G. Hanna, Jr., Eds., Lymphatic Tissue and Germinal Centers in Immune Response, p. 149. New York: Plenum Press, 1969.

6. G. J. Thorbecke, E. B. Jacobson, and R. Asofsky, J. Immunol., 92:734, 1964.

7. M. G. Hanna, Jr., M. W. Francis, and L. C. Peters, Immunology, 15:75, 1968.

8. J. Šterzl and A. M. Silverstein, Advances Immunol., 6:337, 1967.

9. A. M. Silverstein, R. A. Prendergast, and K. L. Kraner,
    J. Exp. Med., 119:955, 1964.

10. A. M. Silverstein, C. J. Parshall, Jr., and J. W. Uhr,
    Science, 154:1675, 1966.

11. A. M. Silverstein, R. A. Prendergast, and C. J. Parshall, Jr.,
    J. Immunol., 104:269, 1970.

12. A. M. Silverstein, C. J. Parshall, Jr., B. I. Osburn, and
    R. A. Prendergast (in preparation).

13. A. M. Silverstein and R. J. Lukes, Lab. Invest., 11:918, 1962.

14. G. J. Thorbecke, H. A. Gordon, B. Wostman, M. Wagner, and
    J. A. Reyniers, J. Inf. Dis., 101:237, 1957.

DISCUSSION TO SESSION 1

CHAIRMAN, A. M. SILVERSTEIN, CO-CHAIRMAN, W. H. HILDEMAN

Co-chairman's remarks: To a considerable extent ontogeny does indeed appear to recapitulate phylogeny. However, our ignorance concerning the phylogeny of immunological characteristics is still
profound. Perhaps the most exciting recent discovery is that certain invertebrates have at least a primitive immunological capacity
with some memory. This is certainly true among the annelids.
There is suggestive evidence that Tunicates may also have some capacity for cellular immunity as indicated by allograft reactions.
Of course, these animals have no thymus. Indeed, the cell infiltrate one sees in allograft rejection has predominantly macrophage
or histiocytic character rather than lymphoid. There is no compelling evidence at the moment that any specific immunoglobulin
antibodies can be made by any invertebrate, but I think we ought
to bear in mind that there has been very little investigative work
done. The very earliest manifestations of specific immunologic
capacity may be found among certain of the invertebrates. This is
an exciting area for future work. Among the most primitive vertebrates, the Agnathans, hagfish and lampreys are not only capable of
rejecting grafts, but of giving vigorous IgM-type antibody responses
to both cellular and soluble antigens. Whether they are capable of
making more than one class of immunoglobulins remains to be demonstrated. We still know little about the cellular bases of their
immunity. Hagfish, for example, may lack a thymus as such, but we
have yet to look at some very young animals, as opposed to adults.
Peripheral lymphoid tissue in hagfish is scarce. Yet, in the peripheral blood we find a whole spectrum of cell types, including
abundant lymphocytes, that one would expect to find in an immunologically competent animal.

Beginning with the sharks and rays, well-organized central as
well as peripheral lymphoid tissue, but no lymph nodes, are found
and there is still the capacity to make only IgM-type antibody.
The Teleosts or bony fishes are a particularly interesting transition group, because it is here that we first find two distinctive
classes of antibody. Australian lungfish quite clearly make two
molecular classes of antibody, whereas goldfish seem to make only
two subclasses that are similar but electrophoretically distinct.
We need to look closely at other fishes, but very interesting
changes are apparent at the Teleost level. The amphibians, as you
have learned from E.L. Cooper this morning, first show if not peripheral lymph nodes, at least lymph glands which are clearly responsible for serum antibody production. Here we definitely have two
major classes of antibody made, as is also true in at least certain
reptiles. We know now that lymph nodes of simple structure occur
in turtles. At the familiar level of birds and mammals, perhaps
the most clear manifestation of evolution is the ability to make
five or more molecular classes of antibody with distinctive func-

43

tions. Probably we should not be calling the similar antibodies
in the lower vertebrates IgM or IgG, but rather IgM-type or IgG-
type in relation to their major characteristics.

There are lots of question marks in our current knowledge of
immunologic phylogeny. Even the answers we have at the avian and
mammalian level are perhaps too heavily biased toward chicken and
rodents. We may well encounter some revealing surprises as we look
further to other species.

J.F.A.P. Miller: Dr Silverstein has shown some very interesting
results on the sequential appearance of the capacity of the fetal
lamb to respond to different antigens. I wonder to which extent
this hierarchy of responsiveness can be attributed to the sensitivity of the technique used for assaying the antibody response and
perhaps also to the mode of presentation of the antigen and the
evolution of certain antigen concentrating mechanisms which may be
required for an effective antibody response. My other point is
concerned with the lack of effect of thymectomy in the fetal lamb.
There is a syndrome in human infants called the "di George syndrome",
in which the thymus does not develop from the branchial clefts. Some
of these children have apparently no thymus whatsoever and they have
no capacity for undertaking cell-mediated immunity. I was very
interested by Dr. Raff´s findings that in a day-old mouse there is
already a definite proportion of θ-positive cells in peripheral
blood and in lymph nodes. This suggests to me that it is very difficult indeed to perform a complete thymectomy even in the mouse
and that there will always be some thymus-derived cells that have
escaped prior to the time of operation. I think we should keep
this in mind when we consider the effects of thymectomy.

J. Shields: How many are aware of the fact that the bursa of Fabricius may well be a gill equivalent? The turtle actually uses
the bursa as a gill for breathing when submerged. Lying inactive
on the bottom, it rhythmically takes in and expels water via the
cloaca, thus perfusing its cloacal gill.

Secondly, I believe that the effect of food, at least protein,
in the gut is an extremely important factor in lymphoid differentiation in this area. In the adult, during starvation for 48 hours,
at least 58% loss of lymphoid tissue mass in the small gut occurs.
Within a few hours after feeding the mass is rapidly restituted
with increased mitotic activity. Would Dr. Nieuwenhuis comment on
his studies on the effect of feeding on the appendix?

P. Nieuwenhuis: No, we did not do any experiments on the effect of
feeding on the gut-associated lymphoid tissue.

M.D. Cooper: That antibody responses are not abolished in fetal
sheep by removing the gut following the development of antibody

forming capability is not inconsistent with the idea that gut-associated lymphoid tissues are the mammalian equivalent of the avian bursa. Deficient development of Peyer's patches after ligation of the upper small intestine is consistent with earlier results of similar experiments in rabbits. Furthermore, the bursa of Fabricius in chickens also is unable to maintain its lymphopoietic capability when implanted away from the gut. The statement that gut-associated lymphoid tissues, such as Peyer's patches, do not develop until well after immunoglobulin-producing cells occur elsewhere seems particularly damaging to the idea that the antibody producing cells are derived from Peyer's patches. In order to examine this question, Drs. Harold Chapman, John Johnson (NIH, Bethesda) and I have examined the relationship between the development of Peyer's patches and the appearance of immunoglobulin-containing cells elsewhere in fetal pigs. We find immunoglobulin-containing cells in the spleen and in the thymus of pig fetuses around 12 cm long, at 60 to 65 days of fetal life. For a long time, we could find absolutely no lymphoid development along the gut of young fetuses by gross examination and by randomly obtaining tissues for histologic examination. But before we concluded that this was indeed the correct temporal sequence of development, we rolled up the small intestine like a firehose, and serially sectioned it. One can then find follicular lymphoid development along the gut in a pig fetus 12 cm long. Thus it may not be valid to conclude that follicular lymphoid development along the intestine is a relatively late developmental event until one has made a very careful search.

K.E. Fichtelius: It is amazing what animals can do without lymphocytes, as we heard from the remarks of Dr. Silverstein and Dr. Hildeman. I would just like to mention the mere existence of symbiont organs in the insects: epithelial organs, rather complex, which have originated from an interaction between epithelium and bacteria. No lymphocytes are found there whatsoever (Lymphology, 3:50, 1970).

A.M. Silverstein: First my apologies to Dr. Nieuwenhuis. I thought I was careful not to identify his affiliation in the war centered around the role of the central lymphoid control organs. With respect to Dr. Miller's comment on the sensitivity of the serologic tests as possibly being responsible for the apparent hierarchical development: this seems not to be the case. Even in our original paper with Jonathan Uhr, we pointed out that this could not be the explanation. I might make two comments about congenital thymic alymphoplasia and other immunological deficiency diseases. These may not be simple defects, but rather multiple defects in several systems. I don't think this question is arguable at the present time. Secondly, I tried to make the point earlier that there is impressive species variation in immunologic maturation and control, and thus would not attempt to extend specific data from the sheep to another species. The general results, however, are pertinent to any generalizations that might be made about all mammals.

E.L. Cooper: I would like to return to phylogenetic perspective and comment on Dr. Shields´ question. I didn´t know that peripheral lymphoid structures in turtles could act as accessory gills. Dr. Borysenko and I have searched for peripheral lymphoid organs in the turtle and have seen in the intestine and in the cloacal region what we think is something structurally equivalent to the bursa, but there is no indication of gill activity. If you remember the slides I presented earlier, I think that the lymph gland in the tadpole may be a larval anuran equivalent to the bursa which is also attached to the gills. I raise the question: Can you tell us a little more about the structure you have seen in turtles, equivalent to the bursa, with gill activity?

M. Raff: I would like to comment on Dr. Warner´s hypothesis that only L-chains are expressed on the surface of thymus-derived lymphocytes. Drs. Mel Greaves and Nancy Hogg at Mill Hill have been able to inhibit the majority of θ-bearing rosette-forming cells (against SRBC) with some anti-μ sera as well as anti-light-chain sera. I think it is very likely that at least some thymus-derived lymphocytes have both μ and L chain determinants on their surface.

J.W. Uhr: I have a question for Dr. M.D. Cooper and a comment concerning Dr. Warner´s paper. Dr. Cooper discussed the important question of whether there is a "switch-over" in IgM-producing cells to IgG production. He presented two types of data: immunofluorescent and serologic. Immunofluorescent studies have a subjective element and I cannot comment on that portion of the data. I think the serologic data are more important. In this regard, I was puzzled by the use of bursectomy in the experimental plan. Bursectomy which may have effects other than preventing migration of precursor cells complicates interpretation of the results. It seems to me that the very elegant, specific anti-μ serum you prepared should have been sufficient to do the job. By analogy with the studies of Dray in rabbits, one would expect IgM production to be suppressed by administration of anti-μ for a considerable period of time. Have you done any experiments in which you have used antibody to IgM only, and if necessary, given it repeatedly?

I have one comment concerning Dr. Warner´s paper and the interesting comment of Dr. Raff. I think that negative results with antiserum do not allow significant interpretations. The immunoglobulin receptors in question are not free in solution to interact with antibody. They are bound to the plasma membrane in a manner which is not understood. Thus, there may be two types of problems: 1) steric hindrance by the membrane antibody binding to a particular determinant, 2) conformational change of the bound Ig molecule resulting in "loss" of a particular antigenic determinant. Thus, a positive experiment can be interpreted, but a negative experiment cannot.

J. Sterzl: My comment concerns the studies on development of immunological response in fetuses. To estimate the onset of the response
to different antigens, some other factors could be involved, not
only the maturity of the fetus itself. Our experimental data prove
that relatively large dose of antigen is necessary for the induction
of primary response in fetuses (H. Tlaskalová, J. Sterzl et al.,
in: Developmental Aspects of Antibody Formation and Structure, Proc.
Symp., p. 767; Academia, and Academic Press, 1970). Already non-
toxic antigens, like sheep red blood cells and phages, injected in
minimal critical amounts, are harmful to early embryos. Of course,
this is even more true about bacterial antigens. To avoid these
difficulties, the lymphoid cells are isolated from the fetal liver
and a primary response is induced in tissue culture according to
Mishell and Dutton. In these experiments it was possible to detect,
by the plaque method, antibody formation in 35-day-old pig embryos
(gestation period 115 days). In some experiments, positive results
were obtained even with cells isolated from the yolk sac. Since
at that very early stage the thymus is not yet in function, the
induction of antibody formation resembles the antibody formation
in phylogenetically low animals with not yet organized thymus.

H. Lischner: The syndrome of congenital absence of the thymus should
not be confused with that of thymic alymphoplasia mentioned by Dr.
Silverstein in which there is an unexplained defect in stem cell
production. In congenital absence of the thymus it is difficult to
imagine a primary defect other than in the thymus which might be
immunologically related. The other defects are related to the
heart, the great vessels, the parathyroids, the skeleton, the face
and such. The role of infections secondary to the immunologic
deficiency is probably not different from animals. A second comment: Dr. Dale Huff, Dr. Angelo Di George and I have tried to find
human models that would relate to the role of lymphoid structures
in the gut in the development of the humoral immune system in man.
Many cases in which absence of the appendix was an incidental finding are described in the literature. No susceptibility to infection or immunologic defect has been reported in those patients, but
this was not looked for specifically. We have looked at one infant
in whom absence of the appendix was discovered at surgery. At four
months and at one year of age response to oral polio and diphtheria-
tetanus immunisation was normal and immunoglobulin levels were normal. We have looked at the autopsy material from three infants who
had congenital absence of the appendix as well as absence of the
major portion of the small and part of the large gut. Their guts
were about one fifth to one eighth of the normal length. In these
infants all of the lymphoid structures were comparable to those of
normal infants of the same age. Plasma cells were present. A few
follicles and rare small germinal centers were present. Their
frequency and appearance were similar to that seen in the tissues
of 50 control autopsies in the same age range. Lymphocytes were
present in the remaining gut wall in normal numbers.

M. Cooper: In response to Dr. Uhr´s question: Yes, we examined the
effects of injections of anti-μ antibodies without bursectomy. Both
IgM and IgG levels were suppressed in these birds but the suppression lasted only a few weeks after hatching in most.

J. Shields: The bursa of Fabricius in the turtle does not, as far
as I know, have much lymphoid tissue surrounding the bursal epithelium. In the chicken, the epithelium invaginates, becomes stranded
and surrounded by lymphoid tissue to become a lymphoepithelial organ histologically very similar to the thymus.

N.L. Warner: I am sympathetic to the viewpoint of Dr. Uhr on this
question of tackling the nature of a surface receptor, by simply
interfering with the site by blocking antibodies. This is why I am
stressing methods, which involve synthesis, using C^{14} amino acid
incorporation. There are some thymomas and lymphoid leukemias
which seem to be synthesising free light chains. There is also the
point, that in certain assay systems where there is no secretion,
such as the rosette-forming assay, anti-μ chain serum does block
the reaction, whereas in the cellular immunity assays it does not.
However, if we are going to say that this latter cell is synthesising IgM there are other problems of interpretation. Firstly, by
amino acid incorporation studies we have shown that neither the
mammalian nor the avian thymus synthesize IgM. And yet, as Dr. Raff
indicated, these organs do contain immuno-competent cells as measured
by GVH reaction. The absence of detectable IgM synthesis occurs at
a time when the five day mouse mesenteric lymph node, for example,
does show detectable IgM synthesis. So I think the only evidence
for IgM presence on T-cells is the inhibition of rosette-forming
cells by anti-IgM, and I would point out that Dr. Schlesinger showed
that these background rosette-forming cells are not inhibited by
anti-theta.

A.H. Coons: I wanted to point out that in Dr. Silverstein´s experiments,which are most interesting and elegant, there is one thing
he cannot remove from the fetus and that is the mother. And it may
be that part of the difficulty in reconciling the human situation
with the thymectomised sheep fetus is the fact that there is a hormonal effect from the mother.

E.L. Cooper: Dr. Yoffey some years ago suggested the term "lymphomyeloid complex" to describe in broad terms the reticuloendothelial
system of lower vertebrates. It was only later in evolution,
especially exemplified in mammals, that true separation of lymphoid
and myeloid elements occurred. Perhaps we can return to Yoffey´s
terminology in view of current findings on thymus and bone-marrow
derived lymphocytes. Distinct separation does not seem so apparent
presently.

M. Raff: I am not sure it is fair to compare Ig synthesis in mesen-

teric lymph node with that in thymus, as there are Ig secreting
cells in lymph node while it is doubtful if this is the case in
thymus. Can you be sure that you could detect μ chain synthesis
in cells synthesizing small amounts of Ig destined solely for the
cell surface?

N.L. Warner: There is no question at all that this method can detect
synthesis without secretion. We have numerous non-secreting plasma
cell tumor mutant lines which show intense synthesis when we specifically analyse the disrupted cultured cells versus the original
supernatant culture fluid by the method of Dr. Thorbecke. It is
also true that the lymphoid leukemias, all but one, showed only
synthesis in the frozen disrupted cells, rather than in the supernatant fluid.

B.D. Jankovic: In connection with the last remark made by Dr. Raff,
I would like to add that Dr. Törö and his group in Budapest proved
that thymus has a secretory function. They used light microscope,
electronmicroscope and histochemical methods to prove this. Clark
(1966) also showed that many epithelial cells in the thymic medulla
contain a mucoid secretory product.

STUDIES ON THE TRANSFER OF NATURAL E. COLI ANTIBODY

PRODUCTION IN RATS

K. Merétey, E. Elekes, V. Várteresz, L. Kocsár

"Frédéric Joliot-Curie" National Research Institute for

Radiobiology and Radiohygiene, Budapest, Hungary

Bone marrow transplantation into heavily irradiated recipients is an extensively used method to follow the function of antibody forming progenitor cells of bone marrow origin in the immune response. However, only sporadic data are available on the production of natural antibodies in radiation chimeras (1, 2, 3). The present studies were undertaken to investigate the kinetics of natural E. coli 0 26 antibody production and its memory in a bone marrow transfer system.

"R" inbred conventional rats of 150 to 200 g body weight were used. In previous experiments the frequency of natural antibodies, demonstrable in adult "R" inbred rats, has been investigated. As it is shown in Fig. 1, almost all of the rats contained sheep red blood cell (SRBC) haemolysin, but only half of the sera did contain antibodies to E. coli 0 26. In the spleens of rats with SRBC haemolysin in the sera, SRBC plaque forming cells (PFCs) were always found. However, a measurable quantity of anti E. coli 0 26 splenic PFCs was observed only in 86% of the animals with E. coli 0 26 antibodies in their sera. It is evident that in certain cases only the extrasplenic sites are responsible for E. coli 0 26 antibody production. The demonstrability of E. coli antibody was found to increase with the ageing of the rats, suggesting that no genetic failure is responsible for the absence of antibodies in young adult animals.

According to the E. coli 0 26 haemagglutinin content of their sera, rats were divided into groups ("coli positive" and "coli negative" animals). Selected "coli positive" and "coli negative" rats were exposed to 780 R co-60 γ-irradiation at a dose

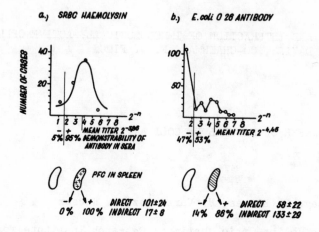

Legend to Figure 1.: (a) Distribution of natural SRBC haemolysin
titers in the sera of rats; direct and indirect PFC counts in the
spleen. (b) The same parameters of the natural E. coli O 26 haem -
agglutinin production.

rate of 180 R/min. Bone marrow and spleen cells were obtained also
from selected rats (See Fig.4.). 5.10^7 nucleated cells were in -
jected i.v. within 3 hours after the completion of irradiation. The
cumulative mortality data showed that, under our experimental con -
ditions, the dose of 780 R was an approximate $LD_{95}/30$ days for the
animals. When transferring bone marrow or spleen cells, the mor -
tality was reduced to 10 to 20 %. The cause of death of trans -
planted animals was lung infection in most of the cases. The re -
lative spleen weights of rats killed at intervals after the trans -
fer showed no differences, irrespective of the origin of the
transferred cells.

    Blood samples were collected at various intervals after the
transfer and antibody titers of the sera were determined by
passive haemagglutination. The following results were obtained:In
irradiated "coli positive" rats (Fig.2.) the antibody titer in the
sera decreased. When transplanting "coli positive" cells into "co -
li positive" animals, a titer increase was observed early after
the transfer. Antibodies did appear in the sera of "coli negative"
irradiated rats given "coli positive" cells. The titers observed
following the eleventh day after the transfer were as high as
found in "coli positive" rats without any treatment. Injecting
cells from rats showing no E. coli O 26 antibody production into
"coli positive" animals, a slight and long-lasting decrease could
be observed in the serum titer. "Coli negative" animals irradiated
or irradiated and transplanted with "coli negative" cells failed

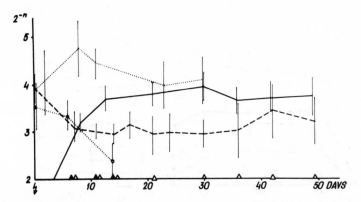

Legend to Figure 2. Changes in E. coli O 26 antibody titer in the sera of irradiated rats after bone marrow or spleen cell trans - plantation. Ordinate: E. coli O 26 haemagglutinin titer (2^{-n}); abscissa: time after irradiation and transfer. Solid line:positive into negative, broken line: negative into positive, dotted line: positive into positive transfer experiment. Dotted line with open circles: irradiated positive control group. Open triangles: ne - gative into negative transfer experiment; closed triangles: ir - radiated negative control group.

to show any antibody activity in their sera during the experimental period.

The kinetics of antibody titers in irradiated "coli negative" animals, given "coli positive" bone marrow cells, were compared with those obtained in the animals transplanted with spleen cells (Fig.3.). An earlier and more pronounced rise of antibody titer occurred in the sera of spleen-cell transplanted than in the sera of bone marrow transplanted rats. The bone marrow and spleen cells used derived from donors producing both 2-mercaptoethanol-re- sistant (MER) and 2-mercaptoethanol-sensitive (MES) E. coli O 26 antibodies (4). It has been proved in former experiments (5,6) that MER antibodies occur not only during the early period of primary immune response but also as natural antibodies. MER antibodies were demonstrable early after the transfer, too. Their level showed parallel changes with the MER+MES antibody titers.

The PFC counts in the spleens of animals used in the transfer experiments were also determined. The Jerne method and Dresser's indirect PFC counting method were used (7,8). PFC count was de -

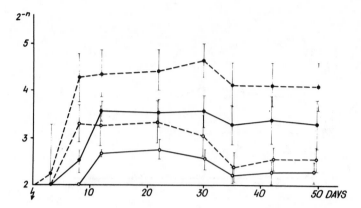

Legend to Figure 3: Transfer of E. coli O 26 haemagglutinin production by bone marrow or spleen cells. For co-ordinates see Fig.2.
Solid line:bone marrow transfer; broken line: spleen cell transfer; lines with closed circles: MES+MER titers; lines with open
circles: MER antibody level.

Table 1. Indirect E. coli O 26 PFC count per spleen of bone marrow-
or spleen cell treated irradiated rats.

Groups* D R	Days after 780 R	Bone marrow	Spleen cell
		t r a n s f e r	
− −	11		−**
	30	−	
− +	30	−	−
	56	−	−
+ +	30		1141±328
+ −	11	819±287	7562±2084
	30	2321±810	
	56	48±14	140±71

Key: *Donors /D/ and recipients /R/ were previously selected ac -
cording to the presence /+/ or absence /-/ of E. coli antibodies
in their sera. Means of five counts ± S.E.
** PFC count per spleen lower than 20.

termined both with SRBCs alone and with SRBCs sensitized by Boivin-
type extract of E.coli O 26 bacteria. PFCs specific to E. coli O
26 were calculated by deducing the SRBC PFCs from the respective
sensitized ones. As SRBC indirect PFC count was almost negligible,
(See Fig.1.), the indirect E. coli PFC count followed more sensi-
tively the minute changes in this natural antibody production.

The highest PFC count was found in the animals given "coli
positive" bone marrow or spleen cells. These values exceeded those
obtained in normal "coli positive" rats (See Fig.1.) and were much
higher than PFC count in irradiated "coli positive" animals
(52±43). The count of PFCs showed a close parallelism with the an -
tibody titers found. The only exception was the result obtained
with the transfer of "coli negative" cells into "coli-positive"
animals, where practically no PFCs were found, in spite of a relatively high antibody titer in the sera.T his finding suggests a
more pronounced effect of transfer on the splenic than on the ex -
trasplenic sites of antibody production. **Table I.**

Fig.4. shows a summarized schema of our results.

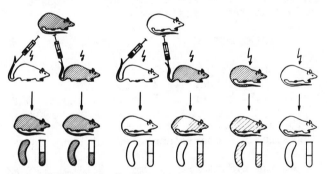

Legend to Figure 4. Experimental schema of results obtained with a
natural antibody transfer system. Open animal-, spleen- and serum -
symbols represent the negative coli-type; hatched symbols the E.
coli O 26 antibody producing activity.

The irradiated but nontransplanted rats did not change their
E. coli O 26 type. The effect of bone marrow or spleen cell transplantation into irradiated animals depended on the coli type in the
donors used. When transferring "coli negative" cells into "coli -

negative" animals no antibody production occurred. E. coli O 26 antibodies and PFCs were demonstrated in all animals given positive cells. "Coli positive" animals given "coli negative" cells stayed positive, as confirmed by the serum titers, though their splenic PFCs disappeared.

The so-called natural antibody production is supposed to be a reaction to the continuous antigen stimulus, mostly of intestinal origin (9,10). As far as our results show, the continuity of the antigen stimulus is not a prerequisite of maintaining the anti - body level. It seems improbable that the adopted coli antibody production should be the consequence of the antigen stored in the transferred cells. The preformed antibodies (11) and the proli - ferating capacity of the lymphoid system (12) might be also es - sential to assure the steady state of natural antibody production. Consequently, the amount of antigen is not the only factor that plays a regulating role.

As suggested by our results, bone marrow and spleen contain progenitor cells committed to natural antibody production that can home to the spleen. Supposing a similar kinetics for the pro - duction of many other natural antibodies, such progenitor-derived cells may constitute a non-negligible part of splenic cells in radiation chimeras.

The authors express their appreciation to Dr.A.J.S. Davies for his helpful suggestions and to Mrs.I.Lipóczky and Miss E. Bagdy for their excellent technical assistance.

REFERENCES

1.) Trentin J. et al.: J.Immunol. 98:1326-1337, 1967.
2.) Shearer G.M. et al.: J.Exptl.Med. 128:437-457, 1968.
3.) Mitchell G.F. and J.F.A.P. Miller: J. Exptl.Med. 128:821-837, 1968.
4.) Hege J.S. and L.J.Cole: J.Immunol. 95:559-569, 1965.
5.) Merétey K., E.Elekes and L.Kocsar: Annal.Immunol.Hung. 11: 157-164, 1968.
6.) Merétey K., E.Elekes and L.Bertok:Inf. Immun. 1:135-136, 1970.
7.) Jerne N.K., A.A.Nordin and C.Henry: p. 109-125. in B.Amos and N.Koprowsky (ed.), Cell-bound antibodies. Wistar Institute Press, Philadelphia 1963.
8.) Dresser D.W. and H.H.Wortis: Nature 208:859, 1966.
9.) Boyden S.V.: Advances Immun. 5: 1-28, 1966.
10.)Sterzl J. and A.M.Silverstein:Advances Immun. 6:375-380, 1967
11.)Pearlman D.S.: J.Exptl.Med. 126:127-148, 1967.
12.)Taliaferro W.H. and L.G.Taliaferro: Proc.Nat.Acad.Sci. 53:139-146, 1965.

LYMPHOID CELLS REACTING AGAINST 'SELF' AND THEIR POSSIBLE ROLE IN IMMUNE RESPONSES

H.S. Micklem and Catherine Asfi

Immunobiology Unit, Department of Zoology

University of Edinburgh

It has repeatedly been shown that an apparent termination of tolerance to protein antigens may be brought about by injection of an antigen structurally related to the tolerogen (1-5). If, for example, dinitrophenyl-BSA is injected into BSA-tolerant rabbits, some antibodies are formed which react with native BSA. The average affinity of these antibodies is lower for native BSA than for BSA modified by the attachment of dinitrophenol (4). One implication of such findings is that the artificial induction of tolerance does not destroy, or irreversibly inactivate, all cells potentially capable of reacting detectably against the tolerogen; some remain or regenerate, and a certain proportion of them can presumably be activated by exposure to any related antigenic structure. We may suppose, following the argument of Smithies (6), that this population, or more probably populations (7,8), carries a spectrum of receptors which react with the tolerogen too weakly to be activated by contact with it, but which may under suitable conditions be activated by contact with a related substance with which they react at sufficiently high affinity. There is much indirect evidence that a similar situation exists in natural 'self'-tolerance, since antigens which may be construed as resembling 'self' have been shown to evoke autoantibody formation (9-12). The present experiments provide a direct demonstration of the existence in normal mice of cells carrying receptors for autochthonous erythrocyte antigens.

MATERIALS AND METHODS

CBA/H mice, 3-5 months old, were used. Cell suspensions were prepared from the lymph nodes, thymus, bone marrow, spleen and

Peyers patches, and washed three times in Hanks solution. Mouse,
sheep and chicken erythrocytes were prepared by washing heparinized
blood cells three times in saline. Receptor-carrying cells were
detected by a modification of the cluster (rosette) technique (13-
15). Six million lymphoid cells and 15×10^6 erythrocytes were
suspended together in 1ml phosphate-buffered saline, pH 7.2,
containing 5% foetal calf serum, and were incubated overnight in
siliconized tubes at 6°C. The cells were resuspended, between
$0.9\mu l$ and $200\mu l$ of the suspension was scanned in a haemocytometer or
larger chamber, and the number of cluster-forming cells (CFC) per
million nucleated cells, and in the whole tissue, was calculated
(15). Three tightly adherent erythrocytes around a single cell
were the minimum criterion for a cluster. Autochthonous and
syngeneic erythrocytes were found to give similar results, and cells
binding either are referred to as syncluster-forming cells (SFC).
Two antisera to mouse immunoglobulins giving strong lines of
precipitation with all five classes of immunoglobulin, and with L-
chains, but lacking precipitating antibodies to any other serum
component, were inactivated and absorbed twice at 2°C with an equal
volume of washed mouse erythrocytes. For control experiments the
same sera were used after removal of all anti-mouse antibodies by
passage through a column of Sepharose 4B (Pharmacia) to which whole
mouse serum had been conjugated (16).

RESULTS AND DISCUSSION

    Table 1 shows the incidence of synclusters in normal CBA mice.
They are significantly more frequent in the thymus than in the bone
marrow or lymph nodes. More than 80% of the CFC are typical small
lymphocytes, the remainder being only marginally larger and with a
slightly greater amount of basophilic cytoplasm. Experiments were
undertaken to determine the nature and specificity of the receptors
on the lymphocyte surface, to identify the population(s) of
lymphocytes involved and to study the possible effects of incidental
or deliberate antigenic stimulation on the number of CFC in the
tissues. Lymphoid cell suspensions were incubated with a 1/10
dilution of rabbit anti-mouse-Ig serum for 30 mins. at 37°C before
addition of erythrocytes. The same concentration of antiserum was
maintained in the medium during the subsequent overnight incubation
at 6°C. A control sample of each suspension was incubated with
Sepharose-absorbed antiserum. Treatment with antiserum regularly
reduced the number of clusters formed (Table 2). Although the

Table 1. Log_{10} SFC/10^6 nucleated cells in CBA mice (mean ± s.e.)

Lymph nodes (53 mice)	3.3254 ± 0.1014	P<0.001
Thymus (34 mice)	3.8223 ± 0.0849	
Bone marrow (23 mice)	3.3565 ± 0.1616	P<0.01

Table 2. Reduction of SFC number by incubation with anti-Ig serum

Tissue	Reduction in:-	Percent reduction
Lymph nodes	17/17	84.74 ± 3.44
Thymus	12/12	34.67 ± 4.79
Bone marrow	14/14	48.29 ± 6.83

reduction approached complete suppression in the lymph nodes, it was less marked in the bone marrow and thymus. These results suggest that the receptors for syngeneic erythrocytes are probably related antigenically to immunoglobulins.

To test the specificity of cluster formation, lymphoid cells were incubated with a mixture of equal numbers of syngeneic mouse and chicken erythrocytes. Less than 0.5% of the clusters were mixed (Table 3). In other experiments it was shown that there was no correspondence between the numbers of clusters formed with syngeneic and with sheep erythrocytes in the different tissues. Thus it seems impossible to attribute syncluster-formation to any non-specific adhesion between erythrocytes and mononuclear cells.

It is possible to distinguish two functionally different populations of lymphocytes, one characterized by a period of residence in the thymus and the other not (7,8). SFC are present in both bone marrow and thymus, as well as in the lymph nodes. The origin of SFC in the peripheral lymphoid tissues has been investigated in two experiments. Fourteen CBA mice deprived of thymus-processed cells by a regime of thymectomy, lethal X-irradiation and bone marrow restoration (17) were kindly provided by Dr. A.J.S. Davies. Seventy-four days after irradiation 6 mice were injected intravenously with 5 x 10^7 syngeneic thymus cells, and 31-39 days later the mice were killed and the synclusters in marrow, spleen, lymph nodes and Peyers patches were enumerated. The thymus-deprived mice had frequencies of SFC which did not differ significantly from those in normal mice. Thus, SFC could develop

Table 3. Specific and non-specific clusters in preparations containing syngeneic and chicken erythrocytes

Tissue	Number of clusters observed containing:-		
	Mouse RBC	Chicken RBC	Mixed RBC
Bone marrow	13	50	2
Spleen	48	184	0
Lymph nodes	63	212	2
Thymus	288	30	0
TOTAL	412	476	4

in normal numbers without the intervention of the thymus or the
participation of thymus-processed cells.   Injection of thymus cells
did not significantly affect the frequency of SFC in any tissue.
However, current experiments with congenitally thymus-less (18) NuNu
mice indicate that these animals possess significantly fewer SFC
than do normal littermate controls.   This suggests that two
populations of SFC may be present, one of which is thymus-processed,
and that removal of the latter may be to some extent compensated by
an increase in the thymus-independent population.

Germ-free and conventional CBA mice harbour very similar
numbers of SFC (19).   The background SFC level is therefore not
determined by previous infection with microorganisms carrying cross-
reacting antigens, although dead microorganisms and endotoxins in
the diet may have an effect.   The effects of stimulation with
various antigens upon the numbers of SFC in conventional mice are
being investigated.   As reported elsewhere (15,20), skin allograft
elicits an increased number of SFC, while a syngeneic graft does not.

The demonstration in normal animals of cells carrying receptors
for 'self' constituents was predictable from experiments on the
circumvention of artificial and natural tolerance (1-5,8,10-12).
The fact that CFC show specificity, and other considerations (15),
render it likely that the receptors are made by the cell itself and
not acquired passively.   It is interesting that SFC were more
numerous in the thymus than in the peripheral lymphoid tissues -
the reverse of the situation with other antigens (21-23; and see
Table 3).   The evidence suggests that SFC in the thymus, as
elsewhere, function as such by virtue of immunoglobulin-like
receptors;   whatever the receptors, they are specific at least to
the extent of distinguishing between mouse and chicken erythrocytes.
It is important, if the physiological role of SFC is to be clarified,
to characterize the antigenic targets on the erythrocyte membrane.
There are two kinds of function which auto-receptor-carrying cells
could plausibly fulfil.   The first is related to the phagocytosis
and disposal of aged autochthonous cells.   There is some evidence
implicating opsonic or cytophilic antibody specific for some
determinant present on aged erythrocytes (24).   If that is correct,
the cell population responsible for such antibodies would
presumably include cells capable of specifically binding aged or
damaged erythrocytes.   This is open to test.   Meanwhile, however,
the presence of large numbers of SFC in the thymus makes this
interpretation seem relatively unattractive, and at the same time
points towards a hypothesis of more fundamental interest.   It is
possible to envisage an evolutionary advantage in the possession of
low-affinity self-reactive lymphocytes.   As we argue elsewhere (25)
an effective surveillance mechanism (26) would practically require
the existence of such cells if it were to have a reasonable
likelihood of detecting an antigenic deviant soon after its
appearance.   If, as suggested by Burnet (26), surveillance was the

primary <u>raison d'être</u> of the vertebrate immune system in evolution, then autoreactive cells may be one of the primitive features of the system.   It may be envisaged that a cell population consisting of individuals reacting at varying affinity with the whole range of autologous 'antigens', would contain occasional cells reactive at high affinity with a vast range of biological configurations. Selection and proliferation of the appropriate clones would endow the population with a wide immunological repertoire.   It may be, therefore, that immunity to microorganisms, as well as to the whole gamut of antigens to which modern animals are exposed in the laboratory, evolved as a result of high-affinity cross-reactions between these antigens and cellular receptors which were originally generated to react with self.   In ontogeny, too, the primary immunological process may be a generation of autoreactive cells. Any that react with self at sufficiently high affinity presumably suffer Burnettian elimination or inactivation.   The remainder constitute the normal pool of lymphocytes available to react against exogenous antigens.   This might be described as a 'heteroclitic' (27) view of immunology.

A tacit assumption in the above argument is that 'self' patterns within an individual are consistent and that deviants arising by somatic mutation are relatively quickly eliminated.   Burnet (28) has recently argued that the soma is likely to be a mosaic of different mutants which continually arise from the basic pattern in all rapidly proliferating tissues and which may only evoke a destructive level of immune response if they form large clones.   There are certain points of resemblance between Burnet's scheme and the present one: both imply that the diversity of lymphocyte receptor patterns is the indirect (evolutionary) or direct (ontogenetic) result of the diversity of cell membrane antigens within the species and the individual respectively; and both explain the unexpectedly large number of immunocytes which often appear to partake in graft-versus-host reactions.

The relative roles of the bone marrow and the thymus are at present difficult to assess.   Although the ratio of cluster-formers to total nucleated cells in the bone marrow is lower than in the thymus, the ratio to total <u>lymphocytes</u> is probably higher.   Since the thymus is itself populated by cells derived from the bone marrow (29), and since normal numbers of SFC can be produced in the absence of the thymus, it seems probable that they arise (in the adult) primarily in the bone marrow, the thymus being involved in the differentiation of a long-lived sub-population.

ACKNOWLEDGEMENT

This work was supported by the Medical Research Council.

REFERENCES

1. W.D. Linscott, and W.O. Weigle, J. Immunol., 95:546, 1965.
2. D. Nachtigal, R. Eschel-Zussman, and M. Feldman, Immunology, 9:543, 1965.
3. F.M. Dietrich, J. Immunol., 97:216, 1966.
4. W.E. Paul, G.W. Siskind, and B. Benacerraf, Immunology, 13:147, 1967.
5. J.E.M. St. Rose, and B. Cinader, J. exp. Med. 125:1031, 1967.
6. O. Smithies in Regulation of the Antibody Response, ed. B. Cinader, C.C. Thomas, 1968, p.363.
7. J.F.A.P. Miller, ed G.F. Mitchell, Transplantation Revs. 1:3, 1969.
8. R.B. Taylor, Transplantation Revs., 1:114, 1969.
9. P. Grabar, Ann Inst. Pasteur, 118:393, 1970.
10. A.E. Bussard in La Greffe des Cellules Hematopoietiques Allogeniques, C.N.R.S., Paris, 1965, p.157.
11. K. Rajewsky, Immunochemistry, 3:487, 1966.
12. W.O. Weigle, J. exp. Med. 121:289, 1966.
13. G. Biozzi, C. Stiffel, D. Mouton, M. Liacopoules-Briot, C. Decreusefond, and Y. Bouthillier, Ann. Inst. Pasteur, 110:7, 1966.
14. O.B. Zaalberg, V.A. van der Meul, and M.J. van Twisk, Nature, 210:544, 1966.
15. H.S. Micklem, C. Asfi, N.A. Staines, and N. Anderson, Nature, 1970, in press.
16. J. Porath, R. Axen and S. Ernback, Nature, 215:1491, 1967.
17. A.J.S. Davies. Transplantation Revs. 1:43, 1969.
18. E.M. Pantelouris, Nature, 217:370, 1968.
19. H.S. Micklem, and J.-C. Salomon. In preparation.
20. H.S. Micklem, C. Asfi, and N.A. Staines. Transplantation Proceedings. In press.
21. R. Laskov, Nature, 219:973, 1966.
22. P. Byrt and G.L. Ada, Immunology 17:503, 1969.
23. J.H. Humphrey and H.V. Keller. Symposium on Developmental Aspects of Antibody Formation, Prague, 1969. In press.
24. D.S. Nelson. Macrophages and Immunity. North-Holland, 1969, p.266-268.
25. H.S. Micklem and C. Asfi. Arch. Zool. Exp. Gen. In press.
26. F.M. Burnet, Cellular Immunology, Cambridge, 1969.
27. O. Makela, J. Immunol. 94:378, 1965.
28. F.M. Burnet, Nature, 226:123, 1970.
29. H.S. Micklem, C.E. Ford, E.P. Evans, and J. Gray, Proc. Roy. Soc. B 165:78, 1966.

IN VITRO INTERACTION BETWEEN BONE MARROW-DERIVED AND THYMUS CELLS[1]

G. Doria, G. Agarossi, and S. Di Pietro

CNEN-Euratom Immunogenetics Group, Animal Radiobiology

Laboratory, C.S.N. Casaccia, Rome, Italy

It has been suggested that the immune response of mice to sheep red blood cells (RBC) depends on interaction between cells of bone marrow and thymus origin, as antibody production can be induced only if both cell types are present (1). Proliferation of thymus-derived cells and antibody synthesis in bone marrow-derived cells have been found to occur after sheep RBC injection in mice which have been thymectomized in adult life, irradiated, and reconstituted by thymus and bone marrow grafts (2). The finding of these cellular events triggered by antigen has been confirmed (3) and extended to neonatally thymectomized mice reconstituted by injection of thymus cells (4). It has also been shown that thymus cells have to react with antigen before the cooperation with bone marrow-derived cells can take place *in vivo* (5). However, the nature of the interactions among antigen and these cells is not understood.

The observations described below demonstrate that the interaction between bone marrow-derived and thymus cells can occur *in vitro*, for a primary immune response could be induced *in vitro* only when both cell types were cultured with sheep RBC. Furthermore, this *in vitro* system appears suitable to investigate possible mechanisms of cell cooperation in the immune response.

Spleen cells from normal or thymectomized (Tx) mice and thymus cells were cultured according to the technique of Mishell and Dutton (6). *In vitro* primary immune response to sheep RBC was evaluated by

---

[1]Supported by CNEN-Euratom Association Contract. Publication No. 620 of the Euratom Biology Division.

the Jerne technique (7) and expressed as number of hemolytic plaque forming cells (PFC) per culture dish. Thymectomized mice, radiation chimeras, suspensions of bone marrow, spleen, or thymus cells, and separate or mixed cell cultures were prepared as previously described (8,9,10).

In one series of experiments with C3HeB/FeJ inbred mice, the addition of sheep RBC to mixed cell cultures of both thymus cells from normal mice and spleen cells from mice thymectomized in adult life, irradiated, and reconstituted by isogenic bone marrow cells, elicited an immune response comparable to that of normal spleen cells. As shown in Table I, the response in mixed cell cultures was much greater than in separate cultures of either spleen cells from Tx-chimeras or thymus cells. In no instance were more than 100 PFC observed in cell cultures without antigen. These results illustrate that antibody production *in vitro* arises from interaction between bone marrow-derived and thymus cells.

A similar interaction was observed in another series of experiments with (C57Bl/10xDBA/2J)Fl hybrid mice. As shown in Table II, the immune response in mixed cell cultures of thymus cells from normal mice and spleen cells from neonatally Tx-mice was several fold greater than in separate cultures of either cell type.

Table I. *In vitro* primary immune response
(PFC per culture) to sheep RBC

Origin of cells in culture	Days of culture			
	3	4	5	6
Tx-Spleen + Thymus	258	380	970	900
Tx-Spleen	60	75	30	25
Thymus	0	0	0	0
Spleen	162	750	560	230

Tx = adult thymectomy, followed by irradiation and bone marrow transplantation.

Table II. *In vitro* immune primary response
(PFC per culture) to sheep RBC

Origin of cells in culture	Days of culture			
	4	5	6	7
Tx-Spleen + Thymus	410	1558	2193	750
Tx-Spleen	77	85	95	64
Thymus	0	0	0	0
Spleen	520	1540	2025	980

Tx = neonatal thymectomy.

The results obtained in the two series of experiments open the possibility of studying *in vitro* the mechanism of interaction between thymus cells and bone marrow-derived cells such as the spleen cells from Tx-animals. Several mechanisms have been proposed (5).

A) Nonspecific. 1. Thymus cells supply nucleic acid precursors for proliferation of Tx-spleen cells with specific receptor sites.
2. Thymus cells are precursors of macrophages that process antigen for stimulation of Tx-spleen cells with specific receptor sites.
B) Specific. 1. Upon specific binding with antigen thymus cells secrete a factor that triggers proliferation of Tx-spleen cells with specific receptor sites. 2. Thymus cell-bound specific receptor sites fix antigen and present it properly to Tx-spleen cell receptor sites. 3. Thymus cells secrete specific receptors that fix antigen and concentrate it for Tx-spleen cell specific receptor sites.

The nonspecific mechanisms either lack direct support (11,12) or are inconsistent with experimental evidence (13). The specific mechanisms are sustained by the results of retransplantation of thymus-derived cells from normal or immune donors in irradiated recipients (5) and of reconstitution of Tx-recipients with thymus-derived cells from tolerant donors (14).

Specific mechanisms imply the existence of specific receptors on both thymus and Tx-spleen cells. Receptors need not be identical on both cell types. If receptors are molecules also present in normal serum, antisera from rabbits immunized with mouse serum may contain

Table III. Effect of pretreatment of normal spleen cells on *in vitro* primary immune response (PFC per culture) to sheep RBC

Pretreatment of normal spleen cells	Days of culture		
	4	5	6
Medium	431	1870	710
Rabbit normal serum	341	2190	690
Rabbit antiserum anti-mouse serum	33	56	170

antibodies directed against mouse cell receptors. Normal spleen cells from hybrid mice were incubated with rabbit antiserum anti-mouse serum for 4 hours at 4°C, washed, and cultured with sheep RBC. As shown in Table III, the immune response of these cells was much lower as compared to controls. This finding suggests the existence of spleen cell receptors antigenically identical or similar to constituents of the normal serum. In cell mixed experiments with hybrid mice, thymus cells from normal mice and spleen cells from neonatally Tx-mice were separately incubated with the same rabbit sera and under the same conditions as in the preceding experiment. After washing, thymus and Tx-spleen cells were mixed and cultured with sheep RBC. Table IV indicates that receptor sites detected by this rabbit antiserum are localized only on Tx-spleen cells. Inference that thymus cells lack these receptors need not conflict with the slight difference in response between cultures in which both cell types or only Tx-spleen cells were pretreated with antiserum. In the two series of cultures, all PFC values but 245 are indeed within the range observed in control cultures without antigen.

All the specific and nonspecific mechanisms of cell interaction outlined above are based on the hypothesis that bone marrow-derived cells involved in antibody formation are provided with specific receptor sites. Indirect tests of this hypothesis have given controversial results. In fact, recovery of the specific immunologic capacity of irradiated recipients injected with both thymus cells from normal donors and bone marrow cells from tolerant donors has been observed by Taylor (15) but could not be confirmed by Habicht *et al.* (16). The present findings uphold the existence on bone marrow-derived cells of specific receptor sites with antigenic determinants common to molecules of the normal serum. These receptors seem to be absent from thymus cells, as the interaction could not be prevented by thymus cell pretreatment with the rabbit antiserum.

Table IV. Effect of pretreatment of Tx-spleen cells and thymus cells on *in vitro* primary immune response (PFC per culture) to sheep RBC

Origin of cells in culture	Days of culture			
	4	5	6	7
Tx-Spleen (NS) + Thymus (NS)	480	920	1165	125
Tx-Spleen (NS) + Thymus (AS)	213	690	1135	300
Tx-Spleen (AS) + Thymus (NS)	8	80	245	48
Tx-Spleen (AS) + Thymus (AS)	7	10	15	5

Tx = neonatal thymectomy.

(NS) = cell pretreatment with rabbit normal serum.

(AS) = cell pretreatment with rabbit antiserum anti-mouse serum.

On the other hand, these receptors may be present and yet be irrelevant to cell cooperation, as thymus cells may interact with bone marrow-derived cells by other receptors antigenically different from components of the normal serum or through some other entangled mechanism.

REFERENCES

1. H. N. Claman, E. A. Chaperon, and R. F. Triplett, J. Immunol., 97:828, 1966.

2. A. J. S. Davies, E. Leuchars, V. Wallis, R. Marchant, and E. V. Elliot, Transplantation, 5:222, 1967.

3. G. F. Mitchell and J. F. A. P. Miller, J. Exp. Med., 128:821, 1968.

4. J. F. A. P. Miller and G. F. Mitchell, J. Exp. Med., 128:801, 1968.

5. J. F. A. P. Miller and G. F. Mitchell, Transplant. Rev.,
    1:3, 1969.

6. R. I. Mishell and R. W. Dutton, Science, 153:1004, 1966.

7. N. K. Jerne and A. A. Nordin, Science, 140:405, 1963.

8. G. Doria and G. Agarossi, Transplantation, 6:218, 1968.

9. G. Doria and G. Agarossi, Nature, 221:871, 1969.

10. G. Doria, M. Martinozzi, G. Agarossi, and S. Di Pietro,
    Experientia, 26:410, 1970.

11. S. H. Robinson and G. Brecher, Science, 142:392, 1963.

12. M. Virolainen, J. Exp. Med., 127:943, 1968.

13. D. E. Mosier, F. W. Fitch, D. A. Rowley, and A. J. S. Davies,
    Nature, 225:276, 1970.

14. J. F. A. P. Miller and G. F. Mitchell, Advan. Exptl. Med. Biol.,
    5:455, 1969.

15. R. B. Taylor, Nature, 220:611, 1968.

16. G. S. Habicht, J. M. Chiller, and W. O. Weigle, in: Symposium
    on Developmental Aspects of Antibody Formation and Structure,
    Praha: Czech. Acad. Sci. Press, 1970, in press.

CELL INTERACTIONS IN THE IN VITRO PRODUCTION OF ANTIBODIES

TO CHEMICALLY DEFINED ANTIGENS*

S. Segal, S. Kunin, A. Globerson, G. Shearer** and M. Feldman

Departments of Cell Biology and Chemical Immunology

The Weizmann Institute of Science, Rehovot, Israel

Antibody production to a number of antigens appears to be determined by a bicellular interaction (1-5). In mice each of the interacting cells seems to be of a different ontogenetic origin, manifesting distinct functional properties. With regard to RBC antigens one of the cooperating cells was shown to derive from the thymus, the other from the bone marrow. Although both seem to be capable of recognizing antigenic determinants of the immunogen, only the bone marrow cell can produce antibodies (6,7). Such a bicellular mechanism was inferred also from experiments of the secondary response to hapten protein conjugates (8-11). Cells recognizing antigeneic determinants of the carrier molecule seem to interact with cells recognizing the hapten determinants, and capable of producing anti-hapten antibodies.

Our objective in the present study was to analyze the bicellular basis of the *in vitro* induction of primary response to chemically defined antigens. We employed the millipore filter well technique for organ cultures of spleen explants (12) in which a primary response to DNP was previously achieved by us, using DNP-protein or DNP-poly-L-lysine as immunogens (13). DNP-conjugated T4 bacteriophage was applied for assaying antibodies produced *in vitro* to DNP (14).

We studied the following questions: (1) Does the primary immune response to DNA-carrier conjugates depend on the recognition of both hapten and carrier determinants? (2) Are the receptors for these

*This work was supported by a grant from the Max and Ida Hillson Foundation, New York, and from DGRST, France.

**Post-doctoral fellow of the American Cancer Society.

determinants located on distinct cells which cooperate in the process of antibody production? (3) What is the origin of these cells?

MATERIALS AND METHODS

Mice. Female (BALB/c X C57Bl/6)F_1 mice, 8-10 weeks old, were used throughout these experiments.

Culture technique. The millipore filter well technique for the induction of antibody response *in vitro* was employed as previously described for sheep red blood cells (SRBC) (12) and adapted for haptens (13).

Immunogens. The dinitrophenyl (DNP) determinant was used as the hapten in this study. The free hapten was employed as DNP-lysine (DNP-lys). The following proteins were used as carriers: (1) Rabbit serum albumin, fraction V (RSA) obtained from Nutritional Biochemical Co. (2) Hemocyanin from *Calinectes sapidus* (Hyc) (13). In some experiments keyhole-limpet hemocyanin (Hcy-KLH, Nutritional Biochemical Co.) was used.

DNP was attached to the carrier RSA at a molecular ratio of 5 molecules DNP to each molecule of carrier (designated as DNP-RSA). The conjugate of the DNP with Hcy (DNP-Hcy, DNP-Hcy(KLH)) was made at a molecular ratio of 7:1.

The chemically defined synthetic antigens used were: (1) Poly-L-lysine (PLL) of an average molecular weight of 5000 (15) was obtained by the courtesy of Dr. Arie Yaron; α-DNP-poly-L-lysine (DNP-PLL) was used as the hapten carrier conjugate (13).

Immunization. (a) *in vivo*: Mice received a single intraperitoneal injection of 0.2 mg of the appropriate antigen in complete Freund's adjuvant. (b) *in vitro*: Explants within the millipore filter well were overlayed with 0.01 ml of medium containing 50 µg of antigen per milliliter. Forty-eight hours later the culture medium was replaced by antigen-free medium. Medium samples were subsequently collected at different time intervals, replaced completely by fresh medium and assayed for the presence of antibodies.

Induction of tolerance. Tolerance was induced in adult mice by 9 weekly intraperitoneal injections of 10 mg RSA in PBS (16,17).

Antibody assay. Antibody assay was carried out by using the modified T4 bacteriophage (2,4-dinitrophenyl bacteriophage T4 (DNP-T4)) technique, as previously described (13,14).

Vinblastine-sulfate (Velbe) (Eli Lilly and Co.) was injected intravenously, at a dose of 0.1 mg.

Reconstituted spleens. Mice were exposed to 750 R total body irradiation. Thymus cells from 6-8 week-old syngeneic donors were inoculated intravenously at doses of 10 X 10⁷ cells per recipient either 1 or 8 days following exposure (see Experimental). Bone marrow (from 6-8 week-old donors) was similarly inoculated at doses of 3.5 X 10⁷ cells per recipient (18). The spleens of the re-colonized animals were explanted 10 days following exposure to X-rays.

EXPERIMENTAL AND DISCUSSION

The first series of experiments aimed at testing whether the primary immune response to DNP, following the application of DNP-poly-L-lysine is determined by the recognition of the hapten via a cell receptor for the DNP. If such receptors have to react with the DNP determinant of the immunogen, then the application of

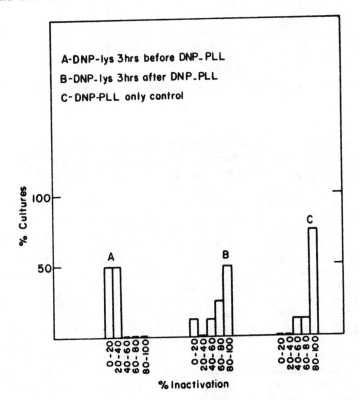

Fig. 1. Effect of DNP-lys on the *in vitro* induction of response to DNP by DNP-PLL.

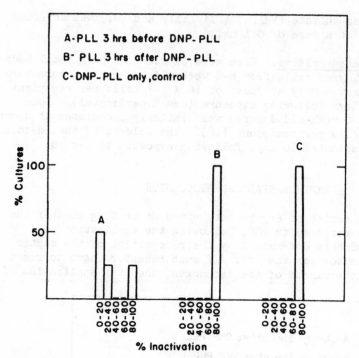

Fig. 2.   Effect of PLL on the *in vitro* induction of response to DNP by DNP-PLL.

free DNP-lysine prior to the stimulation with DNP-poly-L-lysine should inhibit the primary production of antibodies to DNP since free hapten would compete with the immunogen for the specific cell receptors.   Figure 1 demonstrates that the DNP-lysine applied 3 hours prior to the immunogen DNP-poly-L-lysine, did in fact inhibit the production of antibodies to DNP.   Is the response to the hapten determined also by the recognition of the antigenic determinant of the carrier?   To test this we examined the effect of free carrier on the induction of a response to DNP.   It was found that cultures incubated with poly-L-lysine 3 hours before application of DNP-poly-lysine failed to form antibodies to DNP (Fig. 2).   Hence, the production of hapten specific antibodies involves the reaction of both hapten and carrier receptors with the corresponding determinants on the immunogenic molecule.   This can be explained on the basis of interaction via the immunogen between cells equipped with receptors for the carrier determinant and cells possessing receptors for the DNP.   If such a bicellular mechanism operates in antibody production, two predictions can be made.   One is, that pre-immunization against the carrier should increase the anti-DNP reactivity of a given

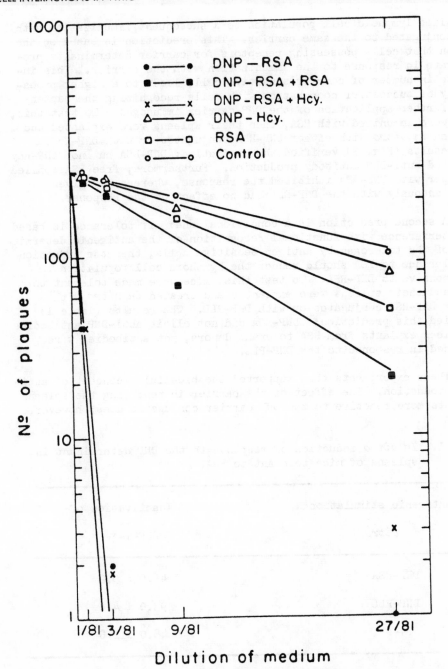

Fig. 3. Inhibition of the carrier effect in the presence of free carrier molecules. Mice were immunized against RSA 14 days before sacrifice.

immunized lymphoid cell population to a subsequent immunization with DNP conjugated to the same carrier. This prediction is based on the notion that cells possessing receptors for carrier determinants proliferate in response to the immunization with the carrier. This increase in number of carrier-sensitive cells leads to a higher probability of successful cooperation with cells recognizing the hapten upon further application of the DNP-carrier immunogen. To test this, mice were immunized with RSA, then their spleens were explanted and treated *in vitro* with either DNP-RSA conjugates or with DNP-Hcy. The results (Fig. 3) verified the prediction: DNP-RSA but not DNP-Hcy elicited anti-DNP antibody production. Furthermore, free RSA applied together with DNP-RSA inhibited the response, whereas Hcy given simultaneously with the DNP-RSA had no effect on the response.

A second prediction is a conditional one: If tolerance is based on interference with functional recognition of the antigenic determinants of the tolerogen by antigen sensitive cells, then the induction of tolerance to RSA should render the lymphoid cell population unresponsive to DNP-RSA. To test this, mice were made tolerant to RSA, and their spleens were explanted and treated *in vitro* with either DNP-RSA conjugates or with DNP-PLL. The results (Table I) verified this prediction: DNP-RSA did not elicit anti-DNP antibodies in spleen explants from RSA tolerant donors, yet antibodies were produced in response to the DNP-PLL.

These experiments thus supported the bicellular concept of antibody production. The effect of the carrier in rendering the spleen explants more reactive to the DNP carrier conjugates does, however,

Table I. *In vitro* induction of response to the DNP determinant in spleens of mice tolerant to RSA.

Antigenic stimulation *in vitro*	% Inactivation of DNP-T4*
DNP-RSA	46.0 ± 9.2
DNP-PLL	93.0 ± 4.8
-	48.0 ±11.8

*Medium samples were diluted 1:9

invite further consideration. The conventional interpretation, as suggested above, would relate the effect to an increase in the population of cells reactive to the carrier. To test whether the effect of priming with RSA is indeed determined by successive replications of RSA-sensitive cells, experiments were designed to prevent cell replication by vinblastine applied at different time intervals following immunization with the carrier, then testing the response of such spleens to DNP-RSA conjugates. The results (Fig. 4) indicated that when vinblastine was injected simultaneously with the carrier, and the spleen explants of such animals were treated *in vitro* with DNP-RSA, no anti-DNP antibodies could be detected. Yet, when vinblastine was applied just 24 hours following immunization with the RSA, the explanted spleens responded to DNP-RSA with a high level of anti-DNP antibodies. These experiments suggest that cell replication is necessary for the carrier effect to manifest itself, but most probably, one cycle of replication is sufficient for its manifestation. Hence, it seems improbably that preimmunization with the carrier enhanced the response to DNP due to the increase in the population of cells reactive with carrier determinants. We suggest that the single cycle of replication was essential in order to produce more receptor molecules per cell. The production of the latter might depend on transcription which could take place only on new DNA strands, which were produced during the single replicating event (19). The increased number of receptors per cell would have led to the same result as the increase in the number of cells sensitive to the carrier determinant.

What is the nature of the cells sensitive to the carrier and the cells sensitive to the hapten and capable of producing anti-hapten antibodies? To test the possibility that the former derive from the thymus, whereas the latter derive from the bone marrow, the following experiments were carried out: We first tested whether the anti-DNP response is thymus dependent. Mice were exposed to 750 R X-irradiation and then repopulated with either thymus cells or bone marrow cells, or both. The animals were immunized *in vivo* with DNP-RSA and their spleens were then cultured and challenged *in vitro* with DNP-RSA. Only spleens of the third group, i.e., of animals treated with both thymus and bone marrow, produced anti-DNP antibodies in response to DNP-protein conjugates (Table II). Thus, the response to DNP requires the interaction of cells originating in the thymus and cells originating in the bone marrow. To test the capacity of recolonized spleens to manifest the carrier effect, animals were exposed to 750 R total body X-irradiation. They were then divided into 3 groups which were inoculated with either thymus and bone marrow cells, or thymus cells, or bone marrow cells only. The animals were then immunized with RSA and their spleens were explanted 10 days later and challenged in culture with DNP-RSA. Only spleens of animals which were inoculated with both thymus and bone marrow cells produced anti-DNP antibodies (Table III). We then designed experiments to test whether the cells

Table II. *In vitro* response to DNP-RSA by spleens of irradiated mice treated with thymus and/or bone marrow cells and injected with DNP-RSA.

Cells injected	Antigen added to culture	% Inactivation of DNP-T4*
Thymus and bone marrow	+	97.4
Thymus and bone marrow	-	19.4
Thymus	+	0
Thymus	-	0
Bone marrow	+	11.0
Bone marrow	-	19.8

*Medium samples were collected on day 8, pooled and diluted 1:3.

Table III. *In vitro* response to DNP-RSA by spleens of irradiated mice treated with thymus and/or bone marrow cells and immunized against the carrier.

Cells injected to spleen donors*	Antigenic stimulation *in vitro*	% Inactivation of DNP-T4**
Thymus and bone marrow	DNP-RSA	96
Thymus and bone marrow	-	0
Thymus	DNP-RSA	26
Thymus	-	36
Bone marrow	DNP-RSA	29
Bone marrow	-	24

*Spleens were explanted 10 days following irradiation.

**Medium samples were collected on days 8 and 9, pooled and diluted 1:3.

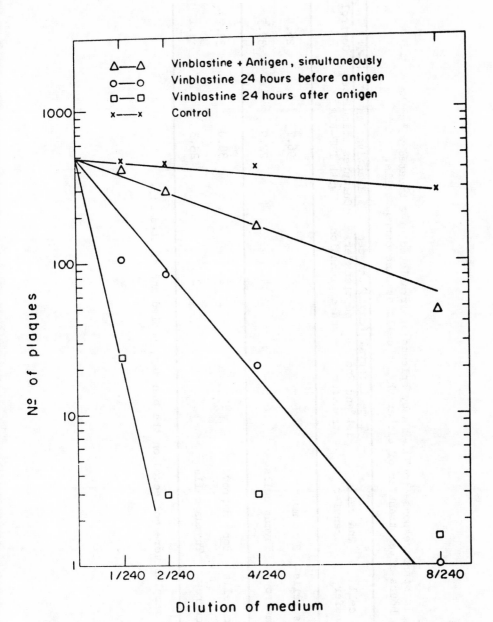

Fig. 4.   Inhibition of cell replication in mice immunized against the carrier.

Table IV. *In vitro* response to DNP–RSA by spleens of irradiated mice treated with the carrier 24 hours after transfer of either thymus cells or bone marrow cells.

Exp. No.	1st cell transfer	2nd cell transfer	Time interval (days) between 1st and 2nd transfer	Time interval (days) between 2nd transfer and explanation	% Inactivation of DNP–T4* Cultures stimulated with DNP–RSA	% Inactivation of DNP–T4* Control
1	Thymus cells	Bone marrow	6	4	96.7	25.9
	Bone marrow	Thymus cells	6	4	22.9	39.5
2	Thymus cells	Bone marrow	8	2	88.0	33.2
	Bone marrow	Thymus cells	8	2	23.3	4.1

*Medium samples were collected on the 8th day, pooled and diluted 1:3.

recognizing the carrier determinants are thymus derived, or whether they are of bone marrow origin. Irradiated mice were divided into two groups: One was inoculated with thymus cells, and the other with bone marrow cells. Both were immunized 24 hours later with RSA. Six days later the thymus-inoculated mice received bone marrow and the marrow-inoculated animals received thymus cells. The spleens were cultured after four additional days and treated with DNP-RSA. Antibodies to DNP were subsequently assayed in the culture medium. The results (Table IV) were that only cultures of the first group, i.e., of spleens from X-irradiated animals which were immunized with the carrier after thymus inoculation, manifested the carrier effect, i.e., the production of anti-DNP antibodies following treatment *in vitro* with DNP-RSA. Spleens of donors which were treated with bone marrow and the carrier before receiving the thymus cells did not manifest antibody production to DNP-RSA in culture. This experiment was repeated with different time intervals: 8 days between first and second cell transfers and 2 days from last transfer to explanation. The results obtained were similar to those of the first experiment (Table IV). These results suggest that the cells reactive to the carrier determinants are of thymic origin. Since it was demonstrated in other experimental systems, using RBC antigens (6,7) that such cells do not actively produce antibodies, it appears that the immune response to hapten-protein conjugates involves a cooperation between two types of cells, distinct in origin and function: a thymus-derived and a bone marrow-derived cell cooperating probably via the immunogenic molecule. The thymus-derived cell functions as an antigen sensitive cell, reacting in the present system with the carrier. Since excess of carrier molecule, or induction of tolerance to the carrier, prevented antibody production it appears that the thymus derived cells are capable of recognizing antigenic determinants of the carrier. The thymus-derived cells have to interact with a bone marrow-derived cell, which is probably also capable of recognition - since the response could be blocked by DNP lysine, but in contrast to the thymus-derived cells it is capable also of producing antibodies.

ACKNOWLEDGMENT

The excellent technical assistance of Mrs. Miriam Shmerling and Miss Miriam Kotler is gratefully acknowledged.

REFERENCES

1. A. J. S. Davies, Transpl. Rev. 1:43, 1969.

2. J. F. A. P. Miller and G. F. Mitchell, Transpl. Rev. 1:3, 1969.

3. H. N. Claman and E. E. Chaperon, Transpl. Rev. 1:92, 1969.

4. R. B. Taylor, Transpl. Rev. 1:114, 1969.

5. A. Globerson and M. Feldman, in: Mononuclear Phagocytes. Blackwell Scientific Publications. In press.

6. A. J. S. Davies, E. Leuchars, V. Wallis, R. Marchant and E. V. Elliot, Transpl. 5:222, 1967.

7. J. F. A. P. Miller and G. F. Mitchell, J. Exp. Med. 131:675, 1970.

8. N. A. Mitchison, in: Cold Spring Harbor Symp. Quant. Biol. 32:431, 1967.

9. Z. Ovary and B. Benacerraf, Proc. Soc. Exp. Biol. Med. 114:72, 1963.

10. N. A. Mitchison, Prog. Bioph. and Mol. Biol. 16:3, 1966.

11. K. Rajewsky, V. Schirrmacher, S. Nase and N. K. Jerne, J. Exp. Med. 123:1311, 1969.

12. A. Globerson and R. Auerbach, J. Exp. Med. 124:1001, 1966.

13. S. Segal, A. Globerson, M. Feldman, J. Haimovich and M. Sela, J. Exp. Med. 131:93, 1970.

14. J. Haimovich and M. Sela, J. Immunol. 97:338, 1966.

15. S. F. Schlossman and H. Levine, J. Immunol. 98:211, 1967.

16. E. Greenberg-Ramon, Studies on the cellular basis of immunological tolerance. Ph.D. thesis, Weizmann Institute of Science, Rehovot, Israel, 1969.

17. N. A. Mitchison, Immunol. 15:509, 1968.

18. G. M. Shearer and G. Cudkowicz, J. Exp. Med. 129:935, 1969.

19. S. D. Barbour, C. Gross and A. Novick, J. Mol. Biol. 33:967, 1968.

CHAIRMAN'S INTRODUCTION TO DISCUSSION

ORIGIN AND INTERACTION OF IMMUNOLOGICALLY ACTIVE CELLS

A. J. S. Davies

Chester Beatty Research Institute, Institute of Cancer

Research, Royal Cancer Hospital, London, S.W.3., England

Biological problems are often intractable in that they present no easy starting point. Usually they require approaches at a number of different levels of organization, results from all of which have to be considered in order to discern the overall picture. Yet even then there is an innate difficulty in arriving at any satisfactory generalizations. These comments are particularly true of the immune response and yet it seems likely that it is from the field of immunity that we shall achieve an entry to the wider problems of differentiation of mammalian cells.

It is sometimes possible in an immune response to define the stimulating antigen in precise biochemical terms and there is a fair chance that the protein antibody which results can similarly be specified. This very fact has led many molecular biologists to consider hopefully that the elegant analyses which have been made in microorganisms, of the mode of gene action, may be repeatable in immunologically reactive cell populations. However, progress in the past has been hampered by lack of clear definition of the responding cell populations. It has been convenient to assume that a single cell lineage is specifically implicated in the development of an antibody producing cell and that other cells simply act in a supportive capacity and are irrelevant to the principal molecular events. This may be an oversimplification and I wish very briefly to review what we know of the origin and interactions of immunologically active cells; they may broadly be thought of as components of the reticulo-endothelial system and as lymphoid cells.

Anatomically many types of cells with phagocytic activity are recognized. For the majority of these we have no clear idea of their origin nor of their participation in immune responses. This is particularly true of the sinusoidal macrophages the distribution and retentive capacities of which can be so prominently revealed in lymphoid organs which receive foreign material.

On the other hand it has been found that at least some of the alveolar macrophages in the lungs and the peritoneal cavities (at least in conditions in which more than usual numbers of cells are induced) can derive from bone marrow (1, 2, 3). This has been most clearly shown in mouse radiation chimaeras but I feel that it is probably valid to suppose that there is a similar source in the intact normal animal. This viewpoint is lent substance from studies made on sterile inflammation in which many of the accumulating macrophages were found to derive from circulating cells almost certainly of bone-marrow origin and with the prior morphology of a blood monocyte (4, 5).

Evidence has been presented that phagocytic cells in the liver, ostensibly Kupffer cells, can under certain circumstances derive from a circulating lymphocyte (6). This finding hints at the possibility that macrophage populations thought to be sessile may have circulating precursors.

Dendritic reticular cells, which seem to exist at the points where germinal centres arise, though not phagocytic cells, have been implicated in immune responses by a number of workers. It is felt that they represent an elaborate antigen trapping mechanism and that their activities are particularly associated with the production of γG_2 antibodies (7). The existence of ectopic germinal centres in a wide variety of disease conditions suggests either that dendritic reticular cells are not a sine qua non of germinal centre production, or that they are a common constituent of reticular tissues or that they have a circulating precursor. Though no direct proof is available the last of these alternatives is preferable.

As far as the immunological properties of macrophages are concerned I shall only exemplify some of the lines of investigation that have been adopted. It has been shown that macrophages may be 'fed' with antigen in vitro and on transfer to suitable recipients antibody is produced (8). It is not supposed that the macrophages themselves produce the antibody but that they act as a source of more or less degraded antigen for cells of the lymphoid series. It is a widely held belief that such a sequence of events is a common pathway in immune responses though we are short of the information which would permit any firm generalizations. It is, however, clear that macrophages completely degrade much of the antigenic material that they engulf and thus they may well act as an antigenic sink in addition to an antigen pool.

Extracts from macrophages which have come in contact with certain antigens in vitro have been found to contain immunogenic material with some of the characteristics of RNA (9). It was claimed that this material was elaborated by the macrophages and that it could impart the specificity to the antibody produced by lymphocytes with which it came in contact. It is not known whether this quite clear-cut finding is of general validity in vivo but it suggests a role for the macrophage in immunity which is active rather than passive.

By way of contrast it has been demonstrated that tumour cells may be killed by macrophages 'armed' with appropriate antibodies (10, 11). Such hostile macrophages may be an important component in the rejection of tissue grafts but the specific reactivity they have is to be thought of as passively acquired.

In a most important series of experiments it has been shown that macrophages of various kinds may develop a heightened capacity for intracellular digestion of certain bacteria during the course of systemic infection (12). As far as can be judged the excitement of these macrophages is not specific but the excitation process probably requires the participation of lymphoid cells the reactivity patterns of which are specific. These findings illustrate the possibility that interaction between immunologically active cells may occur in which macrophages are among the reacting cells.

For many years it has been thought that lymphocytes were a heterogeneous population but the extent and causes of their variability were not precisely known. Two major classes of lymphocyte have now been recognized in mice (13). These two sorts of cells are thought to have (in the adult) a common origin in the bone marrow. Their immediate precursors may also be common but this is a point which has not been verified. It seems that some cells from the bone marrow enter the thymus and there encounter an ill-defined stimulus to differentiate. These 'processed' cells (or more likely their progeny) leave the thymus with properties which appear in a number of significant ways different from lymphocytes which derive from the bone marrow but which have not been processed by the thymus. The thymus processed cells are reasonably designated 'T' cells; the other sort of cell has been termed a 'B' cell (14). T cells in contrast to B cells are thought not to produce antibody. T and B cells have been shown by a number of workers to co-operate in certain humoral immune responses and on various grounds it seems to be likely that such interaction will prove to be a general phenomenon in those immune responses which are thymus dependent. In situations in which an antigen is recognizably of the hapten-carrier variety it

has been found that the T cell population is important in responding to the carrier whereas it appears to be the response of
B cells which determines the specificity of the anti-hapten
response (15).   Other characteristics of T and B cells have been
adduced, for example that they are long and short lived respectively
but such a notion cannot presently be supported by adequate
experimental evidence - it may eventually prove a useful half-truth.
Less controversially it is thought that T cells are a predominantly
recirculating cell population commonly found in the 'thymus-
dependent areas' of lymph nodes and spleen (16).   B cells, in
contrast, seem relatively sessile as a class and to be found
predominantly in the follicular portions of the same organs.

The information which has permitted the delineations of these
populations of lymphocytes and macrophages derives almost entirely
from experiments with small rodents.   It is difficult to apply
some of the cell marker techniques which have been used to obtain
the relevant facts in larger animals and although there is a
considerable body of circumstantial evidence which makes it likely
that the situation is similar in all mammals, nevertheless there
are many areas in which important information is lacking.

For instance, it has been found that the capacity to respond
to different antigenic stimuli not only varies between different
individuals of the same outbred species but also within the same
individual according to its age.   In foetal sheep, the capacity
to produce antibodies against certain bacteriophages is present
at a very early stage of gestation whilst the response to certain
bacterial products can only be elicited after birth some hundred
days later (17).   This maturation cannot presently be associated
with any specific change in the lymphoid system.   The genetic
variability in relation to the capacity to respond to antigenic
stimuli in different members of the same species (or larger taxa)
can occasionally be associated with specific peculiarities of the
lymphoid system but often no such distinction is possible and we
are left uncertain as to the mechanism by which the variation has
developed (18).

It is well known that animals under stress may give unusual
responses to antigenic stimuli.   As it is often difficult to
know, with experimental animals, what is their optimal environment
many results described with perfect honesty may relate to
essentially artefactual situations.   In order to avoid such
hazards which often derive from work with whole animals many
analysts have attempted to demonstrate immunological responses
with cells in vitro.   In some instances they have been successful -
their residual difficulty is then to decide how to relate their
findings to the intact animal.

Thus despite the enthusiasm with which the case for interaction between immunologically active cells is being presented it would be a mistake to suppose that we are other than on the threshold of knowledge of the mechanisms involved in the various co-operative processes.

REFERENCES

1. H.Balner, Transplantation, 1:217, 1963.

2. J.W.Goodman, Blood, 23:18, 1964.

3. M.O.Pinkett, C.R.Cowdrey, and P.C.Nowell, Am.J.Path., 48:859, 1966.

4. A.Volkman, and J.L.Gowans, Brit.J.exp.Path., 46:50, 1965.

5. A.Volkman, and J.L.Gowans, Brit.J.exp.Path., 46:62, 1965.

6. J.G.Howard, G.H.Christie, J.L.Boak, and E.Evans-Anfom, Colloques Internationaux du Centre National de la Recherche Scientifique, No.147. p.95, 1965.

7. R.L.Hunter, R.W.Wissler, and F.W.Fitch, Adv.exp.Med.Biol., 5:101, 1969.

8. A.Cruchaud, and E.R.Unanue, Adv.exp.Med.Biol., 6:

9. M.Fishman, and F.L.Adler, Cold Spring Harb.Symp.quant.Biol., XXXII: 343, 1967.

10. G.A.Granger, and R.S.Weisser, Science,N.Y., 145:1427, 1964.

11. G.A.Granger, and R.S.Weissler, Scienc,N.Y., 151:97, 1966.

12. G.B.Mackaness, J.exp.Med., 129:973, 1969.

13. Transplantation Reviews, vol.1, 1969.

14. I.M.Roitt, M.F.Greaves, G.Torrigiani, J.Brostoff, and J.H.L. Playfair, Lancet, ii:367, 1969.

15. M.C.Raff, Nature, Lond., in press, 1970.

16. D.M.V.Parrott, M.A.B.de Sousa, and J.East, J.exp.Med., 123:191, 1966.

17. A.M.Silverstein, Science, N.Y., 144:1423, 1964.

18. R.T.Smith, P.A.Miescher, and R.A.Good (eds) 'Phylogeny of Immunity', University of Florida Press, Gainesville, 1966.

DISCUSSION TO SESSION 2
CHAIRMAN, A. J. S. DAVIES, CO-CHAIRMAN, F. W. FITCH

H. S. Micklem: Dr. Merétey, there was one thing I did not quite understand about your system. You said if one transfers E. coli positive cells to E. coli negative animals, you get a continuation of antibody formation and plaque cell formation. I think you used that as evidence that continuing antigenic stimulation was not necessary. Does that imply that the E. coli negative rats have actually not got this strain of E. coli in their intestines, or did I miss an important point?

K. Metérey: We followed the appearance of natural antibodies in rats from the birth for a year. We have found that the "positivity" of animals was increased during ageing. In our present studies in the two month period of observation only one untreated control animal became positive, i.e., started to produce natural antibodies to E. coli 0 26 bacteria. It means, that the probability of such spontaneous "positivites" is very low. On the other hand, we had another control group: irradiated "coli negative" animals injected with "coli negative" cells. In this group no positivity did occur.

A. J. S. Davies: Dr. Merétey, if you immunize previously E. coli negative animals with the proper strain of E. coli, presumably you will now produce antibody against E. coli. If you take bone marrow from such an immunized animal and transfer it to an irradiated animal, what happens then?

K. Metérey: Only a few experiments were done along this line. We immunized adult rats with 100 µg E. coli 0 26 endotoxin intravenously. Five days later bone marrow or spleen cells were transplanted from these animals into "coli negative" irradiated rats. We could not achieve better transfer of antibody production by this means. Both PFC count in the spleen and antibody titer in the sera were lower given cells from immunized animals than in the case of natural antibody transfer. Our results concerning the experiments of transfer of immunized cells were similar to the published data on the secondary immune response in radiation chimeras. No antibody production was observed in the recipients given primed cells without secondary antigen injection. It is possible, that the continuous "administration" and processing of the antigen of intestinal origin and some cell migration processes might also account for these positive results in this natural antibody transfer system.

P. Nieuwenhuis: Did you try to inject bone marrow cells from E. coli positive animals to E. coli negative germfree animals, and see whether you get natural antibodies in those animals?

K. Metérey: No, we did not investigate the transfer of natural
antibodies into germfree animals.

C. Rosse: Do you have any idea of the identity of the effective
cells, within the bone marrow?

K. Metérey: We don't know exactly what kind of cells play a role in
this transfer of capacity to produce natural antibodies. It seems
to us that only bone marrow-derived cells participate in it. We
tried to induce an immune response in transplanted animals early
after the transfer. We were unable to immunize the animals after
the transfer of bone marrow cells. After the injection of spleen
cells an immune response occurred to 100 µg E. coli O 26 endotoxin.
The results, that natural antibody transfer was observed both by
bone marrow or spleen cell transplantation, though the active immune
response occurred only after transferring spleen cells, suggests
that different cells interact in these reactions.

M. W. Hess: I have a question related to the questions asked by
Dr. Davies and Dr. Micklem. Can you exclude the possibility that
with transferring cells from E. coli positive animals you transferred
antigen?

K. Merétey: We can't exclude or prove the possibility that we also
injected antigen together with the injected 5×10^7 nucleated cells.
The transferred cells were washed, so that only an extremely little
amount of antigen, if any, could be bound.

J. J. Trentin: I wonder if Dr. Micklem would care to comment on the
possibility that the so called "self" reactive lymphocytes are
reacting with a subpopulation of the erythrocytes that are somehow
antigenically aberrant; perhaps an ageing subpopulation that develops
or exposes new antigens, and that this process might even be part
of the erythrocyte sequestration and elimination process.

H. S. Micklem: We have really just started to look into this question.
I think the first thing to say is that we do have evidence that such
a subpopulation of lymphocytes is involved. If you increase the ratio
of erythrocytes to lymphocytes you do find that there is an increase
in the number of rosettes that you can take out. I think that an
actually similar thing is being described in the anti SRBC system.
Now, it is obviously very important to know what the characteristics
of the subpopulation are. One possibility, as you say, is that this
is an aged suspopulation. We have attempted to test that by substituting heated, "artificially aged" erythrocytes (heated at 50° for
20 minutes) which is a treatment that with human erythrocytes encour-
ages rapid phagocytosis and clearance. We have attempted to compare
erythrocytes treated in this manner with normal erythrocytes and we
found there is no increase in the proportion of erythrocytes that
appear to be taken up into the cluster. However, these are preliminary

experiments and I do not regard them as conclusive. The second possibility is of course a rather more interesting one, and related to the Burnet's recent ideas about the mosaicism which is inherent in every individual. What he suggested roughly was that you had a basic antigenic pattern on the membrane antigens. Arguing from the high mutation rate in the germ line of the histocompatibility antigens, he suggested that in any rapidly proliferating tissue you will get a mosaic of deviants from the self pattern. Of course it would be nice, but we have absolutely no evidence that this is so, if one had a wide variety of subpopulations of lymphocytes which would react with separate subpopulations of erythrocytes, perhaps with overlapping affinities but at least not completely overlapping affinities. These are the lines we are trying to work on at the moment.

W. H. Hildeman: I am really very favorably impressed with the potential sensitivity of your test in being able to pick up all sorts of alloantigens. I am bothered, however, by the fact that you could take CBA mice, immunize them with an A/j skin graft, presumably with a whole series of rather potent H2 antigens; then on testing find a rise in cluster-forming cells, not only against the alloantigens, but apparently against autoantigens as well. If there were sharp quantitative differences, perhaps that would be consistent with the idea of mutant cells and change in ageing, as Trentin has argued. As you recall, several years ago we did quite a lot of work in allo-immunized plaque assay system, but eventually gave up in dismay for using it, with other than H2 antigens, because of a lack of reproducibility of the test. One day it works and the next day it doesn't. Have you actually tried quite unrelated antigens, perhaps rat or chicken or something to see whether there really is specificity in the quantitative rise in cluster forming cells?

H. S. Micklem: The only answer I can give to that is that we have compared the response to an H2 incompatible graft, namely A/j or A/h and an H2 compatible, namely C3H to CBA. The difference that one finds with the C3H is that one gets only the early response. I did not have time to show you the full data on the skin grafting results which are quite extensive, but one gets the early part of the response within about the first 7 days to C3H which is about the same size as it is to the A antigens, but what you get with A is a secondary rise after rejection of the graft, which I think was something you did not find in your experiments. The self-reactive cells fall down to a low level by day 10 when the graft has just been rejected. In the strongly antigenic combination, you get a brisk continuing rise in the antidonor rosette up to about day 15 or 16, and you don't find that in situations where you don't get serum antibodies formed such as the C3H to CBA system. I do not know what the secondary rise means. It may be connected with the precursors of serum antibody formation. I am afraid we do not have any data on more distinctly related combinations. I do not know for sure, but the prediction is that you get a greater stimulation.

M. Feldman: Since the recognition of self antigens might be associated with self tolerance I wonder whether you have measured the incidence of cells in the thymus which can recognize self antigens as a function of age in the fetus and later during the ontogenetic development. Also, I wonder whether these cells are TL positive or TL negative, and I will tell you why I raise this point. In an earlier paper, Dr. Raff has tried to convince us that the second stage of differentiation of thymus cells is associated with a loss of TL antigen and those cells which have lost the antigen will migrate out. We don't have any direct proof for that. One can easily maintain that the TL negative cells which have migrated out of the thymus never contained the TL antigen within the thymus. After all, less than 5% of the cells which are formed within the thymus leave the thymus.

H. S. Micklem: As far as the second question goes, I do not know. First question: I have the impression that there may be a rise with increasing age, but that is really only an impression.

E. Möller: First, a technical point to Dr. Micklem. I wonder if you get "self rosettes" even if you use the McConnell technique of centrifugation and resuspension. There seems to be some data indicating that these rosettes are revealed only after continued incubation. Secondly, as I understand your studies, the presence of rosettes in the thymus was investigated only with syngeneic red cells. Did you study the presence of rosettes with allogeneic red cells? According to Jerne's theory on generation of antibody diversity, one would expect a rather high frequency of such rosettes too.

H. S. Micklem: Yes, we do get rosettes in the McConnell-Coomb's setup. I must say that we have not used this technique a great deal, and when we have used it we have not found it terribly reproducible. But as far as we can see, we can get, at best, equal numbers of rosettes which correspond with those we get with the long incubation technique. There is no problem in demonstrating them. Regarding the incidence of allo-rosettes, we have our most extensive data for allo-rosettes in lymph nodes. With CBA one can generally find that there is a slightly higher incidence of syn-clusters than of allo-clusters in the lymph nodes. Now I am not sure that that is typical of the mouse species as a whole, because in other situations where we have looked rather less extensively, we find the opposite; i.e., that one gets a larger number of allo-rosettes than of syn-rosettes. In the thymus again, we have data on CBA and C51BL and so far the data are a little bit varied, sometimes you get more syn than allo and sometimes you get more allo than syn. One needs a rather large series of observations on these things before one can draw definite conclusions.

G. J. Thorbecke: Recently some evidence has been coming forth from
Dr. Old's laboratory showing that the TL-negative cells in the thymus
are responsible for its graft versus host activity. This suggests
that these cells indeed do arise in the thymus. One more comment on
the cells reactive to transplantation antigens that are present in
the thymus. We have just recently been stimulated by Jerne's
hypothesis to do some mixed lymphocyte reactions with rat thymus.
Dr. Knight found that a very good mixed lymphocyte reactivity is
present in the thymus of neonatal rats to cells of another rat strain,
while reactivity to mouse cells is still lacking at this age.

O. Sjöberg: Dr. Doria, we have studied the inhibition of the immune
response in the Mishell-Dutton system with different antisera. We
found that anti-Fab will inhibit both direct and indirect plaque
forming cells (PFC). Anti-IgM will inhibit direct PFC only and has
no effect on indirect PFC. Antisera against IgG will inhibit indirect
PFC; no effect on direct PFC. Anti-IgA had no effect on the PFC
response at all. Furthermore, it was necessary to have the antisera
in the dishes during the whole culture period. If we just pretreated
the cells before culturing them we got no inhibition.

G. Doria: In our system we looked for direct PFC only, so we don't
have information as to indirect PFC. As to the conditions of cell-
treatment I can say that we got better results when the incubation
was performed during 4 hours than during shorter times prior to
culture.

H. L. Warner: Dr. Doria, with regard to the antisera used for
blocking experiments, rather than asking for evidence of monospecificity, could I ask whether a mouse antiallotype serum is capable of
showing similar blocking. This is the one system in which we can
guarantee that there is no anti-light chain activity.

G. Doria: We did not use anti-allotype antisera. As to the monospecificity of the rabbit antisera which was given to us by Dr. John
Fahey, we tested them against normal mouse serum by immunoelectro-
phoresis and observed in each case only one precipitation band.

L. Fiore-Donati: Dr. Doria, did you try with new born thymus in
comparison with adult thymus to see if there was a difference? Also,
did you get results using bone marrow instead of spleen from thymectomized mice?

G. Doria: We investigated whether normal bone marrow and thymus cells
can interact and produce in vitro PFC to sheep RBC. So far, we have
obtained negative results. We did not look for receptors on thymus
cells from mice younger than 45 days.

INTERACTION BETWEEN T CELLS AND B CELLS IN

HUMORAL ANTIBODY RESPONSES

J. F. A. P. MILLER

Walter and Eliza Hall Institute of Medical Research

c/- Royal Melbourne Hospital P.O. 3050, Australia

Interaction between antigen and two separate classes of lymphocytes is a feature of many antibody responses. Thus, both thymus-
derived "T" cells and non-thymus-derived "B" cells are involved. The
T cells are required to initiate or facilitate antibody production by B
cells in response to certain antigenic determinants. The exact nature
of the interaction is not clear.

IDENTITY AND SOURCE OF T CELLS

The thymus is a source of T cells uncontaminated by B cells.
When thymus lymphocytes (TL) are injected with antigen into a lethally
irradiated host, a proportion of the cells migrate to the spleen where
some differentiate and proliferate to give rise to a progeny of T cells
which differ from the original TL in 2 main characteristics:- (a) they
can behave essentially as recirculating small lymphocytes (1); (b) they
can collaborate with B cells much more effectively than the original TL
(2). T cells do not produce antibody, in the sense of a classical immunoglobulin molecule that is secreted into the serum. Thoracic duct lymphocytes (TDL) seem to contain a much larger proportion of T cells than of
B cells (3). The θ antigen which characterizes TL is also found on some
lymphocytes outside the thymus and preliminary data has suggested that
these were T cells (4). There is, however, no direct evidence to prove
that all T cells have the θ antigen and that no B cells ever exhibit that
antigen.

IDENTITY AND SOURCE OF B CELLS

The bone marrow (BM) is a source of stem cells some of which can differentiate to T cells (thymus-dependent pathway) whilst others can transform to B cells (thymus-independent pathway). When adult mice are thymectomized, given a potentially lethal dose of total body irradiation and protected with BM cells (mice herein after referred to as TxXBM), their lymph nodes and spleen are a source of B cells relatively uncontaminated by T cells. B cells are potentially antibody-forming cells (AFC), are said to lack the θ antigen and cannot, on their own, secrete antibody in response to certain antigenic determinants.

INTERACTION BETWEEN T CELLS AND B CELLS

Claman and colleagues (5) showed that irradiated mice given a mixture of TL and BM produced far more antibody to sheep erythrocytes (SRBC) than if given either TL or BM alone. Since then, evidence of thymus-marrow interactions has been obtained in mice challenged with heterologous erythrocytes, serum proteins and hapten-protein conjugates and it has been unequivocally shown that the AFC are derived from the BM donor and not from the TL given (6). Although mixtures of BM and TL have failed to respond to antigen in vitro, interaction between TL or T cells and spleen from TxXBM mice (i. e. B cells) has been demonstrated in tissue culture with SRBC and hapten protein conjugates (7).

ANTIGEN SPECIFICITY OF T CELLS

Since T cells do not transform to AFC and yet are required to facilitate or initiate the antibody response of B cells, it is important to determine whether they can interact with antigen specifically. There are 4 different experimental designs that have tested for specificity at the level of T cells.

1. The "education" of thymus cells by antigen (Table I) is specific. In this experimental design, two sets of lethally irradiated mice were used. The first received TL intravenously with or without the relevant antigen. After 5-7 days, cells from the spleens of these mice were injected together with BM and the antigen in question (SRBC or fowl immunoglobulin G - FγG - in the examples given in Table I) into the second set of irradiated mice and the antibody generated in these hosts was measured. There was a specific enhancement of the response in irradiated recipients of T cells derived from spleens of irradiated mice given TL and the antigen

Table I. "Education" of thymus lymphocytes by antigen

Cells and antigen given to first irradiated hosts	Cells and antigen given to second irradiated hosts	Peak No. AFC per spleen in second irradiated hosts
1. 10^8 SRBC	one spleen equivalent from first irradiated hosts	1. 310
2. 10^8 TL		2. 248
3. 10^8 TL $+10^8$SRBC	$+ 10^7$ BM $+ 10^8$ SRBC	3. 133
4. 10^8TL$+10^8$SRBC		4. 2103
5. 10^8 TL + FγG	2×10^7 cells from spleens of first irradiated hosts	5. 1130
6. 10^8 TL + BSA		6. 0
7. 10^8 TL	$+ 10^7$ BM + FγG	7. 0

Groups 1-4 give data for direct AFC published in reference (2)
Groups 5-7 give average of indirect AFC values obtained from 8-17
   mice per group - unpublished data of Basten and Miller.

in question (SRBC and not horse erythrocytes - HRBC - in the first
example and FγG and not bovine serum albumin - BSA - in the second
example in Table I). This experimental design for the specific education
of TL by antigen has been widely used (7, 8, 9).

    2. Specific immunological tolerance is a property that can be
linked to TL (10) and to T cells in thoracic duct lymph (11). Thus, for
instance, TDL from mice specifically tolerant of FγG were coated with
the tolerated antigen (in the form of fowl anti-mouse lymphocyte globulin -
FALG - which is not immunosuppressive in mice) in vitro and given to
TxXBM mice.   These failed to respond significantly to FγG although they
could generate AFC to HRBC.   On the other hand, normal TDL coated in
vitro with FALG enhanced the response of TxXBM recipients to both FγG
and HRBC, and the AFC produced were derived, not from the inoculated
TDL, but from the BM cells used to protect the thymectomized mice after
total body irradiation (Table II).   The tolerant TDL population was agglu-
tinated by FALG (just as the normal TDL pool) and the cells must therefore have carried FγG on their surface.   The failure of FALG coated
tolerant TDL to restore reactivity cannot be attributed to an inability to
recirculate normally or penetrate the correct sites in the spleen since
both normal and tolerant FALG-coated TDL preparations were distributed
in an identical way in their hosts as judged by determining the distribution
of Cr^{51}-labelled cells.   The suggestion might be made that T cells have
to proliferate prior to interacting with B cells and that T cells from

Table II.   Effect of inoculating (CBA x C57BL)F_1 TDL coated with FALG on responsiveness of TxXBM CBA mice to FγG and HRBC*

Source of TDL	Antigens given	%^{131}I-FγG serum bound at days[+]			Peak No. AFC per spleen		
					anti-FγG $\mp$		direct HRBC //
		15	22	42	direct	indirect	
none	aggregated FγG and HRBC in vivo	0.5	0.2	1.0	510	2	30
normal	FALG in vitro HRBC in vivo	22.6	17.1	42.0	76980 §	14730 §	24520
FγG-tole-rant	FALG in vitro HRBC in vivo	1.2	1.4	12.1	140	2	35490

* For abbreviations see text.   + 6–19 mice per group. $\mp$ 4–8 mice per group.   // 7–8 mice per group.   § anti-H2 serum treatment of these AFC identified them as CBA.

tolerant donors cannot proliferate in response to the tolerated antigen. If this is so, however, the purpose of this proliferation cannot be ascribed solely to provide a mechanism for increasing the number of T cells capable of transporting the specific antigen and "focussing" it onto those B cells with specificities for the determinants to which the antibody is made. The FγG in the FALG preparations used must have been carried by a vast majority of the inoculated TDL and there must thus have been an ample number of cells able to "focus" the antigen in the correct sites within the spleen. Our findings thus suggest that the role of T cells is linked to a capacity for "recognizing" antigenic determinants and is dependent not simply on the passive transportation of such determinants to B cells, but upon some active process. This presumably involves interaction of the T cell with the determinant and further differentiation of that cell to produce some factor – specific or nonspecific – which plays a role in switching on the B cell to antibody production.

3.   T cells are essential for the expression of specific immunologi-cal memory. TDL from FγG primed mice could adoptively transfer 7S memory responses to irradiated mice even when the cells were exposed in vitro to fluid FγG and extensively washed prior to injection. TDL from normal mice, on the other hand, could not be stimulated by fluid FγG in vitro (Table III). The capacity of primed TDL to transfer memory could be impaired by prior in vitro treatment with an anti-H2 serum directed against the histocompatibility antigens of the TDL donor (7). Neonatally thymectomized CBA mice (which have an impaired response to FγG – reference 12) were given 300 million (CBA x C57BL)F_1 TL during the first

Table III. Role of T cells in the adoptive memory AFC response to FγG in irradiated CBA mice

Source of TDL	In vitro treatment of TDL		Antigen in vivo	Peak 7S AFC per spleen //
	serum	antigen		
normal (CBA x C57BL)F$_1$ *	none	none	aggregated FγG	125
	normal CBA	fluid FγG	none	5
FγG-primed (CBA x C57BL)F$_1$ *	normal CBA	fluid FγG	none	29210
	CBA-anti-C57BL	fluid FγG	none	40
(CBA x C57BL)F$_1$ TL-reconstituted neonatally thymectomized CBA primed to FγG ‡	normal CBA	fluid FγG	none	2250
	CBA-anti-C57BL	fluid FγG	none	80
	CBA-anti-C57BL	none	aggregated FγG +	25

* 10^7 TDL given per irradiated recipient. ‡ 5×10^6 TDL given per irradiated recipient. + 10^7 normal CBA or F$_1$ TDL were given in addition to each irradiated recipient. // 6 - 10 mice per group.

3 weeks of life and then primed to FγG. TDL obtained from these mice 3-4 weeks later could be stimulated in vitro by fluid FγG and successfully transferred 7S AFC responses to irradiated mice. The AFC were shown to be CBA and not F$_1$ by appropriate treatment with anti-H2 sera. Prior treatment of the TDL population from the reconstituted neonatally thymectomized mice in vitro with a CBA-anti-C57BL serum impaired ability to transfer memory and this could not be reversed by injecting in addition, TDL from normal mice and antigen in vivo (Table III). These results indicate (a) that the TDL population of TL-reconstituted thymectomized mice contains both donor type T cells and host type B cells, (b) that both classes of cells are essential for an adoptive memory response, (c) that host type B cells provide the potential 7S AFC and (d) that the ability to induce the memory response is a property linked to T cells from mice specifically primed to the antigen in question and is not a nonspecific property of any population containing T cells.

4. Preliminary evidence indicates that T cells can bind radioactively labelled antigen specifically. Irradiated mice could respond to FγG after receiving mixtures of TL and spleen cells from TxXBM mice, although neither cell population alone could induce the response. When TL had been preincubated with radioactively labelled antigen under conditions

Table IV. Radioactive antigen-induced suicide in T and B cells *

Source of T cells	Source of B cells	Peak No. 7S AFC/ spleen in irradiated mice +	
		anti-FγG	anti-HRBC
normal thymus	spleen from TxXBM mice	16800	89370
TL pretreated in vitro with ^{125}I-FγG	spleen from TxXBM mice	1330 (8%)	36200 (41%)
normal thymus	spleen from TxXBM mice pretreated in vitro with ^{125}I-FγG	1640 (10%)	41300 (47%)

* Unpublished results of Basten and Miller. + 7-9 mice per group.

in which radiation damage to cells could be expected, the recipients gave a poor response to FγG although they did produce a near normal response to HRBC (Table IV). This suggests that in the population of TL, there are cells capable of recognizing and binding antigen specifically and that these very cells are involved in interacting with B cells to allow these to produce a specific antibody response to the antigen in question.

ANTIGEN SPECIFICITY OF B CELLS

The above data, taken as a whole, point to the existence of specificity at the level of antigen recognition by T cells and to an active role in the differentiation of these cells after antigenic stimulation. To date, there is only preliminary experimental evidence suggesting that specificity also exists in the B cell line:

1. Preliminary data outlined in Table IV points to specificity in both T and B cells.

2. Further preliminary data obtained by Chiller et al. (13) suggest that specific immunological tolerance can be linked to both T and B cells - can be induced in both BM and TL.

POSSIBLE MECHANISMS OF COLLABORATION

If we accept that both T and B cells can dictate the specificity of the response, the interaction between them could occur in one of several ways:

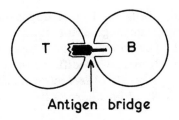

Antigen bridge

Fig. 1. Antigen focussing hypothesis.

1. Antigen focussing: T cells might react with some determinants and focus other determinants on the same antigen molecule onto B cells. Antigen would act as a bridge and the essential element inducing the response may be a twisting of two lymphocytes together, surface to surface (Fig. 1 and reference 9).

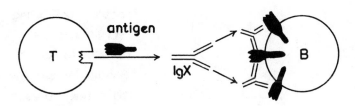

Fig. 2. Antigen concentration via IgX.

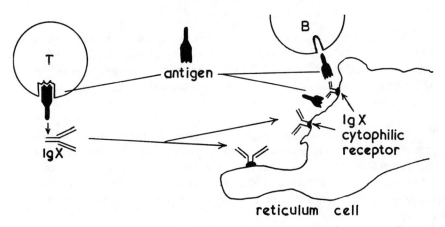

Fig. 3. Antigen concentration via IgX and third-party cell.

2. Antigen concentration via IgX: T cells might interact with some determinants to produce an immunoglobulin molecule, or part of one, which is not secreted in the serum but rapidly absorbed onto other cells - B cells themselves (Fig. 2) or non-specific third-party cells (Fig. 3). The IgX would then concentrate other determinants, on the same antigen molecule, in strategic sites where B cells could be more efficiently stimulated.

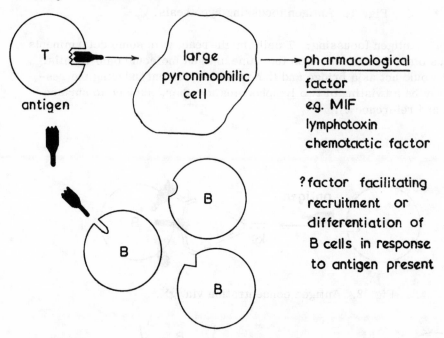

Fig. 4.   Interaction between T and B cells via nonspecific pharmacological factors. Both T and B cells have antigen-binding specificities but recruitment or differentiation of B cell specific for antigen present is facilitated by nonspecific factor elaborated by interaction of T cell with antigen.

3. Production of pharmacological factors: T cells might interact with antigen to produce pharmacological factors. Some such as the migration inhibitory factor, MIF, (14), have been identified and play a role in delayed hypersensitivity reactions. Others might conceivably facilitate the recruitment or differentiation of B cells in response to certain antigens (Fig. 4).

It must be pointed out that, to date, there is no data which would positively and unequivocally exclude any of the above hypotheses. Further work must be directed towards identifying the nature of the antigen binding receptor on T cells, obtaining more extensive data to prove specificity in the B cell line and elucidating the actual mechanism of the interaction that takes place between antigen, T cells and B cells. Finally, it must be determined whether such or similar interactions occur in all antibody responses and in cell-mediated immunity.[15]

REFERENCES

1.   J. F. A. P. Miller, and G. F. Mitchell, In "Lymphatic Tissue and Germinal Centers in Immune Response", L. Fiore-Donati and M. G. Hanna, eds., p. 455, 1969. Plenum, New York.

2.   G. F. Mitchell, and J. F. A. P. Miller, Proc. Nat. Acad. Sci., 59: 296, 1968.

3.   G. F. Mitchell, and J. F. A. P. Miller, J. Exp. Med., 128: 821, 1968.

4.   M. C. Raff, Nature, 224: 378, 1969.

5.   H. N. Claman, and E. A. Chaperon, Transplant. Rev., 1: 92, 1969.

6.   J. F. A. P. Miller, and G. F. Mitchell, Transplant. Rev., 1: 3, 1969.

7.   J. F. A. P. Miller, In Proc. IIIrd Sigrid Juselius Symp., "Collaboration of Different Cells in Immune Responses", Acad. Press, New York, in press.

8.   G. M. Shearer, and G. Cudkowicz, J. Exp. Med., 130: 1243, 1969.

9.   N. A. Mitchison, R. B. Taylor, and K. Rajewski, In "Developmental Aspects of Antibody Formation and Structure", J. Sterzl, ed. Publ. House, Czech Acad. Sci., in press.

10.   R. B. Taylor, Transplant. Rev., 1: 114, 1969.

11.   J. F. A. P. Miller, and G. F. Mitchell, J. Exp. Med., 128: 821, 1970.

12.   J. F. A. P. Miller, and N. L. Warner, Internat. Arch. Allergy Appl. Immunol., in press.

13.   J. M. Chiller, G. S. Habicht, and W. O. Weigle, Proc. Nat. Acad.
        Sci., 65: 551, 1970.

14.   J. R. David, Feder. Proc., 27: 6, 1968.

15.   J. F. A. P. Miller, K. T. Brunner, J. Sprent, and P. J. Russell,
        Transplant. Proc., in press.

DISCUSSION OF DR. MILLER'S PAPER

R. F. Barth: Is the chicken antimouse lymphocyte globulin immunosuppressive in mice?

J. F. Miller: No. I tried to make that point clear. Chicken
antimouse lymphocyte globulin (FALG) does not fix mammalian
complement, nor does it alter the pathway of lymphocyte recirculation.
As you saw from the data, when lymphocytes were coated with FALG
very good responses were obtained provided the cells were normal and
not tolerant. FALG is not immunosuppressive in mice.

W. L. Ford: May I ask about the graft-versus-host activity of the
thymus-derived cells which you recovered from the thoracic duct
lymph of irradiated, allogeneic recipients? Is your finding that
these cells are 50 times as powerful as normal thymus cells an
exception to Simonsen's rule that in strong strain combination, the
"factor of immunisation" is always low, in fact less than 2 in
mice? Have you also compared the GVH activity of these thymus-
derived cells with that of normal thoracic duct lymphocytes?

J. F. Miller: In some experiments, depending on which F-1 hybrid
was used, thymus-derived thoracic duct cells were even more potent,
perhaps even twice as potent as normal thoracic duct cells.

SESSION 3. LYMPHOID CELL MIGRATION
CHAIRMAN, J. LINNA, CO-CHAIRMAN, W. L. FORD

QUANTITATIVE STUDIES OF THYMOCYTOKINETICS

Bernard J. Bryant

Department of Medical Microbiology, University of

California, Davis, California   95616   USA

With the Cold Spring Harbor Symposium on Antibodies in 1967
(1), scholarly opinion shifted away from instruction and toward
clonal selection as the favored immunogenetic theory. A corollary
of this shift, which was brought about largely by the need to explain antibody diversity in relation to chemically defined haptens,
was to significantly reinforce existing data of other types which
had been interpreted as fitting with selective theory. Selective
theory requires elimination of nonmutant potentially self-reactive
cells generated in the thymic immunoglobulin (Ig) diversification
site, and Metcalf's thymocyte kinetic data of 1964 (2), with its
maximum 5% survival of thymocytes in the periphery as long-lived
(presumably mutant nonself-reactive) cells, nicely fitted theory.
However, since that time, a good deal of data on thymocyte fate
has accumulated (3-9), much of it expressing differences of experimental approach that have led to diverse claims for both large and
small scale thymocyte emigration. The exact scale of emigration,
if known quantitatively, would bear not only on selective theory
but on the further question of whether thymic Ig-gene mutational
events take place at ordinary or at hypermutational frequencies.

Of existing experimental approaches, the most obviously amen-
able to in vivo quantitation are those that use radiolabeled precursor incorporation into DNA. This devolves reasonably from the
dogmas of DNA metabolic stability, conservative segregation to progeny cells at mitosis, and dissolution and loss of incorporated label at cell death (10). Tritiated thymidine ($H^3 \cdot TdR$), because of
the specificity of its incorporation into DNA among macromolecules,
has been and remains the DNA precursor of choice for qualitative
cell kinetic and migration studies, but not for quantitative studies. Objections can be raised as to the difficulty of measuring

103

$H^3 \cdot$DNA at the whole-body level (an entire corpse must be DNA-ex-
tracted) and the impossibility of $H^3 \cdot$DNA measurement on the same
material at the three levels (whole-body, organ, and histologic)of
necessary interest for quantitative study. Moreover, the entire
question of quantitation of $H^3 \cdot$DNA is compromized by the extensive
reutilization of $H^3 \cdot$TdR following cell death, approaching 50% of
dead cell $H^3 \cdot$DNA at the whole-body level (11).

It seemed reasonable therefore to devise a technique using
the DNA label concept to advantage but avoiding the usual $H^3 \cdot$TdR
DNA label and its attendant disadvantages for quantitation. The
rationale and results obtained with a new method in a thymocyte
kinetic study are summarized in the following.

METHODS AND MATERIALS

Of tactics of labeling used in studies of thymocyte fate, viz
local labeling without systemically labeled controls, local with
systemic controls, and labeled thymocyte transfusion, the first is
perhaps the most defined, direct, and physiological, provided label reutilization is dealt with effectively. While this is not
possible sensu stricto without continuous post labeling cold precursor infusion, it can be approached using I^{125}-labeled 5-iodo-2'
deoxyuridine ($I^{125} \cdot$UdR), a very poorly reutilized thymidine analog
and specific DNA precursor (12). $I^{125} \cdot$UdR reutilization overall is
thought to approximate the 3 to 4% level of its original whole-
body incorporation into DNA following systemic administration.

The concept of $I^{125} \cdot$UdR locally administered to the thymus is
deficient only in the sense that $I^{125} \cdot$DNA activity cannot be measured without biochemical separation of DNA. However, I^{131} activity from I^{131}-labeled 5-iodouracil ($I^{131} \cdot$U) mixed in the applied
$I^{125} \cdot$UdR solution was found to rapidly equilibrate in all tissues
with <u>degraded</u> I^{125} activity such that sample $I^{125} \cdot$DNA (total I^{125}
less degraded I^{125} determined from I^{131}) could be determined directly by external gamma counting.

This meant that a rationale could be adopted wherein the initial thymus $I^{125} \cdot$DNA counts could be followed quantitatively on
three levels (whole-body, organ distribution, histologic) without
errors of biochemical separation and with considerable economy of
materials. The mathematical analysis formulating an expression for
sample $I^{125} \cdot$DNA was complex, as was the expression itself, and the
mixed isotope data were necessarily processed by computer. Details
of this analysis will be published elsewhere.

The apposite animal for studies of the locally labeled thymus
is the guinea pig. The cervically-located subcutaneous thymus permits surgical mobilization of the organ, clamping of the pedicle
if desired, and most importantly, exposition of the entire ventral

capsular surface. Local labeling has heretofore been accomplished via direct parenchymal injection, but the significant objection can be raised that structural damage of endothelia inevitably ensues, leading to spurious release of labeled living thymocytes to the blood. Injection was therefore avoided and the radiochemical mixture was applied instead to the exposed capsular surface wherefrom it penetrated into the parenchyma by diffusion. Ten to 15 μl volumes containing 10 μCi of both $I^{125} \cdot UdR$ and $I^{131} \cdot U$ (sp. acts., >50 Ci/mM) were applied to the capsules. The animals were housed in a humidified oven at 37^0 C. for one hour to permit transcapsular diffusion of the compounds and their metabolism. The thymus was then swabbed clean of surface activity and reinserted subcutaneously. $I^{125} \cdot UdR$ incorporation was terminated by a one-hour infusion of cold competitor TdR beginning 40 minutes after label application.

Twenty five to 30-day-old individuals of the Hartley strain, adrenalectomized 7 to 10 days previously, were used for local labeling. Intact individuals were systemically labeled by intravenous injection of the radiochemical mixture. All animals were maintained on cold sodium iodide-supplemented diet to minimize radioiodide retention via protein binding.

RESULTS AND DISCUSSION

$I^{125} \cdot UdR$ incorporation into thymus DNA at 2 hours, under conditions of local transcapsular diffusion of $I^{125} \cdot UdR - I^{131} \cdot U$ mixtures, amounted to $10 \pm 4 \times 10^4$ I^{125} cpm. Pedicle clamping during the incorporation period led to no discernable differences in the extent or regression of these $I^{125} \cdot DNA$ counts, compared to non-clamped animals; these groups were therefore combined for data analysis. On the other hand, adrenalectomy was essential, for thymic $I^{125} \cdot DNA$ counts of nonoperated animals frequently regressed rapidly and the associated starry-sky thymic pathology expressed intracortical thymocyte death. The data reported herein for local labeling refer to animals adrenalectomized 7 to 10 days before use.

The regression of $I^{125} \cdot DNA$ in the thymus and whole-body during the first week after local thymus labeling differed insignificantly (Fig. 1). This infers the essential identity of the intrathymic with the whole body survival of the great bulk of the labeled thymocyte progeny. These cells therefore die either in the thymus or elsewhere after a peripheral life of a few minutes or hours and do not transform into other lines of somatic cells. This is the most significant conclusion to be drawn from this study.

Less than 5% of the 2 hour thymus $I^{125} \cdot DNA$ remained in the whole body one week later (Fig. 1). Most of this activity represented label reutilized by proliferating cells throughout the body, as shown by the significant $I^{125} \cdot DNA$ counts recovered in organs rich

I¹²⁵-DNA RETENTION AFTER LOCAL I¹²⁵-UdR LABELING OF THYMUS

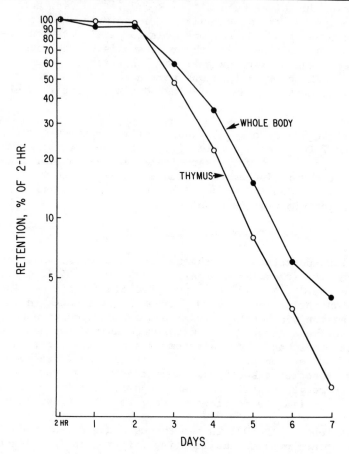

Fig. 1.   I¹²⁵·DNA retention after transcapsular labeling of thymus of adrenalectomized guinea pigs.   The data represent mean values of 6 to 8 animals per time intervals.

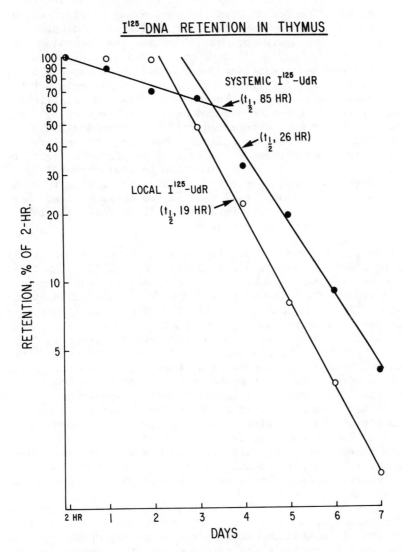

Fig. 2. I^{125}·DNA retention in thymus after transcapsular labeling
of adrenalectomized and systemic labeling of intact guinea pigs.
The data represent mean values of 6 to 8 animals per time interval.

in proliferating cells but not lymphocytes, e.g. testis. Also, the
<5% level coincides remarkably well with the estimated 3 to 4%
whole body level of I^{125}·UdR reutilization following labeled cell
death (vide ante). The actual level of whole-body survival of labeled thymocyte progeny may have been below 1% after one week.
That this was so is suggested by the I^{125}·DNA retention values of
1% found in the whole body at 14 days and of 0.5 to 1.2% found in
pooled cervical and mesenteric lymph nodes and spleen at the 5 day
and later intervals. A definitive estimate of thymic emigrant peripheral survival cannot be made because reutilization contributed
an unknown portion of these counts and because subsequent I^{125} radioautograms of these organs detected only an exceptional labeled
thymic emigrant. Emigrants may well have been present in larger
numbers than suggested by the radioautograms but intervening mitoses (conceivably 6 to 8 divisions after the initial thymus labeling) may have reduced their activity to radioautographically nonde-
tectable levels. On balance, a 1% survival of thymocytes as long-
lived peripheral cells in these immunologically mature animals
seems reasonable as a maximal estimate.

I^{125}·DNA activity in the locally labeled thymus was initially
and remained almost exclusively cortically disposed (Figs. 3 to 6);
the progressive radioautographic grain count decline reflected mitosis of labeled cells. The overall thymic I^{125}·DNA decline at 3
days and later (Fig. 2) therefore reflected loss of labeled cortical thymocytes. The essential agreement between the half time of
this regression (19 hours) and that of the second regression component of the systemically labeled thymus (26 hours) indicates that
the latter regression also represented labeled cortical cell loss.
Cortical thymocytes thus disappeared at approximately a one-day
half time rate. Inferentially, the half time disappearance rate of
labeled medullary lymphocytes is given by the 3½ day first regression component of the systemically labeled thymuses. The absence
of this population in the locally labeled thymuses accounts for the
essential absence therein of this first component (Fig. 2). These
half time estimates are reasonably compatible with overall estimates of thymocyte renewal based on the accession of labeled cells
after H^{3}·TdR labeling (13).

I^{125} radioautograms of locally labeled thymus showed a wave-
like migration of labeled thymocytes from their subcapsular positions at 2 hours (Fig. 3) to the cortico-medullary boundary by 6
hours (Fig. 4). At 6 hours and later (Figs. 4 to 6), they were
seen to be shed across the boundary into the medulla. The number
of such labeled medullary cells was always very small compared to
the labeled cortical population; they were much fewer than suggested
by Figs. 4 to 6, which are not representative in this regard, and
most of them remained in the near vicinity of the boundary. Only
occasionally did they penetrate deep into the medulla and only occasionally did Hassal's corpuscles contain discernable label, although

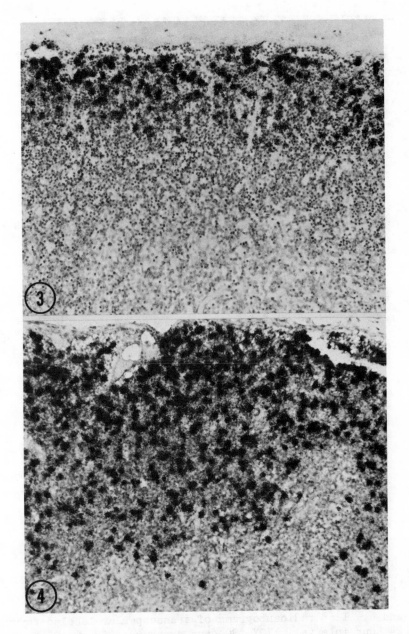

Figs. 3 and 4. I^{125} radioautograms of transcapsular labeled thymuses. Fig. 3, 2 hour interval, 170X, 30 days exposure; Fig. 4, 6 hour interval, 170X, 75 days exposure.

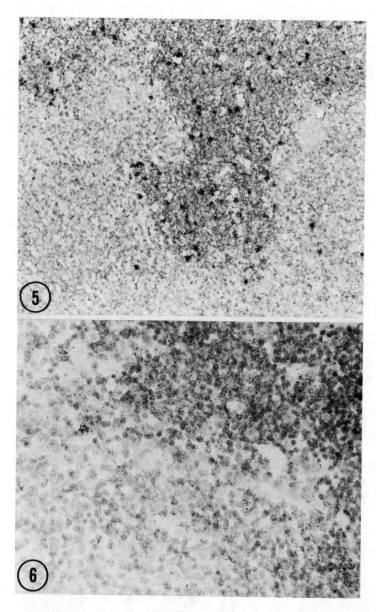

Figs. 5 and 6. I^{125} radioautograms of transcapsular labeled thymuses. Fig. 5, 24 hour interval, 170X, 30 days exposure; Fig. 6, 96 hour interval, 300X, 30 days exposure.

such was found at all times after 6 hours. Their grain count similarity to labeled cells on the cortical side of the boundary and their sparse numbers suggests their random penetration from the cortical interface and their very rapid (minutes) medullary transit time. At this point, it is obscure as to whether they disappeared by emigration into medullary lymphatics and venules, particularly those at the cortical interface, or by explosive intramedullary lysis. There is also the necessary corollary conclusion that the bulk of the medullary lymphocyte population is derived not from the cortex but from stem cells of its own or from an extrathymic source.

SUMMARY

Quantitation of the fate in immunologically mature guinea pigs of proliferating cortical thymocytes, labeled in situ by a method of transcapsular diffusion of $I^{125} \cdot UdR$, indicated that 99% or more of the progeny of these cells die either in the thymus or elsewhere after a peripheral life of minutes or hours. The turnover of thymocytes approximated maximal half-times of 1 day in the cortex and 3½ days in the medulla. The bulk of medullary thymocytes were not cortically derived, although thymocytes of cortical origin penetrated into the medulla shortly before their disappearance.

Acknowledgments. The work was supported by grants from Cancer Research Funds of the University of California and from Syntex Corporation.

REFERENCES

1. Cold Spring Harbor Symposia on Quantitative Biology 23: Antibodies. Cold Spring Harbor Press, N. Y., 1967.

2. D. Metcalf. Wistar Institute Symposium Monograph 2: The Thymus. Wistar Institute Press, Philadelphia, 1964, pp. 53-74.

3. R. Murray and P. Woods. Anat. Rec. 150:113-128, 1964.

4. M. Matsuyama, M. Wiadrowski and D. Metcalf. J. Exp. Med. 123: 559-576, 1966.

5. M. Kotani, K. Seiki, A. Yamashita and I. Horii. Blood 27:511-520, 1966.

6. J. Linna and J. Stillström. Acta Path. et Microbiol. Scandinav. 68:465-475, 1966.

7. J. Linna. Int. Arch. Allergy 31:313-337, 1967.

8. B. Larsson. Acta Path. et Microbiol. Scandinav. <u>70</u>:390-397, 1967.

9. I Weissman, J. Exptl. Med. <u>126</u>:291-304, 1967.

10. W. Hughes, V. Bond, G. Brecher, E. Cronkite, R. Painter, H. Quastler and F. Sherman. Proc. Nat. Acad. Sci. 44:476-483, 1958.

11. L. Feinendegen, V. Bond, E. Cronkite, W. Hughes. Proceedings of the Symposium on the Use of Tritium in Hematological Research, IXth Congress of the European Society of Hematology, Lisboa, 1963.

MIGRATION OF THYMIC LYMPHOCYTES: IMMUNOFLUORESCENCE AND ^{3}HTdR LABELING STUDIES [*+]

A.D. Chanana, E.P. Cronkite, D.D. Joel, R.M.Williams[‡],

and B.H. Waksman

Medical Dept., Brookhaven Nat'l Lab., Upton, N.Y. and

Dept. of Microbiology, Yale U., New Haven, Conn.

Studies utilizing both, continuous in-situ labeling and thymus specific antigen as markers were designed to further clarify some points about thymocyte migration.

MATERIAL AND METHODS

Holstein calves 91-285 days of age were used. The surgical anatomy, the technique of continuous intra-arterial (I.A.) infusion of the bovine thymus with tritiated thymidine (^{3}HTdR) and the technique for measuring the distribution of thymic migrants in tissue sections, have been described (1,2). Following cannulation of the thymic artery in 3 calves continuous I.A. infusion of ^{3}HTdR (Sp.A. 1.9 Ci/mM) was maintained at the rate of 150 µCi/hr. for 2, 7 and 8 days respectively. Twins of 2 experimental calves received comparable amounts of ^{3}HTdR via an indwelling venous cannula for 2 and 8 days respectively. The ratio of the concentrations for ^{3}HTdR perfusing the thymus to concentration perfusing the total body was calculated on the basis of ^{3}HTdR clearance and degradation rates (3). The ratio of thymic

---

[*] Research supported by U.S. Atomic Energy Commission and USPHS grants AI 06112 and AI 06455.
[+] Correspondence: Dr. A. D. Chanana, Medical Dept., Brookhaven Nat'l. Lab., Upton, N.Y. 11973.
[‡] Present Address: Harvard Medical School, Boston, Mass.

artery to total body concentration per gram varied from 100-200: 1.

Cell suspensions were obtained by teasing the tissues in autologous serum. Autoradiograms were processed according to standard techniques and developed after 28 days exposure. Cell suspensions were stained with Giemsa 1:20 at pH 5.75. A Model F Coulter Counter was used for blood and lymph cell counts. Nuclear sizing of smears was done with a particle size micrometer and analyser. Cells with 30 or more grains/cell (heavily labeled cells) in tissue sections following I.A. infusion were considered to be thymic migrants (2). There were no heavily labeled cells

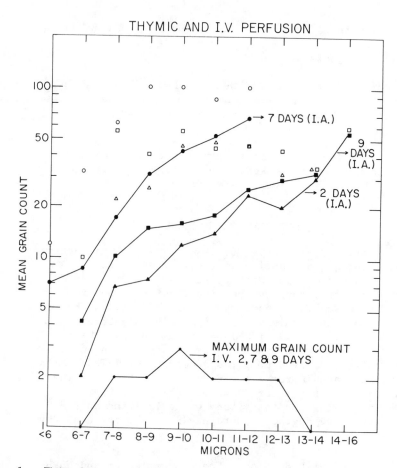

Fig. 1. This figure shows the mean and maximum grain count distribution (closed and open symbols respectively -I.A. infusions) in thymus cells according to the nuclear diameters, following I.A. infusions. The average maximum grain count distribution following I.V. infusions in 3 calves is also shown.

following I.V. infusion (Fig. 1). Such differences in labeling
would be predictable on the basis of the differences in the ratios
of concentrations of ^{3}HTdR perfusing the thymus and total body.
Similarly with cell suspensions, cells with more than 14 grains/
cell were defined as heavily labeled.

Anti-calf thymus serum was prepared in individual rabbits with
thymus cells from a specific calf. Prior to use, the heat inactivated serum was absorbed repeatedly with peripheral lymph node
cells from the thymus cell donor. Cell suspension were incubated
with a 1:50 dilution of absorbed anti-calf thymus serum, washed
twice, and treated with fluorescein-conjugated goat anti-rabbit
IgG. The cells were washed twice more and percentages of fluorescent cells were calculated after examining 200 or more living cells.
Experimental details will be published elsewhere (4).

RESULTS AND DISCUSSION

Thymic cells in smears with a nuclear diameter greater than
9 μ were considered to be large. Approximately 84% of the thymic
lymphocytes were small according to this arbitrary classification.
The percentage of heavily labeled small and large thymic lymphocytes following 2, 7 and 8 days of I.A. infusion ranged from 40.1-
50.6 and 78.9-87.1 respectively.

Anatomic Distribution of Thymic Migrants

For determining the anatomic distribution of thymic migrants,
schematic diagrams of the spleen and lymph nodes sections were
divided into 3 zones. In the lymph node, Zone A corresponds to
the superficial cortex excluding germinal centers, and is characterized by densely packed lymphocytes, Zone B corresponds to
the deep and mix cortex (paracortex) and Zone C represents the
medulla. In the spleen, Zone A represents the dense white pulp
(peri-arteriolar sheath excluding follicles), Zone B the loose
white pulp in calves corresponds to an area outside the marginal
zone possibly representing routes of migration for blood lymphocytes within the spleen (5,6) and Zone C the red pulp. The results
are summarized in Table 1. Briefly, the majority of heavily
labeled cells appeared in the paracortex of lymph nodes and loose
white pulp of the spleen. The density was greater in the spleen.
Thymic migrants were also found in the red pulp of the spleen,
dense white pulp of the spleen, and the medulla and superficial
cortex of the lymph nodes. This finding is in contrast to the
experience of Parrott et al. (7) and Weissman (8), but confirms
the results of other workers (9,10). The total absence of heavily
labeled cells and the paucity of lightly labeled cells in the bone
marrow suggest that bovine thymic cells rarely migrate to the bone
marrow.

Table 1. Distribution of heavily labeled (^{3}HTdR) thymus cells.

Calf No.*	Perfusion (Days)	Zone+	% of total heavily labeled cells	
			Spleen	Lymph Nodes
351	2	A	8	32
		B	68	59
		C	24	9
362	7	A	14	13
		B	62	77
		C	24	10
382	8	A	13	8
		B	52	76
		C	35	16

*   Thymic artery perfusion.
+   For details, see text.

Routes of Migration, Recirculation, and Life Span

The percentage of heavily labeled cells in thymic vein blood and in thymic lymph following continuous I.A. infusion was higher than in jugular or carotid blood (Table 2). Thymic cell migration via lymphatics and veins is in agreement with other studies (11, 12). The presence of some heavily labeled cells in the thoracic duct lymph shows that some of the migrants enter the recirculating pool (13). Occasionally a heavily labeled thymic lymphocyte was observed at the cortico-medullary junction of the unperfused contralateral thymus. This observation is compatible with the notion of migration back to the thymus (14).

The thymus cells appear to be short lived or divide rapidly since 96 hours following the termination of thymic artery infusion with ^{3}HTdR, heavily labeled cells had disappeared from the thymus, thymic vein blood, thymic lymph, and peripheral lymphoid tissues.

Thymus Specific Antigen (TSA)

The distributions of ^{3}HTdR labeled and TSA positive thymic cells are shown in Table 2. Thymic vein blood and thymic lymph contained a greater number of TSA positive cells than the carotid artery blood. As with ^{3}HTdR labeling studies, TSA positive cells were not found in the bone marrow. Within the thymus degree of TSA expression showed an inverse relationship to the thymocyte size. 3-8% of cells leaving the thymus continued to express detectible levels of TSA. This observation suggests that these cells have not completed the process of differentiation, and remain in a thymic state. Our observation that peripheral lymphoid tissues contain very few cells with TSA suggests that transition to peripheral state must occur rapidly at the moment of leaving the thymus.

Table 2.   Heavily Labeled Thymus Cells vs Cells with Thymus
           Specific Antigen.

Cell Source	% Positive Cells (Fluorescence or Tritium)	
	Thymus Specific Antigen	3HTdR labeled[+] (heavily labeled)
Thymus	85.4 (74-91)[‡]	71 (59-88)
Thymic Vein	6 (3-8)	6.7 (3.6-11.7)
Systemic Blood	<1	4.7 (2.7-8.4)
Thymic Lymph	4 (3-5)	12.7 (5.9-17.2)
Thoracic Duct	<1	1.8 (0-4)
Lymph Node[#]	3.5 (3-11)	Not Done
Peripheral Nodes	<1	7.2 (2-12.5)
Bone Marrow	0	0

*   Average of data from 2 to 5 calves.
+   Average of data from 3 calves.
‡   Values in parenthesis represent the range.
#   Draining the thymus.

Quantitative Aspects

The figure of 3-8% of TSA positive cells in the thymic vein
blood can be used to make semiquantitative estimates of the thymic
cell migration. The blood flow in bovine thymus as determined by
direct and ultrasonic flow measurements is 1 ml/g/min. Thymic vein
blood on the average has 6×10^6 lymphocytes/ml. Average weight of
thymus in g/kg body wt. = 1.97. If each TSA positive cell in the
thymic vein blood was produced in the thymus and if one uses .06
as the fraction with TSA in thymic vein blood minus fraction in the
arterial blood, then the number produced/day/kg body weight would
be: 1.02×10^9. Since the blood of calves contains about $0.3 \times
10^9$ small lymphocytes/kg, the daily output of lymphocytes from the
thymus is 3.4 times greater than the number of small lymphocytes
in the blood close to the estimate of 3.7 times per day in the
guinea pig (12). The tissue pool of recirculating small lymphocytes that enters through the thoracic duct of the calf has been
estimated to be 4.8×10^9/Kg (15). Thus the venous output of TSA
positive cells is sufficient to replace this pool every 4.7 days.
However one must also consider the possibility that blood lymphocytes may enter the thymus and pick up a coating of thymus specific
antigen.

SUMMARY

By labeling bovine thymus with [3]HTdR via an indwelling
arterial cannula, the high mitotic rate of thymocytes and the
seeding of thymic migrants to the peripheral lymphoid tissues

have been confirmed. A majority of the thymic migrants were
found in the paracortex of lymph nodes and loose white pulp of
the spleen, areas endowed with suitable vasculature for lymphocyte recirculation. The longer duration of these studies allowed significant numbers of migrants to be seen in the superficial
cortex and medulla of lymph nodes and red pulp of the spleen.
The density of migrants was higher in the spleen than in lymph
nodes. Thymic migrants either have a very short life or divide
rapidly. The routes of migration were shown to be via the thymic
veins and thymic lymphatics. Studies with thymus specific
antigen (TSA) supported the evidence obtained following ^{3}HTdR
labeling and in particularly the lack of migration to the marrow.
Within the thymus, expression of TSA was inversely related to the
cell size. About 3-8% of cells leaving the thymus were TSA positive and it was suggested that transition to peripheral state of
these cells must occur rapidly at the moment of leaving the
thymus.

1. Chanana, A.D., Cronkite, E.P. & Joel, D.D. (1967) Amer. J. Vet.
      Res. 28, 1591.
2. Iorio, R.J., Chanana, A.D., Cronkite, E.P. & Joel, D.D. (1970)
      Cell & Tissue Kinetics 3, 161.
3. Rubini, J.R., Cronkite, E.P., Bond, V.P. & Fliedner, T.M.
      (1960) J. Clin. Invest. 39, 909.
4. Williams, R.M., Chanana, A.D., Cronkite, E.P. & Waksman, B.H.,
      in preparation.
5. Ruchti, C., Cottier, H., Cronkite, E.P., Jansen, C.R. & Rai,
      K.R. (1970) Cell & Tissue Kinetics, in press.
6. Ford, W.L. (1969) Cell & Tissue Kinetics 2, 171.
7. Parrott, D.M.V., DeSousa, M.A.B. & East J. (1966a) J. Exp.
      Med. 123, 191.
8. Weissman, I.L. (1967) J. Exp. Med. 126, 291.
9. Goldschneider, I. & McGregor, D.D. (1968) J. Exp. Med. 127,
      155.
10. Nossal, G.J.V. (1964) Ann. N.Y. Acad. 120, 171.
11. Kotani, M., Seiki, K., Yamashita, A. & Horii, I. (1966) Blood,
      27, 511.
12. Ernström, U. & Larsson, B. (1967) Acta path. Microbiol.
      Scandinav. 70, 371.
13. Goldschneider, I. & McGregor, D.D. (1968) Lab. Invest. 18, 397.
14. Field, E.O. & Stanley, E.M. (1966) Acta haemat. 35, 221.
15. Cronkite, E.P., Chanana, A.D., Joel, D.D., Rai, K.R. & Schiffer,
      L.M. (1968) in Effects of Radiation in Cellular Prolifer-
      ation; pp. 307-326. International Atomic Energy Agency,
      Wien, Austria.

HOMING OF CELLS FROM THE BURSA OF FABRICIUS TO GERMINAL CENTERS IN THE CHICKEN SPLEEN

H.G. Durkin, G.A. Theis and G.J. Thorbecke

Department of Pathology, New York University

School of Medicine, New York, N.Y.

The ability of the chicken to produce humoral immune responses is dependent upon the presence, during ontogeny, of the bursa of Fabricius (1,2). Presence of the other central lymphoid organ, the thymus, is necessary for development of delayed hypersensitivity and of the ability to reject homografts (1,2). It also has been noted that adult chickens, hormonally or surgically bursectomized in ovo, may be completely agammaglobulinemic (3,4) and lack both plasma cells and germinal centers in their lymphoid tissues (5). In addition, inoculation of chickens with avian lymphoid leukosis virus causes initial lesions in bursa follicles, followed by the appearance of enlarged,abnormal germinal centers in the spleen (6). This evidence suggests that the bursa produces precursor cells for the germinal center and plasma cell series of differentiation, as is also supported by the fact that bursa cells are able to produce immunoglobulins earlier than spleen cells during embryogenesis (7).

In mammalian spleen and lymph nodes, areas have been designated as thymus-dependent, partially because they become depleted of small lymphocytes after thymectomy (8), and also because labeled thymus cells and recirculating long-lived lymphocytes tend to home to such areas (9,10). Such studies have not been reported for the avian spleen. It is known that in the chicken the spleen exhibits a much less distinct division between white and red pulp areas. There also may be a different relationship between follicular and periarteriolar lymphoid areas, since the dense mantle zone of lymphocytes around germinal centers present in mammals is completely lacking. An attempt to define the bursa-dependent and thymus-dependent areas of the avian spleen therefore would be of interest.

119

In addition, it appears important to determine where, in the spleen, bursa cells will "home."

To this end, bursa and thymus cells were incubated for 1 hour at 37°C with ^{3}H-adenosine (10 uc/ml; 1 c/mmole, Schwarz Bioresearch, Inc., Orangeburg, N.Y.) in MEM Spinner Medium - Eagle (Microbiological Associates, Bethesda, Md.) containing 5% normal chicken serum. After incubation, the cells were carefully washed in Hanks' Balanced Salt Solution with 2% serum, and injected (1 to 3 x 10^8 cells/recipient; approximately 500,000 counts/minute) into x-irradiated (500-600 R) recipients. More than 90% of donor cells showed variable degrees of labeling by this method. Donors and recipients were 4-6 week old White Leghorn F_1 hybrid chickens of line #96 (Hy-Line Poultry Farm, Johnston, Iowa), homozygous for the major histocompatibility B locus (11). In most experiments, recipients were immunized by 2 weekly intraperitoneal injections of killed B. abortus bacteria (~6 x 10^8 organisms, supplied by the United States Department of Agriculture) in order to ensure the presence of readily distinguishable germinal centers in recipient spleens, even after whole body x-irradiation. Recipients were killed at 6, 24 and 48 hours after intravenous injections of labeled bursa or thymus cells and samples of spleen, liver, lungs, bursa, thymus and intestinal lymphoid tissue (trident-lymphoid nodule) were removed for histological examination. Tissues were fixed in Carnoy's solution and autoradiographs of donor cell smears and tissue sections were prepared using Kodak NTB-3 emulsion. The exposure time was 3 weeks and sections were stained through the emulsion with methyl green pyronin. In addition, weighed segments of each tissue were dissolved in 1-2 ml NCS Solubilizer (Amersham-Searle Corp., Des Plaines, Illinois) and counted in a Packard Tri-Carb Liquid Scintillation Spectrometer. Radioactivity was calculated per gram of tissue.

FATE OF ^{3}H-ADENOSINE LABELED BURSA AND THYMUS CELLS

The amounts of radioactivity found in spleen tissue are shown in Figure 1. When thymus cells were injected, a higher percentage of injected radioactivity was recovered from the spleen than after injection of bursa cells. With both cell types, the ^{3}H-adenosine label appeared to diminish rapidly within the first 2 days after injection. Radioactivity per gram of liver always was low when compared with spleen (between 20 and 50%). The lung contained much less radioactivity (approximately 10% of that found in the spleen) with both cell types studied. Twenty-four hours after transfer of bursa cells, both bursa and thymus tissue of the recipients contained about 15% as much radioactivity as did spleen. At a similar time after transfer of thymus cells, bursa tissue contained approximately 5%, and thymus 10 to 15% of the amount in spleen tissue. Both cell types resulted in

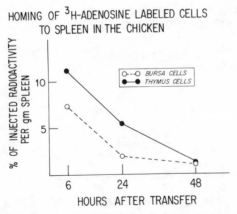

HOMING OF ^{3}H-ADENOSINE LABELED CELLS
TO SPLEEN IN THE CHICKEN

% OF INJECTED RADIOACTIVITY PER gm SPLEEN

O--O BURSA CELLS
●—● THYMUS CELLS

HOURS AFTER TRANSFER

Fig. 1. Radioactivity of spleen samples from recipient chickens, measured as cpm/gm spleen and expressed as percentages of injected radioactivity.

a fair degree of labeling of the trident-lymphoid nodules, varying between 90 and 250 cpm/nodule.

        The location of the labeled cells in autoradiographs of spleen sections was studied by examination (magnification 400 x) of various fields to include a minimum of 50 labeled cells. The percentages of those labeled cells clearly localized within germinal centers are recorded in Figure 2. Thymocytes were rarely observed in such centers, but appeared especially frequent in areas surrounding the central arteries and its branches and often bordered on the slightly basophilic reticulum which accompanied such arteries (Figs. 3 and 4). Small lymphocytes were not abundant in these periarteriolar areas, probably because the recipients had been irradiated. A fair percentage of thymus cells also appeared in the red pulp-like tissue. Bursa cells, on the contrary, preferentially localized within germinal centers (Figs. 5 and 6). As early as 6 hours after injection of bursa cells, a few were seen in germinal centers, although most of the labeled cells were observed in the red pulp-like tissue, often very close to the denser reticulum surrounding central arteries and to Schweigger-Seidel sheaths. At 24 hours after injection, a larger percentage of the labeled bursa cells was found within germinal centers, often several cells per center, forming clusters (Fig.6). Most of the remaining labeled cells were located in or next to Schweigger-Seidel sheaths. By 48 hours, the labeled cells situated within germinal centers appeared to have lost a large part of their radioactivity since several centers were observed with light labeling over a number of cells ("sprinkle of label"). These cells could not be counted accurately and were recorded as single labeled cells for the calculation of percentages. As a

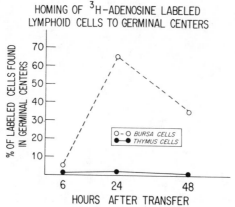

Fig.2. Frequency of localization within germinal centers of intravenously injected ^{3}H-adenosine labeled bursa and thymus cells.
The numbers of cells definitely situated within clearly recognizable germinal centers are expressed as percentages of total numbers of labeled cells counted in spleen sections.

result, since cells outside germinal centers were still clearly
present, again in the vicinity of Schweigger-Seidel sheaths or in
red pulp areas, there was an apparent increase in these cells at
this time (Fig. 2).

PERSISTANCE OF ^{3}H-THYMIDINE LABELED BURSA CELLS

Since the ^{3}H-adenosine radioactivity of in vitro labeled
cells disappeared relatively quickly after transfer, an attempt
was made to study the fate of cells labeled in vivo with ^{3}H-
thymidine 24 to 48 hours previously.

Female inbred White Leghorn F_1 hybrid chickens of line
#96 (Hy-Line Poultry Farm, Johnston, Iowa), homozygous for the
major histocompatibility B locus (11), of approximately 350 grams
body weight, were injected intramuscularly with 100 uc ^{3}H-thymidine
(1.9 c/mmole, Schwarz Bioresearch, Inc., Orangeburg, N.Y.)every
12 hours for 48 hours. Their thymuses and bursas were removed,
teased, washed and injected intravenously (usually 5 x 10^7 cells,
and ranging from 20,000 to 70,000 cpm) into female, immunized
recipients of the same inbred line and size. The amounts of
radioactivity in recipients' tissues were determined on days 1,
7 and 14 after transfer. Spleens of recipients were weighed to
permit calculation of radioactivity for total spleen, as recorded in Figure 7.

A larger percentage of ^{3}H-thymidine labeled cells localized in the spleen than had been seen for the ^{3}H-adenosine labeled

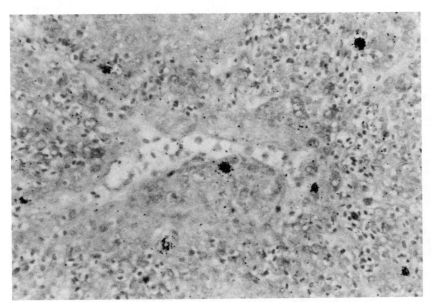

Fig. 3. Autoradiograph of spleen removed from irradiated chicken 6 hours after receiving ^{3}H-adenosine labeled thymus cells. Note accumulation of labeled cells in vicinity of a central artery and its branches. Methyl green pyronin, 400 x.

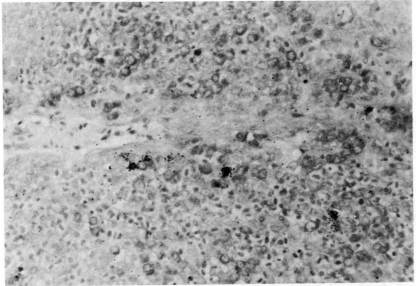

Fig. 4. Autoradiograph of spleen taken from irradiated chicken 20 hours after receiving ^{3}H-adenosine labeled thymus cells. Labeled cells remain concentrated in periarteriolar sheath. Germinal centers (not shown) contained no labeled cells.

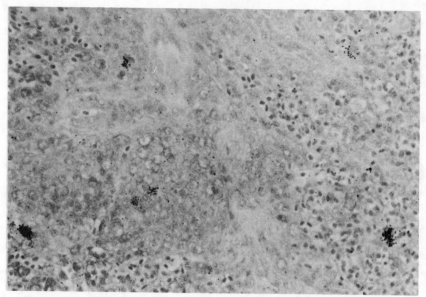

Fig. 5. Autoradiograph of spleen removed from irradiated chicken 6 hours after injection of ^{3}H-adenosine labeled bursa cells. Note that some labeled cells are already present within a germinal center, while the majority are in the surrounding tissue. Methyl green pyronin. 400x.

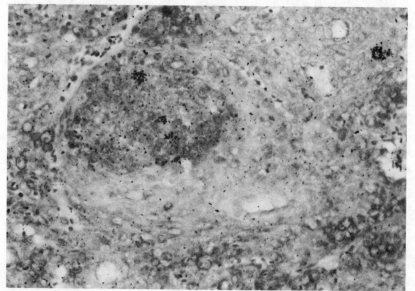

Fig. 6. Autoradiograph of spleen taken from irradiated chicken 20 hours after transfer of ^{3}H-adenosine labeled bursa cells. Note several labeled cells localized within a germinal center, and a single labeled cell adjacent to a Schweigger-Seidel sheath.

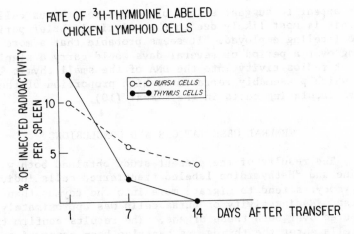

Fig. 7. Radioactivity of spleen samples from recipient chickens, measured as cpm/spleen and expressed as percentages of injected radioactivity.

cells. Again it was found that thymus cells tended to home to the spleen more than did bursa cells. Spleen weights were generally less than 1 gram immediately after transfer, and increased to 1 to 1.5 gram during the following two weeks. The radioactivity attributed to injected thymus cells declined precipitously during the first week, with the single chicken killed two weeks after thymus cell transfer showing no detectable radioactivity in its spleen (Fig.7). A similar decline in radioactivity was observed in the trident-lymphoid nodule.

The radioactivity due to injected bursa cells did not decrease nearly as rapidly, with significant levels of radioactivity remaining two weeks after transfer in both spleen and trident nodule (Fig.7). This pattern of persistence of label after injection of ^{3}H-thymidine labeled bursa cells was observed in all of 3 experiments. In view of the difference in the persistance of the label after giving approximately equal amounts of radioactivity of either thymus or bursa cells, it seems unlikely that reincorporation of ^{3}H-thymidine, locally or systemically, is an important factor in the interpretation of these findings. Thus, the results suggest that the labeled bursa cells themselves or their progeny were long-lived cells.

Localization of the ^{3}H-thymidine labeled cells was not as yet studied since preliminary observations showed that the level of radioactivity per cell obtained with the in vivo method of labeling was not sufficient to be detected on autoradiographs with a 3-week exposure time. More intense labeling and longer exposures of autoradiographs will be needed to determine where these apparently long-lived labeled bursa cells localize. The results appear to suggest a lack of long-lived thymus cells. However, this is most likely due to the relatively brief period of in vivo labeling employed. It seems probable that a more intense labeling over a period of several days would carry a significant amount of radioactivity into the DNA of the small thymic lymphocytes, which presumably represent a high proportion of the long-lived recirculating cells in the mammal (10).

GENERAL OBSERVATIONS AND CONCLUSIONS

The results of the present study obtained both with ^{3}H-adenosine and ^{3}H-thymidine labeled transferred cells indicate that thymocytes tend to migrate more into the thymus than into the bursa. Radioactivity of bursa cells was approximately equally distributed over both these organs. The results confirm that some bursa cells enter the thymus, as has also been observed previously by Woods and Linna (12). Although in rodents lymph node cells have been reported to find their way into the thymus in small numbers (13), thymocytes have not been observed to return to the thymus (14). However, since the normal chicken thymus differs from that of the mammal in other ways as well, such as in the presence of numerous plasma cells and germinal centers (15), it might be expected that its barrier to incoming cells is less complete.

Differences in homing capacity to spleen for ^{3}H-uridine in vitro labeled and ^{3}H-thymidine in vivo labeled cells also have been reported by Austin (16). Warner (17), in comparing the fate of ^{3}H-uridine labeled bursa and thymus cells in the chicken, found that 3.5 to 9.6 as much radioactivity of thymus than of bursa cells localized in the spleen 24 hours after injection. In the present study, this ratio was found to be lower for ^{3}H-adenosine labeled cells (2.8), as well as for ^{3}H-thymidine labeled cells (1.3). This difference in homing capacity may be partly due to the enormous fragility of bursa cells in vitro, particularly in the absence of serum or other viscosity enhancing agents (18). Even though in the present study care was taken to avoid damage to bursa cells, the percentage of viable bursa cells after labeling of the cells in vitro was always at least 20% lower than for thymus cells.

Preferential homing of lymphoid cells to germinal centers has not been previously reported. Thymus cells in the mouse are known to avoid germinal centers (9,19), as was also observed in these experiments in the chicken. Spleen cells are reported to enter germinal centers only rarely (9). Lack of homing of bursa cells to germinal centers was seen by Linna (20) after labeling bursa cells in situ with ^{3}H-thymidine and examining the spleen 48 hours later. This may appear in contrast to the present findings. It should be noted, however, that in our results a striking diminution of the label in germinal centers occurred between 24 and 48 hours, suggesting that the bursa cells localizing in germinal centers participate in the proliferative process locally and dilute their DNA and RNA label accordingly.

SUMMARY

The fate of thymus and bursa cells labeled with ^{3}H-adenosine in vitro, was studied by transfer into x-irradiated syngeneic chickens. Both cell types homed to lymphoid tissue, but differed markedly in their localization patterns. At 24 hours after transfer, the majority of labeled bursa cells in the spleen were localized within germinal centers, whereas thymus cells did not appear in such centers.

Preliminary experiments involving transfer of bursa and thymus cells labeled with ^{3}H-thymidine in vivo, suggest that the bursa of Fabricius may give rise to long-lived cells, but the localization of such cells was not yet determined.

ACKNOWLEDGMENTS

This research was supported by Grant AI-3076 from the United States Public Health Service and by Grant T-524C from the American Cancer Society. HGD-Predoctoral Fellow United States Public Health Service Training Grant #1 T01 AI00392; GAT-Postdoctoral Fellow Arthritis Foundation; GJT-Recipient Career Development Award K3-GM15522 United States Public Health Service.

REFERENCES

1. N.L. Warner, A.Szenberg, and F.M. Burnet. Austral. J. Exp. Biol., 40:373, 1962.

2. R.L. Aspinall, R.K. Meyer, M.A. Graetzer and H.R. Wolfe. J. Immunol., 90: 872, 1963.

3. N.L. Warner, J.W. Uhr, G.J. Thorbecke and Z. Ovary, J. Immunol., 103:1317, 1969.

4. W.A. Cain, M.D. Cooper, P.J. Van Alten, and R.A. Good. Immunol., 102:671, 1969.

5. M.D. Cooper, R.D.A. Peterson, M.A. South and R.A. Good. J. Exp. Med. 123: 75, 1966.

6. R.D.A. Peterson, B.R. Burmester, M.D. Cooper and R.A. Good. in: H. Cottier, N.Odartchenko, R.Schindler and C.C. Congdon,

Eds., Germinal Centers in Immune Responses, p.443. New York: Springer-Verlag, 1967.

7. G.J.Thorbecke, N.L. Warner, G.M. Hochwald, and S.H. Ohanian. Immunol., 15:123, 1968.

8. M.A.B. De Sousa and D.M.V. Parrott. in: H. Cottier, N. Odart-chenko, R.Schindler and C.C.Congdon, Eds., Germinal Centers in Immune Responses, p. 361. New York: Springer-Verlag, 1967.

9. D.M.V. Parrott. in: H. Cottier, N.Odartchenko, R.Schindler and C.C. Congdon, Eds., Germinal Centers in Immune Responses, p. 168. New York: Springer-Verlag, 1967.

10. I. Goldschneider and D.D. McGregor. J. Exp. Med.,127:155,1968.

11. L.W.Schierman and A.W. Nordskog. Science (Washington) 134: 1008, 1961.

12. R.Woods and J. Linna. Acta Path. et Microbiol. Scand., 64: 470, 1965.

13. M. Galton and P.B. Reed. Transplantation 4: 168, 1966.

14. R.G. Murray and A.Murray. Anat. Record, 150:95, 1964.

15. G.J. Thorbecke, H.A. Gordon, B. Wostmann, M. Wagner and J.A. Reyniers. J. Infect. Diseases, 101:237, 1957.

16. C.M. Austin. Austral. J. Exp. Biol. and Med.Sci., 46:581, 1968.

17. N.L. Warner. Aust. J. Exp. Biol and Med. Sci. 43:440, 1965.

18. W.P. McArthur and G.J. Thorbecke. Unpublished observations.

19. D.V.M. Parrott. J. Exp. Med., 123: 191, 1966.

20. T.J. Linna, T. Brenning and E. Hemmingsson. in: L. Fiore-Donati and M.G. Hanna, Jr., Eds., Lymphatic Tissue and Germinal Centers in Immune Responses, p. 133. New York: Plenum Press, 1969.

IMMUNE COMPETENCE OF CELLS DERIVED FROM HEMOPOIETIC LIVER AFTER TRAFFIC TO THYMUS [1]

Osias Stutman and Robert A. Good

Departments of Laboratory Medicine, Pathology and
Pediatrics, University of Minnesota Medical School,
Minneapolis, Minnesota, U. S. A.

We have shown in a previous communication that hemopoietic
liver cells from 17-19 day old mouse embryos are capable of migration to thymus and bone marrow (1). Since a similar traffic
pattern has been demonstrated for bone marrow cells (2) it seemed
of interest to study the behavior of the embryonic cells in more
detail, since the liver is a major source of hemopoietic elements
during early embryonation and first days after birth in the mouse
(3). Interest in these studies resided in the possibility that
traffic to and from the thymus represented a true maturation
process, leading to the production of immunocompetent cells.

The experimental models were: I) 45-day old neonatally
thymectomized CBA/H mice grafted intraperitoneally (IP) or subcutaneously (SC) with a thymus graft from newborn CBA/HT6 donors
and injected IP with embryonic or newborn liver or adult bone
marrow cells from CBA/HT6T6 donors (cell dosage usually 5 x 10^7).
Twenty to 90 days after treatment, chromosome preparations were
made of the thymus grafts and other lympho-hemopoietic tissues of
the hosts. Cells in division from any of the three origins (host,
thymus graft and injected cells) could be recognized due to particular chromosome markers (for details on these syngeneic sublines,
see 2). II) 45-day old neonatally thymectomized CBA/H secondary
hosts grafted SC or IP with a thymus graft from the experimental
model I. This graft, 15 to 20 days after cell injection, contains
CBA/HT6T6 migrating cells in transit (1). Twenty to 90 days after

[1] Research supported by USPHS grants CA-10445, AI.00798, AI.08677 and
National Foundation, March of Dimes. O.S. is a research associate
of the American Cancer Society.

regrafting of the thymus, chromosome preparations were made of lymph nodes and other lympho-hemopoietic tissues of the secondary hosts. In this model the only source of CBA/HT6T6 cells was the graft itself. III) Similar to II but lymph nodes of the secondary hosts were tested for response to phytohemagglutinin (PHA) or allogeneic cells in vitro. After 48-72 hours in culture for PHA and after 6 days in culture with C57BL cells for the mixed leukocyte cultures, mitotic arrest was induced and the karyotype of the responding cells determined. Model I is capable of showing the traffic pattern to thymus of the hemopoietic cells and the thymus-dependency of the migration of these cells to lymph nodes; model II shows that after traffic to thymus the hemopoietic cells are capable of migration to lymph nodes and model III shows that cells derived from the injected hemopoietic cells, after thymus traffic, are capable of immune responses in the lymph nodes.

Table 1 shows experiments using model I. It can be seen that in the thymectomized host, liver cells (from 17-19 day old embryos or newborn donors) were detected only in bone marrow (approximately 1% of the metaphases scored) but not in lymph nodes. On the other hand, 20 days after treatment in the presence of a thymus graft, liver type cells could be detected in the lymph nodes (approximately 10% of the metaphases scored). The proportion of liver type metaphases in lymph nodes increased with time (17 to 20%, 60 days after treatment) only in the animals that had received a thymus graft.

Table 1

Chromosome Analysis of Lymphoid Tissues from Neonatally
Thymectomized CBA/H Mice (45-day old), 20 Days After
CBA/HT6T6 Liver Cells with or without a CBA/HT6 Thymus Graft

Experimental group[*]	Liver cells	"Liver-Type" metaphases per total		
		NODES	SPLEEN	MARROW
Thymec.	newb.	1/249	0/229	3/310
Thymec.	emb.	0/221	0/456	3/301
Thymec. + Thymus	newb.	14/194 (7%)	3/490	3/298
Thymec. + Thymus	emb.	19/201 (10%)	3/429	3/306

[*] All animals received 5 x 10^7 liver cells from 17-19 day old embryos or newborn CBA/HT6T6 donors, IP. Thymus graft from newborn CBA/HT6 donors implanted IP.

The percentage of liver type metaphases in the thymus graft itself 20 days after treatment was 14% and 13% for embryonic and newborn liver cells (from a total of 466 and 550 metaphases scored respectively). Table 2 shows a similar type of experiment but indicating that a viable thymus graft and not a thymus within a cell-impenetrable chamber is required for the establishment of the "liver-type" population in the lymph nodes of the thymectomized hosts. In summary, these experiments indicate that hemopoietic liver cells of embryonic or newborn origin are capable of traffic to thymus and bone marrow and that they require a viable thymus graft to establish a population of cells capable of migration to lymph nodes.

Table 3 shows experiments with model II. It can be seen that approximately 3% of the dividing cells in the lymph nodes of the secondary hosts, 60 days after thymus grafting, are derived from hemopoietic cells in transit within the thymus graft itself (the source of the hemopoietic cells in the primary host was 17-19 day old embryonic or newborn liver or adult, 60-day old bone marrow).

Table 4 indicates the results obtained with model III and shows that 27% of the cells responding to PHA in the lymph nodes of the secondary hosts, indeed, were derived from the hemopoietic precursors present in the thymus graft. Eleven percent of the cells responding to allogeneic cells in the lymph nodes were also derived from the hemopoietic cells in transit within the thymus graft.

Table 2

Chromosome Analysis of Lymphoid Tissues from Neonatally Thymectomized CBA/H Mice (45-day old), 20 Days After CBA/HT6T6 Liver Cells with or without a CBA/HT6 Thymus

Experimental group	"Liver-Type" metaphases per total	
	NODES	MARROW
Thymec.	0/380	3/301 (1%)
Thymec. + Thymus graft*	29/270 (10%)	3/255 (1%)
Thymec. + Thymus in DC*	1/432	4/312 (1%)

* Thymus graft implanted intraperitoneally. Diffusion chambers (0.1 μ pore size) implanted intraperitoneally. All animals received 5 x 10^7 liver cells from 17-19 day old CBA/HT6T6 embryos.

Table 3
Chromosome Analysis of Tissues from Neonatally Thymectomized
CBA/H Secondary Hosts Grafted with CBA/HT6 Retransplanted
Thymus "Containing" CBA/HT6T6 Cells

Type of CBA/HT6T6 cells in primary host	"Liver" or "Marrow" type metaphases in tissues of secondary hosts		
	NODES	SPLEEN	MARROW
Embryonic liver	54/1180 (4%)	2/1116	1/1441
Newborn liver	20/640 (3%)	1/446	1/801
Adult bone marrow	36/1160 (3%)	1/879	1/1109
Nothing	0/690 16/* (2%)	0/512 2/*	0/619 0/*

* Thymus type metaphases. Tests performed 60 days after
   IP grafting of the thymus.

Table 4
Chromosome Analysis of PHA or Mixed Leukocyte Culture
Response of Lymph Nodes Derived from Neonatally Thymectomized CBA/H Secondary Hosts Grafted with Thymus Containing CBA/HT6T6 Liver Cells. (60 days after grafting)

Experiment	Number of CBA/HT6T6 (Liver-type) cells per total metaphases
PHA*	664/2467 (27%)
Mixed leukocyte culture (unidirectional)**	90/899 (11%)

*   Response stopped after 48 hours in culture.
** Response against mytomycin-treated C57BL cells,
    6 days after culture.

These results indicate: 1) that hemopoietic cells from embryonic and newborn liver contain precursors capable of undergoing a traffic to thymus; 2) after thymus traffic these precursors acquire the capacity to migrate to lymph nodes; 3) the progeny of the precursors contained in hemopoietic liver that are detected in lymph nodes after thymus traffic are capable of response to PHA and allogeneic cells in vitro; 4) the presence of viable thymic stroma is essential for the development of this population of cells.

From these studies we can infer that direct evidence is now available to establish the existence of a hemopoietic stem cell in the embryonic liver which after complex traffic patterns to thymus and lymph nodes establishes a population of cells capable of immunological response. We have shown that a similar stem cell is present in hemopoietic yolk sac cells from 10-13 day old embryos and is also circulating and detectable in embryonic blood (4). This type of cell that requires thymic traffic for the development of immunological functions was shown to be insensitive to the humoral activity of the thymus and has been termed prethymic (5).

References

1. O. Stutman and R. A. Good. Exptl. Hematol. 19: 12, 1969.
2. C. E. Ford, in: Ciba Foundation Symp. The Thymus, G. E. Wolstenholme and R. Porter, Eds., p. 131. Little, Brown and Co., 1966.
3. R. B. Taylor. Brit. J. Exptl. Path. 46: 376, 1965.
4. O. Stutman and R. A. Good. Transplant. Proc. In press.
5. O. Stutman, E. J. Yunis and R. A. Good. J. Exptl. Med. 132: 601, 1970.

THE FATE OF LYMPH-BORNE IMMUNOBLASTS

Marilyn E. Smith and J. G. Hall

Chester Beatty Research Institute: Institute of

Cancer Research, Belmont, Sutton, Surrey, England

The efferent lymph from a single lymph node of a sheep consists of 98% small lymphocytes, the occasional eosinophil and a background resting level of 2% of immunoblasts. About three days after antigenic stimulation of the lymph node, by injecting, for instance a bacterial suspension subcutaneously into the drainage area of the node, the output of lymphocytes has doubled and immunoblasts constitute up to 40% of that output (1). Similar basophilic blast cells form up to 15% of the cells in the thoracic duct lymph of rats about three days after antigen has been injected subcutaneously to the drainage area of superficial nodes which contribute their efferent lymph to the thoracic duct (2).

Immunoblasts are one and one-half to three times the size of small lymphocytes and have a basophilic and pyroninophilic cytoplasm. The cytoplasm is packed with polyribosomes but no organized endoplasmic reticulum. Despite this lack of endoplasmic reticulum, they are producing specific antibody (1,3,4,5), and are specifically cytotoxic to their target cells in vitro (6). A characteristic, seen when live cells are viewed by phase-contrast microscopy, is the extremely energetic and motile behavior of these large, mitotically active cells (2,5).

Immunoblasts have been shown to turn into plasma cells (7) and to be important in the propogation and amplification of a systemic immune response (5). However, the fate of these cells, once they have entered the blood via the main lymphatic trunks, is still in question. Gowans and Knight in 1964 (8) noted that 'large lymphocytes' from rat thoracic duct lymph, unlike small lymphocytes, did not recirculate into efferent lymph but settled in the lamina propria of the small intestine. Because immunoblasts are released in large numbers before antibodies appear in the blood serum, it has been suggested that their most important function is to extravasate into the tissues, and so provide, by local synthesis, the antibody that the blood is unable to supply (9).

The fate of immunoblasts was investigated in two ways: A) Immunoblasts in the efferent lymph from a single lymph node of a sheep were labelled *in vitro* with radioactive DNA precursors, and injected intravenously into the same sheep. The specific radioactivity of blood and lymph lymphocytes was followed during the next 24 hours both by scintillation counting and autoradiography. B) Immunoblasts in the thoracic duct lymph of inbred, immunized donor rats were labelled *in vitro* with radioactive DNA precursors and injected intravenously to syngeneic recipients. The recipients were killed at various times after injection and the quantitative distribution of labelled cells in various organs determined by scintillation counting. The fate of the labelled cells was also followed by autoradiographic studies.

Distribution of Labelled Immunoblasts between Blood and Lymph of a Sheep

A twelve-hour collection of efferent lymph from a single stimulated node of a sheep was incubated in TC199 with 1 µc/ml of ^{3}H thymidine or its analogue I^{125}deoxyuridine for one hour at 38°C. The cells were washed twice and injected intravenously to the autochthonous animal by direct injection into the jugular vein or through an indwelling catheter. An injection sample was saved so that the total activity injected and its theoretical dilution, assuming that no labelled cells left the blood, could be calculated. The first blood sample was withdrawn from the jugular vein four minutes after the injection and further blood and lymph samples were obtained at intervals during the next 24 hours. White blood cell samples were prepared from the blood by the method of Dain and Hall, 1967 (10). I^{125} was counted in a Packard Auto-gamma Spectrometer.

The first blood sample consistently had a specific activity lower than 4% of the theoretical dilution; thereafter the specific activity fluctuated, never reaching a steady state, and had practically disappeared by 24 hours. Negligible activity appeared in efferent lymph. The results of scintillation counting were confirmed by autoradiography of blood and lymph smears from an animal which had received immunoblasts labelled with ^{3}H thymidine. The short circulatory half-life of immunoblasts must be compared with the results of similar experiments where small lymphocytes from the efferent lymph of unstimulated nodes were labelled with Cr^{51} or ^{3}H cytidine and injected intravenously. The initial specific radioactivity of blood lymphocytes was about 15% of the theoretical value and activity appeared in efferent lymph by three hours after the injection. By twelve hours, the labelled small lymphocytes had 'equilibrated' between blood and lymph; the activity decayed away slowly from a plateau of 6% of the theoretical dilution.

Distribution of Thoracic Duct Immunoblasts Labelled *in vitro*, in the Tissues of Syngeneic Rats after Intravenous Injection

Pure-line SPF hooded male rats weighing about 220g were used. Donor rats were immunized by subcutaneous injections of an antigen into the hind foot pads, blutei, inner surface of the thighs and flanks. The antigens used were Brucella Abortus, BCG, sheep red cells or irradiated syngeneic sarcomata. Three days later the thoracic ducts of four to six donor animals were cannulated and the lymph collected. The number of lymphocytes and the percentage of immunoblasts in a pooled lymph collection of not more than twelve hours' duration, were determined and the cells incubated at $38°C$ for one hour with 1 µc/ml of ^3H thymidine or I^{125}deoxyuridine. The cells were washed twice and injected intravenously to syngeneic recipients. An aliquot of the injection was saved for autoradiographic or radio-assay. Usually 2 x 10^8 lymphoid cells were injected of which 15-20% would be labelled immunoblasts. At various times after the injection the recipients were exsanguinated, illed, and the viscera fixed in 10% formal saline.

The quantitative distribution of the injected cells among the tissues was determined by scintillation counting of organs from rats which had received immunoblasts labelled with I^{125}deoxyuridine in a Packard Auto-gamma Spectrometer. This thymidine analogue is not 're-utilized' and the isotope is easily and accurately counted (11). The results were expressed as the percentage of total activity injected and as the specific radioactivity as counts/min/g wet weight.

Table I. The distribution of radioactivity in various organs 24 hr after the intravenous injection of 3.5 x 10^7 syngeneic immunoblasts labelled with I^{125}deoxyuridine.

Tissue	Percentage of total activity injected	Specific radio-activity (c/m/g)
Lung	0.4	247
Liver	1.1	82
Spleen	2.1	3835
Small gut	34.1	6350
Large gut	3.7	1745
Peyer's patches	4.4	10600
Mesenteric lymph nodes	0.7	2540
Peripheral lymph nodes	0.6	1860
Thymus	0.08	284

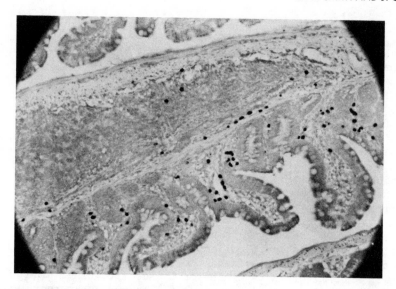

Photomicrograph of an autoradiograph of a 4 μm section cut from the
small gut of a rat 20 hr after the intravenous injection of syngeneic
immunoblasts that have been labelled *in vitro* with ^{3}H thymidine.

The distribution of labelled cells was the same whatever the
antigen that had been used to stimulate the donor animals. Immediately after the injection, many labelled cells were retained in the
lung, liver and spleen but thereafter the radioactivity in these
organs declined as activity appeared in the small intestine. The
distribution pattern found at 24 hr was well-established at 5 hr.

The microanatomical location of the injected cells was determined by autoradiography of sections of tissues from rats which had
received immunoblasts labelled with ^{3}H thymidine. In all rats killed
at 5 hr or more after injection, the small gut always contained most
of the recoverable radioactivity, sometimes as much as 40% of the
injected dose. This was confirmed by autoradiography. Sections of
the small gut showed a massive infiltration of the lamina propria
by labelled cells which were extravascular and present both at the
bottom of the crypts and well up into the villi. Very few labelled
cells gained entry to the Peyer's patches; the high specific activity
of Peyer's patches, cut from the full thickness of the gut, from
scintillation counting was because of a higher concentration of
labelled cells in the shorter villi overlying an aggregation of
lymphoid tissue. The total number of labelled cells in all other
organs, including the organized lymphoid tissue, spleen, lymph nodes

and thymus, never exceeded 20% of that in the small gut. However, every organ examined contained some activity and labelled cells were seen in the mucosa of the trachea, the parenchyma of the lung, in the kidney and in the salivary glands (11).

Electron microscope studies of the labelled cells in the gut have shown that the injected cells develop an endoplasmic reticulum, not present in the immunoblasts injected, within 24 hr of settling in the extravascular spaces in the lamina propria of the small intestine (12). Most immunoblasts, generated to varied antigenic stimuli in lymphoid tissue remote from the gut, are destined to enter the lamina propria of the small intestine. Many of these cells are probably plasmablasts and may be particularly concerned with providing the immunoglobulins, especially IgA (13), which protect the mucous surfaces and are contained in the external secretions. Although most of the transferred cells are entering the gut, the adoptive transfer of humoral antibody production can be determined (12). This antibody production is presumably by the cells that settle in the recognized lymphoid tissue. An assessment of the cellular economy of an immune response must include the antibody production in the mucosa and external secretions as well as the humoral antibody production by plasma cells in the recognized lymphoid tissue.

REFERENCES

1. J. G. Hall and B. Morris, Quart. J. Exp. Physiol., 48:235, 1963.

2. E. J. Delorme, J. Hodgett, J. G. Hall, and P. Alexander, Proc. Roy. Soc., B, 174:229, 1969.

3. A. J. Cunningham, J. B. Smith, and E. H. Mercer, J. Exp. Med., 124:701, 1966.

4. J. G. Hall, Ann. Rev. Scientific Basis of Medicine, in press.

5. J. G. Hall, B. Morris, G. D. Moreno, and M. C. Bessis, J. Exp. Med., 125:91, 1967.

6. S. Denham, J. G. Hall, A. Wolf, and P. Alexander, Transplantation, 7:194, 1969.

7. M. S. C. Birbeck and J. G. Hall, Nature, 214:183, 1967.

8. J. L. Gowans and E. J. Knight, Proc. Roy. Soc., B, 159:257, 1964.

9. J. G. Hall, Lancet, i 125, 1969.

10. A. R. Dain and J. G. Hall, Vox. Sang., 13:281, 1967.

11. J. G. Hall and M. E. Smith, Nature, 226:262, 1970.

12. M. E. Smith, to be published.

13. D. R. Tourville, R. H. Adler, J. Bienenstock, and T. B. Tomasi,
     J. Exp. Med., 129:411, 1969.

MASSIVE MIGRATION OF THYMIC LYMPHOCYTES TO PEYER'S PATCHES IN NEONATAL MICE

D.D. Joel, M.W. Hess and H. Cottier
Department of Pathology, University of Bern,
Switzerland, and
Medical Research Center, Brookhaven National
Laboratory, Upton, L.I., N.Y. 11973, U.S.A.

Although migration of cells from the thymus to intestinal lymphoid tissues has been demonstrated in young
animals (1-3), the magnitude of this process remains to
be clarified, particularly during the early development
of these tissues. Neonatal mice are useful experimental
animals in which to study this problem. The Peyer's
patches of newborn mice are poorly developed at birth
and contain only a small number of lymphoid cells (4),
however, within 2 or 3 days after birth, the number of
lymphoid cells increases markedly. Kinetic studies suggest that during this same developmental period there
is an extensive emigration of thymic lymphoid cells (5-
7). Systemic labeling data in newborn mice have provided
evidence for a substantial immigration of lymphocytes
into Peyer's patches (8). These observations focus on
the question of whether the gut associated lymphoid
tissue in mice is a "primary" lymphoid organ as was proposed for the bursa of Fabricius in birds (9,10,11) or
a "secondary" organ whose immunological development is,
at least in part, thymus-dependent. This report provides
direct evidence for the thymic origin of the majority
of lymphocytes in the developing Peyer's patches of newborn mice.

MATERIALS AND METHODS

One-day old Charles River mice (mean body weight =

2,0 g, mean thymus weight = 6,2 mg) were anesthetized
with ether until respiration had momentarily ceased.
With the aid of a stereomicroscope the thymus was exposed
and ^{3}H-thymidine (specific activity 1.9 Ci/mmole; concentration 20 µCi/ml) was injected subcapsularly with a
glass microcapillary (1 µl/thymus). This dose of thymidine is below that known to cause radiotoxicity. Groups
of 5 mice each were sacrificed at 1 h, 2 h, 1, 2, and
3 days after injection. Animals in which there was leakage of thymidine or visible thymic damage and those
which did not exhibit normal weight gains were excluded
from the experiment. Thymus, spleen, Peyer's patches and
mesenteric lymph nodes were fixed in Bouin's solution,
embedded in paraffin, sectioned at 5 µ and dipped in
NTB-2 emulsion (Kodak, Rochester, N.Y.). The slides were
exposed for 57 days at 4°C, developed and stained with
nuclear fast red. To correct for systemic labeling which
might have resulted from the passage of ^{3}H-thymidine into the blood during injection, background was established
by counting grains over proliferating erythroblasts and
intestinal crypt cells. An average of 1 per 500 of these
cells had 3 grains over the nucleus with the vast majority of cells showing no label. Based on these counts,
cells with 3 or more grains over the nucleus were considered to have been labeled in the thymic area. Autoradiographic studies with ^{3}H-thymidine in newborn mice
suggest that thymic lymphoid cells migrate from the outer cortical zone to the cortico-medullary junction at
which time emigration commences (8). Therefore, the
thymic labeling index was determinated by counting cortical lymphocytes near the cortico-medullary junction
from 3 different areas of the thymus.

RESULTS

Labeling indices of thymic cortical lymphocytes and
Peyer's patch lymphocytes are shown in Fig. 1. The labeling index of thymic cortical lymphocytes at the cortico-medullary junction increased steadily reaching a
peak of 17% on day 2. This is consistent with migration
of cells from the outer cortex, which initially had a
higher labeling index and intensity, to the inner cortex.
No labeled cells were observed in Peyer's patches 1 or
2 hours after intrathymic injection, however, by day 1
the labeling index of Peyer's patch lymphocytes was

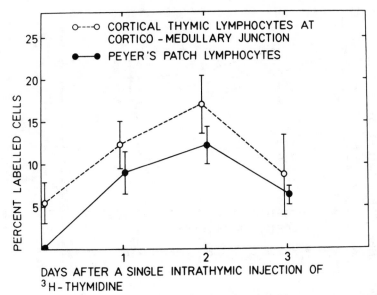

Fig. 1. Labeling indices of thymic cortical lymphocytes and Peyer's patch lymphocytes as a function of
time following a single intrathymic injection of tritiated thymidine. Lymphoid cells with 3 or more grains
over the nucleus were considered labeled. Points represent the mean and standard deviation obtained from 5
mice.

approximately 75% of the labeling index of thymic cortical cells. A further increase in labeling index, paralle-
ling that of the thymic cortex, was seen between days 1
and 2. The labeling index then decreased in both organs
but to a somewhat greater degree in the thymus so that
on day 3 the labeling index in 2 of 5 mice was greater
in Peyer's patch lymphocytes, than in thymic cortical
lymphocytes. The labeling pattern in mesenteric lymph-
nodes was similar to that in Peyer's patches.

Fig. 2 illustrates the mean grain counts of labeled
thymic cortical and Peyer's patch lymphocytes. The mean
grain count of thymic lymphocytes decreased progressive-

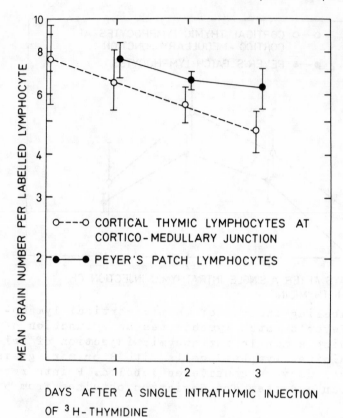

Fig. 2. Mean grain count of labeled thymic cortical
lymphocytes and Peyer's patch lymphocytes as a function
of time after a single intrathymic injection of tritiated thymidine. Cells with 3 or more grains were considered labeled. Points represent the mean and standard deviation obtained from 5 mice.

ly, however, the mean grain count of Peyer's patch lymphocytes deviated from a single negative exponential function and on day 3 was significantly higher than that of
thymic cortical cells. Heavily labeled cells (>15 grains)
constituted 6 to 7 per cent of the labeled lymphocytes
in Peyer's patches on day 3, but less than 1 per cent in
the thymus.

DISCUSSION

Although migration of thymus cells to Peyer's patches has been repeatedly demonstrated by the technique
of local labeling of the thymus, the magnitude of this
migration has generally been reported to be quite low
(1-3). It should be emphasized, however, that these experiments have usually been performed at a time when the
gut-associated lymphoid tissues are well developed and
contain a large number of pre-existant lymphocytes, and
that only heavily labeled cells have been considered as
thymus-derived. The latter point may be quite significant
since the vast majority of thymic cortical cells at the
cortico-medullary junction (the proposed site of migration) have a relatively low labeling intensity mainly
due to dilution of label by cell division in the outer
cortex.

In the present study neonatal mice were used because of the rapid development of gut-associated lymphoid
tissues which takes place during the first few days after
birth. In addition, all cells were considered labeled
which had more grains than the number possibly attributable to initial systemic labeling. The labeling index of
lymphoid cells present in Peyer's patches 1 and 2 days
following the intrathymic injection of ^{3}H-thymidine was
between 60 and 75 per cent of the labeling index of
thymic cortical lymphocytes. Assuming that non-labeled
cells migrate in the same manner as labeled cells, it
can be concluded from these data that the majority of
lymphocytes in the Peyer's patches of newborn mice had
their origin in the thymus. This magnitude of migration
is much greater than has been previously reported with the
technique of local thymus labeling, but is in agreement
with the degree of migration suggested by systemic labeling studies in newborn mice (8). The origin of Peyer's
patch lymphocytes at the time of intrathymic injection
is not known. There is suggestive evidence, however,
that thymic migration begins prior to this time (5-7).

These findings are thus not in support of the concept that gut-associated lymphoid tissue is a "primary"
lymphoid organ, as was proposed for the bursa of Fabricius (12). Furthermore, the magnitude of thymic cell
migration was essentially the same to both the mesenteric lymph node, a recognized "secondary" lymphoid organ,

and the Peyer's patches.

The possibility that some lymphocytes in Peyer's patches became labeled through reutilization of labeled nucleoside from degenerating migrants cannot be ruled but seems unlikely to be of appreciable importance for the following reasons: (a) Other proliferating cell populations in the Peyer's patches, such as reticulum cells, histiocytic cells and epithelial crypt cells did not become labeled throughout the course of the experiment; (b) evidence of cellular degeneration, i.e. pyknotic nuclei, within the intestinal lymphoid tissue was rarely seen.

At all time intervals the mean grain count of labeled lymphoid cells in Peyer's patches was higher than that of thymic cortical cells. This may have been due, in part, to cells which after migration did not enter immediately into a proliferative phase. The high proportion of heavily labeled cells ($>$15 grains) found in Peyer's patches on day 3, at a time when these cells were rarely seen in the thymus, would support this view. Higher mean grain counts in Peyer's patches could also have resulted from cellular emigration from the thymus medulla which initially had a labeling intensity higher than the inner cortex. The actual proportion of migrants which originated in the medulla cannot be determined, however, the labeling pattern of lymphoid cells in Peyer's patches more closely resembled that in the thymic cortex.

This work was supported by the Swiss National Foundation for Scientific Research and the US Atomic Energy Commission.

REFERENCES

1.   G.J.V. Nossal, Ann. N.Y. Acad. Sci., 120:171, 1964.

2.   T.J. Linna, Blood, 31:727, 1968.

3.   R.J. Iorio, A.D. Chanana, E.P. Cronkite and D.D. Joel,Cell Tissue Kinet., 3:161, 1970.

4.   J.J. Miller, Lab. Invest., 21:484, 1969.

5. H. Cottier, Méd. Hyg., 23:794, 1965.

6. M.W. Hess, R.D. Stoner and H. Cottier, Nature, 215: 426, 1967.

7. W.D. Michalke, M.W. Hess, H. Riedwyl, R.D. Stoner and H. Cottier, Blood, 33:541, 1969.

8. J. Köbberling, Z. Zellforsch., 68:631, 1965.

9. N.L. Warner, A. Szenberg and F.M. Burnet, J. exp. Biol. med. Sci., 40:373, 1962.

10. O.K. Archer, B.W. Papermaster and R.A. Good, in: R.A. Good and A.E. Gabrielsen, Eds., The Thymus in Immunobiology, p. 414. New York: Hoeber-Harper, 1964.

11. K.E. Fichtelius, Exp. Cell Res., 46:231, 1967.

12. M.D. Cooper, D.Y. Perey, A.E. Gabrielsen, D.E.R. Sutherland, M.F. McKneally and R.A. Good, Int. Arch. Allergy, 33:65, 1968.

CHAIRMAN'S INTRODUCTION TO THE DISCUSSION

LYMPHOID CELL MIGRATION

T. Juhani Linna, Rune Bäck and Erik Hemmingsson

Department of Histology, Institute of Human Anatomy

University of Uppsala, Uppsala, Sweden

The current interest in lymphoid cell migration is mainly concentrated in four fields:
1. Stem cell problems, pioneered by Ford and collaborators (1,2) and evaluated by Stutman and Good in this session (3).
2. Central lymphoid organ function; the question of the function of the thymus, of the bursa of Fabricius and of the bone marrow through cell export to peripheral lymphoid organs, and the mapping of the traffic patterns and functions of these cells. These questions have been in the focus in the presentation by Bryant (4), by Chanana et al. (5), by Durkin et al. (6) and by Stutman and Good (3).
3. The sequence of events on the cellular level in the immune reaction, from antigenic stimulation to antibody formation or the cellular immune response. The paper by Hall and Smith (7) has dealt with this issue.
4. Recirculation of lymphoid cells. This has not been the main subject of any of the sessions's speakers, although it has been briefly discussed in many of the papers.

These four fields are obviously closely related. Lymphoid cell recirculation has been recently extensively reviewed (8,9) and will not be taken up at length in this presentation.

There are some facts which are very basic but may still be useful to bring up for the discussion: When we sample a lymphoid organ in any experiment, we get the mixed population of cells which happen to be in that organ at that moment; the natives, the immigrants and the visitors. Cell traffic studies show that there is an immigration of cells not only to the so called peripheral lymphoid organs, but from other lymphoid organs to the thymus as well (10,11,12,13,14). There are also thymus-derived cells in the bone marrow (15,16).

The demonstrations of interaction between two or more cells of different origin in the immune reaction, at least in the sheep erythrocyte response in the mouse (17,18,19) and in the model just presented by Miller (20), need to be complemented by cell traffic studies showing that the thymus-derived cell and the bone marrow-derived cell actually meet each other in a situation which does not involve cell transfer and, ultimately, that these cells cooperate. In other words, it is necessary to show not only that the cells are able to perform certain functions but also that these cells have the chance to meet and cooperate in the normal situation. We know that the white pulp of the spleen contains thymus-derived and bone marrow-derived cells (21,22), and could thus be one of their meeting places.

When we sample a cell population, label the cells in one way or another and transfer them to another animal, the cells are bound to "home" somewhere, and the homing of these injected cells does not necessarily reflect the normal homing pattern. Such studies can provide us with useful information, but this limitation has made it necessary to work out other techniques in cell migration studies.

The perfect experiment would be to be able to label a stem cell for the lymphoid cell line and to follow that cell and its progeny through all the phases of life of the cells, map their participation in immunological and other events, and to be able to do it in the intact animal which has formed the stem cell and its progeny. Our laboratory approximations of this perfect experiment have brought us different techniques, all with their advantages and limitations. These have been discussed somewhat in this session and extensively in the literature.

Chromosome markers, such as the sex chromosomes in the chicken and the mouse T6 chromosome have provided much information on cell traffic, starting on the stem cell level. The chromosome markers have the advantage and the limitation that the traffic of a few cells can be detected if the immigrant cells with the marker proliferate rapidly. The marker is present in all the progeny and can be detected in metaphase preparations, and only in metaphase preparations. This means that the traffic of resting cell populations can not be detected with this technique. It is obvious that this technique does not give quantitative information.

Stutman and Good (3) have given us a very interesting sequence of events of cell colonization, from the hemopoietic stem cell source to the thymus and thereafter to the peripheral lymphoid organs. They have also shown that these cells which are present in the periphery and are carrying the stem cell source derived T6 marker are also functioning as we expect a thymus-derived cell population to function, but only if the cells have had the chance to pass the thymus. These cells are susceptible to antiserum against the θ antigen, indicating that they have acquired normal surface characteristics of thymic and post-thymic cells.

The current view of cell traffic from the bone marrow to the thymus is founded mainly on studies using the T6 chromosome marker. It is of interest that we (22) have not been able to trace bone marrow cells to the thymus with the local labelling technique. This can mean 1) that very few cells actually migrate from the bone marrow to the thymus in normal animals and/or 2) that these prethymic cells are not in DNA synthesis while in the bone marrow and are therefore not labelled at the local labelling injection with the DNA-precursor. Few immigrating bone marrow-derived cells could then acquire a high mitotic activity in the thymus and many T6-labelled cells in metaphase preparations of thymus and peripheral lymphoid organs would be found. The confirmation of the finding of bone marrow cell traffic to the thymus and the quantitation of this traffic with an independent technique in a normal animal seems important.

Other techniques than the T6-marker have been useful in studies of thymic cell emigration. One way to study this question is to count the number of lymphoid cells entering and leaving the thymus. We know from the work of Ernström et al. (23,24) that a great number of lymphocytes are leaving the thymus through the blood, and we know also that many cells are leaving through the lymphatics (25). This significant emigration is emphasized by Dr Chanana et al. (5). The actual figures on thymus cell emigration with these techniques are very high. The best way to combine these figures and figures on normal lymphocyte levels in blood, lymph and tissues is given to us by Bryant (4) and by Chanana et al. (5): the great majority of these emigrating cells may be very shortlived.

It is possible to label many lymphoid cells in certain lymphoid organs by local application of radioactively labelled DNA precursors and to follow these cells in the same animal which has formed them. We know from these studies that thymic lymphocytes do emigrate to other lymphoid organs (26,27,28), and that they do so in quantitatively significant amounts (15,29). It has also been established that the thymus contributes heavily to the lymphocyte population of developing "peripheral" lymphoid organs (30,31,32,33), maybe as the main original lymphocyte source of these organs (33), while the thymic contribution can also be detected in adult animals but is not quantitatively significant (30,31). Participation of thymus-derived cells in immune reactions will be taken up below. This labelling technique in its different forms gives the possibility to study traffic patterns of those cells which have been in DNA synthesis at the time of the application of the isotope. Thus, all figures on cell emigration obtained with this technique and autoradiography are minimum figures; emigrating non-labelled and weakly labelled cells escape detection, as do part of the heavily labelled emigrants which proliferate rapidly.

Bryant (4) has demonstrated that it is possible to label thymic cortical lymphocytes selectively, and his method also gives us the unusual possibility to study the same animal at different times after labelling. Bryant's difficulty to find thymus-derived lymphocytes in the peripheral lymphoid organs may, at least partly, be explained by the fact that the lymphatic system of month-old guinea pigs is already functionally faily mature, (34,35) and thus more comparable to adult animals of other species.

Chanana et al. (5) have shown in the calf, as it has been shown in the quinea pig (21), that the thymus-derived cells home not only to the paracortical areas, but also to other areas in the lymph nodes and that they can also home in other areas than the so called thymus dependent ones in the spleen. Thus, it is not possible to define a strictly thymus-dependent area in peripheral lymphatic organs in terms of cell migration.

Chanana et al. (5) have also used an antigenic marker, the thymus specific antigen (TSA), for the detection of thymus-derived lymphocytes. Raff (36) and others (37) have presented data on the TL antigen and the Θ antigen in the mouse. These antigenic markers, especially the Θ antigen, seem to provide us with a good tool for the detection and the quantitation of thymus-derived cells in the periphery. However, it seems possible that an emigrating cell may change surface characteristics, including the loss of the Θ antigen, which would mean that even with this method we are studying minimum figures. Thus, we are still looking for the perfect marker system for the study of cell traffic from the thymus and from other organs.

The chicken is a unique experimental animal because of the functional delineation of the immune system in a bursa-dependent part responsible for humoral immunity and a thymus-dependent part mainly concerned with cellular immune reactions. (38,39). Since germinal centers are absent in chickens lacking humoral immunity (39,40), these structures have been regarded as bursa-dependent, maybe bursa-derived. Dr. Durkin et al. have demonstrated that in vitro ³H-adenosine labelled bursa cells have the capacity to home a.o. to the germinal centers, when given to an irradiated immunized recipient.

We (41) have done an ontogenetic study on thymus and bursa cell emigration in the chicken. We have obtained good local labelling of the bursal or of the thymic cells by local injections of small amounts of ³H-thymidine directly into the parenchyma of the organ. There is inevitable leakage of isotope at every labelling injection. The way we have chosen to deal with leakage has been to accept it and control for it, using control animals labelled intravenously with ³H-thymidine. The animals have been killed and different organs sampled 48 hours after isotope administration. We have used two different methods to obtain the results, a radiochemical method and autoradiography. In the radiochemical studies, nucleic acids were extracted from the organs (42) and DNA (43) and tritium (44,15) measured. The specific activity (spec. act.) of each organ was calculated. Since intestinal epithelium is dividing very rapidly, it is labelled almost exclusively by leaking ^{3}H-thymidine at the local labelling injection. Therefore, we have calculated the ratio between the spec. act. of an organ and the spec. act. of duodenum of the same animal in the locally and intravenously labelled animals. We call this ratio relative activity (rel. act.). Significant cell migration from the locally labelled organ to another organ is reflected by a significantly higher rel. act. for that organ in the locally labelled animals than in their intravenously labelled controls. This radiochemical method gives quantitative information about the magnitude of transport of labelled cells from the locally labelled organ (Table 1 and 2). With autoradiography we have looked for the localization of heavily labelled cells, i.e. cells with a higher grain count than what can be maximally found in the intravenously labelled animals.

We have studied chickens of four different ages: 1) newly hatched; 2) 9-day-old, when we find the first foci of lymphocytes in the peripheral lymphatic organs; 3) 6-week-old, which are fully immunologically competent and have a morphologically well developed bursa of Fabricius; and 4) 14-week-old, with beginning bursal involution. The radiochemical data showed that in the immediate posthatching period there was already quantitatively significant cell traffic from the bursa to other lymphoid organs, including the thymus (Table 1). This was also the case in 9-day-old and 6-week-old chickens. In 14-week-old animals, a good local labelling could still be obtained, but cell traffic could not be demonstrated longer in quantitative terms. Autoradiographic studies on localization of heavily labelled cells in 6-week-old animals showed that 96 % of these bursa-derived cells were found in the thymic medulla, while 4 % were found in the cortex. Thus, these data and earlier studies (10,14) show that bursa cells migrate to the thymus to a quantitatively significant extent, suggesting that the lymphoid organ delineation in the chicken may be more complex than was initially thought. In the spleen, 83 % of the cells were found in or immediately adjacent to the white pulp. We were not able to find any heavily labelled bursa-derived cells in the germinal centers of any peripheral lymphoid organ at any age in the chickens we have studied. This result is in contrast to that reported by Durkin et al. (6), but it must also be pointed out that the study by Durkin et al. is a cell transfer study using immunized recipients and it is therefore difficult to compare our results. We are presently studying cell traffic in immunized animals using the local labelling technique (16). Because of our cell traffic data and other data on the mechanism of germinal center formation (45), we suggest that germinal centers are formed by another mechanism than cell traffic from the bursa or the bursa equivalent.

Table 1. Ontogenic data on bursa cell traffic in the chicken. Means ± S.E. of the means of rel. act.[x] of chickens labelled intrabursally or intravenously with ^{3}H-thymidine. Significant cell migration from the locally labelled bursa to another organ is reflected by a significantly higher rel. act. for that organ in the locally labelled group than in the intravenously labelled controls. Such migration occurred already in the newly hatched period and continued in the older age groups but was not quantitatively significant in the 14-week-old animals.

Age of the animals	Route of injection of ^{3}H-thymidine	Organ				
		Thymus	Spleen	Tonsilla caecalis	Bursa of Fabricius	Bone Marrow
< 24h	Intrabursal (n=13)	0.36 ± 0.03	2.19 ± 0.16	2.27 ± 0.14	29.90 ± 2.60	0.82 ± 0.04
	Intravenous (n=14)	0.25 ± 0.01	1.27 ± 0.08	1.22 ± 0.05	0.32 ± 0.02	0.69 ± 0.05
	Probability (P <)	0.005	0.001	0.001	0.001	——
9d	Intrabursal (n=15)	0.42 ± 0.04	3.50 ± 0.30	3.90 ± 0.40	49.00 ± 8.00	0.88 ± 0.09
	Intravenous (n=16)	0.17 ± 0.01	1.05 ± 0.06	1.36 ± 0.09	0.32 ± 0.02	0.78 ± 0.04
	Probability (P <)	0.001	0.001	0.001	0.001	——
6w	Intrabursal (n=16)	0.18 ± 0.01	1.09 ± 0.06	1.06 ± 0.10	16.00 ± 2.00	1.20 ± 0.06
	Intravenous (n=17)	0.15 ± 0.01	0.83 ± 0.05	0.73 ± 0.06	0.42 ± 0.03	1.08 ± 0.07
	Probability (P <)	0.05	0.005	0.01	0.001	——
14w	Intrabursal (n=9)	0.20 ± 0.01	0.58 ± 0.05	0.62 ± 0.03	11.00 ± 2.70	1.32 ± 0.05
	Intravenous (n=10)	0.17 ± 0.01	0.48 ± 0.04	0.68 ± 0.08	0.50 ± 0.06	1.30 ± 0.10
	Probability (P <)	——	——	——	0.005	——

Table 2. Ontogenic data on thymus cell traffic in the chicken. Quantitatively significant migration did not occur in the newly hatched period, but could be demonstrated in 9-day-old animals, 6-week-old animals and in 14-week-old animals.

Age of the animals	Route of injection of ^{3}H-thymidine	Organ				
		Thymus	Spleen	Tonsilla caecalis	Bursa of Fabricius	Bone Marrow
< 24h	Intra thymus (n=11)	11.00 ± 1.70	1.58 ± 0.12	1.44 ± 0.11	0.45 ± 0.03	0.72 ± 0.13
	Intravenous (n=12)	0.21 ± 0.02	1.35 ± 0.12	1.25 ± 0.07	0.51 ± 0.04	0.69 ± 0.05
	Probability (P <)	0.001	——	——	——	——
9d	Intra thymus (n=17)	18.00 ± 1.80	1.29 ± 0.05	1.26 ± 0.08	0.39 ± 0.02	0.80 ± 0.03
	Intravenous (n=13)	0.14 ± 0.01	1.04 ± 0.04	0.88 ± 0.05	0.40 ± 0.03	0.63 ± 0.06
	Probability (P <)	0.001	0.005	0.001	——	0.025
6w	Intra thymus (n=17)	11.00 ± 2.00	0.93 ± 0.04	0.78 ± 0.06	0.41 ± 0.03	0.99 ± 0.07
	Intravenous (n=17)	0.14 ± 0.01	0.79 ± 0.03	0.67 ± 0.04	0.39 ± 0.02	0.97 ± 0.08
	Probability (P <)	0.001	0.025	——	——	——
14w	Intra thymus (n=9)	10.00 ± 3.30	0.60 ± 0.06	0.78 ± 0.07	0.53 ± 0.09	1.02 ± 0.08
	Intravenous (n=12)	0.19 ± 0.01	0.44 ± 0.03	0.67 ± 0.08	0.65 ± 0.14	1.14 ± 0.11
	Probability (P <)	0.005	0.025	——	——	——

[x] Rel. act. is defined as spec. act. of an organ divided by spec. act. of duodenum of the same animal.

The radiochemical data on thymus cell traffic (Table 2) show that significant numbers of thymus-derived cells could not be found in other lymphoid organs with this method in the newly hatched period, while quantitatively significant transport of label, presumably as labelled cells from the thymus, was found to the spleen and other organs in 9-day-old animals and to the spleen in the 6-week-old and 14-week-old animals. The thymus-derived heavily labelled cells in the spleens were found mainly in or adjacent to the white pulp (92 %). Also the thymus-derived cells avoided the germinal centers in the spleens and in other lymphoid organs. We have not been able to demonstrate thymus-derived cells in the bursa, neither with the radiochemical technique nor with autoradiography.

Hall and Smith (7) have given us interesting data on the sequence of events following antigenic stimulation, and recent reviews (see e.g. 46) cover more of the same subject. Hall and Smith describe profound changes in immunoblast formation and traffic after an antigenic stimulation. It is also clear that cell traffic from central lymphoid organs is influenced by antigenic stimulation. There is a significant increase in cell migration from the thymus to the lymph node local to the sensitized skin area in the early phase of the sensitization in delayed hypersensitivity (21), supporting the hypothesis that antigen-sensitive cells in delayed allergy are thymus-derived. It is well documented that the majority of the mononuclear cells present in the skin at the height of the delayed allergic reaction are derived from the bone marrow (47,48), but bone marrow derived cells are not found more frequently in the lymph node local to the skin reaction than in the contralateral node (47). This lack of capacity to recognize the lymph node local to the skin reaction supports the idea that the bone marrow derived cells are unspecific effector cells in delayed allery (47,48).

We (16) are also studying the early changes caused by antigenic stimulation on lymphoid cell traffic patterns in the chicken. 6-week-old chickens were immunized intravenously with human serum albumen (HSA) and different groups were labelled 24 hours later in the thymus, in the bone marrow or in the bursa by local injections of small amounts of ^{3}H-thymidine. The control animals were given saline intravenously and labelled locally 24 hours later as described above. All animals were killed and organs sampled 48 hours after local labelling. Specific activity of each sampled organ was calculated after extraction of nucleic acids and measurement of DNA and of tritium. The ratio between the spec. act. of an organ and that of the sum of the spec. act. of all sampled organs except the locally labelled one was calculated for each animal in the HSA- and saline-treated groups. This figure gives the distribution of label (transport + leakage), for each animal. Since leakage is obviously not influenced by an earlier antigen administration, a significantly higher figure obtained in this way for an organ in the HSA-treated group than

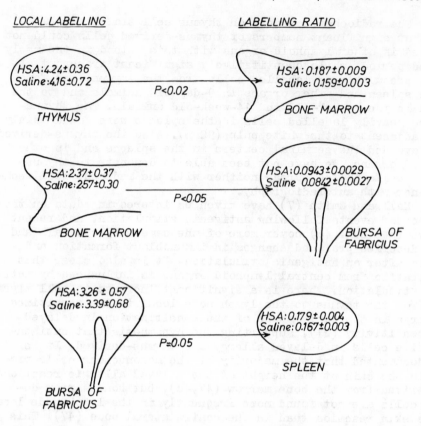

Fig. 1. Labelling ratio[x] (means $\pm$ S.E. of the means) of different lymphoid organs after local labelling with ^{3}H-thymidine of the thymus, of the bursa and of the bone marrow of antigen (HSA) and saline injected chickens. Local labelling was performed 24 hours after administration of HSA or saline, and organs were sampled 48 hours after local labelling. The figure shows that antigen administration causes quantitatively significant transport of label, presumably by cells, from the thymus to the bone marrow, from the bone marrow to the bursa and increases the normal transport of label from the bursa to the spleen.

---

[x] Labelling ratio = $\dfrac{\text{spec. act. of an organ}}{\begin{array}{l}\text{sum of spec. act. of sampled organs except}\\ \text{the locally labelled one of the same animal}\end{array}}$

in the corresponding saline treated group means that a greater
fraction of the total radioactivity found in the sampled organs
is transported to that organ from the locally labelled organ,
presumably by trafficing cells. We sampled thymus, bone marrow,
bursa, spleen, cecal tonsil and intestine from each animal in
each group. We could find (Fig. 1) that HSA administration caused
1) a quantitatively significant export of thymus cells to the
bone marrow ($p < 0.02$) (the intrathymically labelled groups),
2) a quantitatively significant export of bone marrow cells to
the bursa ($p < 0.05$) (the bone marrow labelled groups), and 3)
significantly increased cell traffic from the bursa to the spleen
($p \approx 0.05$) (the intrabursally labelled groups) (Fig. 1). We have
no good explanation at the present time for the cell traffic
from thymus to bone marrow as a result of antigenic stimulation.
Such traffic has also been demonstrated in the rabbit (15). The
existence of a thymus-derived cell population in the bone marrow
after antigenic stimulation is of interest in the present discussion on qualitatively different functions of thymus-derived
and bone marrow-derived cells. We interpret the cell traffic
from the bone marrow to the bursa as the result of a possibly
increased demand of bursa cell precursors due to the antigenic
stimulation. At this stage we find it reasonable to assume that
the increase in bursa cell traffic to the spleen reflects migration of antibody forming cell precursors.

ACKNOWLEDGEMENTS

This work was supported by the Swedish Medical Research
Council and the Regnell Fund.

REFERENCES

1. C. E. Ford, and H.S. Micklem, Lancet, I:359,1963.
2. H. S. Micklem, C.E. Ford, E.P. Evans, and J. Gray, Proc. Roy. Soc.
   (London), Ser. B, 165:78,1966.
3. O. Stutman, and R.A. Good, in: K. Lindahl-Kiessling, M. G. Hanna,
   Jr., and G.V. Alm, Eds., Morphologic and Functional Aspects of
   Immunity, p.129. New York: Plenum Press, 1971.
4. B. J. Bryant, in: K. Lindahl-Kiessling, M. G. Hanna, Jr., and
   G. V. Alm, Eds., Morphologic and Functional Aspects of Immunity,
   p.103. New York: Plenum Press, 1971.
5. A. D. Chanana, E. P. Cronkite, D. D. Joel, B. H. Waksman, and
   R. M. Williams, in: K. Lindahl-Kiessling, M.G. Hanna, Jr., and
   G. V. Alm, Eds., Morphologic and Functional Aspects of Immunity,
   p.113. New York: Plenum Press, 1971.
6. H. G. Durkin, G. A. Theis, and G. J. Thorbecke, in: K. Lïndahl-
   Kiessling, M. G. Hanna, Jr., and G. V. Alm, Eds., Morphologic and

Functional Aspects of Immunity,p.119.New York: Plenum Press,1971.

7. J. G. Hall, and M.E. Smith, in: K. Lindahl-Kiessling, M. G. Hanna, Jr., and G.V. Alm, Eds., Morphologic and Functional Aspects of Immunity,p.135. New York: Plenum Press, 1971.

8. W. L. Ford, and J.L. Gowans, Seminars in Hematology, 6:67, 1969.

9. K. E. Fichtelius, and O. Bäck, in: K. Lennert, and D. Harms, Eds., The Spleen, p. 118 New York: Springer-Verlag, 1970.

10. R. Woods, and T.J. Linna, Acta Pathol. Microbiol. Scand., 64:470, 1965.

11. E. O. Field, and E. M. Stanley, Acta haematol., 35:221,1966.

12. M. Galton and P.B. Reed, Transplantation, 4:168, 1966.

13. M. Brumby, and D. Metcalf, Proc. Soc. Exptl. Biol. Med., 124: 99, 1967.

14. T. J. Linna, T. Brenning, and E. Hemmingsson, in: L. Fiore-Donati, and M.G. Hanna, Jr., Eds., Lymphatic Tissue and Germinal Centers in Immune Response, p. 133 New York: Plenum Press, 1969.

15. T. J. Linna, Intern. Arch. Allergy Appl. Immunol., 31:313, 1967.

16. R. Bäck, and T.J. Linna, to be published.

17. H. N. Claman, E. A. Chaperon, and R. E. Triplett, Proc. Soc. Exp. Biol. Med., 122:1167, 1966.

18. A. J. S. Davies, E. Leuchars, V. Wallis, R. Marchant, and E. V. Elliott, Transplantation, 5:222, 1967.

19. G. F. Mitchell, and J.F. A. P. Miller, J. Exptl. Med., 128:821, 1968.

20. J. F. A. P. Miller, in: K. Lindahl-Kiessling, M. G. Hanna, Jr., and G. V. Alm, Eds., Morphologic and Functional Aspects of Immunity, p.93. New York: Plenum Press, 1971.

21. T. J. Linna, Intern. Arch. Allergy Appl. Immunol., 38:230, 1970.

22. T. J. Linna, and S. Lidén, Int. Arch. Allergy Appl. Immunol. 35: 35, 1969.

23. U. Ernström, L. Gyllensten, and B. Larsson, Nature, 207:540,1965.

24. U. Ernström, and G. Sandberg, Acta Pathol. Microbiol. Scand., Sect. A, 78:362, 1970.

25. M. Kotani, K. Seiki, A. Yamashida, and J. Horii, Blood, 27:511, 1966.

26. G. J. V. Nossal, and J. Gorrie, in: R. A. Good, and A. E. Gabrielsen, Eds., The Thymus in Immunobiology: Structure, Function, and Role in Disease, p. 288 New York-Evanston-London: Hoeber, 1964.

27. R. G. Murray, and P. A. Woods, Anat. Record 150: 113, 1964.

28. G. J. V. Nossal, Ann.N.Y. Acad. Sci., 120:171, 1964.

29. T. J. Linna, and J. Stillström, Acta Pathol. Microbiol. Scand., 68:465, 1966.

30. T. J. Linna, Acta Universitatis Upsaliensis. Abstracts of Uppsala Dissertations in Medicine, 42, 1967.

31. T. J. Linna, Blood, 31:727, 1968.

32. I. L. Weissman, J. Exptl. Med., 126:291, 1967.

33. D. D. Joel, M. Hess, and H. Cottier, in: K. Lindahl-Kiessling, M. G. Hanna, Jr., and G. V. Alm, Eds., Morphologic and Functional Aspects of Immunity, p.141. New York: Plenum Press, 1971.

34. L. Gyllensten, Acta Anat., suppl. 18-1 ad Vol. 17, 1953.

35. U. Ernström, Acta Pathol. Microbiol. Scand., 65:192, 1965.

36. M. C. Raff, and J. J. T. Owen, in: K. Lindahl-Kiessling, M. G. Hanna, Jr., and G. V. Alm, Eds., Morphologic and Functional Aspects of Immunity, p.11. New York: Plenum Press, 1971.

37. T. Aoki, U. Hämmerling, E. de Harven, E. A. Boyse, and L. J. Old, J. Exptl. Med., 130:979, 1969.

38. N. L. Warner, A. Szenberg, and F. M. Burnet, Austral. J. Exptl. Biol. Sci., 40:373, 1962.

39. M. D. Cooper, R. D. A. Peterson, M. A. South, and R. A. Good, J. Exptl. Med., 123:75, 1966.

40. T. J. Linna, D. Frommel, and R. A. Good, Fed. Proc., 29:825,1970.

41. E. Hemmingsson, and T. J. Linna, to be published.

42. W. C. Schneider, J. Biol. Chem., 161:293, 1945.

43. K. Burton, Biochem. J., 62:315, 1956.

44. G. A. Bray, Analyt. Biochem., 1:279, 1960.

45. T. Mariani, T. J. Linna, and R. A. Good, in: K. Lindahl-Kiessling, M. G. Hanna, Jr., and G. V. Alm, Eds., Morphologic and Functional Aspects of Immunity, p.625. New York: Plenum Press, 1971.

46. J. Hall, Rev. Europ. Études Clin. et Biol., 15:145, 1970.

47. D. M. Lubaroff, and B. H. Waksman, Science, 157:322, 1967.

48. S. Lidén, and T. J. Linna, Int. Arch. Allergy Appl. Immunol., 35:47,1969.

DISCUSSION TO SESSION 3
CHAIRMAN, J. LINNA, CO-CHAIRMAN, W. L. FORD

J.F.A.P. Miller: Just a point of clarification: Dr. Bryant, did you or did anybody else find thymus cell migrants in the bone marrow following in situ thymus labelling?

B. Bryant: In my material, the one-month-old guinea-pig, which certainly is an immunologically mature animal, I found very few definitive cortical thymic emigrants in the marrow or in any of the peripheral lymphatic tissue sites. The general conclusion of my studies was that fewer than one percent of the total thymocyte production survive in the periphery as long-lived cells. The other 99 per cent or more, regardless of their site of death, whether in the thymus or in the periphery, constitute a short-lived population.

J. Linna: In answer to Dr. Miller's question, we can trace thymic cells to the bone marrow in the antigen stimulated chicken. I have data in the rabbit that thymus cells go to the bone marrow. It is very difficult to say how much with the technique we are using, but we can say it is a quantitatively significant amount of label, presumably labelled cells, that is going there.

A.J.S. Davies: There are some thymus cells in the bone marrow, as has been shown by Doenhoff et al. by transfer experiments. He could not quantitate exactly how many there are, but probably less than five per cent of the total number of cells.

C. Rosse: Does Dr. Bryant consider the cells he labelled representative of the whole thymic population? His preparations showed only a narrow band of labelled cells confined to the cortex.

M.W. Hess: Dr. Bryant, can you exclude the possibility that your dose of IUdR was killing thymocytes by radiotoxicity?

B. Bryant: The answer has several parts. First of all the initially labelled cells were purely cortically disposed, so any conclusions from these experiments relate exclusively to the fate of cortical thymocytes. Second, after the initial labeling of these cells the radioautographic grain count progressively drops, indicating the labeled cells are healthy enough to go through several mitotic stages during several days following the initial labeling. Thirdly, the I^{125} UdR used had a specific activity in excess of 50 curies per millimole. The amount in biochemical terms of IUdR actually applied to the thymus was therefore very small (less than 0.06 µg) and was below the level necessary to bring about autoradiosensitisations of the tissue. The amount of I^{125} UdR applied in terms of radioactivity was 10 microcuries which is a standard dosage of precursor to apply in this kind of situation. Finally, the regression of thymic I^{125} DNA after local labeling was essentially identical to that of systemically labeled controls.

I.L. Weissman: One question, Dr. Chanana. You stated that a number of the emigrating cells found in the thymic lymph and thymic vein were medium and large lymphocytes that were labelled within the thymus. What about immigrant cells in the tissues, in the lymph nodes and spleen?

A.D. Chanana: I confined my remarks to the lymph and the venous blood because here you don't have to be brutal with the cells, which can therefore be sized reliably. My impression is that we do find medium thymocytes in the tissues.

R.K. Gershon: Dr. Chanana suggested that 3 to 8 per cent of the lymphocytes leaving the thymus, that contain thymus specific antigen will mature rapidly and lose that antigen. An alternate explanation is that this antigen could act as a marker and that rather than cells losing the antigen, cells bearing it are eliminated. Most of the cells from a thymus-cell suspension will migrate to the liver. It is possible that these are the cells with the thymus-specific antigen and this is the mechanism by which the excess cells, that are normally made in the thymus, are eliminated.

E.M. Lance: In contrast to theta antigen, TL antigen, in the normal mouse, is expressed in some strength only on thymocytes and is never expressed in the periphery. If thymocytes are to peripheralize and become members of the recirculating lymphocyte pool there must be a mechanism for a repression of the antigenic cell surface. The methods that were used to investigate this problem involved the in vitro labelling of cells with radiochromium and their subsequent injection into mice. The amount of migration was assessed by radioactivity measurements on lymphoid tissues obtained at various times after injection. Normally, thymocytes, approximately 1.5% of the injected cells, localize in the recipient lymph nodes while more than 20% accumulate in the spleen. The lymph node localizing thymocytes are interesting in that they represent those cells which have already acquired the property of recirculation. They are also the cells which are resistant to cortisone, and which can initiate graft-versus-host disease. At various times after injection, secondary cell suspensions were made from the recipient lymph nodes or spleen and the cells were tested for the presence of TL antigen by the addition of complement and the appropriate alloantisera. Since the cell transfer system used different strains as donor and recipient, antisera detecting the H-2 type of the donor provides an additional marker. Controls consisted of A strain lymph node cells which were handled in precisely the same manner as thymocytes.

At no time after migration was significant radioactivity released from lymph node cells which settled either in recipient lymph node or spleen by the addition of antisera detecting TL, whereas antisera detecting H-2 consistently caused release of radioactivity equivalent to that found after incubation with unmigrated A strain lymph node cells. This, of course, is precisely what might be expected since peripheral lymphocytes do not express TL antigen. On the other hand, the susceptibility of thymocytes to anti-TL depended upon whether they had migrated to recipient lymph node or spleen. Those thymocytes localizing in recipient lymph node were TL negative at all times after migration, whereas those cells which localized in the spleen initially expressed TL. With the passage of time, the spleen localizing thymocytes also became less susceptible to TL. Both populations of thymocytes remained fully susceptible to the action of anti-H-2 antisera.

We interpret these results to indicate that thymocytes which have already acquired the property of recirculation in situ, i.e. those migrating to recipient lymph nodes, have also undergone considerable modification of their cell surface membrane. Therefore, loss of TL occurs pari passu with the acquisition of recirculation and, we infer, maturation. The mechanisms controlling the maturation of thymocytes including change in cell surface antigens which are the product of selective gene action are, at present, completely unknown.

H.L. Langevoort: Dr. Thorbecke, you start with stimulated germinal centers, and you find a homing of bursal cells to the germinal centers. The germinal centers can be considered as reactive structures, reactive to the antigen you give. Your experiments make the impression of trying to find where immunologists home in Europe. To answer this question you organize a germinal center conference in Uppsala. Now count the number of immunologists that home in Uppsala. I think you will find a large number of them there. So the first question I would like to ask is: Is there a clean control in which you find bursal cells in non-stimulated spleens, at least spleens with non-stimulated germinal centers? My second question is - and you can draw the comparison with the immunologists a little bit further - do you have the impression that the bursal cells which you find in your germinal centers home there, because there is something attractive for them?

G.J. Thorbecke: In fact, we tried to quantitate if there was a difference between irradiated, normal and immunized recipients in the homing capacity of bursa cells to their spleens, and we found too much variation between animals to establish whether there was a difference. In normal animals we see the cells also in many of the germinal centers that we can recognize. What puzzles me is the large number of germinal centers that, after immunization with the one antigen (Brucella) contains these bursa cells. The cells are taken from relatively young donors and should not have a large proportion with reactivity to this antigen, so I doubt very much that it´s the antigen in the germinal centers that is attracting the

bursa cells. I think there is another interesting possibility.
We have recently found that we can kill a large percentage of bursa
cells with antiimmunoglobulin determinants on their surface, it might
be that surface receptors on reticulum cells or antibody complexes
containing complement are important in detaining these cells in
germinal centers.

B.D. Jankovic: Dr. Thorbecke, I'm not fully convinced that the
bursa cells you transferred preferentially locate in the germinal
centers of the chicken spleen. Your microphotographs undoubtedly
show that there are labelled cells also in the area which we call
red pulp. This is quite understandable because the bursa function
concerns both germinal centers and the plasma cellular elements of
the chicken spleen.

G.J. Thorbecke: I certainly don't want to make the impression that
all the bursa cells went there, because we also saw this peculiar
localization next to Schweiger-Seidel sheaths, which we don't see
for thymus cells. I have not studied the route by which bursal
cells enter germinal centers.

H. Cottier: Dr. Stutman, your experiments seem to indicate that
thymus-derived cells are able to migrate to lymph nodes, but that
hemopoietic cells which have not resided in the thymus, apparently
lack this ability. We will have to reconcile this view with the
presently held theory that bone-marrow-derived cells are precursors
of antibody producers and thymus-derived cells are not. I wonder
whether anybody in this audience can give quantitative data on the
magnitude of migration of non-committed immunocompetent cells from
bone marrow to lymph nodes, for instance in newborn mice.

O. Stutman: In mouse radiation chimeras all the dividing cells in
the lymph node are derived from bone marrow and repopulation seems
to be thymus-dependent.

P. Niewenhuis: In answer to the question about the number of cells
derived from bone-marrow in peripheral lymphoid tissues it has been
demonstrated by thymectomy combined with whole-body X-irradiation
that the whole cortical system and all follicular structures throughout the lymphoid tissues are not thymus-derived and thus may be
bone-marrow-derived. This is in sharp contrast to the population
of the lymphocyte sheaths and the paracortical areas and the interfollicular areas of the appendix which have been demonstrated to be
thymus-derived. It seems possible that part of the population in
the non-thymus-derived follicular structures may not be directly
bone-marrow-derived but are derived from germinal centers in other
follicular structures.

I.L. Weissman: Dr. Stutman, in your experiments it was mitogen or
antigen induced mitosis you were looking at, so you would not

necessarily see the bone-marrow-derived cells. My results also suggest that the whole follicular structure is not thymus-derived, but bone-marrow-derived.

W.H. Hildemann: If indeed there are two major lymphocyte populations in the kinetic sense, long-lived versus short-lived, I am not clear about the life spans of thymus-derived and marrow-derived cells. What do the short-lived lymphocytes do? I've heard nothing today concerning studies with bone marrow cells fractionated by density-gradient or albumin-gradient techniques. We talk glibly about 'bone-marrow cells'. I think of the marrow as a source of most if not all circulating cell types, but only a sub-population of these cells should be involved in antibody production.

D.G. Osmond: For the past 5 years we have used a technique of selective bone marrow labelling in vivo to study the migration and extramyeloid localisation of lymphocytes produced in the marrow (Osmond, Proc. 8th int. Congr. Anat., 1965; Osmond, Anat. Rec. 154:397, 1966; Brahim and Osmond, Proc. Can. Fed. Biol. Soc., 1967). In the following experiments with Mr. F. Brahim thymidine-H[3] was injected directly into the femoral and tibial marrow of guinea pigs while the hind limb circulation was arrested for 30 minutes and non-radioactive thymidine was administered systematically.

Radioautographic labelling was localised at first to the DNA-synthesising cells in femoral and tibial marrow. The local marrow small lymphocytes subsequently showed a wave of labelling increasing from 5 hours to 2 days. In the blood, well-labelled small lympho-cytes appeared from 12 hours to 5 days. Their maximal labelling indices at 3-4 days were one third to one half as high as those reached by blood granulocytes.

Sections of both spleen and mesenteric lymph node showed nu-merous well-labelled small lymphocytes from 12 hours onwards, reach-ing maximal numbers per unit area at 4-5 days and declining rapidly from 5 to 12 days. Such cells were rarely seen either in the thymus or in humeral marrow.

In the spleen the labelled small lymphocytes occurred predo-minantly throughout the red pulp cords and sinusoids at first. How-ever, by 4-5 days a large proportion (40%) became concentrated in areas of white pulp where their maximal labelling index (10.7 per 1,000 small lymphocytes) exceeded that in the red pulp (2.5 per 1,000 small lymphocytes). Some labelled small lymphocytes were found within periarteriolar lymphoid sheaths, and in a few instances within germinal centers, but the majority occurred randomly through-out the lymphoid follicles.

In the mesenteric lymph node labeled small lymphocytes were seen mainly in the cortex initially but from 3 days onwards their

numbers per unit area of cortex and medulla were approximately
equal. Cortical marrow-derived small lymphocytes occurred in the
subcapsular sinus, in the walls and lumen of postcapillary venules,
and around but not within germinal centres, but were principally
scattered randomly throughout both the superficial and deep cortex.
Some well-labelled small lymphocytes appeared within sinuses and
efferent hilar lymphatics (0.6-3.6/1,000 small lymphocytes) of
mesenteric lymph node medulla, and within thoracic duct lymph
collected at 2-3 days (0.2/1,000 small lymphocytes).

These studies have demonstrated that 1) bone marrow is an active
site of production and export of small lymphocytes, 2) a significant
proportion of circulating newly-formed small lymphocytes are marrow-
derived, 3) many small lymphocytes produced in the bone marrow
migrate rapidly and selectively to both the spleen and mesenteric
lymph nodes where their localisation overlaps the "thymus-dependent
zones", 4) some marrow-derived small lymphocytes recirculate from
blood to lymph but their rapid disappearance from the tissues
suggests that most have a short extramyeloid life span in the normal
animal.

K.E. Fichtelius: My remarks are not only related to Dr. Smith´s
paper but also to session 2 and to Dr. Miller´s paper. Most workers
in the field of cell-to-cell interaction in the immune response talk
only about different kinds of lymphocytes and macrophages. I think
it is time to consider also the relationship between epithelial
cells and lymphocytes in connection with cell-to-cell interaction
in the immune response. The reason for this is based on some hard
facts; first lymphocytes migrate to the gut epithelium; second,
these migrating lymphocytes constitute a selection of cells that
synthesize DNA to a surprisingly high extent; third, some of the
lymphocytes leave the gut epithelium for lamina propria. They do
not leave the organism, but they go back again. The fourth point
is that the presence of the intestinal content is important to the
appearance of lymphocytes in the epithelium.

The function of the epithelial cells can only be guessed at.
They may process antigen in the same way as macrophages do, or they
may be educating the lymphocytes in the way the thymic and bursal
epithelial cells are supposed to do.

R. Wissler: I was interested in the excellent autoradiographs of
the gut in the rat experiments and I wonder if you have any observations as to how many of these cells are small lymphocytes as
compared to larger pyroninophilic cells.

M. Smith: The cells to be injected were labelled in vitro as immunoblasts and since the material for autoradiographs was taken between
10 and 20 hrs after intravenous injection, I would think, although
I have not done an actual count, that the labelled cells have re-

mained large pyroninophilic cells or developed to plasma cells rather than reverting to small lymphocytes.

C. Griscelli: I would like to make a very short comment on migration, circulation and transformation of the rat lymph node immunoblasts labelled in vitro with tritiated thymidine and injected intravenously in syngeneic recipients.

1) The large pyroninophilic cell (immunoblast) homes in the lymph node through the postcapillary venule. That can indicate that the large cells can reach the deep cortex of the lymph node like the small lymphocytes (according to the studies of Gowans).

2) 24 hours after intravenous transfer it is possible to find large pyroninophilic cells in the thoracic duct lymph. This finding means that some immunoblasts may recirculate as small lymphocytes do.

3) I would like to make another comment about the transformation of immunoblast into plasma cells in rat lymphoid organs. We can see plasma cells in autoradiographic preparations. These labelled plasma cells are found 48 h after an intravenous transfer of mesenteric or axillary and popliteal labelled immunoblasts in the red pulp of the spleen, the liver and the lung. But it is impossible to find plasma cells in the lymph node. However, when we transfer mesenteric lymph node labelled cells it is possible to observe many labelled plasma cells in the lamina propria of the gut.

To answer Dr. Wissler's question about the proportion of different kinds of cells found in the gut, according to our results, I think that 40% of the labelled cells observed in the lamina propria of the gut 48 hours after the transfer are plasma cells, 20% are still large pyroninophilic cells and 40% are small lymphocytes or medium lymphocytes.

SESSION 4. LYMPHATIC TISSUE AND GERMINAL CENTERS IN RELATION
TO ANTIBODY PRODUCTION
CHAIRMAN, H. COTTIER, CO-CHAIRMAN, A. FAGRAEUS

HISTOLOGICAL CHANGES OF LYMPHOID TISSUES IN RELATION TO THE ONTOGENY OF THE IMMUNE RESPONSE IN GERMFREE PIGLETS [1]

Yoon Berm Kim and Dennis W. Watson

Department of Microbiology, University of Minnesota

School of Medicine, Minneapolis, Minnesota USA

Germfree, colostrum-deprived piglets obtained by aseptic hysterectomy 3 to 5 days prior to term were devoid of immunoglobulins
and their tissues were free of "background" antibody forming cells.
They were immunologically "virgin"; however, they were highly immunologically competent as demonstrated by an excellent immune response upon antigenic stimulation (1,2,3). In the "true" primary
immune response, the first antibody formed was 19S$^{\gamma}$G followed by
7S$^{\gamma}$G-immunoglobulins (4). These immunologically "virgin" piglets
were used to investigate the cellular origin of the sequential synthesis of 19S to 7S antibody in the ontogeny of the immune response.
This report presents briefly the histological changes of the lymphoid
tissues in relation to the "true" primary immune response (5,6).

MATERIALS AND METHODS

Germfree colostrum-deprived piglets (1) were randomly divided
into four groups. Group A received a single injection of 10^{12}
purified actinophage (MSP-2), 1 ml, i.p., or 1 ml of 20% sheep
erythrocytes (SRC) i.p., within 4 hrs after hysterectomy. Group B
were uninjected littermate controls. Each group was divided into
two subgroups: One-half of each group was maintained germfree and
fed an "antigen-free" diet of sterile pyrogen-free distilled water
for short term experiments (72 hrs). The other half of each group
was maintained germfree and fed Mullsoy-Diet (Borden Co., Pharma-
ceutical Division, New York) for prolonged observation. Antibody

1 Research supported by USPHS grant No. AI-03439. Y.B. Kim is the
recipient of RCDA K3-AI-37,388, USPHS.

responses and histological changes of the spleen and various lymph
nodes were examined at given intervals. In addition, embryos in
varying stages of development, ranging from 45 days of gestation to
term (114 days), were examined for the development of lymphoid
tissues. Conventional pigs and sow lymphoid tissues were also
examined for comparison. Antibody responses were measured by actinophage neutralization for anti-MSP-2 (1) and hemolytic plaque assay
for anti-SRC forming cells (7). For histological examination, tissues
were fixed in 6% formalin-60% alcohol for 24 to 48 hrs; paraffin
sections were stained with methyl green-pyronin, hematoxylin-eosin
and Gridley's silver stain for reticulum.

RESULTS

Histology of Lymphoid Tissues of Immunologically "Virgin" Piglets

The histology of lymphoid tissues of the spleen and lymph nodes
of germfree colostrum-deprived piglets on the day of hysterectomy
(109-112 days of gestation) are shown in Fig. 1.

Spleen. There are discrete thin periarteriolar lymphatic sheaths
composed of uniformly small non-pyroninophilic lymphoid cells having
scanty cytoplasm loosely filled in the networks of reticulum cells
surrounding the arterioles in the spleen (Fig. 1A,B). These sheaths
comprise the only elements in the white pulp of the spleen of these
piglets. In contrast, the white pulp of the "normal" adult spleen
is made up of thick periarteriolar lymphatic sheaths and lymphoid
follicles with germinal centers. Gridley's silver stain for reticulum demonstrates clearly that germinal centers are not present in
immunologically "virgin" piglets, but are present in conventional
"normal" adult pigs. In pre- and neo-natal spleens there were abundant erythroid cells (hemopoietic cells) in varying stages of differentiation. These erythroid cells in the red pulp decreased
rapidly after 3 days of life.

Lymph Nodes. A representative structure of the lymph nodes of
immunologically "virgin" piglets on the day of hysterectomy is shown
in Fig. 1C,D. The mesenteric lymph nodes have well developed cortex
and medulla; in contrast to adult lymph nodes, there were neither
germinal centers nor mature plasma cells. The cortex with primary
follicles were loosely filled with small and medium sized lymphoid
cells. Occasional weak pyroninophilic cells similar to those of
the thymus, spleen and bone marrow were scattered in the cortex.
These cells appear to be distinct from the large pyroninophilic
cells arising in response to antigenic stimulation. The position
of cortex and medulla is inverted in contrast to most other species
(8,9); the cortex, including primary follicles, is located in the
central position and usually develops along the trabeculae, while

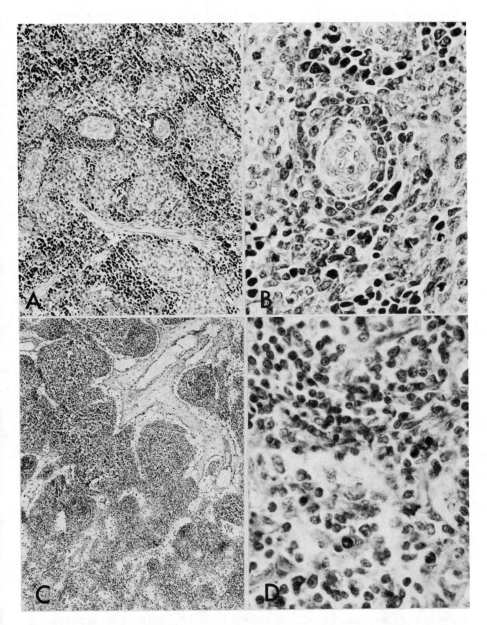

Fig. 1. Spleen (A,B) and mesenteric lymph nodes (C,D) of a germ-free colostrum-deprived piglet on the day of hysterectomy. Stained with methyl green-pyronin, (A) 150x, (B) 600x, (C) 60x, (D) 600x.

the loosely arranged "medullary" area is located in the periphery
of the nodes which is the subcapsular area.

Histological Changes of the Spleen
during the "True" Primary Immune Response

Histological examinations of the spleens were performed on the
piglets 1, 1-1/2, 2,3,6,8,10,14, and 16 days after injection of
MSP-2. For controls, uninjected littermates of the same ages were
used. Cellular changes in the periarteriolar lymphatic sheaths--
including the appearance of large pyroninophilic cells and a slight
increase in small lymphoid cells--were detected within 24 hrs after
the injection of antigen. However, the one-day old control piglets
maintained on an "antigen-free" diet were essentially similar to
those of the 0-day control. The number of large pyroninophilic
cells in the periarteriolar lymphatic sheaths increased on day 2
and further increased on day 3 in the spleen of the antigen-injected
animals (Fig. 2B), while uninjected littermate controls remained
unchanged (Fig. 2A). In contrast, in the early so-called "primary"
immune response in 4-month-old piglets, the number of pyroninophilic
cells increased markedly, not only in the periarteriolar lymphatic
sheaths but also in the germinal centers and red pulp. On the 6th
and 8th days after injection of antigen, the number of large pyroninophilic cells and small lymphoid cells increased further in the
sheaths which correlated with an increase in 19S antibody response.
On the 14th and 16th days after injection of antigen, the numerical
increase of pyroninophilic cells was even more striking. These cells
tended to aggregate at the margin of the lymphatic sheaths; thus a
group of the pyroninophilic cells could be seen separate from a
group of small lymphoid cells surrounding the same arterioles. This
may be the initial site of germinal center formation. In the uninjected littermate controls fed with Mullsoy-Diet, there was a very
slow, gradual increase in the number of small lymphoid cells as
well as pyroninophilic cells in the lymphatic sheaths. No germinal
centers developed in these animals. These results correlate with a
low "background" antibody response in the control animals.

Histological Changes of Lymph Nodes
during the "True" Primary Immune Response

Cellular changes within the cortex and follicles were detected
within 24 hrs after the injection of antigen including the appearance
of large pyroninophilic cells and an increase in small lymphoid
cells, while the one-day old control piglets maintained on an "antigen free" diet were essentially similar to those of the 0-day control. The onset and degree of the early cellular response in the
nodes appeared in the following order: Substernal > mesenteric >
submaxillary > deep neck > axillary > superficial neck lymph nodes.

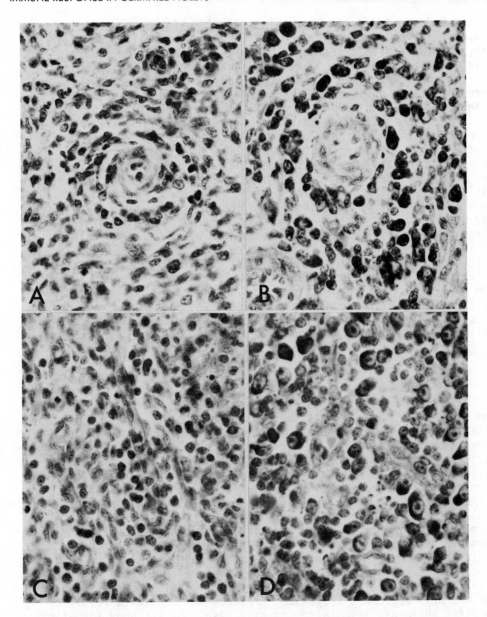

Fig. 2. Spleen (A,B) and mesenteric lymph nodes (C,D) of 3-day-
         old germfree colostrum-deprived piglet: (A) and (C) are
         unstimulated controls. (B) and (D) are injected with 10^{12}
         MSP-2 i.p. on the day of hysterectomy. Note the large
         pyroninophilic cells in the periarteriolar lymphatic sheaths
         of the spleen (B) and in the cortex of the nodes (D) in the
         stimulated animal. Stained with methyl green-pyronin, 600x.

On the 2nd and 3rd days after injection of antigen, the cellular
response increased and included the large pyroninophilic cells in
varying stages of maturation (Fig. 2D). The uninjected controls
were unchanged due to the absence of antigenic stimulation (Fig. 2C).
On the other hand, when piglets were fed with Mullsoy-Diet there
were some large pyroninophilic and small lymphoid cells responses
within 48 hrs in the cortex and follicles, especially in the mesenteric and submaxillary or pharyngeal lymph nodes. However, no
changes were seen in the superficial neck and axillary lymph nodes
until 72 hrs. These results suggest that Mullsoy-Diet contains
antigens which are absorbed through the oro-gastrointestinal tract
and stimulate the regional lymph nodes. The number of large pyroninophilic cells in the cortex of lymph nodes reached a maximum at 4
days after injection of antigen, and then decreased gradually. On
day 6, there was a greater proportion of small lymphoid cells than
large pyroninophilic cells. These changes may be due not only to
cellular migrations (10) but also to cellular differentiation, proliferation and maturation of the nodes. On the 14th day after the
injection of antigen, cortical areas were greatly increased including
the development of "germinal centers" and immature and mature plasma
cells in the cortico-medullary junction. Uninjected controls showed
less response than antigen-injected animals; however significant
cellular changes were observed in response to antigens in the diet.

                                DISCUSSION

        There have been numerous studies (11,12) on the development
and function of lymphoid tissues. However, the initial reaction
site after antigenic stimulation and the development and role of
germinal centers have not been completely resolved (13-18). It is
well established that most animals, including germfree, have so-
called "natural" or "normal" antibodies and "background" antibody-
forming cells to many antigens. These animals are chronically
stimulated by ubiquitous antigens in the diet and the environment
(19) resulting in formation of antibodies as well as formation of
germinal centers and cellular reactions including the appearance of
immature and mature plasma cells in the spleen and lymph nodes.
As in the ontogeny of the humoral antibody response (1,2), it is
important to know whether the germinal centers and plasma cell-series
develop spontaneously without antigenic stimulation or are required
for the primary immune response. Are they acquired as a result of
specific antigenic stimulation or as a result of antibody formation?
This information is essential for the interpretation of results pertaining to the primary immune response and ultimately to understand
the cellular origin and mechanism of the immune response.

        Study of the histogenesis of antibody-forming cells in the "true"
primary immune response requires antigenically unstimulated "virgin"
lymphoid tissues as well as the absence of pre-existing antibodies.

Because the germfree colostrum-deprived piglets obtained by aseptic
hysterectomy 3 to 5 days prior to term from specific pathogen-free
Minnesota miniature sows are immunologically "virgin" (1), they
provided the ideal conditions for such studies. The immunologically
"virgin" piglets on the day of hysterectomy have developed discrete
periarteriolar lymphatic sheaths within the spleen and a cortex with
primary follicles in the lymph nodes, but there are neither plasma
cells nor typical germinal centers in the spleen and lymph nodes.
The absence of "background" plasma cells and germinal centers is
consistent with the lack of immunoglobulins and antibody-forming
cells, and supports our contention that these animals are indeed
immunologically "virgin".

Large pyroninophilic cells with large pale nuclei and distinct
nucleoli are first detected in the periarteriolar lymphatic sheaths
of the spleen and the cortex and primary follicles of lymph nodes
within 24 hrs after the injection of antigen. These cells increased
on day 2 and markedly increased on day 3 with varying stages of
maturation (Fig. 2B,D). These observations are consistent with the
earlier reports by Langevoort (16) and Movat and Fernando (20) on
the rabbit and Fitch et al. (21) on the rat. These histological
changes of the lymphoid tissues were in response to antigenic stimulation, but preceded the detection of antibodies. The circulating
19S antibodies and antibody-forming cells (direct plaque) were detected within 48 hrs. In contrast, there were no pyroninophilic
cell responses in unstimulated animals within these periods (Fig.
2A,C). The appearance of numerous large pyroninophilic cells in
the spleen and the lymph nodes within 24 hrs after the injection of
antigen suggests that these antigen-responding cells are non-specific
or multipotential. These observations are not incompatible with the
hypothesis that the immunologically "virgin" piglets may have uncommitted "multi-potential" immunocompetent cells (2). These cells become committed "monopotential" upon initial antigenic exposure.

When the piglets were fed Mullsoy-Diet there was a slight pyroninophilic and small lymphoid cell response within 48 hrs, especially in the mesenteric and submaxillary lymph nodes; yet no
changes were seen in the superficial neck and axillary nodes until
72 hrs. This indicates that Mullsoy-Diet contains antigens, which
are absorbed through the oro-gastrointestinal tract and stimulate
regional lymph nodes. It is obvious that so-called "normal" animals
are chronically stimulated by ubiquitous antigens. Therefore, when
these "normal" animals are used for studying the "primary" immune
response, reactions observed will be a mixture of primary and secondary responses depending upon the immunological state of the host
to the antigens used. This is illustrated when the 4-month-old
pigs were injected with the MSP-2; there was a marked increase in
the number of pyroninophilic cells in germinal centers, in periarteriolar lymphatic sheaths as well as in the red pulp of the spleen.
These results explain the controversial reports in the past (13-17).

On the 6th day after the injection of antigen, there was a
further increase in the number of both small lymphoid cells and
large pyroninophilic cells which correlated with the increase in 19S
antibody response. Thereafter further increase of these cells and
the occurrence of plasma cells paralleled the appearance of 7S antibody. Thus, cellular responses including differentiation and proliferation of lymphoid cells and pyroninophilic cells in the cortex
of lymph nodes as well as the periarteriolar lymphatic sheaths of
the spleen correlate well with sequential synthesis of 19S and
7S antibody formation in the "true" primary immune response.
Antigenic and multi-cellular interactions (22-24) must take place
in these areas initially in order to induce antibody formation.
Furthermore, in the "true" primary immune response germinal centers
apparently are not required for either 19S or 7S antibody formation,
but they are formed as a result of this primary response and may
play a more important role in the secondary immune response (25,26).

SUMMARY

1. Germfree colostrum-deprived piglets are immunologically
"virgin" animals which have neither plasma cells nor germinal
centers in their spleens and lymph nodes.
2. The large pyroninophilic cell-response in the periarteriolar
lymphatic sheaths as well as in the cortex and primary follicles of
the lymph nodes of the piglets results from antigenic stimulation,
but precedes the detection of antibody-forming cells or circulating
antibodies.
3. Cellular responses including differentiation and proliferation of lymphoid cells and pyroninophilic cells in the periarteriolar
lymphatic sheaths of the spleen and in the cortex and follicles of
lymph nodes correlate well with the sequential synthesis of 19S and
7S antibodies in the "true" primary immune response.
4. It is suggested that uncommitted "multipotential" immunocompetent cells may become committed "monopotent" cells upon initial
antigenic exposure in the "true" primary immune response.
5. It appears that germinal centers are not required for the
"true" primary immune response, but are formed as a result of this
primary response and may play a role in the secondary immune response.

REFERENCES

1.   Y.B. Kim, S.G. Bradley, and D.W. Watson, J. Immunol. 97:52, 1966.
2.   Y.B. Kim, and D.W. Watson, Adv. Exp. Med. and Biol. 3:259,
     Plenum Press, N.Y., 1969.
3.   J. Sterzl, J. Vesely, M. Jilek, and L. Mandel, In: J. Sterzl and
     co-workers, Eds., Molecular and Cellular Basis of Antibody
     Formation, p. 463, Publishing House of the Czechoslovak
     Academy of Science, Prague, 1965.

4.   Y.B.Kim, S. G. Bradley, and D.W. Watson, J. Immunol. 101:224,
      1968.
5.   Y.B. Kim, J.H. Sung, and D.W. Watson, Fed. Proc. 28:813, 1969.
6.   K.Y. Chang, Y.B. Kim, and D.W. Watson, Bact. Proc. 70:85, 1970.
7.   N.K. Jerne, A.A. Nordin, and C. Henry, In: B. Amos and H. Kop-
      rowski, Eds., Cell-Bound Antibodies, p. 109, Wistar Institute
      Press, Philadelphia, 1963.
8.   A. Trautmann, and J. Fiebiger, In: Fundamentals of the Histology
      of Domestic Animals. Translated and revised from 1949 German
      edition by R.E. Habel and E.L. Biberstein, p. 126, Comstock
      Publishing Associates, Ithaca, N.Y., 1952.
9.   R.M. Binns and J.G. Hall, Brit. J. Exp. Path. 47:275, 1966.
10.   J.L. Gowans and E.J. Knight, Proc. Roy. Soc. (B) 159:257, 1964.
11.   H. Cottier, N. Odartchenko, R. Schindler and C.C. Congdon, Eds.,
      Germinal Centers in Immune Responses, Springer-Verlag, N.Y.,
      1967.
12.   L. Fiore-Donati, and M.G. Hanna, Jr., Eds., Lymphatic Tissue
      and Germinal Centers in Immune Response, Plenum Press, N.Y., 1969.
13.   R.W. Wissler, F.W. Fitch, M.F. LaVia, and C.H. Gunderson,
      J. Cell Comp. Physiol. 50: Suppl. 1, 265, 1957.
14.   P. Ward, A.G. Johnson, and M.R. Abell, J. Exp. Med. 109:463,
      1959.
15.   G.J. Thorbecke, R.M. Asofsky, G.M. Hochwald, and G.W. Siskind.
      J. Exp. Med. 116:295, 1962.
16.   H.L. Langevoort, Lab. Invest. 12:106, 1963.
17.   M.G. Hanna, Jr., Int. Arch. Allergy 26:230, 1965.
18.   B. Sordat, M. Sordat, M.W. Hess, R.D. Stoner, and H. Cottier,
      J. Exp. Med. 131:77, 1970.
19.   G.F. Springer, Angew. Chem. (Eng.), 5:909, 1966.
20.   H.Z. Movat and N.V.P. Fernando, Exp. Mol. Path. 4:155, 1965.
21.   F.W. Fitch, R. Stejskal, and D.A. Rowley, In: L. Fiore-Donati
      and M.G. Hanna, Jr., Eds., Lymphatic Tissue and Germinal Cen-
      ters in Immune Response, p. 223, Plenum Press, N.Y., 1969.
22.   G.J.V. Nossal, G.L. Ada and C.M. Austin, Aust. J. Exp. Biol.
      Med. Sci. 42:311, 1964.
23.   R.I. Mishell and R.W. Dutton. J. Exp. Med. 126:427, 1967.
24.   G.F. Mitchell and J.F.A.P. Miller, J. Exp. Med. 128:821, 1968.
25.   E.B. Jacobson and G.J. Thorbecke, Lab. Invest. 6:635, 1968.
26.   R.A. Good, W.A. Cain, D.Y. Perey, P.B. Dent, H.J. Meuwissen,
      G.E. Rodey, and M.D. Cooper, In: L. Fiore-Donati, and M.G.
      Hanna, Jr., Lymphatic Tissues and Germinal Centers in Immune
      Response, p. 33, Plenum Press, N.Y., 1969.

SITES OF SPECIFIC ANTIBODY PRODUCTION AFTER INJECTION OF HUMAN

SERUM ALBUMIN (HSA) IN COMPLETE FREUND-TYPE ADJUVANT IN THE CHICKEN

V.I. French, J.M. Stark and R.G. White

Department of Bacteriology and Immunology

University of Glasgow, Scotland

This work was undertaken during an investigation into the effects of various adjuvants on the immune response in the chicken following intravenous or intramuscular injection of Human Serum Albumin (HSA). Site of antibody formation in various tissues were examined in relation to the circulating antibody response.

Experiments were set up in which batches of 4 - 5 chickens were injected intramuscularly with 40 µg of HSA. Each batch was injected with HSA in one of three forms, either as complete Freund-type adjuvant i.e. a water-in-oil emulsion with 1 - 5 mg heat-killed Mycobacterium tuberculosis, or as a simple water-in-oil emulsion, or as a solution in 0.15M saline. The birds were bled at intervals after injection and the Farr technique (1) used to determine the antigen binding capacity of the serum as a measure of its antibody content.

It should be made clear that only one injection of HSA was given to each bird and that the pattern of the primary circulating antibody response in birds to HSA and other antigens differs from that of mammals. In that the response is very rapid in onset, it more closely resembles a mammalian secondary response. In general free circulating antibody is not detectable before the 4th day after injection and the peak level is reached between the 8 - 12th days. Thereafter the level rapidly falls until low levels are reached by the 18th day. This pattern of response was fairly constant whether HSA was injected in Freund-type adjuvant, water-in-oil emulsion or saline. The main peak level of antibody response during this phase was not found to be higher in birds receiving Freund-type adjuvant and it would appear that water-in-oil emulsions with or without added Mycobacteria exert very little effect on the primary response. However from the 21st day onwards antibody levels again started to rise in birds given complete Freund-type adjuvant and very high levels were reached between the 40 - 60th days after injection. These were several hundred fold greater than that found at the first peak. To a lesser extent water-in-oil emulsion produced a second rise also. (Fig. 1).

During the first phase of the primary response anti-HSA production takes place mainly in the spleen after intramuscular or intravenous injection. There was proliferation of cells of the plasma cell series in the red pulp and many cells containing anti-HSA could be demonstrated using the fluorescent antibody technique (Fig. 2). The initial appearance of these cells preceded the detection of circulating antibody by 3 days and their total disappearance by the 12th day coincided with the onset of a fall in circulating antibody from the primary peak (2).

Splenectomy does not abolish the circulating anti-HSA response but the response is reduced and delayed (3). Although other sites of production during the primary response must exist the spleen is a major site of production. However during the second rise in anti-HSA levels in birds given HSA in complete Freund-type adjuvant no antibody containing plasma cells were found in the red pulp of the spleen at any time. Cells with the morphology of medium lymphocytes containing anti-HSA in their cytoplasm were seen in a few of the germinal centers of the spleen from the 22nd day of the response onwards (Fig. 3). The number of these cells was quite small and would seem inadequate to account for the very high levels of circulating antibody. A search in other tissues was made with the fluorescent antibody technique, for cells producing anti-HSA. None were found, but for technical reasons the fluorescent antibody technique was not satisfactory for the bone marrow and granuloma. Extracts from various organs were therefore made by alternate freezing and thawing and ultrasonication. The antibody content of the extracts was then measured using the Farr technique. The only tissue found to contain an appreciable amount of anti-HSA was the granuloma (Table I).

The granulomata produced at the site of injection of Freund-type adjuvant were detectable by palpation by the 21st day after injection and subsequently increased in size so that a visible swelling was produced by the 40th day after injection (Fig. 4). Microscopically on the 6th day of the primary response many small lymphocytes were seen at the site of injection of HSA in complete Freund-type adjuvant but few cells with the morphology of mature plasma cells. This is in marked contrast to the red pulp of the spleen at this time in which many immature and mature plasma cells containing anti-HSA were found. But by the 40th day many plasma

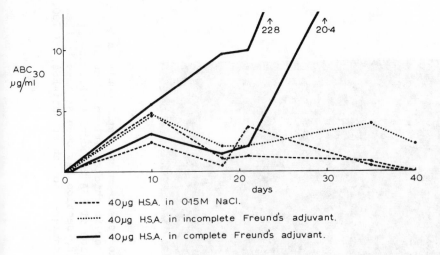

Fig. 1. Circulating antibody production in chickens after immunization with HSA in complete Freund-type adjuvant, water-in-oil emulsion,
or 0.15M NaCl.

Table I. Anti-HSA content of tissue extracts obtained from chickens
53-55 days after injection of 40 µg HSA in complete Freund-type
adjuvant.

Tissue	Antibody content (ABC$_{30}$ mg/g tissue or mg/ml serum)		
	53 days Chicken 143	54 days Chicken 145	55 days Chicken 146
Granuloma	132.0	1200.0	120.0
Cecum	28.0	17.0	1.62
Bursa	8.3	20.8	-
Spleen	6.7	11.8	2.95
Lung	26.7	-	-
Liver	20.8	19.0	-
Thymus	-	14.4	5.1
Skin	-	41.8	23.8
Bone marrow	-	17.0	15.2
Serum	48.0	780.0	21.0

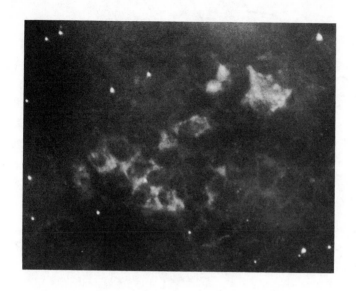
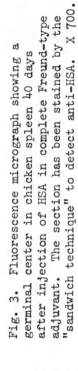

Fig. 3. Fluorescence micrograph showing a germinal center in chicken spleen 40 days after injection of HSA in complete Freund-type adjuvant. The section has been stained by the "sandwich technique" to detect anti-HSA. X 700.

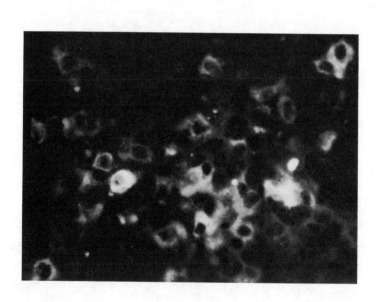

Fig. 2. Fluorescence micrograph showing the red pulp of chicken spleen 4 days after intravenous injection of HSA. The section has been stained by the "sandwich technique" to detect anti-HSA. X 700.

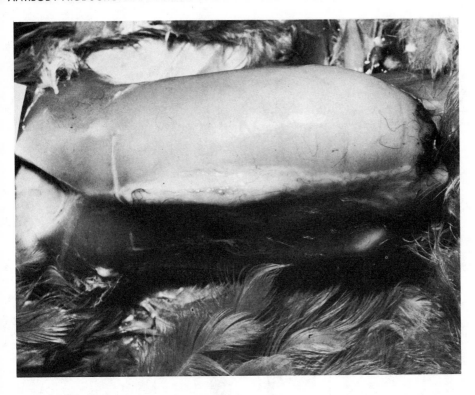

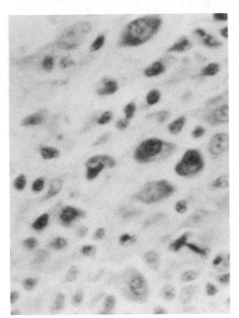

Fig. 5. Photomicrograph of the granuloma at the site of injection of HSA in complete Freund-type adjuvant 40 days after injection. There are many mature and immature plasma cells present (arrowed). X 1000.

Fig. 4. Pectoralis muscle of a chicken 40 days after intramuscular injection of complete Freund-type adjuvant into the L. breast. The left pectoralis contains a granuloma.

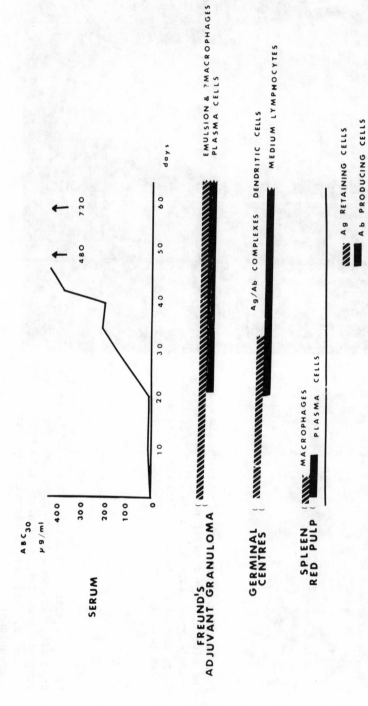

Fig. 6. Sites of antigen retention and antibody production after immunisation using complete Freund-type adjuvant in chickens.

cells were found in the granuloma (Fig. 5).

It is unlikely that the high content of anti-HSA found in the granuloma was the result of extravascular exudation of plasma proteins due to a non-specific inflammatory response, as in all birds the serum level was appreciably below that in a comparable weight of granuloma. It is also unlikely that it was present mainly in the form of antigen-antibody complexes held in the granuloma by the HSA depot and which were dissociated during the extraction process; the antigen binding capacity of the granuloma extract was considerably greater than that required to bind all the injected HSA (40 µg). On this and the histological evidence it is probable that anti-HSA was produced in the granulomata in quite large amounts (4).

These findings are summarised in Figure 6. It can be seen that the first phase of antibody production is associated with a response in the red pulp of the spleen. The onset of the second phase of the response corresponds with the development of anti-HSA containing plasma cells in germinal centers and with the development of a granuloma at the site of injection of Freund-type adjuvant.

Sites of specific antibody production are related to sites of antigen retention. The uptake of HSA by the splenic red pulp macrophages is associated with production of anti-HSA by plasma cells in the red pulp. The presence of HSA-anti-HSA complexes on germinal center dendritic cells is later followed by anti HSA production in germinal centers, and retention of HSA in the water-in-oil emulsion at the site of injection is also associated with antibody production at that site.

We should like to relate these findings to the hypothesis that germinal centers are sites in which "memory" cells responsible for secondary responses are stimulated to proliferate (5). It is clear that specific antibody producing or containing lymphocytes are present in some germinal centers during the second phase of the response. The striking absence of specific antibody producing cells from the red pulp of the spleen suggests that almost all HSA sensitive cells are present either in germinal centers or the granuloma. It is tempting to postulate a migration of immunologic-ally competent cells from germinal centers to the site of continuing antigenic stimulation, the granuloma.

ACKNOWLEDGMENTS

We thank Mrs. Sheila McLaren for technical help.
V.I.F. was in receipt of a grant from the Scottish Hospitals Endowment Research Trust.

REFERENCES

1. R.S. Farr, J. Infect. Dis., 103:239, 1958.

2. R.G. White, V.I. Fench, and J.M. Stark, J. Med. Microbiol., 3:65, 1970.

3. G.L. Rosenquist, and H.R. Wolfe, Immunology, 5:211, 1962.

4. V.I. French, J.M. Stark, and R.G. White. Immunology, 18:645, 1970.

5. R.G. White, in Mechanisms of antibody formation. M. Holub and L. Jaroskova Ed., p. 29. Prague 1960.

FATE AND IMMUNOGENICITY OF ANTIGENS ENDOCYTOSED BY MACROPHAGES[1]

André Cruchaud[2] and Emil R. Unanue[3]

Department of Experimental Pathology, Scripps Clinic and

Research Foundation, La Jolla, California USA

Soluble and particulate antigens taken up by macrophages are immunogenic. The immunogenicity of macrophage-associated antigens has been tested in several experimental system. In one such system live macrophages - after exposure to the antigen - are transferred into mice; the immune response of the mice to the antigen associated with live macrophages is then studied (1-7). The immunogenicity of soluble proteins bound to macrophages has been attributed mostly to molecules of non pinocytosed antigen retained on the plasma membrane of macrophages (6,8). On the other hand, the pathway by which particulate or heavily aggregated antigens are presented to lymphocytes for immunological recognition has not been elucidated. These large antigens are totally endocytosed following their binding to the membrane of the macrophages and presumably may be submitted to the action of enzymes from intracellular vesicles.

Antigens endocytosed by macrophages may suffer different fates depending upon their physicochemical properties. For instance,

---

[1]This is publication No. 450 from the Department of Experimental Pathology, Scripps Clinic and Research Foundation, La Jolla, California. This research was supported by U.S. Public Health Service Grant AI 07007.

[2]Present address: Laboratory of Immunology, Department of Medicine, Hôpital Cantonal, Geneva, Switzerland.

[3]Supported by an American Cancer Society fellowship. Present address: Department of Pathology, Harvard Medical School.

Table I.   Handling of ^{125}I-SRBC by macrophages after
various periods in culture

	Time after initiation of culture		
	1 hr	18 hrs	42 hrs
^{125}I in supernatant	11.1	74.1	93.6
-non protein-bound I	8.8	63.1	78.9
-protein-bound I	2.3	11.0	14.7
^{125}I bound to macrophages	88.9	25.9	6.4
-membrane-bound I	14.9	5.7	1.5

Macrophages and ^{125}I-SRBC were reacted in suspension for 1 hr.
Following elimination of nonendocytosed SRBC the macrophages were
planted in tissue culture dishes. After 1, 18 and 42 hrs the
supernatant of 2 to 3 culture dishes was harvested and treated with
trichloracetic acid. The macrophages were then incubated with
trypsin for 15 min. to remove membrane-bound material. The
trypsinized supernatant was collected and the cells were harvested
with a rubber policeman. Results are expressed as percentage of
the total initial radioactivity. The data are combined results
from two experiments.

human serum albumin and hemocyanins are extensively degraded by
proteolytic enzymes to the level of aminoacids (3,9); in contrast,
pneumococcal polysaccharides (10) and synthetic polypeptides made
up of D-aminoacids (11) are not catabolized and may be slowly
released from tissues.

In this paper we report attempts to study the fate and immunogenicity of sheep red blood cells (SRBC) and rabbit IgG after endocytosis by macrophages. It has been found that part of these antigens
are incompletely degraded; some are released into the extracellular
medium, and some become associated with the plasma membrane of
macrophages. Most of the immune response to SRBC ingested by macrophages appears to be directed against antigens bound to the surface
of the macrophages.

EXPERIMENTAL APPROACH

Peritoneal macrophages from (CBA x A)F$_1$ hybrid mice were exposed,
in vitro, to SRBC (labeled with ^{51}Cr or ^{125}I) opsonized with mouse
anti-SRBC serum. In some experiments, SRBC were coated with ^{125}I-
rabbit anti-SRBC IgG prior to incubation with macrophages. After
1 hr, the macrophages had taken up about 10-15% of the SRBC. The

Table II. Immunogenicity of M-SRBC

| M-SRBC | | | | |
Number of macrophages (x 10^{-6})	Content of SRBC (x 10^{-6})	SRBC (x 10^{-6})	Recipients	Antibody titer* Day 6
1.2	5.0	-	N	4.0
1.2	5.0	-	X-irrad.**	0.0
-	-	5.0	N	6.5
-	-	2.0	N	3.8
-	-	2.0 (opsonized)	N	5.1

Macrophages containing SRBC were transferred into normal or X-irradiated syngeneic recipients. The hemagglutinin titer of these animals was compared with the immune response of recipients injected with untreated SRBC or SRBC previously incubated with mouse anti-SRBC serum.

*Hemagglutinin titers are geometric means of groups of 5-10 mice.

**X-irradiated mice received 660 R of whole body irradiation 2 hrs prior to cell transfer.

SRBC that were not phagocytized were eliminated by lysing them in hypotonic media. The content of SRBC in macrophages was then determined by radioactive counting of either ^{51}Cr or ^{125}I. Macrophages containing SRBC (M-SRBC) were cultured for various periods of time in plastic dishes or siliconized flasks and/or were transferred into syngeneic recipients to assay for immunogenicity.

The catabolism of ^{125}I-SRBC and ^{125}I-rabbit anti-SRBC-IgG following endocytosis was studied by counting the radioactivity of the cells and of the media after various time periods in culture. It had been previously established that in the case of ^{125}I-labeled SRBC, at least 3/4 of the radioactivity was tightly bound to some proteins of the SRBC stromata. The degradation products of IgG were studied using sucrose density gradient analysis and double diffusion in agar.

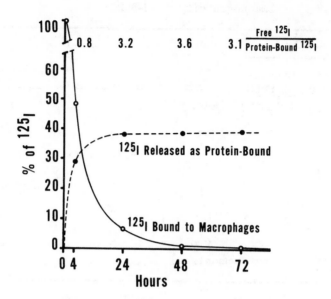

Fig. 1.   Fate of ^{125}I-rabbit anti-SRBC-IgG taken up by macrophages.
SRBC were incubated with ^{125}I-rabbit anti-SRBC-IgG, and then reacted
with macrophages.   After elimination of nonphagocytized SRBC, M-SRBC
were cultured on 8 plastic dishes.   After 4 hrs, the supernatant of
all dishes was collected, and the cells of 2 dishes were harvested.
Fresh medium was added to the remaining dishes and the culture was
continued.   The same procedure was repeated after 24, 48 and 72 hrs.
The supernatant collected at each time was pooled and treated with
trichloracetic acid.   Top figures represent the ratio of non-protein-
bound vs protein-bound I in the different supernatants.

Hemagglutinin titer was determined in recipients 6 days after
transfer of M-SRBC as well as 10 days after a booster injection of
2×10^6 erythrocytes (given on day 20).   Antibodies to IgG were
determined by a modification of the Farr technique (12).

RESULTS

The ^{125}I-SRBC were extensively catabolized after their ingestion
by macrophages.   Note in Table I the amount of I-label remaining with
the macrophages at different times of culture.   Two points should be
stressed: 1) that some of the label released into the supernatant
was bound to protein (i.e., most likely represented incompletely

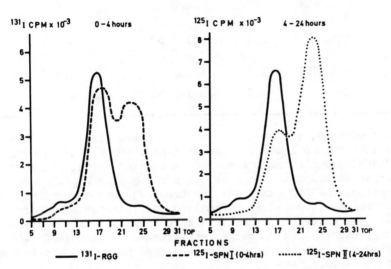

Fig. 2.   Sucrose density gradient analysis of supernatant of cultures
of macrophages containing SRBC coated with ^{125}I-rabbit anti-SRBC-IgG.
Supernatants of several culture dishes were collected after 4 hrs
and pooled; fresh medium was added to the cultures, and supernatants
were harvested again after 24 hrs.   Free ^{125}I was eliminated by dial-
ysis against buffered saline; the supernatants were concentrated and,
after addition of a small amount of ^{131}I rabbit-IgG, they were run
at 114.000 G for 22 hrs in a Beckman L 3-40 preparative ultracentrifuge.   Fractions of 10 drops were collected, and both ^{131}I and ^{125}I
were counted simultaneously using a differential counting procedure.

Table III. Effect of anti-SRBC antibody on the immunogenicity of M-SRBC

M-SRBC +		Normal macrophages		Ab titer
Number (x 10^{-6})	Treatment	Number (x 10^{-6})	Treatment	Day 6
1. 1.0	Anti-SRBC + NMS	1.0	None	1.6
1.3	None	1.3	Anti-SRBC + NMS	4.1
2. 1.3	Anti-SRBC	1.3	None	3.0
0.8	None	0.8	Anti-SRBC	6.5

20×10^6 macrophages, either normal or containing SRBC, were incubated at 4°C for 1 hr with 0.1 ml of mouse anti-SRBC serum. In experiment 1, the media also contained a five-fold excess of normal mouse serum (NMS) in order to minimize the possible non-specific binding of anti-SRBC serum. M-SRBC (untreated or treated) were then mixed with normal macrophages (treated or untreated) and injected into normal recipients. The number of M-SRBC was adjusted to provide 5×10^6 SRBC. Hemagglutinin titers are geometric means of groups of 6-8 mice. Differences between groups in each experiment are statistically significant (P <0.01).

degraded material), and 2) that some protein-bound ^{125}I was associated with the macrophage membrane (i.e., it was removed by treatment with trypsin).

The fate of ^{125}I-rabbit anti-SRBC-IgG attached to SRBC after endocytosis is shown in the experiments of Fig. 1. More than 90% of the label was released into the extracellular medium within 24 hrs. Some of the material was protein-bound. The ratio of non protein-bound/protein-bound I varied with the time of incubation.

The size of the ^{125}I-IgG released from the macrophages was studied by sucrose density gradient analysis (Fig. 2). Some of the released IgG was of size comparable to monomeric IgG. However, there was also lighter sedimenting material that most likely represents a fragment of the IgG molecule. The amount of small molecular weight material increased with time of culture.

Table IV. Effect of trypsin on the immunogenicity of M-SRBC

M-SRBC		Ab titer
Number (x 10^{-6})	Treatment	Day 7
2.0	None	3.4
2.0	Trypsin	0.1

M-SRBC were cultured for 18 hrs, and then treated with trypsin (0.2 mg of enzyme to 10^7 macrophages for 30 minutes at 37°C). Untreated and treated M-SRBC were then injected i.p. in recipients. Hemagglutinin titers are geometric means of groups of 7 mice.

Immunogenicity of SRBC and Rabbit IgG following Endocytosis

Phagocytized SRBC retained immunogenicity as shown in Table II. The immune response in the recipients was not due to synthesis of antibodies by the macrophages or by the lymphocytes contaminating peritoneal exudate cells. This was proven by the absence of detectable antibody in X-irradiated recipients of M-SRBC.

The immune response was mainly directed to SRBC antigens associated with macrophages. Thus, in one experiment, the macrophages that had ingested SRBC were cultured for several hours. At different times, the macrophages, as well as the culture supernatant, were each injected into mice to assay for immunogenicity. The mice injected with macrophages made a strong anti-SRBC response, while those injected with supernatants made a feeble immune response.

Further experiments suggested that some of the immunogen associated with macrophages was bound to their plasma membrane. Thus M-SRBC incubated in vitro with mouse anti-SRBC serum - in order to cover surface immunogens - were indeed less immunogenic than untreated M-SRBC (Table III). Note in the experiment of Table III that treatment of normal macrophages with antibodies did not abrogate the anti-SRBC response to M-SRBC transferred simultaneously. This suggested that the abrogation of the response by treatment of M-SRBC with antibodies was the result of specific binding to antigenic determinants during the in vivo incubation. Furthermore, in other experiments, treatment of M-SRBC with trypsin resulted in a significant decrease of the immune response (Table IV). Trypsin most likely removed SRBC antigens from the plasma membrane of the macrophages.

Mice injected with macrophages containing 1 µg of endocytosed rabbit IgG developed a weak primary response to the Fc fragment but no response to the Fab fragment.

DISCUSSION

Our results demonstrate that endocytosed SRBC were immunogenic after ingestion by macrophages. The immunogen(s) after endocytosis became associated with the plasma membrane of macrophages where it was held for some periods of time. Hence, the surface membrane becomes the main site where the macrophage presents the antigen to the lymphocytes. In the case of soluble proteins (6,8) the surface bound antigen was mainly represented by non pinocytosed molecules. In the case now studied with SRBC, the surface antigen derives from molecules that have followed an intracellular pathway. It became clear from the tissue culture experiments that SRBC and IgG after their endocytosis were not completely catabolized and that some non-degraded material was in fact liberated from the cells and appeared in the culture fluid as well as on the plasma membrane of the cells. The pathway that the antigens follow from the intracellular vesicles to the surface membrane is not clear and requires further study. Perhaps the immunogenic material is first released into the extracellular medium, and then immediately adsorbed on the membrane of macrophages.

Hence, it may be that one function of macrophages during the inductive process consists in the concentration of immunogenic molecules on their plasma membrane. The surface bound molecules are therefore accessible to immunocompetent cells. The macrophages may then contribute in bringing together at one point antigen and lymphocytes.

REFERENCES

1. R. Gallily and M. Feldman, Immunology, 12:197, 1967.

2. B. F. Argyris, J. Immunol., 99:744, 1967.

3. E. R. Unanue and B. A. Askonas, J. Exp. Med., 127:915, 1968.

4. E. R. Unanue and B. A. Askonas, Immunology, 15:287, 1968.

5. N. A. Mitchison, Immunology, 16:1, 1969.

6. E. R. Unanue and J. C. Cerottini, J. Exp. Med., 131:711, 1970.

7. A. Cruchaud, J. P. Despont, J. P. Girard, and B. Mach, J. Immunol., 104:1256, 1970.

8. E. R. Unanue, J. C. Cerottini, and M. Bedford, Nature, 222:1193, 1969.

9. B. A. Ehrenreich and Z. A. Cohn, J. Exp. Med., 126:941, 1967.

10. L. D. Felton, B. Prescott, G. Kauffmann, and D. Ottinger, J. Immunol., 74:204, 1955.

11. C. A. Janeway, Jr. and J. H. Humphrey, Immunology, 14:225, 1968.

12. J. C. Cerottini, J. Immunol., 101:433, 1968.

CELLULAR AND IMMUNOLOGICAL EVENTS FOLLOWING INJECTION

OF ANTIGEN INTO THE CHICKEN THYMUS

B. D. Janković, Katarina Isaković and Spomenka Petrović

Microbiological Institute, Faculty of Pharmacy, University
of Belgrade; Department of Experimental Immunology,
Institute of Immunology and Virology, and Immunology Unit,
Institute for Biological Research, Belgrade, Yugoslavia

It seems generally accepted that the thymus, as a "central" or
primary lymphoid organ (1), is not capable of taking a direct part
in the realization of immune reactions. So far as avian species are
concerned, the thymus plays a role in the development of cell mediated
immunity, whereas it does not interfere with the antibody-producing
capacity of the immune system, the latter capacity being dependent
on the function of the bursa of Fabricius. However, experimental
observations made in our laboratory imply that the chicken thymus is
capable of participating directly in immune responses. Consequently,
chicken thymus shares some characteristics with so-called "peripheral"
or secondary lymphoid tissues. Besides, it seems that the avian
thymus may be engaged in antibody production.

The previous findings gathered in our laboratory during several
years of experimentation support the concept that the chicken thymus
is active in antibody production. Here is the previous evidence:

(a) About 15% of normal chickens have germinal centers and
cells of plasmacytic series in the thymus (2).

(b) There is an increase in the number of germinal centers
and plasma cells in the thymus after hyperimmunization of chickens
by systemic routes (2).

(c) Formation of germinal centers and proliferation of plasma-
cellular elements in the thymus can be induced in chicken by means
of *in ovo* grafting with allogeneic bursal tissue (3).

(d) Specific fluorescent cells are regularly present in the thymus of chickens hyperimmunized with a soluble antigen (4).

(e) Production of specific antibodies and proliferation of plasma cells occurs in 7 to 14-day-old chickens which were grafted during the embryonic life with allogeneic thymus from adult immune donors (5).

(f) Antibody production is suppressed in chickens repeatedly injected with rabbit anti-chicken thymus globulin (6).

The present communication is an outline of experiments which deal with the production of circulating antibody and cellular changes in lymphoid tissues of the chicken following introduction of a soluble antigen directly into the thymic parenchyma.

MATERIALS AND METHODS

Crystallized bovine serum albumin (BSA) was used as antigen. The first group of New Hampshire 8-week-old chickens was injected into the six thymic lobes with BSA (10 mg of BSA/0.02 ml/thymic lobe). Contralateral lobes served as controls. The second group of birds received a single intravenous injection of BSA (60 mg of BSA/1 ml). The third group was injected intrathymically with saline alone (0.02 ml of saline/thymic lobe). Chickens of all groups were bled at various time intervals after immunization, and mercaptoethanol-sensitive and mercaptoethanol-resistant antibodies were determined by means of a passive hemagglutination technique (7). Histological examination of injected and noninjected thymus lobes, spleen and bursa was performed on chickens of experimental and control groups.

RESULTS

Changes in the spleen after intrathymic injection of BSA. Spleens from chickens injected into the thymus with BSA or with saline alone, and spleens from birds immunized by intravenous route were taken 3 days after antigenic stimulation and examined histologically. The results are shown in Table I.

There was a decrease in the number of small lymphocytes only in the periarterial areas of the chickens injected into the vein. At that time blastic proliferation (transformation) occurred in birds injected either intrathymically or intravenously with BSA, the proliferation being more pronounced in chickens of the latter group.

Table I.   Differential counts* of cells in splenic periarterial area of chickens 3 days after intrathymic injection of BSA.

Group	Small lymphocytes	Blasts	Plasma cells	Other cells
Intrathymic injection of saline	50.0 ± 1.37	4.1 ± 0.47	6.1 ± 0.82	39.8 ± 1.02
Intrathymic injection of BSA	51.1 ± 1.51	8.8 ± 1.03	5.8 ± 1.03	34.3 ± 0.84
Intravenous injection of BSA	47.9 ± 0.49	19.3 ± 1.50	5.4 ± 0.41	27.4 ± 3.91

Five chickens in each group.

*Based on 785-1430 counted cells per spleen section.

Changes in the bursa after intrachymic injection of BSA.   The administration of antigen directly into the thymic parenchyma induced profound changes in the cellular make-up of the bursa 3 days after challenge.   There was a significant reduction in the size of bursal follicles and a proliferation of interfollicular connective tissue. Changes within the follicles were characterized by a marked depletion of lymphocytes in the medulla, disappearance of the cortical area, an increase in the number of strongly basophilic cells in the medulla, and occurrence of cystic formations.   The number of pyronin-positive cells in interfollicular connective tissue was also augmented.

Changes in the thymus after intrathymic injection of BSA. Blastic proliferation (transformation) in the medulla of thymic lobes injected with BSA occurred within 24 hours of the administration of antigen.   This proliferation reached its peak about the 5th day both in thymic lobes injected with BSA and in noninjected lobes of the contralateral side.   The plasma cell population in the thymus was bigger in chickens injected with antigen into the thymus than in birds that received intravenously BSA or intrathymically saline.   A general increase in the number of medullary lymphocytes of all sizes appeared between the 1st and 7th day after intrathymic immunization.

Antibody production following injection of BSA into the thymus. Circulating anti-BSA antibodies appeared within 24 hours of the injection of antigen into the thymus, and increased in the following

Table II.　Antibody production following intrathymic injection of BSA.

Group	No. of chickens	Mean antibody titer ($\log_2$)			
		Days after immunization			
		1	3	5	7
Intrathymic injection of BSA	5	2.4 (0)	4.6 (3.4)	5.2 (3.4)	8.8 (5.2)
Intravenous injection of BSA	12	0	0	7.5 (6.3)	8.6 (6.7)

In parenthesis:　mean titer ($\log_2$) of mercaptoethanol-resistant anti-BSA.

days (Table II).　The mercaptoethanol-resistant antibody also made its appearance first in birds which received BSA by the intrathymic route.　The first detectable amount of anti-BSA antibody in intravenously injected birds was recorded after the third day of immunization.

Short Comment

The results reported in this paper show that a proliferation of blasts and plasma cells occurs in the thymus medulla following administration of bovine serum albumin directly into the thymic parenchyma. This provides further support for the belief that the chicken thymus is capable of participating in immune reactions, in this case in the production of antibody.

The question arises, however, as to which cells are reacting in the injected thymus.　Since the thymus is a composite organ, built of cells of different origin, including cells of nonthymic source, one would not expect the cells which responded to antigen to be proper thymic cells.　We believe, however, that reacting cells in the thymus are of thymus origin and/or uncommitted bone marrow cells that migrated to the thymus and acquired immunocompetence in the thymus.　In this respect, the thymus is similar to other "peripheral" or secondary lymphoid tissues which are also of a composite nature being made up of cells from different sources.　Therefore, if the composite nature of a secondary lymphoid tissue allows its effector activity in immune reactions, the same would hold for the thymus. Some embryological findings related to the maturation of lymphoid tissues (8) undoubtedly support the possibility that the chicken thymus may, under certain experimental conditions, exhibit the qualities of a secondary lymphoid organ.

In conclusion, previous evidence and results obtained in this experiment strongly suggests that the chicken thymus possesses not only the properties of a primary, but also some characteristics of a secondary lymphoid tissue.

ACKNOWLEDGMENT

This research was aided by grants from the Federal Scientific Fund, Belgrade.

REFERENCES

1. World Health Organization Technical Report Series, No. 448, "Factors Regulating the Immune Response," Geneva, 1970.

2. K. Isaković and B. D. Janković, in: H. Cottier, N. Odartchenko, R. Schindler and C. C Congdon, Eds., Germinal Centers in Immune Responses, p. 379. New York: Springer-Verlag, 1967.

3. B. D. Janković, K. Isaković, and D. Vujić, in: L. Fiore-Donati and M. G. Hanna, Jr., Eds., Lymphoid Tissue and Germinal Centers in Immune Response, Adv. Exp. Med. Biol., p. 269, New York: Plenum Press, 1969.

4. B. D. Janković and K. Mitrović, Folia Biol., 13:406, 1967.

5. B. D. Janković and K. Isaković, Experientia, 24:1272, 1968.

6. B. D. Janković, K. Isaković, S. Petrović, D. Vujić, and J. Horvat, Clin. Exp. Immunol., 7:709, 1970.

7. E. Orlans, Immunology, 14:61, 1968.

8. A. Romanoff, in: The Avian Embryo, p. 571. New York, Macmillan, 1960.

CHAIRMAN'S INTRODUCTION TO THE DISCUSSION

LYMPHATIC TISSUE AND GERMINAL CENTERS IN RELATION TO

ANTIBODY PRODUCTION

H. Cottier and B. Sordat

Department of Pathology, University of Bern

Bern, Switzerland

This introductory outline is an attempt to consider
some general ideas on lymphatic tissue and, in particular,
germinal centers, in relation to the complex process of
antibody production within the intact mammalian organism.
Little mention will be made of topics discussed in other
sessions, such as origin and interaction of immunologically active cells, cell kinetics, regulation of lymphatic
tissue function and tolerance. In the four years that
have elapsed since the first Conference in Bern, several
hypotheses regarding the role of lymph follicles have
come into clearer focus. We will first try to summarize
the essentials of the present knowledge in this field,
and then direct our interest to problems that are still
unresolved.

Comparative phylogenetic studies by Good and his associates (review: 1) have indicated that fishes equiped
with a thymus, but having no germinal centers, can produce plasma cells and synthesize both large (19S) and
small (7S) immunoglobulins that are probably most closely
related to IgM. The capacity to form 7S IgG in addition
to IgM type immunoglobulins is definitely established
in amphibians in which the first appearance of germinal
centers has been reported. This developmental correlation
may be regarded as suggestive evidence linking the germinal center system with synthesis and release of IgG type
of immunoglobulins. In mammals, germinal centers are
formed in lymphoreticular tissue in response to antigenic

stimulation as evidenced from early de novo formation
and rapid growth of these structures following secondary
antigenic stimulation (2). In contrast, newly formed
germinal centers appear only late in the course of a true
primary antibody response to non-complexed antigen (3,4).
Sequential studies on the ontogeny of antibody formation
in germfree piglets further emphasize the view that, in
a true primary response, germinal center formation is
not a prerequisit for either 19S or 7S antibody production
(5). Rather it would appear that germinal centers origin-
ate from presensitized and/or complex-stimulated cells
and represent sites of rapid multiplication of these
elements (3).

Since in a secondary antibody response extensive
lymphoid germinal center cell proliferation preceeds the
log phase of humoral antibody production, one wonders
what other function germinoblasts could have except that
of precursors which may ultimately develop into antibody forming cells. This notion, in order to be reasonable, would imply 1) that germinoblasts or germinocytes
migrate out of centers and reach other sites of the
lymphoreticular or other tissues and develop into plasma
cells and/or memory cells (6), and 2) that it may be
possible, at least during a certain phase of the process,
to detect small amounts of antibody within lymphoid germinal center cells. Migration of lymphoid germinal center
cells from the densely populated and heavily proliferating portion to the more loosely structured area of the
centers (7) and out into the adjacent lymphoid tissue (8)
has been demonstrated using tritiated thymidine as a cell
marker. Immunohistochemical and electron microscopic
studies on the human tonsil suggested differentiation
towards antibody-producing cells along this migrational
pathway in at least a fraction of the cells produced by
basal germinoblasts (9). With regard to the second postulate, although the presence of immunoglobulins within
germinal centers has long been noticed (10), their origin
is still controversial. White and his colleagues (review:
11) described antibody-containing cells within germinal
centers of chicken spleen from between 14 to 28 days following a primary intravenous injection of human serum albumin. In contrast, other authors (12) maintained that
in mammals,such as the rabbit, at least for 20 days after
either primary or secondary antigenic stimulation, immunoglobulins are not synthesized by cells in the germinal
centers but are deposited there as antigen-antibody

complexes with β_{1C}-globulin.

   To further elucidate this problem, we made use of
the antigenic and catalytic properties of plant enzymes
such as horseradish peroxidase (13) which retains most
of its enzymatic activity after combination with specific
antibody. This enzyme (HRP) can be used to visualize in
tissues and cells antigen or the corresponding antibody
by either light or electron microscopy. It was found that
lymphoid germinal center cells of popliteal lymph nodes
in mice contained anti-HRP antibody from 17 to 26 days
after primary injection of aluminum phosphate-adsorbed
HRP into the hind leg footpads (Fig. 1). Intercellular
anti-HRP, localized between dendritic reticular cells
and germinoblasts was not observed prior to the appearance
of intracellular antibody in lymphoid germinal center
cells. Both HRP and corresponding antibody persisted in
intercellular spaces for the rest of the observation
period, i.e. 35 days, while intracellular anti-HRP was
not detected later than 26 days after primary stimulation
(14,15). The presence, within the same stimulated lymph
node, of germinal centers which are either positive or

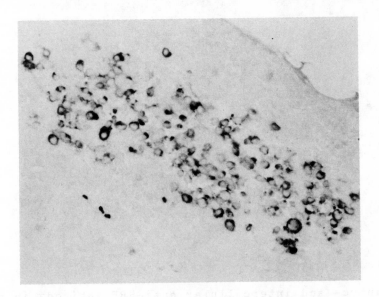

Fig. 1. Presence of anti-horseradish peroxidase (HRP) antibody in
lymphoid germinal center cells of a mouse popliteal lymph node,
20 days after primary stimulation with aluminum phosphate-
adsorbed HRP via the hind leg footpads. 250 x.

negative with regard to specific intracellular anti-HRP
antibody suggests monospecificity of individual centers,
at least for a certain period of time. In more recent
experiments, appearance of intracellular anti-HRP in
lymphoid germinal center cells during the anamnestic
antibody response was seen as early as 6 days following
booster injection into the hind leg footpads of mice
primed via the same route 77 days earlier (Fig. 2). Intercellular localization of antibody was again found to
be concomitant with intracellular anti-HRP (Fig. 3),
and persisted as long as 75 days. This reaction pattern
of germinal centers was paralleled by an increase in
numbers of anti-HRP positive plasma cells, particularly
in the medullary cords.

When HRP was incubated with the cut surface of lymph
node sections obtained from freeze-substitution, anti-
HRP antibody appeared to be evenly distributed throughout the cytoplasm of positive lymphoid germinal center
cells, whereas in electron microscopic preparations, antibody was most often confined to the perinuclear space.

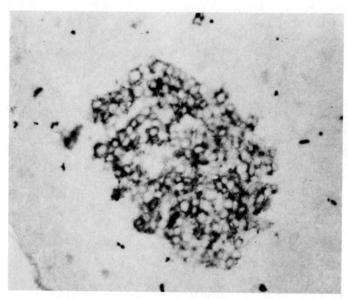

Fig. 2.   Intra- and intercellular anti-HRP antibody in a
germinal center of a mouse popliteal lymph node, 10 days
after a secondary injection of fluid antigen into the
hind leg footpads. The animal had been given a primary
stimulation as described in Fig. 1 87 days earlier. 400 x.

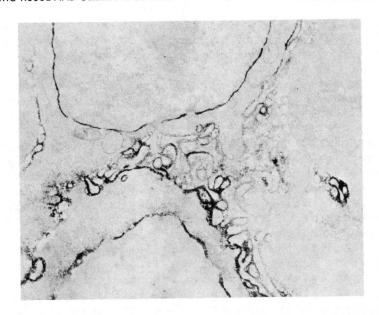

Fig. 3. Electron micrograph showing anti-HRP antibody
in the perinuclear space of lymphoid germinal center
cells and in the intercellular spaces between the former
and dendritic reticular cells. The popliteal lymph node
was obtained 17 days after a secondary stimulation via
the hind leg footpad. 20 000 x.

As discussed previously (15), the latter finding probably
does not reflect the true situation, in the sense that
HRP diffusion through tissue blocks prefixed with glutaraldehyde may be hindered by material or structures
such as intercellular antibody or surface and intracellular membranes. In addition, prefixation with glutaraldehyde may cause partial denaturation of immunoglobulins
(16).

    Since these findings strongly suggest antibody form-
ation by lymphoid germinal center cells, at least during
a certain phase of the antibody response, the phenomenon
of antigen-trapping in these structures (17) may well be
initiated and/or enhanced through corresponding antibody locally produced by lymphoid germinal center cells
(15). In addition, the well known sensitivity of the
mechanism responsible for antigen trapping in germinal
centers towards ionizing radiation (18,19,20) and other

immunosuppressive agents (21) may, at least in part, be
linked with destruction or repression of antibody-producing lymphoid germinal center cells.

It is probable that only a fraction of the antibody contained within germinal centers is produced locally by germinoblasts since strong evidence points towards entry of circulating immunoglobulins into the intercellular spaces of these structures (22). The view that
lymphoid germinal center cells are more important as precursors of plasma cells than as active antibody producing
elements has received additional support from irradiation
experiments indicating different degrees of radiosensitivity of germinoblasts as compared to immature and mature
plasma cells. Stoner and Hale (23) reported that secondary tetanus antitoxin responses in mice were abolished
when whole body radiation in doses of 650 and 800 rads
were delivered by short term exposure three hours before
to one day after the booster injection of antigen. Nearly
normal secondary responses were obtained, however, if the
same radiation doses were given 4 days after secondary antigenic stimulation, and the sera were titrated 6 days later.
It could be demonstrated in addition that tritiated L-
histidine was readily incorporated into antitoxin produced during secondary responses when injected repeatedly from days 4 to 7 after booster stimulation with tetanus
toxoid, i.e. 1 to 3 days following whole body irradiation.
Sera obtained 10 days after the second stimulus under
these conditions showed no difference between irradiated
mice and controls with regard to tritium activity of
washed antigen-antibody precipitates. These results indicated that during this period antibody was actively
produced in irradiated animals at the same rate as in
controls, and was not merely released from damaged cells.
We have correlated these findings with cellular and
histological changes and with autoradiographs of lymph
nodes regional to the site of secondary antigenic stimulation. Lymphoid germinal center cells that were newly
formed after the booster injection of antigen rapidly
disintegrated after radiation on day 4 and remnant germinal center areas remained devoid of germinoblasts throughout a period of at least 3 days following radiation exposure. Good survival of cells was observed, however,
in the medullary cords where numerous plasmocytoid precursors and plasma cells had resisted the radiation
damage. If under the same conditions, sera for titration
were obtained not on the 10th but on the 32nd day after

the second stimulus, tetanus antitoxin concentration in
the blood of irradiated animals was only half that of
unirradiated controls. It appears, therefore, that pratic-
ally all the antibody produced in irradiated animals between 4 and 7 days after secondary stimulation, i.e. 1
to 3 days after radiation, originated from plasmocytoid
cells outside germinal centers, but that with time a
lack of antibody producing elements became apparent. It
is conceivable that radiation-induced destruction of
lymphoid germinal center cells may ultimately lead to an
insufficient supply of plasma cell precursors.

Although much evidence associates or even identifies
lymphoid germinal center cells with immature precursors
of antibody producing cell lines, many problems related
to their origin, behavior and role remain unresolved.
The following is meant to be a sketchy catalogue of
questions which will have to be answered by further experimentation.

Why do germinal centers form where they do, i.e. in
mammals usually within primary lymphoid follicles of
spleen, lymph nodes and other lymphoreticular organs or
at ectopic sites in other tissues? Is this phenomenon
associated with, and subsequent to, fixation of antigen
on the surface of particular dendritic reticulum cells;
to prefenrential channels or other ways of access and
retention of antigen; to special patterns of diffusion
within lymphoreticular tissue; or a combination of such
and other factors?

What triggers the germinal center system to grow in
the course of a true primary antibody response? Is it
possible that the presence of complexed antigen is a prerequisit for this cell line to multiply and differentiate
into antibody-producing elements?

Do germinoblasts within one and the same germinal
center represent true clones originating from a single
cell or is a center formed by initial aggregation of
lymphoid cells? We have no kinetic data answering this
question.

Are antigen-containing lymphoid cells within one and
the same germinal center monospecific with regard to the
antigen that stimulated their growth? There is evidence
that materials and proteins other than one specific

antibody and complement may enter and be retained in intercellular spaces of the centers.

Does antibody contained within germinoblasts of one and the same germinal center belong to one, or more than one, subclass of immunoglobulins? If the latter is true, would this mean that germinal centers are not real clones, or that cells of the same line may switch from the production of one type of immunoglobulin to that of other types?

What are the causes of cell death within germinal centers? To what extent does this phenomenon prevent newly formed cells from leaving the centers during an immune response, and what possible meaning could there be in this close topographic relation of cell proliferation and disintegration?

Why can intracellular antibody, such as anti-HRP, in germinoblasts be detected only during certain phases of germinal center development? Is this phenomenon related to shifts in the degree of cellular differentiation; to changing turnover rates of antibody within cells; to repression of antibody synthesis by excess antibody in the surrounding intercellular spaces; to varying affinity of antibody; or a combination of such and other mechanisms?

What is the ultimate fate of emigrating lymphoid germinal center cells? Do they in fact reach the lymph, blood and other sites of the body to develop into plasma cells or memory cells? Final evidence to support this view is still lacking.

SUMMARY

Some of the evidence identifying or associating germinal center cells with immature precursors of certain antibody producing cell lines is reviewed, and an account is given of unresolved problems which may be clarified by further experimentation.

This work was supported by the Swiss National Foundation for Scientific Research and the US Atomic Energy Commission.

REFERENCES

1. R.A. Gatti, O. Stutman and R.A. Good, Ann. Rev. Physiol., 32:529, 1970.

2. H. Cottier, N. Odartchenko, G. Keiser, M. Hess and R.D. Stoner, Ann. N.Y. Acad. Sci., 113:612, 1964.

3. H. Cottier, G. Keiser, N. Odartchenko, M. Hess and R.D. Stoner, in: H. Cottier, N. Odartchenko, R. Schindler and C.C. Congdon, Eds., Germinal Centers in Immune Responses, p. 270. Berlin-Heidelberg-New York: Springer 1967.

4. J. Laissue, R.D. Stoner, M.W. Hess and H. Cottier, in: Proc. 3rd Internat. Conference on Lymphatic Tissue and Germinal Centers in Immune Reactions, Uppsala, 1970 (in press).

5. Y.B. Kim and D.W. Watson, in: Proc. 3rd Internat. Conference on Lymphatic Tissue and Germinal Centers in Immune Reactions, Uppsala, 1970.

6. G.J. Thorbecke, R. Asofsky, G.M. Hochwald and G.W. Siskind, Fed. Proc., 20:25, 1961.

7. M.G. Hanna, Jr., Lab. Invest., 13:95, 1964.

8. E. Koburg, in: H. Cottier, N. Odartchenko, R. Schindler and C.C. Congdon, Eds., Germinal Centers in Immune Responses, p. 176. Berlin-Heidelberg-New York: Springer 1967.

9. B. Sordat, R. Moser, H. Gerber and H. Cottier, in: L. Fiore-Donati and M.G. Hanna, Jr., Eds., Lymphatic Tissue and Germinal Centers in Immune Response, p. 73. New York: Plenum Press, 1969.

10. A.H. Coons, E.H. Leduc and J.M. Connolly, Fed. Proc., 12:439, 1953.

11. R.G. White, V.I. French and J.M. Stark, in: H. Cottier, N. Odartchenko, R. Schindler and C.C. Congdon, Eds., Germinal Centers in Immune Responses, p. 131. Berlin-Heidelberg-New York: Springer 1967.

12. K.J. Gajl-Peczalska, A.J. Fish, H.J. Meuwissen, D. Frommel and R.A. Good, J. exp. Med., 130:1367, 1969.

13. S. Avrameas and G. Lespinats, C.R. Acad. Sci. Paris, 265:302, 1967.

14. B. Sordat, M. Sordat and H. Cottier, C.R. Acad. Sci. Paris, 268:1556, 1969.

15. B. Sordat, M. Sordat, M.W. Hess, R.D. Stoner and H. Cottier, J. exp. Med., 131:77, 1970.

16. J.P. Kraehenbuhl and M.A. Campiche, J. Cell Biol., 42:345, 1969.

17. G.J.V. Nossal, G.L. Ada and C.M. Austin, Aust. J. exp. Biol. Med. Sci., 42:311, 1964.

18. B.N. Jaroslow and G.J.V. Nossal, Fed. Proc., 25:612, 1966.

19. R.L. Hunter, R.W. Wissler and F.W. Fitch, in: L. Fiore-Donati and M.G. Hanna, Jr., Eds., Lymphatic Tissue and Germinal Centers in Immune Response, p. 101. New York: Plenum Press 1969.

20. P. Nettesheim and M.G. Hanna, Jr., in: L. Fiore-Donati and M.G. Hanna, Jr., Eds., Lymphatic Tissue and Germinal Centers in Immune Response, p.167. New York: Plenum Press, 1969.

21. P. Nettesheim and A.S. Hammons, Proc. Soc. exp. Biol. Med., 133:696, 1970.

22. B. Pernis, G. Chiappino, A. Kelus and P.G.H. Gell, J. exp. Med., 122:853, 1965.

23. R.D. Stoner and W.M. Hale, N.Y.St. J. Med., 63:691, 1963.

M. Feldman: I think one should distinguish between the germinal centers as an organized structure and the individual germinal center cells. Dr. Cottier, do you need the organized structure of the germinal centers to get a primary immune response, immunological memory and a secondary response or any other immune response? After all we can induce immune responses in cell suspensions in vitro under conditions where no germinal centers form.

H. Cottier: There is no evidence showing that germinal center formation is a prerequisite for the production of a particular class or subclass of immunoglobulins. However, in intact animals it just happens that some of the cells that proliferate in response to antigenic stimulation do so in a rather closed area. This phenomenon is concomitant with the ability of the organism to give very efficient anamnestic antibody responses. Since we know that in a true primary response the germinal center development occurs only late in the process, i.e. considerably later than antibodies are first being formed, it appears that this type of reaction is more closely related to secondary antibody responses than to primary responses. As far as the type of immunoglobulin produced in these structures are concerned, several observations seem to indicate that in the human it may be particularly 7S IgG antibody, and in mice maybe the γ_2 antibody. These suggestions, however, await further confirmation.

M.G. Hanna: I would like to comment on Dr. Feldman's question. We have raised this point several times at the two previous meetings. The answer probably rests in the recent data that demonstrate antibody production in in vitro systems. When unprimed spleen cells are stimulated with antigen, either in the Mishell-Dutton system or in Millipore diffusion chambers, one gets good IgM responses but feeble or absent IgG_2 production. With primed cells IgG_2 production is achieved. This may stress the requirement for tissue organisation, such as germinal centers, for a complete primary immune response with development of immunologic memory.

R.K. Gershon: There is one form of the immune response that as far as I know has never taken place in the absence of germinal center formation; that is the maturation to high affinity antibodies that occurs in the immune response.

J. Linna: You can also get germinal center formation as a non-immunological phenomenon within a few hours after endotoxin administration, probably without any cell proliferation. There may be germinal centers of different kinds, we are not speaking of a single structure with a single function.

213

W. Pierpaoli: If you perform neonatal thymectomy in certain strains
of mice you have a diminished response to SRBC and you have no
germinal center formation in the spleen. If you perform early
gonadectomy of these mice, you prevent the effects of some hormones
which antagonistically to other hormones regulate the formation of
lymphoid tissue. You then observe the formation of gigantic lymphoid
follicles and germinal centers in the spleen, of these thymectomized
and gonadectomized mice, but you don't reconstitute the immune
capacity of these animals. Therefore the function of germinal centers
could be to amplify the immune response once the cells are available.
Otherwise it can be simply expressed as cell proliferation under
other non-specific circumstances when the right cells are not available, as after neonatal thymectomy.

M.D. Cooper: Some agammaglobulinemic patients have been seen who
make germinal centers but lack any antibody forming cells detectable
with immunofluorescent techniques. Morphologically these germinal
centers are not distinguishable from normal germinal centers, at
least at the light microscopic level. These observations suggest
that cells can respond by proliferating in the usual germinal center
configuration and location in the absence of antibody and without
the capability of making detectable amounts of antibody themselves.

H. Cottier: I would go along with this statement and add the trivial
remark that not every structure that is round and contains proliferating blasts is necessarily a germinal center. One would have to
know what the potential differentiation pathways of these cells are.
Therefore, it is important to show that lymphoid germinal center
cells do contain specific antibody, at least during a certain phase
of the antibody response.

     As to the precursor cells which form the germinal centers they
may well be presensitized cells and/or, as Dr. Laissue will discuss
later, cells stimulated by immune complexes instead of antigen only.
The question arises as to whether or not the presence of immune
complexes is a prerequisite for germinal center development to occur.

N.R. Sinclair: Dr. Cottier, what differences have you obtained between the localization of antigen or antibody in these germinal
centers?

H. Cottier: If one looks only for the presence of antigen, there
are small groups of HRP-positive particles between germinal center
cells and dendritic reticular elements and not this nice covering
and outlining of dendritic cell surfaces that you find when you
stain for anti-HRP antibody.

M. Smith: As Dr. Kim said, the pig lymph node is inside out when
compared to those of other animals. The pig is also unusual, in
that, as Drs. Haland Binns showed three or four years ago, there

are very few lymphocytes in the efferent lymph. The pig is different to other animals in that very few lymphocytes are returned to
the blood via the lymph. The "recirculation" of lymphocytes occurs
within the loosely organized structure of the lymph node blood
vessels.

Y.B. Kim: I agree. Pigs also have high numbers of lymphocytes in
the circulation: more than 60-70% of the white blood cells are
lymphocytes.

A.G. Jonson: Dr. Kim, do your piglets respond with delayed hypersensitivity reactions to actinophage and if so, how can you differentiate the reactions you have shown from those in delayed hypersensitivity?

Y.B. Kim: Recently we used highly purified pneumococcal polysaccharide and Vi antigen which, known to give only humoral antibody
response, gave similar results. This indicates that the cellular
response is related to the humoral antibody response, but any combination with delayed hypersensitivity cannot be completely ruled
out.

Furthermore, when we used foci assay for specific antibody
formation according to Dr. Fitch et al. (ref. No. 21), the periarteriolar sheaths coincide with the antibody producing foci. Also
in our preliminary observations on the fine structure of the immune
response, we found that some of the pyroninophilic cells in the
periarteriolar sheaths and the single cells by the plaque assay for
antibody-forming cells are similar. Therefore, there are antibody-
forming cells in the periarteriolar sheaths.

O. Mäkelä: Dr. Kim, are colostrum-deprived piglets healthy? I seem
to remember that colostrum-deprived calves die within a few weeks.

Y.B. Kim: Colostrum-deprived piglets all die within five days when
kept in conventional environment. Without colostrum they are highly
susceptible to environmental micro-organisms. That is why they
are kept in germ-free isolators.

R. Gallily: Dr. French, how do you explain the fall of the antibody
titre 12 days after the injection of the antigen with Freund´s
complete adjuvans? Did you inject higher doses of the antigen and
receive the same fall of antibody titres?

V. French: We have used various doses, the highest dose used was
40 mg and the lowest dose 40 µg. While the peak response is higher
the final pattern is the same. You get the fall again after the
12th day. This peak is very constant whether you vary the dose or
whether you use Freund´s adjuvans. I have no explanation for it.

V. Stejskal: Did you find any differences in the molecular types of
antibodies in chickens which have been immunized with HSA with or
without Freund´s adjuvans? Did you use also another method that is
more sensitive for detecting IgM antibodies, e.g. passive haemagglutination? It is well known that Farr´s antigen-binding technique
detects preferentially IgG types of antibodies.

V. French: We have not investigated in great detail the type of
antibody produced after Freund´s adjuvant. As far as we can tell
it is mainly IgG type whether you put the antigen in Freund´s or
saline. I take issue with you on the failure to detect IgM antibody by the Farr technique. You can increase the sensitivity for
IgM antibody by decreasing the amount of the antigen added. We
have done this on occasion. We feel we detect all types of antibody.

H. Friedman: Your data show that late in the primary antibody
response, when the granuloma tissue contains high levels of antibody and the spleen very low amounts, the bursa and the thymus contain 2-3 times more extractable antibody than the spleen. Have you
looked for antibody-forming cells in these organs as did Dr. Jankovic?

V. French: We found no antibody-forming cells in the bursa and the
thymus, using the fluorescent antibody technique. The difference
in the antibody content may be associated with the blood supply to
these organs. The thymus and bursa do not contain nearly as much
antibody as the granuloma.

H.L. Langevoort: One of the early features of the germinal center
reaction is the appearance of tingible bodies and macrophages. You
could say that with your granuloma you create an artificial germinal
center. Have you studied the histology of the granuloma with regard
to the appearance of tingible bodies?

V. French: No, but we would like to do so.

M. Feldman: When an antigen is injected into an organism many processes are initiated. They may be classified in three categories:
1) One category of processes that determine whether or not antibody
will be formed. 2) Processes associated with the control of the
quantitative levels of antibody. 3) Processes that take place, but
are irrelevant to antibody production. Dr. Cruchaud, in what category would you classify the interaction between macrophages and red
blood cells?

A. Cruchaud: In the in vitro induction of the immune response to
sheep red blood cells at least two populations of cells are necessary.
These are lymphoid cells and macrophages. The handling of red blood
cells by macrophages seems to be a necessary step. This does not

imply that in any situation the uptake and handling of antigen by macrophages result in an immune response. It is entirely possible, for instance, that the uncompletely degraded product released by macrophages following endocytosis may be tolerogenic rather than immunogenic.

R. Gallily: Dr. Cruchaud, do you exclude the possibility that antigen might be stored in the vesicles or other cellular compartments of the macrophage without being catabolized by lysosomal enzymes. In addition to its effect on the plasma membrane, does trypsin treatment alter some function of the macrophages, thereby reducing antigen immunogenicity in them?

A. Cruchaud: We trypsinized the macrophages containing sheep red cells after one hour in culture and then again after 18 hours, or only after 18 hours. Most of the material present on the plasma membrane was released within the first hour and only a small amount in the following hours. The total amount of material released from the plasma membrane by two trypsinizations after 1 and 18 hours was the same as the amount released by one trypsinization at 18 hrs. Thus we assume that treatment with trypsin did not influence the behaviour of material present in the phagocytic vacuoles.

M.W. Hess: Dr. Cruchaud, do the macrophages in your transfer experiments have to be alive?

A. Cruchaud: We did not transfer dead macrophages. Other workers have, however. In my laboratory in Geneva, for instance, Dr. Jean-Pierre Despont has tried to induce an immune response in mice by transferring macrophages first incubated with human gammaglobulin and then killed by freezing and thawing. The response elicited with dead macrophages was much smaller than with live macrophages.

A.G. Johnson: We have done similar experiments. If you render the cells non-viable with actinomycin D, you prevent the response. Does the material excreted or the second peak you observe after catabolism contain detectable amounts of bound RNA?

A. Cruchaud: We did not assay for RNA in the supernatant of cultures of macrophages containing sheep red cells. The material released in the supernatant was slightly immunogenic. It did not induce a primary response in recipients, but it primed them for a secondary response. After RNA-ase treatment, this material still primed for a secondary response. Therefore, in our system, an association between immunogenic material and RNA was not a prerequisite for priming.

J.F.A.P. Miller: Dr. Jankovic, did you have evidence to show that the cytological changes which occur in your chicken thymuses are in fact the result of antigen-induced differentiation of thymus

cells? Could they not be the result of differentiation of cells
coming from elsewhere: say bursa-derived cells? Do these changes
occur in bursectomized birds? Has anyone before found such remarkable changes in the chicken thymus after antigenic stimulation?

B.D. Jankovic: You suggest that cells reacting in the thymus following intrathymic administration of antigen are immigrants. Then you
do not take into account that not only the thymus but also other
lymphoid organs, in particular the spleen and bursa, are of composite
nature. Dr. Fichtelius has suggested that the thymus, as well as
other lymphoid organs are in fact "epithelial-mesenchymal symbioses".
Furthermore, the traffic of lymphoid cells is so extensive that it
would be rather unwise to attribute the characteristic of being a
composite organ to the thymus, and to use this as an argument against
the possibility that the thymus is capable of taking a direct part
in immune reactions. Indeed, why is it that the composite nature
of the spleen, for example, enables its engagement in the immune
response while the composite nature of the thymus prevents its
direct participation in immune reactions? With respect to this, it
seems to me that the importance attaches more to the question,
which cell is immunologically reactive, not which organ. So far
as bursectomized chickens are concerned, the experiments are in
progress in our laboratory.

M.G. Hanna: Dr. Miller, I will show later that by intrathymic injection of Gross virus, germinal centers are induced in the thymus
of 12 weeks old AKR mice. These changes were essentially like those
described by Metcalf as pre-leukaemic, occurring in 8 weeks old
AKR mice. The follicles form around the dendritic reticulum cells
which have trapped the virus extracellularly. I must point out,
however, that these follicles were extrathymic but within the
medulla.

J. Linna: Dr. Miller, the presence of germinal centers in the normal
thymus is a fairly normal feature in the older chicken. They are
presumably part of the bursa-derived thymus cell population.

M.L. Warner: I would like to strongly take issue with Dr. Jankovic´s
implication that the thymus is acting in a sense as a central organ
for inducing the differentiation of antibody-producing cells. We
have to distinguish between several interpretations of the function
of a primary organ. I think the only valid interpretation is that
it is the site of induced differentiation of the true immunocompetent cell. Later on, that cell may possibly collaborate in the
Miller and Mitchell collaboration sense, following antigenic stimulation. It is also possible that later in life the primary organ
may receive peripheral cells. As Dr. Thorbecke showed 13 years ago,
the thymus can develop germinal centers, but only after a few months
of life. The essential point is that the young chicken thymus, in
the embryo and during the neonatal period, shows no germinal centers

and no evidence of immunoglobulin synthesis. When immunoglobulin synthesis does start in the thymus, it is of G-type and not M-type which suggests that an immigration of a population of cells into the thymus has occurred. I think the parameters that you have taken to indicate that the thymus is involved in antibody production, are all explicable in terms of entry of antigen and immigrant cells. The only data that is out of line with this interpretation is your point concerning anti-chicken thymus globulin. The intriguing possibility arises that in chickens "T" cells are also involved in antibody synthesis. Even if they are, this still does not make the thymus a primary organ in terms of antibody production. Are your antisera, used for eliminating "T" cells in chickens, completely unreactive against bursal cells and against antibody-producing cells?

B.D. Jankovic: Thymus cells derived from sensitized thymus, i.e. thymus injected with antigen, were fully capable of passively transferring antibody production in normal chickens. Further, the intrathymic injection of human 0 red blood cells induced the appearance of a large number of plaque-forming cells in the thymus, bursa and spleen.

According to our concept, the thymus is not only a "central" lymphoid organ, but also takes a direct part in immune responses like "peripheral" lymphoid tissues. We think that the formidable augmentation of plasma cells in the thymus following appropriate stimulation, cannot be attributed exclusively to the proliferation of cells of non-thymic origin. In the embryo the bone marrow, which is the chief place of both red and white blood cell formation in adult chickens, is the last tissue in which lymphocytopoiesis begins. On the other hand, the thymus is the first functioning lymphoid organ in the chicken embryo. Therefore, the first lymphoid cells that occur in the thymus are not of bone marrow origin.

Finally, both rabbit anti-chicken thymus and anti-bursa sera exhibited very similar serological activity when tested by leucoagglutination, passive haemagglutination and cytotoxic reaction. However, they differed substantially when injected into the chicken. For example, anti-thymus globulin suppressed the development of experimental allergic encephalomyelitis whereas anti-bursa globulin failed to affect this autoallergic disease.

SESSION 5. LOCALIZATION OF ANTIGEN AND IMMUNE COMPLEXES IN
LYMPHATIC TISSUE WITH SPECIAL REFERENCE TO GERMINAL CENTERS
CHAIRMAN, M. G. HANNA, JR., CO-CHAIRMAN, R. L. HUNTER

THE MECHANISM OF ANTIGEN LOCALIZATION IN LYMPHOID FOLLICLES AND THE

PATTERNS OF LOCALIZATION OF TOLERANCE-INDUCING FLAGELLAR PROTEINS

C. R. Parish and G. L. Ada

Department of Microbiology, John Curtin School of

Medical Research, Canberra, A.C.T., Australia

If an antigenic protein is labelled to high specific
activity with a suitable isotope, such as iodine-125, and either
injected subcutaneously into an animal and the localization
pattern of the label in the draining lymph examined, or reacted
in vitro with a cell suspension prepared from spleen or lymph
node, three main types of cells can be seen to have reacted with
the antigen.   These cells are (1) macrophages, such as those
lining the medullary sinuses in lymph nodes; (2) the dendritic
cell as it occurs in the primary lymphoid follicle of lymph
nodes (in vivo only); and (3) lymphocytes.   Of these, only
one type of cell is fundamentally concerned in the process of
antibody production and tolerance.   This is the lymphocyte
as shown beyond reasonable doubt by the recent work of Shortman,
Diener, Russell and Armstrong (1970).   As far as the two
processes - antibody production and tolerance - are concerned,
it now seems most unlikely that antigen located in lymphoid
follicles is active in a way that cannot be duplicated in tissue
culture where this anatomical structure is not present.   Thus,
if we ask the question - what is the special function of antigen
localized in lymphoid follicles? - it is unlikely that we will
get a clear cut answer indicating a unique function.   Such an
answer might have been for example, that only antigen in
lymphoid follicles can induce either antibody formation or
tolerance, or even that this type of localization ensures that
one or the other of these results will occur.   Rather, what we
may find is that antigen held on the surface of dendritic cells
in lymphoid follicles may be more efficient at carrying out a
particular function than is unfixed or circulating antigen.   To
establish such a role, however, will not be easy.

221

MECHANISM OF ANTIGEN LOCALIZATION IN LYMPHOID FOLLICLES

To investigate the phenomenon of follicular localization of antigen, a first step was to establish the mechanism of interaction between antigen and dendritic cells. This work has mainly been described elsewhere (e.g. Nossal and Ada, 1970) and the main points will merely be summarized here.

1. As far as we are aware, all antigens will localize in lymphoid follicles if antibody is present. This antibody may be either "natural" antibody or specific antibody occurring as a result of sensitization by that antigen. In fact, it has been proposed by others (e.g. Humphrey and Frank, 1967) and we entirely concur, that follicular localization is an extremely sensitive test for the presence of antibody.

2. Antigen-antibody complexes, using syngeneic, allogeneic or xenogeneic antibody, localize in lymphoid follicles of rats, rabbits and mice (Lang and Ada, 1967a). It might be thought that the follicle is simply a means of trapping particulate material. This is not so. A soluble antigen which, upon injection, does not localize in follicles still does not localize there after injection in an aggregated form (Lang and Ada, 1967b).

3. IgG, either syngeneic, allogeneic or xenogeneic, will localize in lymphoid follicles of rats or rabbits. When fragments of rabbit IgG were injected into rats, only those fragments which contained the Fc portion of the molecule (Fc, heavy chain) localized in the lymphoid follicles. However, rabbit Fab localized in the follicles of rabbit nodes and rat Fab in the follicles of rat nodes. This suggested the presence of an anti-globulin antibody reacting with syngeneic Fab (Herd and Ada, 1969).

4. Human serum albumin (HSA) complexed with rabbit anti-HSA IgG localized in rat lymphoid follicles. HSA complexed with Fab, prepared from rabbit anti-HSA IgG, did not (Herd and Ada, 1969).

These results are consistent with the notion that antibody acts as the bridge between the dendritic cell membrane and antigen. It may be that occasionally a substance will be found to localize in lymphoid follicles, and antibody cannot be implicated in the process. Further work is needed here. We stress our opinion however, that antibody mediated localization is the mechanism of physiological importance.

A POSSIBLE ROLE FOR ANTIGEN LOCALIZED IN LYMPHOID FOLLICLES

If the prime mechanism of follicular localization of antigen

is antibody-mediated, it seems not unreasonable to postulate
that there may be some connection between this process and the
biological effects caused by the presence of antibody.   The
latter has been reviewed by Uhr and Möller (1968).   The principle
effects are (1) Injection of antigen with specific antibody
usually inhibits a primary antibody response.   (2) It is much
more difficult to inhibit a secondary antibody response in this
way.   (3) It appears that antibody may react in two ways.
The first is the masking of an antigenic determinant because
of its reaction with the specific antibody.   The second, more
recent evidence, which seems to be completely clear cut (Feldman
and Diener, 1970), is that antigen in the presence of specific
antibody, inactivates antigen-reactive cells (tolerance).   Two
years ago, we suggested (Ada and Parish, 1968) that an important
role for antigen localized in lymphoid follicles was to induce
tolerance (inactivation of antigen reactive cells).   More
recent evidence is consistent with this hypothesis and we would
like to conclude by referring to it here.

In discussing the mechanism of immunological paralysis,
Dresser and Mitchison (1968) refer to a category of antigens which
they term non-immunogenic.   The principle example in this
category is IgG.   In the absence of adjuvant, this globulin
induces tolerance but not antibody production.   Furthermore, the
threshold dose for tolerance induction is low (Mitchison, 1964).
As we have seen, IgG localizes well in lymphoid follicles of
several species.

The second aspect which favoured this notion was the
localization pattern of flagellar antigens.   Three such antigens,
prepared from the flagella from Salmonella adelaide were
available.   They were the monomeric flagellin molecule
(molecular weight, 40,000), a linear polymer of this, polymerized
flagellin, and a fragment of the monomer (fragment A) which had
a molecular weight of 18,000 and retained most if not all of the
serological properties of the monomer (Parish and Ada, 1969).   The
in vivo properties of these materials were interesting.   When
placed in a hierarchy in terms of their immunogenicity (injection
in saline into adult rats) the following sequence was found: -
polymerized flagellin > flagellin > fragment A, the latter being
almost non-immunogenic.   When tested for their ability to induce
tolerance in adult rats (injection in multiple doses during a
4 week period), the reverse was found.   Only fragment A was
effective at inducing tolerance, the doses given being 100 µg per
day.   When the response of adult rats to different doses of
fragment A was studied, another dose range was found where partial
tolerance occurred (low zone tolerance).   The dose level was
100 femtograms per day or about 10^8 molecules of fragment A
during a 4 week injection schedule.   As the adult rat contains
> 10^9 lymphocytes and as only a small portion of the injected

fragment A would lodge in the lymphoid organs, it seemed
mandatory to suppose that fragment A was selectively and
effectively concentrated in the body in a location where it
could contact circulating lymphocytes.   The follicular-type
of localization seemed well suited for this.   Upon investigation
fragment A, as did both the monomer and polymer, was seen to
localize well in follicles but in contrast to the other two,
poorly in the medulla.   More recently it has been found (Parish,
in preparation) that if flagellin is heavily substituted with
acetoacetyl groups, the resulting product has almost no
immunogenicity, but is an excellent tolerogen, a single
injection in saline of as little as 1 μg into adult rats causing
an almost complete suppression of antibody formation after a
subsequent injection of flagellin.   As well as causing this
type of tolerance however, rats so treated have an enhanced
susceptibility to delayed type hypersensitivity.   We do not
wish at this stage to discuss the possible inter-relationship
of these two types of activities but merely to point out that
these substituted flagellins, upon labelling with isotope
injection into rats, also predominantly localize in lymphoid
follicles.

The last piece of evidence concerning the role of antigen in
follicles to tolerance induction I wish to mention comes from
the work of Diener and Feldman (1970).   In their in vitro
tissue culture system, they have shown that whereas polymerized
flagellin and flagellin may cause either immunity or tolerance,
according to the dose of antigen used, fragment A causes neither.
However, in the presence of a given amount of specific antibody,
fragment A causes specific tolerance.   These authors consider
that the antibody helps to focus the antigen onto the surface of
the antigen reactive cell and tolerance ensues.   It is simple
to point out the similarity of the two patterns.   Follicular
localization can be represented thus;   dendritic cell membrane-
antibody-antigen, the latter reacting with the receptors of
appropriate lymphocytes: and in vitro, the pattern would be;
antibody-antigen-lymphocyte receptor.

It has become clear that the decision between antibody
production or tolerance is essentially a matter of antigen
presentation at the lymphocyte surface.   The arguments we have
used above do not preclude antigen localized in follicles having
a role other than tolerance induction.   In view of the known
difficulty of inhibiting a secondary immune response by added
antibody, antigen in the follicle may be well placed to stimulate
primed cells, as distinct from unprimed cells.

In conclusion, these results do not prove that antigen in
lymphoid follicles specifically induces tolerance.   They present
supporting but indirect evidence.   What is needed is for

Pharmacia to prepare giant size Sephadex beads or cylinders of
internal pore size about 50 microns.   If these were lined with
antibody and then antigen, we would have a synthetic follicle
through which we could slowly circulate cells.   Cells so
treated could then be tested for their biological activity.

REFERENCES

Ada, G.L. and Parish, C.R. (1968). Proc. Nat. Acad. Sci. 61, 556.
Diener, E. and Feldman, M. (1970). J. exp. Med. In press.
Dresser, D.W. and Mitchison, N.A. (1968). Adv. Immunol. 8, 129.
Feldman, M. and Diener, E. (1970). J. exp. Med. 131, 247.
Herd, Z.L. and Ada, G.L. (1969). Aust. J. exp. Biol. med. Sci.
    47, 73.
Humphrey, J.H. and Frank, M.M. (1967). Immunology, 13, 87.
Lang, P.G. and Ada, G.L. (1967a). Immunology, 13, 523.
Lang, P.G. and Ada, G.L. (1967b). Aust. J. exp. Biol. med. Sci.
    45, 445.
Mitchison, N.A. (1964). Proc. Roy. Soc. B161, 275.
Nossal, G.J.V. and Ada, G.L. (1970). In "Antigens, Lymphoid
    Cells and the Immune Response" Academic Press. New York. In
    press.
Parish, C.R. and Ada, G.L. (1969). Immunology 17, 153.
Shortman, K.D., Diener, E., Russell, P. and Armstrong, W.D. (1970).
    J. exp. Med. 131, 461.
Uhr, J.W. and Moller, G. (1968). Adv. Immunol. 8, 81.

ACCELERATED AND ENHANCED GERMINAL CENTER DEVELOPMENT IN REGIONAL LYMPH NODES OF MICE FOLLOWING PRIMARY STIMULATION WITH ANTIGEN-ANTIBODY COMPLEXES AS COMPARED TO ANTIGEN ONLY

J.Laissue, R.D.Stoner*, M.W.Hess and H.Cottier
Institute of Pathology, University of Bern,
Switzerland
* Medical Research Center, Brookhaven National
Laboratory, Upton, L.I., N.Y. 11973, U.S.A.

In earlier studies (1,2) enhanced primary tetanus antitoxin responses were obtained in mice immunized with antigen-antibody complexes at equivalence, as compared to antibody responses following antigenic stimulation with the same amount of fluid tetanus toxoid only. In an attempt to correlate potentiated antibody formation with morphological changes, the appearance and growth of germinal centers in lymph nodes regional to the site of a primary injection of either immune complexes or antigen only were analyzed. Such a comparison appeared to be of interest in the light of present views regarding lymphoid germinal center cells as proliferating immature antibody forming elements (review: 3).

MATERIALS AND METHODS

Specific pathogen-free female Swiss albino mice of the Hale-Stoner, BNL strain were used. At the age of 8 to 12 weeks, 2 groups of 90 mice each were stimulated by a primary injection of antigen via both hindleg footpads. The first group of animals was given a dose of fluid tetanus toxoid corresponding to 20 000 MLD of active toxin. The second group received the same amount of antigen in complex with isologous antitoxin at equivalence. Ten nonstimulated mice served as controls.

Ten mice of each group were killed 4,8,12,16,20,24,

227

28,32 and 36 days after primary antigenic stimulation.
Antitoxin titers of the pooled sera were determined by
a toxin neutralization test according to Ehrlich. All
animals received a single i.v. injection of ^{3}H-thymidine
(Schwarz BioResearch Laboratories, specific activity
1.9 Ci/mmole, dose 1 μCi/g body weight, administered as
an isotonic saline solution with a concentration of
100 μCi/ml) 1 hour before sacrifice. Popliteal lymph
nodes were removed and processed for histology and autoradiography. Cut surfaces of germinal centers were measured in serial cross sections of lymph nodes as described
previously (4).

Autoradiographs were obtained after an exposure time
of 200 days. Following correction for background, germinal center cells with more than 3 grains over their nucleus
were registered as labeled.

Statistical evaluation of the data was based on a
χ^2-test modified by Smirnow and Dunin-Barkowski (5).

RESULTS

Enhanced antitoxin production in mice following
stimulation with antigen in complex with isologous antitoxin appears to be correlated with the development of
germinal centers in lymph nodes regional to the site of
antigen injection.

Histometric evaluation of popliteal lymph node cross
sections revealed that the total cut surface occupied by
germinal centers increased in size earlier and reached
significantly higher values in animals stimulated with
immune complexes than in mice which were given antigen
only.

As demonstrated in Fig. 1, complex-stimulated animals showed an earlier onset of antitoxin production and
higher antitoxin titers in the serum than did mice given
antigen only.

As evident from Figs. 1 and 2, the acceleration and
enhancement of antibody formation in animals stimulated
with antigen in complex was in parallel with an increase
in number of individual germinal centers in regional

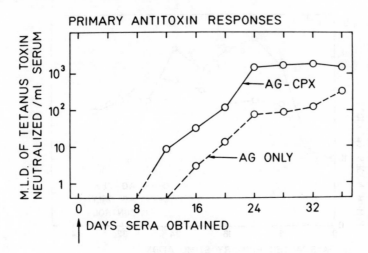

Fig. 1. Primary antitoxin responses in mice given an injection of tetanus toxoid only (AG only) or of the same dose of toxoid complexed with isologous antitoxin at equivalence (AG-CPX).

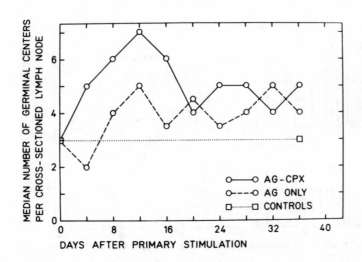

Fig. 2. Median number of germinal centers per cross-section of popliteal lymph nodes as a function of time after injection of either antigen-antibody complexes (AG-CPX) or antigen only (AG only) into the hind leg footpads.

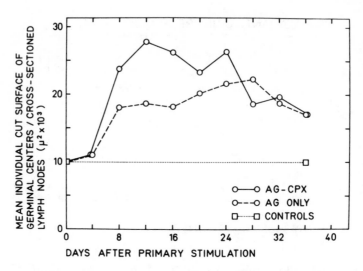

Fig. 3. Mean size of individual germinal centers in cross sectioned popliteal lymph nodes as a function of time following primary stimulation with immune complexes (AG-CPX) or with antigen only (AG only) via the hind leg footpads.

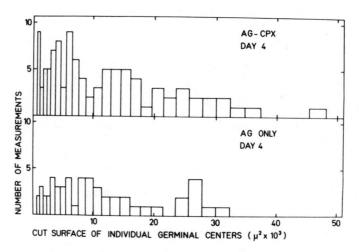

Fig. 4. Frequency distribution of individual germinal center size in cross sectioned popliteal lymph nodes 4 days after primary injection of either immune complexes (AG-CPX) or antigen only (AG only) into the hind leg footpads.

lymph nodes. The median number of germinal centers per cross section of popliteal lymph nodes exceeded that obtained in nonstimulated controls already 4 days after primary antigenic stimulation with antigen-antibody complexes, at a time when the number of germinal centers in corresponding lymph node sections of mice given antigen only had not yet increased. Peak values in both groups of stimulated mice were reached 12 days after injection of antigen. It should be emphasized, however, that after subtraction of control values the median number of germinal centers per cross section of popliteal lymph nodes of animals stimulated with immune complexes was higher than that in mice given antigen only by a factor of approximately 2.

The size of individual germinal centers (Fig. 3), as determined 12 days after primary stimulation with antigen in complex, was significantly larger than in animals stimulated with antigen only (P<.01). With both forms of antigen, germinal centers were larger than those measured in nonstimulated controls (P<.01).

An analysis of the size distribution of germinal centers in the early phase of the immune response (day 4) following stimulation with antigen in complex indicated the presence of more small, presumably newly formed, germinal centers as compared to values obtained in animals stimulated with antigen only (Fig. 4).

No significant difference was observed between mice given antigen only and those stimulated with antigen-antibody complexes in respect to initial labeling indices of lymphoid germinal center cells 4, 12 and 20 days after primary stimulation.

DISCUSSION

Acceleration and enhancement of humoral antibody formation after a primary stimulation with tetanus toxoid in complex with isologous antitoxin at equivalence as compared to antigen only (1) was confirmed by the present study. Circulating antibody titers in animals given a primary stimulation with antigen in complex rose earlier and reached higher levels than in animals stimulated with tetanus toxoid only.

The time course of germinal center development in animals stimulated with tetanus toxoid only was in good agreement with results reported previously (6). Precocity of antitoxin responses in mice following primary stimulation with antigen in complex as compared to antigen only was paralleled by the earlier appearance of additional, presumably newly formed, germinal centers in regional lymph nodes. The enhancement of antibody production following primary injection of complexed antigen was reflected in a more pronounced germinal center growth with regard to both number and size of these structures.

Since the germinal center system appears to be intimately associated with the capacity of the organism to respond to antigenic stimulation in an anamnestic manner, it is interesting to note that in the present study complex-induced de novo germinal center growth was observed prior to the rise of serum antibody titers. This sequence is typical for anamnestic reactions but not for pure primary responses elicited with antigen only (6). It should be mentioned, however, that antibody responses develop even faster, and produce higher serum antitoxin titers, following secondary stimulation with fluid tetanus toxoid only than after primary injection of the complexed antigen.

The question arises as to whether or not the presence of immune complexes is required for the induction of germinal center development, and whether or not the magnitude of such a response is related to the amount of complexed antigen present. Since marked enhancement of primary responses occured after either in vivo or in vitro mixing of complexes (1), the anamnestic type of immune response might be induced by antigen-antibody complexes formed in vivo.

It was suggested from earlier studies (3,6,7) that lymphoid germinal center cells represent precursor cells which, during and after a period of proliferation and differentiation, develop the capacity for antibody production, in mice possibly of the γ_2 variety (8). More experimentation is necessary to test the hypothesis that the cell system responsible for this response, i.e. possibly precursors of lymphoid germinal center cells, is triggered by antigen-antibody complexes also after primary stimulation with antigen only.

SUMMARY

     In an earlier study (1) an enhancement of primary
antibody responses was demonstrated when mice were immunized with a complex prepared at equivalence with mouse
antitoxin and tetanus toxoid. Since germinal centers may
be directly concerned with antibody formation, we attempted to correlate the appearance and growth of these
structures with the rise in antibody titers following a
primary injection of tetanus toxoid complexed with autologous antitoxin at equivalence as compared to the injection of an equal dose of fluid antigen only. The increase in number and size of germinal centers in lymph
nodes regional to the site of antigenic stimulation was
found to begin earlier and to reach higher values in
animals showing complex-induced acceleration of the antibody response than in those injected with the antigen
only. The de novo formation and growth of germinal
centers preceded the log phase of enhanced antibody
response. Possible mechanisms responsible for triggering
the germinal center system following primary stimulation
with antigen-antibody complexes are discussed.

     This work was supported by the Swiss National Found-
ation for Scientific Research and the US Atomic Energy
Commission.

REFERENCES

1.   R.D. Stoner and G. Terres, J. Immunol., 91:761, 1963.

2.   M.W. Hess, G. Terres and R.D. Stoner, Radiat. Res.,
     25:655, 1965.

3.   B. Sordat, M. Sordat, M.W. Hess, R.D. Stoner and
     H. Cottier, J. exp. Med., 131:77, 1970.

4.   J. Laissue, M.W. Hess, R.D. Stoner, H. Riedwyl and
     H. Cottier, in: L. Fiore-Donati and M.G. Hanna, Jr.,
     Eds., Lymphatic tissue and germinal centers in im-
     mune response, p. 285. New York: Plenum Press, 1969.

5.   N.W. Smirnow and I.W. Dunin-Barkowski, in: Mathema-
     tische Statistik in der Technik, p. 236. Berlin:
     VEB Deutscher Verlag der Wissenschaften, 1963.

6. H. Cottier, G. Keiser, N. Odartchenko, M. Hess and
    R.D. Stoner, in: H. Cottier, N. Odartchenko, R. Schind-
    ler and C.C. Congdon, Eds., Germinal centers in im-
    mune responses, p. 270. New York: Springer 1967.

7. M.G. Hanna, Jr., A.K. Szakal and H.E. Walburg, Jr.,
    in: L. Fiore-Donati and M.G. Hanna, Jr., Eds.,
    Lymphatic tissue and germinal centers in immune
    response, p. 149. New York: Plenum Press, 1969.

8. R. Asofsky, N.S. Ikari and M.B. Hylton, Fed. Proc.,
    25:547, 1966.

LYMPH NODE RESPONSE TO ANTIGEN-ANTIBODY COMPLEXES AND THE FATE OF INJECTED PRIMED LYMPHOCYTES IN A TOLERANT HOST

B. M. Balfour, D. M. V. Parrott, J. H. Humphrey and
M. de Sousa

Department of Bacteriology & Immunology, Glasgow University,
National Institute for Medical Research, London N.W. 7

The object of the present experiments was to investigate the origin of germinal center blast cells and to see whether an antigen trapped in germinal centers during an immune response played any part in the recruitment of cells from outside the primary nodule. We hoped to demonstrate this process, if indeed it had any reality, by taking lymph node cells from a donor primed against an antigen A (HSA) and transferring them into a recipient in whom that antigen, in the form of antigen-antibody complexes, had localized in the germinal centers of a particular lymph node. Furthermore, we arranged to have another antigen B (lysozyme) localized in the germinal centers of the contralateral node. In this situation we would expect the HSA primed cells to gather round the HSA and not the lysozyme complexes. Conversely, if we took cells primed against lysozyme they would gather round the lysozyme complexes (Fig. 1). In order to ensure that no host cells would interfere with this phenomenon, we decided to use animals made tolerant to the antigen against which the cells had been primed.

EXPERIMENTAL DESIGN

Tolerance was maintained by repeated injections of high doses of antigen from birth. Thus, we had mice tolerant to HSA that received HSA primed cells, and were injected with HSA containing complexes into the right front foot pad and lysozyme containing complexes into the left front foot pad. Another group of mice was made tolerant to lysozyme, and received lysozyme primed cells; this group had also injections of HSA and lysozyme containing complexes in the right and left front foot pads, respectively. In order to

235

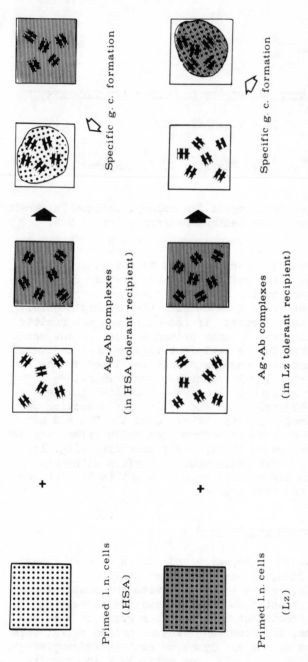

Fig. 1. General design of experiment and expected result. The circular black dots on a white background represent lymphoid cells in a donor primed against HSA, the black triangles on a striped background, lymphoid cells in a donor primed against Lysozyme. Antigen–antibody complexes shown on a white background contained HSA, whereas complexes shown on a striped background contained Lysozyme. HSA primed cells transferred to an HSA tolerant host who had received complexes containing HSA and Lysozyme were expected to gather round the HSA containing complexes, whereas Lysozyme primed cells transferred to a Lysozyme tolerant host who had also been given both complexes were expected to gather round the Lysozyme containing complexes.

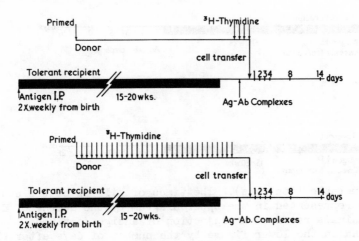

Fig. 2. Timetable (Main Experimental Groups). The end of the solid black line represents the point at which the tolerogenic injections were stopped: the times of killing of the experimental animals are represented by the number of days after the animals received a cell transfer.

trace the fate of the transferred cells both donor groups were injected with ³H-thymidine (see below). The timetable of the experiment has been represented diagramatically in Fig. 2.

The donor mice were primed with the appropriate antigen 31 days before cell transfer, each group was further subdivided according to the ³H-thymidine labelling schedule. In one schedule (the short-term labelling) the mice received a 3 day course of injections 28 days after priming and just before cell transfer. In the other group (the long-term labelling) the mice were given the ³H-thymidine injections immediately after priming and these were continued daily until 3 days before transfer. The two labelling schedules were adopted to obtain labelled short-lived and long-lived populations.

In addition to the two main experimental groups there were a number of control groups, two of which are represented in Fig. 3. One consisting of animals who had been made tolerant to HSA or lysozyme, who were given the two injections of complex but no primed cell transfer, another similar group was given neither cell transfer or injections of complexes. Other tolerant animals were given injections of complex followed by a normal cell transfer.

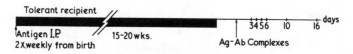

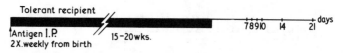

Fig. 3.   Timetable (Controls). The times of killing of the control
animals are represented in the upper diagram by the number of days
after the animals received an injection of antigen/antibody
complexes and in the lower figure by the number of days after they
received the last of the tolerogenic injections.

METHODS

A number of tissues including the apical axillary, mesenteric
lymph nodes, also pieces of spleen and thymus were removed from most
animals. Sections were stained for HSA and lysozyme and for antibody to these two proteins and for mouse gammaglobulin by the
fluorescent antibody technique. The position of the antigen-antibody
complexes and of the cells containing antibody to either antigen was
recorded by photography and the sections were later coated with
photographic emulsion and autoradiographs prepared. The number and
position of labelled cells was determined and their relationship to
the antigen-antibody complexes or to antibody containing cells was
checked. The sera of all animals were collected and assayed for the
presence of antibody to HSA or lysozyme or both antigens, by the
Farr test.

RESULTS

The antibody response of the donor mice to the priming antigen,
whether HSA or lysozyme, suggested that continuous injections of
^{3}H-thymidine impair the immunological performance of the animal.
In both cases the mice receiving the short-term labelling schedule
responded better (Table I).

All the tolerant mice remained tolerant throughout the period
of observation, that is to say they did not produce any circulating
antibody to the tolerogenic antigen, but from the 8th day after cell

Table I. Ag binding capacity of donors (µg/ml)

Labelling	HSA	Lys
Short term	8.7	3.6
	(5.6 - 11)	(2.7 - 4.0)
Long term	3.2	1.3
	(1.9 - 5.5)	(0.3 - 2.2)

transfer a few antibody containing cells were found in the lymph nodes draining the site of injection of the complexes, rather more in the lysozyme than in the HSA tolerant group. The HSA tolerant animals who had received a transfer of HSA primed cells all made a definite response to lysozyme and again those who received cells from the short term tritium labelled group of donors responded better than those who received cells from the long term labelled donors; the control group who received a transfer of cells from normal animals made no response to lysozyme, nor did the HSA tolerant animals who received injections of complex but no cell transfer. Not one of the lysozyme tolerant animals made any response to HSA, though a few antibody containing cells were found in lymph nodes draining the site of injection of the HSA containing complexes. Four hundred antibody containing cells, mostly those containing antibody to lysozyme were checked under the fluorescent microscope against the corresponding autoradiographs, and not a single one was found to be labelled. In fact, the transferred labelled cells did not do any of the things which might have been expected of them. There was no concentration of labelled cells in the germinal centers of any of the nodes examined. The proportion of the labelled primed cells in the HSA and lysozyme draining nodes was completely random in all groups, 85 to 90% of the cells were in the thymus-dependent area. Nor could there have been any accumulation of unlabelled donor cells in the germinal centers containing the appropriate antigen since these centers were almost devoid of blast cells and had very few surrounding lymphocytes.

In many cases all that we could find was a squashed collection of dendritic cells near the surface of the node with an occasional blast cell nearby. The dendritic cells can easily be identified by the lacey pattern of their processes and in adjacent sections the antigen was found to be localized in the same area. In many cases the primary nodules had largely disappeared.

CONCLUSIONS

We concluded from the behaviour of the transferred lymph node cells that the majority of them were thymus-derived and perhaps not likely to be precursors of germinal center blast cells. On the other hand, they might include precursors of other elements in germinal centers, such as mantle lymphocytes, but again these cells were mostly absent from the germinal centers of the draining nodes and almost none of them were labelled. We are therefore fairly sure that thymus-derived lymphocytes taken from animals primed against HSA or lysozyme are not attracted away from their recirculatory pathway through a node by the mere presence in that lymph node of the appropriate antigen localized in a germinal center.

We wondered if there might not be another reason why the homing of germinal center cells is particularly difficult to demonstrate. Supposing that their route of access to the center was not direct from the blood stream via the post-capillary venules but from the peripheral tissues via the afferent lymphatics, one might expect their appearance in germinal centers to be delayed, as in a normal response. This possibility has now been tested in experiments in the rabbit (1), in which the afferent lymphatic coming from an antigen depot has been cannulated, the afferent lymph cells collected, labelled in vitro with ^{3}H-adenosine and returned to the same lymphatic. The fate of the afferent lymph labelled cells in the draining node was followed by means of autoradiography and it appears that following the injection of antigens which provoke a germinal center response, the number of blast cells in the afferent lymph draining from the site of injection increases sharply on the 4th and 5th day, and that a high proportion of these cells does localize in germinal centers in the draining node.

We were puzzled by the changes which we observed in the draining nodes taken from the animals in the two main experimental groups. In many cases the primary nodules had almost disappeared and there were no germinal centers except the peculiar remnants described above. At first we thought that these changes were due to the high dose tolerogenic injections and such changes are actually found in young animals receiving large amounts of antigen (2) but both in the tolerant group that received neither complexes nor cells, and in the group that received complexes but no cells, the draining nodes were found to contain germinal centers.

We therefore concluded that the transferred cells were partly responsible for the disappearance of pre-existing germinal centers and that they also prevented the growth of new centers in response to the injections of antigen-antibody complexes.

REFERENCES

1. R. Kelly, Nature, 227:510, 1970.

2. M. de Sousa, J. H. Humphrey, and B. M. Balfour, these
    Proceedings, p. 481.

MECHANISM OF INTERACTION BETWEEN IMMUNE COMPLEXES AND RECEPTORS

FOR ANTIBODY ON MACROPHAGES

Julia M. Phillips-Quagliata, B. B. Levine, F. Quagliata,

and J. W. Uhr, Depts. of Pathology and Medicine

New York University School of Medicine, New York 10016

Follicular localization of antigen depends on the presence of antibody (1-3). It has been suggested (1) that one of the cells involved in trapping of antigen-antibody complexes is the dendritic macrophage. This cell is similar to the circulating monocyte and macrophage, and it is possible that, like them, it possesses separate surface receptors for antibody and for modified complement (4-6). Either or both of these receptors may be necessary for antigen localization.

We have been studying interaction between receptors for antibody on macrophages and antigen-antibody complexes in vitro. It has been shown both by ourselves and by others (7-10) that antigen-antibody complexes bind to the surfaces of macrophages even when little or no binding of antibody alone is demonstrable. Binding is known to be mediated by the Fc region of the antibody molecule (8) and is inhibited by Fc but not $F(ab')_2$ fragments (11). We have been trying to elucidate the mechanism involved. One hypothesis is that complex formation might cause an allosteric change in the antibody molecule, resulting in exposure of a binding site for the macrophage surface. There is considerable evidence for conformational changes in antibody molecules upon combination with antigen (12-17), however no function has yet been definitely assigned to them. An alternative hypothesis is that "free" antibody molecules already have a binding site for the macrophage surface, but binding is weak. Formation of complexes containing more than one antibody molecule and thus more than one potential site of attachment might increase the strength of binding. A divalent antigen is a minimal requirement for formation of such complexes, whereas combination with monovalent antigen might be sufficient to provoke an allosteric change in the antibody molecule.

We have investigated the binding of labelled, purified anti-hapten antibody to macrophages alone and in the presence of monovalent, divalent and polyvalent haptens. Our results support the hypothesis that the enhancement of antibody binding to macrophages in the presence of antigen is due to increased energy of binding resulting from summation of individual binding sites, rather than to the occurrence of allosteric change.

MATERIALS AND METHODS

Washed rabbit alveolar or peritoneal macrophages at a concentration of 2×10^7/ml in Medium 1066 containing 20% fetal calf serum, Iodine-125 labelled, purified rabbit anti-benzyl penicilloyl 7S IgG (I-125 anti-BPO) and the following haptens: monovalent, BPO_1-propylamine (BPO_1 Prop), divalent, BPO_2-hexamethylenediamine (BPO_2HMD) oligovalent, $BPO_6Lysine_7$ (BPO_6Lys_7) and polyvalent, succinylated $BPO_{93}poly$-L-$lysine_{402}$ ($BPO_{93}PLL_{402}S$), were prepared as previously described (18-21). The cells were incubated at $37^{\circ}C$ for 10 minutes or at $4^{\circ}C$ for 20 minutes with 2 micrograms of I-125 anti-BPO with or without hapten and/or normal rabbit gamma globulin (RGG), in a final volume of 1.2 or 1.3 ml. Both I-125 anti-BPO and RGG were ultracentrifuged to remove aggregates immediately before use. Control tubes contained medium without cells or an equal packed volume of sheep erythrocytes. After incubation, the reaction mixtures were diluted with cold medium, centrifuged and the supernatants discarded. The tubes were then washed four times and the remaining radioactivity counted in an autogamma counter. Control values were subtracted. Reactions were carried out in duplicate or triplicate and the results averaged.

RESULTS

When 2×10^7 macrophages were incubated either at $4^{\circ}C$ or $37^{\circ}C$ with I-125 anti-BPO alone, significant quantities remained bound after washing. The amount varied from .006 to .033 μg in seven experiments, that is between 0.3 and 1.6% of the I-125 anti-BPO available. A typical experiment is shown in Table I. Binding was markedly enhanced by the addition of either divalent or polyvalent hapten at equivalence; the presence of excess hapten resulted in less

Enhancement of binding of I-125 anti-BPO to macrophages by hapten

H added	0	$BPO_{93}PLL_{402}S$		BPO_2HMD		BPO_1Prop		$BPO_{93}PLL_{402}S$ (0.02)* +	
								BPO_2HMD	BPO_1Prop
H/Ab mol. ratio		0.02*	2.0	1.0*	1000	2.0*	2000	1000	2000
μg Ab bd.	.031	.171	.083	.129	.083	.032	.033	.062	.092

*Hapten/antibody molar ratio at equivalence.

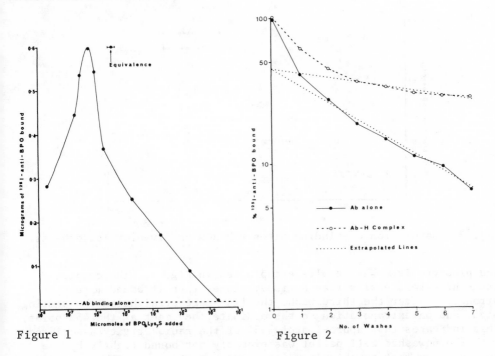

Figure 1   Figure 2

Fig. 1 - Effect of concentration of oligovalent hapten on binding
        of I-125 anti-BPO to rabbit alveolar macrophages.
Fig. 2 - Elution of antibody and BPO_6Lys_7-antibody complex from
        macrophages

enhancement. Monovalent hapten did not enhance binding at any concentration ratio tried; furthermore, excess of both monovalent and
divalent hapten inhibited the enhancement due to polyvalent hapten
at equivalence.

    In the next experiment, the effect of various concentrations of
hapten were tried (Fig. 1). An oligovalent hapten was used, as it
gave a sharp equivalence point in precipitin reactions with rabbit
antibody (22). Binding was optimal in the region of slight antibody
excess; at extreme antigen excess, it was not enhanced. These
results support the idea that lattice formation is essential for enhancement of binding; the monovalent hapten and the oligovalent hapten in antigen excess should have been able to induce the hypothetical allosteric change, but they did not enhance binding.

    We next investigated the possibility that antigen-antibody com-
plexes might bind more strongly to macrophages than antibody alone,
by studying their elution during different numbers of washes. The
reaction and washes were carried out at $4^{\circ}C$ to minimize phagocytosis

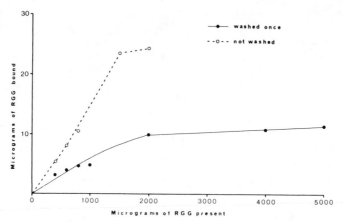

Fig. 3 - Saturation of binding sites for RGG on alveolar macrophages.

and pinocytosis. The results are plotted in Fig. 2. The complex
was eluted less easily than antibody alone, thus it bound more
strongly. After the third wash, the lines are straight on the semilog
plot, and on extrapolation to the ordinate, they meet at the 45% point.
This indicates that approximately 55% of the radioactivity associated
with the unwashed cell pellet was probably not bound tightly by the
membrane, or that the binding sites were heterogenous with respect to
affinity for antibody.

Our results so far have shown that (a) uncomplexed I-125 anti-
BPO has a binding site, (b) lattice formation is necessary for enhancement of binding, (c) complexes bind more strongly than
uncomplexed antibody.

To show that even normal, uncomplexed rabbit gamma globulin has a
binding site for the macrophage surface, we carried out inhibition
experiments using ultracentrifuged RGG at various concentrations to
inhibit binding of BPO_6Lys_7-I-125 anti-BPO complex. Almost complete
inhibition of binding occurred in the presence of sufficient RGG, and
only 50 μg were necessary for 50% inhibition. Thus it was concluded
that unaggregated RGG molecules have an exposed binding site for
macrophages.

An experiment in which I-125 anti-BPO was thrice absorbed with
2×10^8 packed macrophages was done to determine whether all, or only
some IgG molecules have the binding site. Approximately the same proportion of the available antibody was removed at each absorption.
This result is consistent with the presence of the binding site at
least on the majority of the antibody molecules.

Finally, we made a rough estimate of the number of binding

sites for IgG on macrophages by saturating them with high concentrations of IgG and then calculating how much was bound. I-125 anti-BPO
was mixed with various concentrations of RGG and incubated with the
cells at 4°C. In one experiment we then washed the cells once, in
the other we drained the cells without washing them. The radioactivity in the cell pellets was counted and the bound IgG calculated from
the initial concentration added per tube. The results are plotted
in Fig. 3. At high IgG concentrations, plateaux of antibody bound
were observed. At the highest points on the plateaux, 24.3 and 11.3
μg of IgG were associated with the cells. From the extrapolated
lines in the washing experiment (Fig. 2), we derived correction
factors to find the proportions of these bound strongly to unwashed
cells. Thus, by multiplying 24.3 x 45/100 and 11.4 x 45/41, it was
found that 10.9 and 12.5 μg of IgG could be bound by 2×10^7 macrophages. From these figures approximately 2 million molecules were
calculated to be bound per cell.

DISCUSSION

Our evidence supports the concept that the increased binding of
antibody to macrophages in the presence of antigen is due to a summation effect and not to exposure of new binding sites on the antibody
molecule as a result of allosteric change. The evidence consists of
the observations that (1) both I-125 anti-BPO and RGG have binding
sites, (2) antigen-antibody interaction per se did not enhance binding
since neither monovalent nor excess polyvalent hapten was effective:
lattice formation was necessary, (3) complexes were less easily dissociated from the cell surface than antibody alone, and thus may be
considered to bind more strongly.

We cannot exclude the possibility that an allosteric change may
take place within a complex thus exposing additional binding sites.
The fact that both RGG and labelled antibody display binding suggests
that new binding sites are not essential. This is not to deny that
conformational changes take place in antibody molecules upon combination with antigen (12-17) the question is whether they have any significance for the binding of antibody to macrophages.

We have no information pertaining to the suggestion that such
conformational changes of cell bound antibody are important in the
induction of immunity or paralysis in lymphocytes (24). It is not
known whether the macrophage receptors for antibody are the same as
those which display endogenous antibody on some lymphocytes. In connection with in vivo effects of antigen-antibody complex, however, the
observation that sufficient antigen excess prevents enhancement of
antibody binding to the cell surface may be of significance in phenomena such as high dose tolerance. Perhaps localization can be prevented by this means.

We attempted to determine whether all, or only a sub-population of rabbit IgG molecules can bind to macrophages. While our results supported the idea that they can, the point was not proved. However, assuming both homogeneity of antibody with respect to ability to bind to macrophages and binding sites on all macrophages, we calculated that there are approximately 2 million per cell.

The function of these binding sites has not been established. It has been shown that though phagocytosis of antigen-7S antibody complexes takes place in the absence of complement, it is markedly enhanced when complement is added. This suggests that unphagocytosed antigen on the surface of macrophages within lymphoid tissue may be localized there by means of receptors for antibody rather than for complement. However, it may well be that the antibody molecules involved are IgM (5) rather than IgG. This would be particularly likely in a primary response since most "natural" antibodies are IgM.

SUMMARY

The mechanism of binding of immune complexes to macrophages was investigated using purified anti-hapten antibody and haptens of different valences. The results support the hypothesis that the enhancement of antibody binding after complex formation is due to an increase in the energy of binding from summation of individual binding sites rather than to exposure of new binding sites as a result of allosteric change in the antibody molecule.

ACKNOWLEDGEMENTS

Supported by grants from the National Institutes of Health (AI-09647, 5-T01-AM05064, and AI-0834) and by Contract Da-DA 17-16-7119 from the U.S. Army Medical Research and Development Command. F.Q. is an Arthritis Foundation post-doctoral fellow.

REFERENCES

1. J. Mitchell and A. Abbot, Nature (Lond.), 208:500, 1965.

2. G.J.V. Nossal, G.L. Ada, C.M. Austin and J. Pye, Immunology, 9:349, 1965.

3. J.H. Humphrey and M.M. Frank, Immunology, 13:87, 1967.

4. H. Huber, M. Polley, W.D. Linscott, H.H. Fudenberg and H.J. Muller-Eberhard, Science, 162:1281, 1968.

5. W.H. Lay and V. Nussenzweig, J. Immunol., 102:1172, 1968.

6. W.H. Lay and V. Nussenzweig, J. Exptl. Med., 128:911, 1968.

7. J.W. Uhr, Proc. Nat. Acad. Sci., 54:1599, 1965.

8. J.W. Uhr and J.M. Phillips, Ann. N.Y. Acad. Sci., 129:793, 1966.

9. J.M. Phillips and J.W. Uhr, Fed. Proc., 25:728, 1966.

10. A. Berken and B. Benacerraf, J. Exptl. Med., 123:119, 1966.

11. C. Inchley, H.M. Grey and J.W. Uhr, J. Immunol., in press, 1970.

12. A. Feinstein and A.J. Rowe, Nature (Lond.), 205:147, 1965.

13. R.C. Valentine and N.M. Green, J. Mol. Biol., 27:615, 1967.

14. K. Ishizaka and D.H. Campbell, J. Immunol., 83:318, 1959.

15. C. Warner, V. Schimaker and F. Karush, Biochem. Biophys. Res. Comm., 38:125, 1970.

16. C.S. Henney and D.R. Stanworth, Nature (Lond.), 210:1071, 1966.

17. A.L. Grossberg, G. Markus and D. Pressman, Proc. Nat. Acad. Sci., 54:942, 1965.

18. J.M. Phillips-Quagliata, B.B. Levine and J.W. Uhr, Nature (Lond.), 222:1290, 1969.

19. J.M. Phillips-Quagliata, B.B. Levine, F. Quagliata and J.W. Uhr, in press, 1970.

20. B.B. Levine and V. Levytska, J. Immunol., 102:647, 1969.

21. B.B. Levine, M.J. Fellner and V. Levytska, J. Immunol., 96:707, 1966.

22. B.B. Levine, J. Med. Chem., 7:675, 1964.

23. P.A. Bretscher and M. Cohn, Nature (Lond.), 220:444, 1968.

FOLLICULAR LOCALIZATION OF ANTIGEN: POSSIBLE ROLE OF LYMPHOCYTES BEARING A RECEPTOR FOR ANTIGEN-ANTIBODY-COMPLEMENT COMPLEXES[1]

Celso Bianco[2], Peter Dukor and Victor Nussenzweig[3]

Department of Pathology, New York University School of

Medicine, New York, New York 10016 U.S.A.

Follicular localization of antigen (1-6) can be viewed as a mechanism designed to concentrate antigenic material in strategic regions of lymphoid organs, in their pathway for the induction or maintenance of immunity (and/or tolerance). The evidence suggesting that antigen localized in those areas is relevant for the immune process can be summarized as follows: (a) unlike antigen in other locations, membrane bound antigen can be detected in follicles for relatively long periods of time. Protected from digestion by intracellular enzymes, it may be readily available for interaction with membranes of other cells; (b) the sites of follicular localization of antigen coincide with the regions of intense cellular proliferation in some immune responses; (c) the intensity of localization is linked to the immunogenicity of the antigen: only highly antigenic substances are taken up very rapidly in the follicles; follicular localization of antigen is greatly enhanced in primed animals; under conditions of immunological tolerance, however, follicular localization is abolished. The precise mechanism of retention of antigen in those areas is not known. Two questions are obviously of primary importance. Which are the cells involved? How do these cells recognize foreignness? The purpose of this presentation is to summarize

(1) This investigation was supported by a National Institutes of Health grant No. AI08499.
(2) Supported by a training fellowship from the World Health Organization and from the Fundacao de Amparo a Pesquisa, Sao Paulo, Brazil.
(3) Career Investigator of the Health Research Council of the City of New York, Contract I-558.

some recently obtained evidence suggesting that a distinct class
of lymphocytes actively participate in follicular localization of
antigen and that this process may be complement mediated.

Table 1

PROPERTIES, DISTRIBUTION AND ORIGIN OF CRL[1]

I. Properties

    a. Have the morphological appearance of lymphocytes
    b. Are present in different mammalian species, including man
    c. Bind AgAbC complexes probably through C3
    d. Adhere preferentially to nylon wool
    e. Overlap extensively with the lymphocyte sub-population
        which have Ig determinants on the membrane. However,
        the receptor for AgAbC complexes is distinct from the
        membrane bound Ig (11)
    f. Have a relatively lower density than non-CRL
    g. Can be short and long lived

II. Distribution in lymphoid tissues

    a. Are absent from the thymus and present in different propor-
        tions in other lymphoid organs (details in Table 2)
    b. Have a defined histological localization:
        spleen - present in the marginal zone and in the folli-
        cles, absent from periarteriolar lymphocyte sheaths
        lymph nodes - present in the cortical areas, absent
        from paracortical areas
        Peyer's patches - present in follicular areas, absent
        from interfollicular areas
        thymus - absent

III. Origin

    Extrathymic, probably bone marrow derived (12)

(1) This table summarizes data from references 9 to 12.

    The basic finding is that some (but not all) lymphocytes from
many mammalian species including man, can bind antigen-antibody-
complement (AgAbC) complexes to their membranes (7-9). When the
antigen in these complexes is an erythrocyte, the interaction
between the red cells and the lymphocytes is easily visualized
because it leads to the formation of rosettes. Table 1 shows that
these lymphocytes (which we call CRL) have distinct properties and

Table 2

PERCENTAGE OF CELLS BEARING RECEPTORS FOR AgAbC COMPLEXES, Ig DETER-
MINANTS AND θ ANTIGEN AMONG LYMPHOCYTES FROM DIFFERENT ORGANS OF
THE MOUSE

Organ	% of cells bearing		
	receptors for AgAbC[1]	Ig determinants[2]	θ antigen[3]
Thymus	0	0	100
Thoracic duct	10-20	5	80
Lymph node	10-25	15	65
Spleen	25-40	35	35

(1) Based on rosette formation between lymphocytes and sheep red
     blood cells coated with rabbit anti-Forssman antibodies and
     mouse complement (from references 8 and 9)
(2) Determined by immunofluorescence, cytotoxic tests, and reverse
     cytoimmunoadherence (from references 9, 13, 14)
(3) Determined by cytotoxic tests and immunofluorescence (from
     reference 15)

a characteristic distribution in lymphoid organs of the mouse.
CRL thus constitute a separate sub-population of cells. The
frequency of CRL in cell suspensions of different lymphoid organs
of the mouse is seen in Table 2. The proportions of CRL actually
coincide with that of lymphocytes having Ig markers of the membrane, a
fact that suggests that both markers may be present in the same
cell. This is in agreement with our findings that the specific
depletion of CRL induces simultaneous depletion of cells bearing Ig
determinants on their membranes (9). It is also evident from
Table 2 that the proportions of θ bearing cells (which are probably
thymus derived, as reviewed in reference 15) are almost complementary
to the proportions of CRL. We have reasons to believe that CRL are
not thymus derived. Evidence suggesting that this is actually the
case has been recently obtained and is based on the following observations: (a) CRL are histologically localized in areas which are
considered to contain non-thymus derived cells (1); (b) CRL are
present in increased proportions in neonatally thymectomized mice and
their histological distribution is not altered (12); (c) CRL are
present in increased proportions in thymectomized and lethally
irradiated adult mice which receive a bone marrow transplant (12).

It is reasonable to believe that the specific markers identified on the membrane of lymphoid cells are the result of differen-

tiation by selective activation of genes characteristic for these
cells, and probably related to their function. Specific cell
contacts, tissue organization, the stimulation or repression of
unique activities, may be primarily regulated or triggered by interactions with membrane recognition units. In the case of lymphoid
cells, for example, the presence of membrane bound immunoglobulins
has been related to the function of these cells in the immune
response as targets for antigen and/or as antibody producers. The
same reasoning leads us to believe that the presence of multiple
binding sites for AgAbC complexes on the membrane of CRL indicates
that immune complexes may play a role in the life history of these
cells. What is the evidence which associates CRL with the phenomenon of follicular localization of antigen?

(a) Follicular localization of antigen is definitely an antibody
mediated phenomenon (4,5,16). It is enhanced in the presence of
passively administered or actively produced antibody, it is less
efficient in germ-free animals (17) and is increased when antigen
is injected combined with antibodies. The F(c) fragment of immunoglobulins, which mediates complement fixation is necessary for the
retention of AgAb complexes in the follicles (3). Complement
fixation could also be the explanation for the puzzling observation
that heterologous, homologous and even autologous Ig, but no other
serum proteins, localize in the lymphoid follicles (18,19). It
appears likely that aggregates that would fix complement could
contaminate these preparations.

(b) Several investigations have pointed out that lymphoid cells
bind antigen after it is injected into normal or immune animals
and that sometimes a surprisingly large proportion of lymphocytes
contain antigen (reviewed in 20). However, in most instances these
findings were difficult to interpret in relation to the specificity
of the binding and its relevance to the immune process.

(c) The depletion of lymphocytes by thoracic duct drainage reduces
the uptake of antigenic material by primary follicles and antibody
injections only partly restore localization (21).

(d) Using electron microscopy it has been shown that antigen is
associated in part with processes of dendritic reticular cells
(2,3,22). However, in many cases the cells are so densely packed
that it is not possible to decide whether the antigen is bound to
lymphocyte membranes or dendritic processes of reticular cells.
In other instances antigen is seen between lymphoid cells where no
reticular cell processes can be resolved.

(e) The distribution of antigen in the lymphoid follicles coincides
with the histological distribution of CRL which do bind AgAbC
complexes. Moreover, binding of AgAbC complexes to lymphocytes and

reticular cells has been recently demonstrated by electron microscopy (10).

All this evidence strongly suggests that CRL contribute
substantially to the localization of antigen and that complement
participates in this process.

On the other hand, the presence of AgAbC complexes in the
follicles, bound either to lymphocytes or to dendritic cells might
provide an explanation for the trapping and accumulation of CRL in
the follicles. We proposed (10) that CRL could be either bound
to AgAbC complexes previously deposited on the process of the
dendritic cells, or CRL which had previously bound AgAbC to their
membrane while in circulation could be trapped within the reticular
framework of the follicles. In either case, complement would
provide the adhesive responsible for the dense follicular accumulation of specialized lymphocytes in peripheral lymphoid tissues.
It is tempting to postulate that both phenomena, antigen localization and lymphocyte accumulation in the follicles depend on the
same basic mechanism.

Our findings also imply that antigen can bind to certain
lymphocytes (CRL) in two distinct ways: either specifically to
those cells which display the adequate immunoglobulin receptor on
their membranes (clonal selection?), or through receptors for
AgAbC if antibody, natural or immune, is present.

REFERENCES

1.   White, R. G. in The Immunologically Competent Cell, Ciba
      Symposium, ed. S.E.W. Wolstenholme and G.Knight, London,
      Churchill, 1963.
2.   Mitchell, J. and Abbot, A., Nature, 208, 500, 1965.
3.   Ada, G. L., Parish, C. R., Nossal, G. J. V. and Abbot, A.,
      Cold Spring Harbor Symp. Quant. Biol., 32, 381, 1967.
4.   Nossal, G.J.V., Ada, G. L., Austin, C. M. and Pye, J.,
      Immunology, 9, 349, 1965.
5.   Humphrey, J. H. and Frank, M. M., Immunology, 13, 87, 1967.
6.   Balfour, B. M. and Humphrey, J. H., in Germinal Centers in
      Immune Responses, ed. H. Cottier, N. Odartchenko, R.
      Schindler and C. C. Congdon, Springer-Verlag, New York Inc.,
      1967.
7.   Uhr, J. W. and Phillips, J. M., Ann. N.Y. Acad. Sci., 129,
      793, 1966.

8. Lay, W. H. and Nussenzweig, V., J. Exp. Med., _128_, 911, 1968.
9. Bianco, C., Patrick, R. and Nussenzweig, V., J. Exp. Med.,
    in press.
10. Dukor, P., Bianco, C. and Nussenzweig, V., Proc. Nat. Acad.
    Sci., in press.
11. Bianco, C. and Nussenzweig, V., in preparation.
12. Dukor, P., Bianco, C. and Nussenzweig, V., in preparation.
13. Raff, M. C., Sternberg, M. and Taylor, R. B., Nature, _225_,
    553, 1970.
14. Paraskevas, F., Lee, S. and Israels, L. G., Nature, _222_,
    885, 1969.
15. Raff, M. C., presented at the Third Sigrid Juselius Symposium
    on Cell Cooperation in Immune Responses, Helsinki, 1970.
16. Lang, P. G. and Ada, G. L., Immunology, _13_, 523, 1967.
17. Miller, J. J., Johnson, O. and Ada, G. L., Nature, _217_, 1056,
    1968.
18. Ada, G. L., Nossal, G. J. V. and Austin, C. M., Austr. J.
    Exp. Biol. Med. Sci., _42_, 331, 1964.
19. Ada, G. L., Nossal, G. J. V. and Pye, Jr., Austr. J. Exp.
    Biol. Med. Sci., _42_, 295, 1964.
20. Sulitzeanu, D., Bact. Reviews, _32_, 404, 1968.
21. Williams, G. M., Immunology, _11_, 467, 1966.
22. Nossal, G. J. V., Abbot, A., Mitchell, J. and Lumus, Z.,
    J. Exp. Med., _127_, 227, 1967.

CHAIRMAN'S INTRODUCTION TO THE DISCUSSION

LOCALIZATION OF ANTIGEN AND IMMUNE COMPLEXES IN LYMPHATIC

TISSUE, WITH SPECIAL REFERENCE TO GERMINAL CENTERS[1]

M. G. Hanna, Jr., and R. L. Hunter

Carcinogenesis Program, Biology Division, Oak Ridge
National Laboratory, Oak Ridge, Tennessee, and
Department of Pathology, University of Chicago,
Chicago, Illinois USA

The localization of antigen, both cellularly and extracellularly, is an extremely relevant topic to this conference. The subject becomes especially significant in light of current studies which emphasize the role of tissue-retained antigens in the production and maintenance of the immune phenomena (1-3), and of reports suggesting that continuous antigenic stimulation is requisite for the complete differentiation of immunocompetent cells (4-7).

Immunocompetent organs, such as the spleen and lymph nodes, process degradable antigens in two main ways. First, the greatest part of the material is phagocytized and degraded by macrophages, which results in a rapid inactivation of the major portion of the immunogenic capacity of the intricate antigen. Second, a small but significant portion of sequestered antigen is retained in lymphoid tissue for extended periods after its administration, as shown by the localization of immunologically active material in subcellular fractions in the spleen (2,8,9), and by the sustained retention of labeled antigen in lymphoid follicles of the spleen and lymph nodes (10-18).

Correlation of these two processes with the induction of the primary immune response is most difficult, since numerous studies (19-22) have shown that certain antibodies have specificity for the tertiary and quaternary structures of immunogens. This implies that suitably competent cells can be immunologically induced by

---

[1] Research supported jointly by the National Cancer Institute and the
U. S. Atomic Energy Commission under contract with Union Carbide
Corporation.

undegraded and undistorted forms of the immunogen. Also, in many cases, the extracellular localization and its subsequent effects follow the period related to induction of immunologically competent cells. Yet it is reasonable to consider that these processes are related to the maintenance of the developing immunologic capacity, and in this respect antigen localization in lymphoid follicles becomes of interest due to its causal relationship to the proliferation of immunologically active cells in germinal centers. A most intriguing aspect of antigen localization in germinal centers is the fact that it implies the ability to recognize foreignness. Studies by Ada (23) and White (24) clearly show that incorporation of nonantigenic material into germinal centers in no way resembles that of antigen onto dendritic reticular cells.

ANATOMICAL ASPECTS OF ANTIGEN LOCALIZATION IN GERMINAL CENTERS

In general, whether antigen is injected into the footpads of normal rats for study of the popliteal lymph nodes or injected intravenously in normal chickens or mice for study of the spleen, the histologic aspects of its localization are in agreement. It is initially localized in the marginal zone or in medullary macrophages, and eventually a small but significant portion is localized on dendritic reticular cells in germinal centers of the primary follicles. The amount of labeled antigen in the macrophages decreases rapidly, but that on the reticular cells of germinal centers persists for many weeks with a gradual decline of radioactivity.

A significant feature of antigen localization in spleen lymphatic nodules of germfree mice or in popliteal lymph nodes of normal rats is the deposition of antigen in areas in which no active germinal centers were detected (10,25-27). In these experiments active germinal centers formed in these specific regions of the lymphoid follicle during the primary response. Anatomically, the antigen-trapping device in germfree mice corresponds to the germinal center region in conventional mice, and it is reasonable to assume that there is a preexisting reticulum cell stroma capable of localizing antigen and that the characteristic lymphoid germinal center cells are grouped in relation to this structure. Thus, these findings support the contention of Menzies (28) that in lymphoid tissue, the stromal compartment of the secondary follicle, termed the "centron," is constant and preexistant, even though its contained lymphoid population is variable. Further, the reticulum of this constant structure of the germinal center is capable of initially trapping and localizing antigen in the absence of the characteristic pyroninophilic lymphoid (parenchymal) cells of active germinal centers.

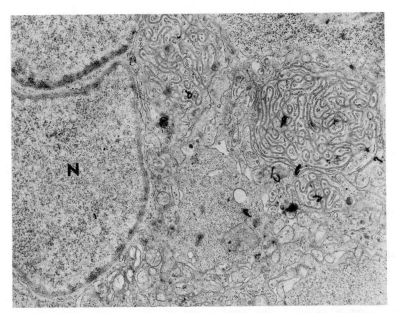

Fig. 1. Microautoradiogram illustrating the distribution of silver grains over the labyrinthine plasma membrane infoldings of antigen-retaining, dendritic reticular cell processes after the initiation of an immune response to ^{125}I-HGG in mouse spleen germinal centers. Note the uniformity of the plasma membrane infoldings and the indented electron-lucent nucleus (N) of the cell. 17,500X.

Dendritic reticular cells, which have been studied at the ultrastructural level in lymph nodes (29,30) and the spleen (31,32), retain antigen at the surface membrane of their extensive plasma membrane infoldings, which are part of the dendritic projections of these cells (Fig. 1). This is in marked contrast to the observed deposition of antigen in phagocytic vacuoles and lysosomes of macrophages.

It has been suggested (24) that antigen is transported from the outer cortex or marginal zone of the primary nodule toward the germinal center region by virtue of its being attached on migrating dendritic cells. It has also been proposed (13,38) that antigen is passively carried through the intercellular spaces between the dendritic processes. Perhaps an equally acceptable alternative, but one that has not been extensively considered, is that antigen is passed from one dendritic cell to another during intimate membrane-membrane contact, as suggested by the process of "membrane-flow" described by Bennett (33).

When antigen is injected into primed animals its localization in macrophages is somewhat increased, and is greatly increased, at least initially, in germinal centers (26,34). A key point of one ultrastructural study of the secondary immune response (32) is the apparent degradation of the plasma membrane infolding during this reaction. The degradation occurred at a time when the majority, if not all, of the antigen was complexed with specific antibody. Using this finding as a basis, the authors proposed that the cytotoxic sequalae described in germinal centers of primed animals could be a result of an excess, high avidity antibody-antigen-complement complex. It is questionable, based on these studies, whether the quality of the complex that persists in germinal centers in the secondary immune response is similar to that in the primary response. In contrast to the long-term persistence of antigen in splenic germinal centers during the primary response, the period of localization during the secondary response was limited to only a few days. It is interesting to speculate that such a mechanism could be essential for the operation of an efficient immune system by preventing, after the development of a large sensitized cell compartment, further contact of immune progenitor cells with the antigen, and thus clear the centers for the development of subsequent immune reactions against other antigens.

REQUIREMENT FOR SPECIFIC ANTIBODY IN ANTIGEN LOCALIZATION

Antigen and specific or cross-reacting antibody have similar distributions when they localize on dendritic reticular cells of germinal centers (12,15). Since this finding was obtained primarily with immunofluorescence techniques, it could not be adequately determined whether in all cases the antibody was locally produced in cells of the germinal center, or whether it was selectively taken up from the surrounding fluids.

Sordat et al. (30), using high-resolution electron microscopy, have recently studied horse radish peroxidase (HRP)-anti-HRP reactions. They observed within lymphoid cells of developing germinal centers, specific anti-HRP in conjunction with extracellular antibody — suggesting that local production of antibody for the fixation of antigen is still in part realistic. According to them, the intercellular fixation within germinal centers of circulating antibodies could in part be interpreted as a secondary phenomenon. It would be assumed that locally produced antibody with low avidity may combine with antigen to form complexes containing free antigenic determinants, and that extraneous antibody may react with these determinants in a later phase. At the ultrastructural level, as shown by Sordat et al. and others (31,32), the dendritic processes of germinal center reticular cells become more prominent and numerous as the amounts of extracellular antibody increase. Thus, it is possible that these cell membrane processes developed as a consequence of the presence of antigen-antibody complexes and were not well developed prior to their involvement with the complexes.

There is little question that antigen-antibody complexes injected into normal animals localize in germinal centers, or that localization of many antigens occurs more readily in the presence of specific antibody (34,35). We must be careful of our interpretation of the functional aspects of this type of localization, however. As described in one study of the secondary response (32), the persistence of complexes in germinal centers and their cytotoxic effect at high concentrations on the developed plasma membrane infoldings of the reticular cells are quite different from localization during the primary response. The functional significance of the immune reaction of enhanced localization in passively immunized animals can also be questioned. It has been demonstrated that specific passive antibody infusion, while enhancing the initial follicular antigen trapping, also results in a marked suppression of antibody-producing cells and a depression in the hyperplasia of the germinal centers during the primary response (7,36).

It may be that a broad generalization about the enhancing effect of antibody on antigen localization is inaccurate and misleading. What may have been overlooked thus far is the determination of the qualitative and functional effectiveness of the type and avidity of the antibody, either as a part of the complex or as specialized receptor sites on the reticular cell. Quantitative differences in possible saturation of a limited number of receptor sites on the reticular cells may also be of importance.

It seems reasonable that an opsonin, perhaps an immunoglobulin, may be involved in antigen localization early in the primary response (prior to detectable serum antibody). We should also emphasize at this point that localization of antigen in germinal centers is not a static phenomenon, but a dynamic process. This conclusion was reached in studies of the effect of competitive injections of specific or non-cross-reacting antigens on localization of the specific antigen in spleen germinal centers (18). Thus, for some antigens there may be opsonins, readily available at the time of injection, which promote initial localization in germinal centers. The continued localization over weeks and months, however, appears to be a function of specific antibody, and continued antigen localization appears to be inversely dependent on the rate of production of the antibody. What is lacking is information concerning which type or types of antibodies are chiefly responsible for functional localization of antigens in these follicles. One could tentatively rule out IgG_1 as being functional in this process, based on the studies of Hunter (37). These experiments demonstrated that hyperimmunized hamsters producing specific IgG_1, but no detectable IgM, IgA, or IgG_2, could not localize ^{125}I-chicken egg albumin antigen in germinal centers. In addition, germinal center hyperplasia was not observed in these animals. These findings correlate with the fact that IgG_1 is a poor opsonin.

The requirement of opsonic factors for the interaction of antigen and/or antigen-antibody complexes on the surface membranes of dendritic reticular cells is in keeping with the functional aspects of this cell class. Phagocytosis by macrophages in these cells is enhanced by opsonic factors, as is pinocytosis (38). One wonders about the inability of this antigen-retaining dendritic reticular cell to either pinocytose or phagocytize the antigenic material in this location of the spleen. It might be assumed that the development of plasma membrane infoldings as a result of antigen contact is a selective function of the cell designed to prevent sequestration of the antigen and provide antigen for surface contact essential to the differentiation and development of immunologically competent cells. In this context, the presence of antigen or antigen-antibody receptor sites on the surface of these specialized reticular cells becomes a most important question.

FACTORS WHICH ALTER ANTIGEN LOCALIZATION IN GERMINAL CENTERS

Age

The decrease with age of the primary and secondary antibody-forming potential has been associated with the reduction of potential antibody-forming cells (39). Also, studies of Legge and Austin (40a) with 1½-year-old mice have demonstrated the failure of the extracellular antigen-trapping mechanism of germinal centers and have correlated it with the loss of stimulation of antibody-forming cells and reduction of immunologic competence in the aged mice. Antigen localization in spleen germinal centers of 2½-year-old $BC3F_1$ mice is an extremely rare event (40b). Animals of this age produce a reasonable 19S response but a very deficient 7S response to sheep erythrocyte antigen (41).

Williams and Nossal (42), and Hunter (43), have demonstrated that newborn rats lack the follicular and medullary antigen-trapping structures characteristic of adult rats. Williams and Nossal (42) show that throughout the development of the lymphoid tissue in rats the increased magnitude of the antibody response parallels the increased ability of lymphoid structures to retain antigen. During the 1st week of life, primitive lymphoid tissue appeared capable of undergoing the initial steps in differentiation toward antibody production in response to neonatal injection of polymerized flagella. Further maturation appeared to be blocked, however, and by 2 weeks of age this had resulted in a complex immunological state

characterized by increased IgM and decreased IgG antibody response
to antigenic challenge. After the 2-week interval, true follicular
antigen-capturing structures appeared in the lymphoid tissue of the
animals. These studies in newborn and aged animals correlate with
descriptions, by Diener and Nossal (44), of the immune response in
the toad *Buffo marinus* after injection of labeled flagella. They
did not observe antigen trapping in lymph node follicles, nor did
they see any germinal center activity in the jugular bodies. There
was a good primary response characterized by the synthesis of IgM,
with little or no memory formation. Both memory and IgG were
lacking in the absence of germinal centers and antigen trapping
from the lymphoid tissue. Similar findings in other lower vertebrates have been discussed by Pollara *et al.* (45).

Radiation

There appears to be some controversy over the radiosensitivity
of the antigen-retaining reticular cells of germinal centers.
Jaroslow and Nossal (46) proposed that the cytoplasmic processes of
these cells, which are responsible for antigen localization in rat
lymph nodes following footpad injection, are radioresistant. Little
damage could be observed with doses of 1,250 R, and it took 8000 R
to destroy the structure completely. However, these investigators
were referring primarily to antigen trapped in the "sub-sinus region"
of the draining node. In the spleen, where antigen arrives essentially as a single pulse after intravenous injection, total retention
was markedly impaired after 450 R of X-radiation.

Nettesheim and Hanna (47) also observed decreased antigen
(HGG)—trapping ability in the spleens of mice after 400 R of
X-radiation. This corresponded to radiation damage to the dendritic
reticular cell plasma membrane processes. Furthermore, they showed
that antigen-trapping radiosensitivity could not be alleviated in
the presence of circulating IgM or IgG. Their studies are supported
by those of Hunter *et al.* (48), in which shielding of one-half of
the spleen during whole-body X-irradiation (600 R) in rats resulted
in a decrease of follicular trapping of flagellin in the unshielded
region. Although demonstrating the radiosensitivity of the antigen-
trapping mechanism, both these studies are incompatible with the
hypothesis that circulating antibody alone, such as that produced
in the shielded part of the spleen, would confer recognition of
foreignness on the dendritic cell.

Immunosuppressive Agents

The effects of actinomycin D, cyclophosphamide, and cortisone
acetate on localization and retention of radioactive antigen have
been studied in the liver and spleen (49). All three drugs

interfered with antigen retention by the spleen and splenic germinal centers, but not with that by the liver; this impairment of splenic antigen retention was more easily induced when the insult was given before the test antigen. At the dose applied, cortisone acetate did not interfere with immune elimination — a sign of early antibody production — but damaged retention of antigen in splenic germinal centers most severely. These data are considered consistent with the hypothesis that antigen depots in germinal centers are of functional significance for late (particularly 7S) antibody production. These experiments further emphasize the dual effect of immunosuppressive drugs on lymphatic tissue: (1) reduction of their immunologically responsive cell population, and (2) impairment of the dendritic reticular cell capacity to capture and retain antigens.

Earlier in this summary, reference was made to the ability of specific antibodies to enhance localization of test antigens in germinal centers. Further, it has been suggested that during the primary immune reaction the persistence of antigen in germinal centers is a dynamic process, sensitive to and altered by the level of free specific antibody. Sahiar and Schwartz (36) have demonstrated that rabbits receiving heterologous passive antibody 1 hr after antigen have a marked decrease in germinal center hyperplasia during later intervals of the primary response. Thus, two parameters reflect antibody-mediated immune suppression: decrease in the size of the 19S and 7S antibody-producing cell compartments, and decreased proliferation of pyroninophilic cells in germinal centers, as reflected by the centers' lack of growth.

Hanna *et al.* (7) considered the relations between germinal center growth and the development of 19S and 7S cellular responses. During the primary response, the growth of direct plaque-forming cell compartments preceded the growth of germinal centers by 24 hr, while the growth of indirect plaque-forming cell compartments coincided with the growth of germinal centers. Isologous passive antibody injection resulted in an inhibition of germinal center growth, whether or not antibody was infused 1, 2, or 4 days after antigen injection. In terms of formation of sensitized cells, marked depression of 7S memory after passive immunization at 24 hr was observed in contrast to enhancement of the 19S memory. This corresponded to the suppressed growth of germinal centers during the primary response. Thus, if the germinal center is, as has been suggested, a site of the proliferative expansion of immunocompetent cells, these data indicate that germinal center growth is related to the 7S cellular response. The functional significance of persisting antigen in these centers, as studied in the presence of specific passive antibody, appears to be more closely related to the 7S antibody response and the development of 7S memory.

The Germfree State and Antigen Competition

To our knowledge there are only two studies comparing antigen localization in germfree and conventional animals. The first of these (50) describes localization of ^{125}I-labeled Salmonella flagella antigen in popliteal lymph nodes of germfree rats. It demonstrates active localization in the lymphoid follicles of the germfree rats; however, the degree of the follicular reaction, as well as the individual follicular concentration of antigen, was somewhat lower than that measured in the conventional animals. Furthermore, the detectable antibody titer in germfree rats was higher than that measured in conventional rats after both the primary and secondary antigen stimulations.

The second study (25) compares localization of ^{125}I-labeled human gamma globulin (HGG) in spleen germinal centers of germfree and conventional mice. In this study antigen was localized in the cortical regions of spleen lymphatic nodules of germfree mice. Although no active germinal centers were detected in these regions prior to antigen injection, it was apparent that they formed later in response to the antigen. Furthermore, the data in germfree mice obtained with HGG and sheep erythrocyte antigen demonstrated that the early hemagglutinin (19S) response can be initiated in the absence of active germinal centers. However, as compared to the conventional mice, an enhanced 7S response (∿4-fold higher after 7 days) in the germfree animals corresponded to a much greater proliferative reaction in germinal centers as measured both by *de novo* formation and surface area changes of the follicles. Thus the data of both of these experiments demonstrate that antigen localization occurs in germfree mice, and that these animals have an increased immune capacity compared to conventional animals. This is in contrast to earlier studies in germfree animals (51,52), which suggested that the immune capacity, as defined either morphologically or serologically, is limited or underdeveloped in comparison to that of conventional animals. Since the level of antigenic background stimulation in the conventional mouse is not controlled, the magnitude of this difference could be expected to vary among experiments.

Studies measuring recovery of the primary immune potential after irradiation in germfree and conventional mice (53) demonstrate that recovery is earlier and 7S antibody-forming potential greater in the germfree animals. One interpretation of these data is that the lack of competition with adventitious antigens allows for total commitment of immunologically competent cells to localized test antigen in the spleens of the germfree mice.

That antigen competition can be a real factor in this system is further supported by studies (54) in which the immune responsiveness to ^{125}I-HGG was measured in animals injected 1 or 3 days

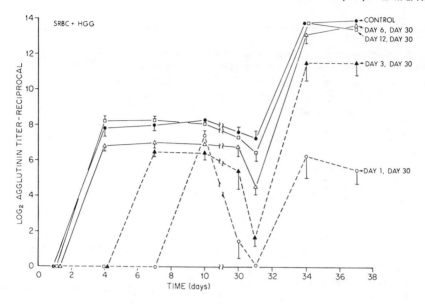

Fig. 2.   Total primary and secondary anti-HGG agglutinin response
in mice primed at various intervals after SRBC immunization:
☐, 1 ml 1.0% SRBC minus 12 days, 0.1 mg aggregated HGG 0 days,
0.1 mg aggregated HGG 30 days; △, 1 ml 1.0% SRBC minus 6 days,
0.1 mg aggregated HGG 0 days, 0.1 mg aggregated HGG 30 days;
▲, 1 ml 1.0% SRBC minus 3 days, 0.1 mg aggregated HGG 0 days,
0.1 mg aggregated HGG 30 days; ○, 1 ml 1.0% SRBC minus 1 day,
0.1 mg aggregated HGG 0 days, 0.1 mg aggregated HGG 30 days;
●, 0.1 mg aggregated HGG 0 days, 0.1 mg aggregated HGG 30 days.
Each point represents a mean of 5 mice ± 1 standard error of the
mean.

previously with SRBC; follicular localization of ^{125}I-HGG was normal,
if not enhanced, while the detectable immunologic reactivity to the
second antigen (HGG) was impaired by antigen competition (Fig. 2).
Thus it is apparent from these studies that dendritic reticular
cells are capable of simultaneously trapping more than one antigen.
However, the impaired immune response to a second antigen during
antigen competition (in the case of SRBC-HGG, a prolonged latent
phase and a deficient primary response to HGG) could be attributable
to a lack of responding immunocompetent progenitor cells. It is
quite possible that such a deficiency is a result of a humoral
factor elaborated in the response to the first antigen (55). As
demonstrated in the SRBC-HGG competition studies, the eventual
recruitment of immunocompetent cells to the second antigen was
limited by the decreased levels of preexisting tissue-associated

antigen and/or free antigen. This system clearly demonstrates that
for some period of time there is a mutual independence of the
antigen-retaining reticular cell from the immunocompetent lymphoid
cells of the follicle, and that the antigen localization by itself
may be a necessary, but not a self-sufficient process for development of some aspects of the primary immune response.

                              Tolerance

    Follicular localization of antigen has been tested in animals
made specifically tolerant to the antigen as newborns. Humphrey
and Frank (17) studied the fate of labeled haemocyanin (HCy) and
human serum albumin (HSA) in the lymph nodes of rabbits made
tolerant as newborns. They found no localization of either antigen
in germinal centers, in a typical dendritic pattern, while the
response of the medullary sinus macrophages was equivalent to that
observed in the nontolerant rabbits. The failure of White *et al.*
(16) to demonstrate localization of crystalline HSA in chickens
rendered specifically immunologically tolerant by neonatal and
continuous injection of antigens lends support to these findings.
These findings are extremely compatible and provide clear evidence
for the participation of some form of specific or cross-reacting
antibody in the initial localization of antigen in germinal centers.

    Somewhat in opposition to these findings are the results of
Ada *et al.* (56,57), which show localization of a prepared digest
of Salmonella flagellin in adult rats previously made tolerant with
high or low dose ranges. It was interpreted from these studies
that follicular localization of the flagellin digest antigen might
act as an amplification mechanism where circulating lymphocytes
react with the antigen, resulting in tolerance.

    Mitchison (58) has shown that mice paralyzed by bovine serum
albumin (BSA) gradually recovered immunologic reactivity. In these
studies recovery from paralysis induced at 1 day of age was markedly
slower than recovery from paralysis induced at 6 weeks of age, but
in general recovery is more rapid in young than in old animals.
In many cases the recovery from paralysis resulted in overshoot of
once paralyzed animals to become responsive. Recovery in these
animals was demonstrated to be a function of stimulatory material
(antigen) in the lymphoid tissue. It is still a possibility that
the antigen localization observed by Ada *et al.* (56) in germinal
centers of adult rats made tolerant to flagella could be functional
in the recovery of the animals from tolerance rather than in the
maintenance of the tolerant state. One could visualize a situation
similar to that described previously in the case of antigen competition between SRBC-HGG. Here the localization occurred in the absence
of functional immunocompetent progenitor cells, but the antigen was

essential for recovery during the restoration or release of
functional immunocompetent cells.

Genetics

There is little information about the influence of genetics
on the ability of animals to localize antigen on dendritic reticular
cells. Hunter (37) has shown a variation of spleen retention of
equivalent doses of antigen among Fischer (F344/N), Marshall (M520)
and outbred Sprague-Dawley rats of similar age, weight, and
environmental background. Autoradiographs confirm that the difference in isotope counts in the spleen were due primarily to differences in the amount of ^{125}I-labeled antigen retained by the dendritic
reticular cells (Fig. 3). Specifically, among the Sprague-Dawley
rats there was a large variation in ability to localize ^{125}I-
Salmonella flagella; whereas the Fischer rats uniformly localized
high levels of antigen, and the Marshall rats uniformly localized
low levels of the antigen. Results of tests with 13 other strains
showed that localization varied greatly among outbred compared to
inbred strains. Further results of this study demonstrate that
both cellular and serologic factors are involved in this genetically
determined variation in antigen retention.

VIRUS LOCALIZATION IN GERMINAL CENTERS:

RELATION TO DISEASE PROCESSES

Germinal centers have been implicated as possible factors in
leukemogenesis. Metcalf (59) demonstrated the abnormal occurrence
of germinal centers in the thymus of aged AKR mice during a preleukemic period. Jerusalem (60) recently demonstrated the relationship of thymic germinal centers to an aleukemic malignant lymphoma
in Swiss mice. He presented evidence of virus particles in thymic
germinal centers and suggested that these particles could influence
the role of the thymus in leukemogenesis. Finally, endogenous
C-type leukemogenic virus particles have been detected in lymphatic
tissue germinal centers of BC3F$_1$, C58, and AKR mice, as well as
normal guinea pigs (61).

Histologic and ultrastructural studies of Hanna et al. (62) on
BALB/c mice infected with Rauscher leukemia virus (RLV) strongly
suggest that one of the earliest detectable tissue sites of C-type
virus localization, as well as replication in immunocompetent
progenitor cells, is in the nonthymus-dependent areas of spleen
lymphatic nodules and lymph nodes, particularly in the germinal
centers. This site of C-type virus replication was observed within
the 1st day after injection and was associated with the capacity of

antigen-trapping reticular cells to localize the virus extracellularly in proximity to parenchymal immunoblasts of this region of the nodule. We attribute the initial localization of the virus primarily to its antigenic quality and not necessarily to its biologic quality. Because of this morphologic study, we concluded that a selective replication of the virus in proliferating cells of the germinal centers causes lymphoblastosis, an early and essential aspect of the splenomegaly associated with Rauscher disease.

It is not unreasonable that RNA viruses would concentrate in germinal centers when one recognizes this region's high mitotic activity and relates this to a general assumption that the cell lesion or malignant transformation of cells by viruses depends on a specific interaction between the viral and the host-cell genome. A replication requirement of the host cell for virus production would limit other cells, such as mature lymphocytes and reticular cells of the nodule, as target cells. Thus, functionally adapted cells, such as the dendritic reticular cells in germinal centers, perform a specialized role in retention and/or processing of antigen, and consequently concentrate a large number of virus particles. The concentration of antigen may be essential to the animal in development of an immune response, but in the case of viruses with biological activity, it may lead to infection of local parenchymal cells that are susceptible to the virus because of their level of maturation. In this way antigen retention in germinal centers may contribute directly to the pathogenesis of the disease (73,31).

A most exciting aspect of virus localization in germinal centers is the recently demonstrated ability to induce, by intrathymic injection of Gross leukemia virus (GLV), germinal centers in the thymus medulla of 12-week-old AKR mice (Fig. 4). Spontaneous formation of germinal centers in the thymus medulla of 8- to 10-month-old AKR mice has been described by Metcalf (59) as a preleukemic change preceding the development of thymomas. As described in the study of Hogg and Hanna (63), the thymus germinal centers in the young adult AKR mice were characteristic of those observed in spleen and lymph nodes and contained numerous cells with developing plasma membrane infoldings that were morphologically indistinguishable from the dendritic reticular cell. Numerous C-type virus particles were detected extracellularly in the plasma membrane infoldings of these cells (Fig. 5). This would tend to correlate the preleukemic germinal centers with the increasing concentration of C-type virus in the aged AKR thymus. Also, a dynamic mobility of the antigen-retaining reticular cells is suggested from these studies, since the germinal centers developed in areas of the medulla in which extrathymic mononuclear cell infiltration had previously occurred. The induced infiltration of antigen-retaining reticular cells with subsequent germinal center formation accounts for ectopic germinal center formation in various autoimmune conditions and situations of

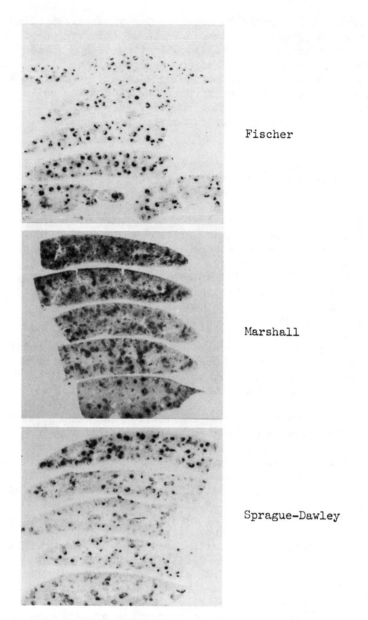

Fischer

Marshall

Sprague-Dawley

Fig. 3. These low power (5X) autoradiographs show the differences
in the retention of ^{125}I-*Salmonella typhi* flagella by the dendritic
macrophages of the three rat strains. The black spots are silver
grains of ^{125}I label over individual lymphoid follicles.

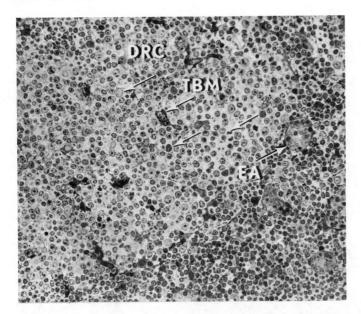

Fig. 4. A thymus germinal center 3 days after the intrathymic
injection of Gross leukemia virus in 3-month-old AKR mice. Note
the epithelial acinar formation (EA) characteristic of the mouse
thymus medulla. The germinal center contains characteristic
tingible body macrophages (TBM), dendritic reticular cells (DRC),
and numerous mitotic figures (→). 450X.

chronic infection. Further, the overall process must correlate
with increasing antigen concentration in the tissue and must be
assumed to be a form of local immune surveillance.

CONCEPTS OF THE ROLE OF ANTIGEN LOCALIZED IN GERMINAL CENTERS

     Neither the peak titers of 2-mercaptoethanol-sensitive antibody
(IgM) nor peak number of direct plaque-forming cells (IgM cellular
response) during the primary immune reaction correlate well with
the amount of antigen localized in dendritic reticular cells or
with the proliferative development of immunocompetent lymphoid
cells of the centers (7,64). This poor correlation is only one
of several reasons to believe that the dendritic reticular cells
and their interaction with antigen-antibody complexes are not
necessary for IgM antibody synthesis. Other correlations mentioned
in this review are: (1) Newborn and aged mice and rats almost
exclusively synthesize IgM antibody before they develop antigen-
retaining reticular cells or after this capacity is lost as a

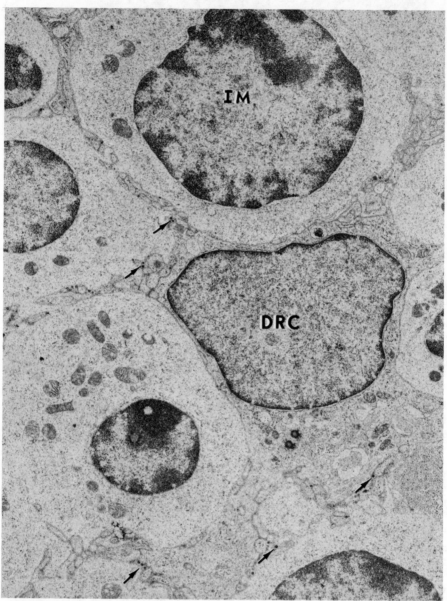

Fig. 5. An electron micrograph of cells in the GLV-induced thymus
germinal center. A dendritic reticulum cell (DRC) containing
numerous C-type virus particles (→) within plasma membrane infoldings
can be seen adjacent to an immunoblast (IM).   16,000X.

degenerative function of senescence. An exception to this condition of newborn mice and rats is the 7S antibody-forming capacity of fetal sheep. As pointed out by Silverstein in these Proceedings, the fetal lymphoid tissue of these animals contains lymphatic germinal centers. (2) In systems where follicular antigen localization has been depressed by X-irradiation or drugs, animals are able to synthesize IgM but have a deficient IgG capacity. (3) In lower vertebrates, no germinal center activity or antigen trapping in lymphoid follicles can be observed in the primitive lymphoid tissue, but there is generally a good primary IgM response with little or no IgG development. These studies suggest that both memory and IgG are essentially lacking when germinal centers are absent from lymphoid tissue.

Studies by Fitch *et al.* (64) of the concentrations of hemolysin-containing cells in lymphatic tissue demonstrate that the localization of these cells in lymphoid follicles during a primary immune response corresponds with IgG rather than IgM antibody response. These data provide additional evidence that lymphoid follicles in germinal centers may act as part of the amplification system characteristic of the IgG response.

It is not difficult to reconcile this requirement of the 7S response for antigen on cell membranes, since principle recruitment of the 7S cellular response occurs after the major sequestration of metabolizable antigen, whereas 19S response recruitment occurs much earlier, at a time when there are high levels of antigen throughout the lymphoid tissue. Also, it is difficult to elaborate situations in which IgG_2 antibody, as well as IgG_2 memory formation, is developed in the absence of the tissue organization associated with functional dendritic reticular cells. The tentative inability to produce an adequate 7S or IgG phase of the primary immune response with unprimed, dissociated spleen or lymph node cells in *in vitro* systems can be used to support this statement.

The basis for a model of the interaction of antigen-antibody complexes on dendritic reticular cells and potential antibody-forming cells might be taken from the concept that antigen has a continuous role in the recruitment and differentiation of antibody-forming cells. The strongest support for this concept is derived from recent studies of passive antibody-mediated suppression (65). Moreover, the immune cell maturation scheme of Sercarz and Coons (66) and the modification of Sterzl (5), commonly referred to as the X-Y-Z model, is based on the requirement of continuous antigenic stimulation in the development and differentiation of antibody-producing cells. As defined, the antigen-sensitive cell (X-cell) is converted to sensitized Y-cells upon stimulation. Recent evidence suggests that this step would require interaction with at least one other cell type (67). Presumably, the Y-cell is not an efficient antibody-producing cell, but acts as a sensitized progenitor cell that is qualitatively distinct from the antigen-sensitive cell. Stimulation of the Y-cell by antigen

results in proliferation of these sensitized cells which then expand
the cell compartment prior to irreversible maturation of Y-cells to
functional antibody-producing Z-cells.

In support of this immune cell model, Byers and Sercarz (68)
suggested that a condition of excess antigen depletes or depresses
the Y-cell compartment. In addition, Hanna et al. (7) have demonstrated, in the in vivo transfer system, that after initial recruitment with antigen-sensitive cells, passive administration of antibody
results in an enlarged Y-cell compartment. It can be considered that
this enlarged sensitized cell compartment is a result of the rescue
of Y-cells from their normal antigen-driven maturation to functional
antibody-forming cells, which is a natural occurrence during the
primary response. Thus, an important correlary to these findings is
the existence of antigen depots in immunologically competent tissue.
These depots, then, could act as a microenvironment in lymphoid
tissue, functioning not only in the expansion or amplification of
the sensitized or memory cell compartment, as has been suggested by
Wakefield and Thorbecke (69), but also in the continued differentiation of primary antibody-forming cells.

This model would require that the population of immunologically
competent effector cells possess membrane receptors for the antigen-
antibody complexes attached to the dendritic reticular cell processes.
This provision of extracellular antigen depots interacting with
lymphocytes that bear specific receptors would be applicable and
essential to the model of antigen-driven selection and replication
during the later stages of the primary response of immunocompetent
cells capable of producing higher affinity antibody, as described
by Siskind and Benacerraf (70).

Dukor et al. (71) and Bianco et al. (72) have demonstrated in
the follicular areas and marginal zone of the spleen, as well as in
the true cortex of lymph nodes, the localization of a subpopulation
of lymphocytes distinguished by a membrane receptor for antibody-
complement complexes. They argue that follicular antigen localization
in vivo has been shown to be antibody-dependent and to involve the
participation of the Fc fragment, which is required for complement
fixation. Their combined evidence, both in vivo and in vitro, demonstrate that a specialized lymphocyte may participate in follicular
antigen trapping, and that the antigen localization in follicles is
mediated by membrane receptors common to both lymphoid and reticular
cells. This specific subpopulation of lymphoid cells was conspicu-
ously absent from the thymus and from the thymus-dependent areas of
spleen, lymph node, and Peyer's patches. This would suggest, therefore, that the lymphocyte subpopulation distinguished by the membrane
receptor for antibody-complement complex is directly derived from
bone marrow. This suggestion fits well with the known compartmenta-
lization of lymphoid tissues into thymic and nonthymic-dependent areas

and the demonstrated immediate independence from the thymus of the parenchymal lymphoid cells which occupy germinal centers.

REFERENCES

1. J. Sterzl, Nature, 183:547, 1959.

2. Robert E. Franzl, Nature, 195:457, 1962.

3. D. H. Campbell and J. Garvey, in: F. J. Dixon and H. G. Kunkel, Eds., Advances in Immunology, Vol. 3, p. 263. New York: Academic Press, 1963.

4. Z. Trnka and J. Sterzl, in: Mechanisms of Antibody Formation, p. 190. New York: Academic Press, 1960.

5. J. Sterzl, Cold Spring Harbor Symp. Quant. Biol., 32:493, 1967.

6. N. K. Jerne, Cold Spring Harbor Symp. Quant. Biol., 32:591, 1967.

7. M. G. Hanna, Jr., P. Nettesheim, and Mary W. Francis, J. Exp. Med., 129:953, 1969.

8. G. L. Ada and J. M. Williams, Immunology, 10:417, 1966.

9. G. L. Ada, C. R. Parish, G. J. V. Nossal, and A. Abbot, Cold Spring Harbor Symp. Quant. Biol., 32:381, 1967.

10. G. L. Ada, G. J. V. Nossal, and J. Pye, Aust. J. Exp. Biol. Med. Sci., 42:295, 1964.

11. L. G. Sweet, G. D. Abrams, and A. G. Johnson, J. Immunol., 94:105, 1965.

12. H. O. McDevitt, Brigitte Askonas, J. H. Humphrey, I. Schecter, and M. Sela, Immunology, 11:337, 1966.

13. G. J. V. Nossal, Caroline M. Austin, J. Pye, and Judith Mitchell, Int. Arch. Allergy, 29:369, 1966.

14. M. G. Hanna, Jr., T. Makinodan, and W. D. Fisher, in: H. Cottier, N. Odartchenko, R. Schindler, and C. C Congdon, Eds., Germinal Centers in Immune Response, p. 86. New York: Springer-Verlag, 1967.

15. B. M. Balfour and J. H. Humphrey, in: Germinal Centers in Immune Response, p. 80.

16. R. G. White, V. I. French, and J. M. Stark, in: Germinal
    Centers in Immune Response, p. 311.

17. J. H. Humphrey and M. M. Frank, Immunology, 13:87, 1967.

18. M. G. Hanna, Jr., Mary W. Francis, and Leona C. Peters,
    Immunology, 15:75, 1968.

19. C. S. Henney, D. R. Stanworth, and G. H. Gell, Nature, 205:1079,
    1965.

20. K. Rajewski, E. Rottlander, G. Peitre, and B. Muller,
    J. Exp. Med., 126:581, 1967.

21. M. J. Crumpton, Nature, 215:17, 1967.

22. M. Seligmann and C. Mihaesco (editorial), Rev. Franc. Études
    Clin. Et. Biol., 12:851, 1967.

23. G. L. Ada, in: Enrico Michich, Ed., Immunity, Cancer and
    Chemotherapy. Basic Relationship on the Cellular Level, p. 17.
    New York: Academic Press, 1967.

24. R. G. White, Antibiotica et Chemotherapia, 15:24 (Karger,
    Basel/New York, 1969).

25. M. G. Hanna, Jr., P. Nettesheim, and H. E. Walburg, Jr., in:
    E. A. Mirand and N. Black, Eds., Germ-Free Biology: Experimental
    and Clinical Aspects, p. 257. Advan. Exp. Med. Biol., Vol. 3,
    New York: Plenum Press, 1969.

26. G. J. V. Nossal, G. L. Ada, Caroline M. Austin, and J. Pye,
    Immunology, 9:349, 1965.

27. G. L. Ada, G. J. V. Nossal, and Caroline M. Austin, Aust. J.
    Exp. Biol. Med. Sci., 42:331, 1964.

28. D. W. Menzies, Nature, 208:163, 1965.

29. G. J. V. Nossal, A. Abbot, Judith Mitchell, and Z. Lummus,
    J. Exp. Med., 127:277, 1968.

30. B. Sordat, M. Sordat, M. Hess, R. D. Stoner, and H. Cottier,
    J. Exp. Med., 131:77, 1970.

31. A. K. Szakal and M. G. Hanna, Jr., Exp. Mol. Pathol., 8:75, 1968.

32. M. G. Hanna, Jr. and A. K. Szakal, J. Immunol., 101:949, 1968.

33. H. S. Bennett, J. Biophys. Biochem, Cytol., 2:99, 1956.

34. P. Gillian Lang and G. L. Ada, Immunology, 13:523, 1967.

35. R. C. Mellors and W. J. Bazosko, J. Exp. Med., 115:891, 1962.

36. K. Sahiar and R. S. Schwartz, Int. Arch. Allergy Appl. Immunol., 29:52, 1966.

37. R. L. Hunter, unpublished data.

38. Z. A. Cohn, in: R. T. Smith and R. A. Good, Eds., Cellular Recognition, p. 34. New York: Appleton-Century-Crofts, 1969.

39. T. Makinodan and W. J. Peterson, J. Immunol., 93:886, 1964.

40a. J. S. Legge and C. M. Austin, Aust. J. Exp. Biol. Med. Sci., 46:361, 1968.

40b. M. G. Hanna, Jr., P. Nettesheim, and M. J. Snodgrass, Nat. Cancer Inst. (in press), 1970.

41. M. G. Hanna, Jr., P. Nettesheim, L. Ogden, and T. Makinodan, Proc. Soc. Exp. Biol. Med., 125:882, 1967.

42. G. M. Williams and G. J. V. Nossal, J. Exp. Med., 124:47, 1966.

43. R. L. Hunter, New Physician, 15(5):111, 1966.

44. E. Diener and G. J. V. Nossal, Immunology, 10:535, 1966.

45. B. Pollara, J. Finstad, and R. A. Good, in: L. Fiore-Donati and M. G. Hanna, Jr., Eds., Lymphatic Tissue and Germinal Centers in Immune Response, Advan. Exp. Med. Biol., Vol. 5, p. 1. New York: Plenum Press, 1969.

46. B. N. Jaroslow and G. J. V. Nossal, Aust. J. Exp. Biol. Med. Sci., 44:609, 1966.

47. P. Nettesheim and M. G. Hanna, Jr., in: Lymphatic Tissue and Germinal Centers in Immune Response, p. 167.

48. R. L. Hunter, R. W. Wissler, and F. W. Fitch, in: Lymphatic Tissue and Germinal Centers in Immune Response, p. 101.

49. P. Nettesheim and Anna S. Hammons, Proc. Soc. Exp. Biol. Med., 133:696, 1970.

50. J. J. Miller III, D. O. Johnsen, and G. L. Ada, Nature, 217:1059, 1968.

51. H. Bauer, R. E. Horowitz, K. C. Watkins, and H. J. Popper,
     J. Amer. Med. Ass., 87:715, 1964.

52. G. B. Olson and B. S. Wustmann, Fed. Proc., 14:1400, 1965.

53. P. Nettesheim, H. E. Walburg, Jr., and M. G. Hanna, Jr.,
     unpublished data.

54. M. G. Hanna, Jr. and Leona C. Peters, J. Immunol., 104:166, 1970.

55. T. Radovich and D. W. Talmadge, Science, 158:512, 1968.

56. G. L. Ada, G. J. V. Nossal, and J. Pye, Aust. J. Exp. Biol.
     Med. Sci., 43:337, 1965.

57. G. L. Ada and C. R. Parish, Proc. Nat. Acad. Sci. U.S.A.,
     61:556, 1968.

58. N. A. Mitchison, Immunology, 9:129, 1965.

59. D. Metcalf, The Thymus. Its Role in Immune Response, Leukemia
     Development and Carcinogenesis. New York: Springer-Verlag, 1966.

60. C. Jerusalem, in: Lymphatic Tissue and Germinal Centers in
     Immune Response, p. 497.

61. D. C. Swartzendruber, B. I. Ma., and W. H. Murphy, in:
     Lymphatic Tissue and Germinal Centers in Immune Response, p. 203.

62. M. G. Hanna, Jr., A. K. Szakal, and R. L. Tyndall, Cancer Res.,
     30:1748, 1970.

63. R. A. Hogg and M. G. Hanna, Jr., unpublished data.

64. F. W. Fitch, R. Stejskal, and D. A. Rowley, in: Lymphatic Tissue
     and Germinal Centers in Immune Response, p. 223.

65. J. W. Uhr and G. Moller, in: Advances in Immunology, Vol. 9,
     p. 81. New York: Academic Press, 1968.

66. E. E. Sercarz and A. H. Coons, in: M. Hasek, A. Lenogerova,
     and M. Vojtiskov, Eds., Mechanisms of Immunological Tolerance,
     p. 73. Prague: Publishing House of the Czechoslovak Academy
     of Sciences, 1962.

67. D. E. Mosier, J. Exp. Med., 127:277, 1969.

68. V. S. Byers and E. E. Sercarz, J. Exp. Med. 127:307, 1968.

69. J. D. Wakefield and G. J. Thorbecke, J. Exp. Med., 128:171, 1968.

70. G. W. Siskind and B. Benacerraf, in: Advances in Immunology, Vol. 10, p. 1. New York: Academic Press, 1969.

71. P. Dukor, C. Birnco, and V. Nussenzweig, Proc. Natl. Acad. Sci. U.S.A. (in press), 1970.

72. C. Bianco, P. Dukor, and V. Nussenzweig, these Proceedings p. 251, 1970.

73. D. C. Swartzendruber, B. I. Ma and W. H. Murphy, Proc. Soc. Exptl. Biol. Med., 126:731, 1967.

DISCUSSION TO SESSION 5
CHAIRMAN, M. G. HANNA, JR., CO-CHAIRMAN, R. L. HUNTER

Co-chairman's remarks: There is abundant evidence that antigen-antibody complexes are involved in the retention of antigen by the dendritic reticular cells (DRC) located in germinal centers. Dr. Hanna has just alluded to evidence that other factors are also involved. I would like to very quickly show two experiments which demonstrate the existance of another factor. Leon Pringle and I have studied the uptake of antigen by the DRC of the rat spleen *in vitro*, in an isolated perfused spleen system (1). Rat spleens were perfused at a constant pressure of 60 mm Hg through the splenic artery with a mixture of Eagles minimal essential media (45%), Dextran 75 (Abbott Laboratories, Chicago, Illinois) (45%), and immune rat serum (10%). ^{125}I-labeled S. typhi flagella were "injected" via the perfusate and the localization and movements of flagella in the spleen were followed by autoradiography. As seen in Figure 1, the antigen was removed from the blood stream by cells in the marginal sinus surrounding the lymphoid follicle. Using this system, we demonstrated that the antigen particles destined for localization in the DRC were first taken up by cells in the marginal sinus and were then carried to the DRC in the lymphoid follicles. Since the adherence of material to the marginal sinus is the first step in the uptake of material by the DRC, this adherence phenomenon might properly be called "antigen recognition" for the DRC.

The work of Stejskal and Fitch has given us an *in vitro* method of studying the adherence of material to the marginal sinus of the spleen (2). In their model, frozen sections of rat spleen were incubated with a suspension of sheep red blood cells. The section was then inverted in a dish of saline and the cells were allowed to settle away. Red cells adhered to the section wherever there was antibody or any other material which bound them. The location of the adherent cells was determined under a microscope. In unimmunized animals, sheep red blood cells characteristically adhered only to the marginal sinus of the spleen. At five days after immunization, red cells adhered, in addition, over much of the red pulp and the white pulp as seen in Figure 2. This adherence over the red and white pulp was almost certainly due to antibody (2,3). Now, if the frozen sections were treated with 0.1 M 2-mercapto-ethanol, before adding the red cells, the adherence of cells over the red pulp and the white pulp was destroyed, but that over the marginal sinus remained undisturbed, Figure 3. In contrast, if the sections were heated to 56°C for 30 minutes, the adherence of material to the marginal sinus was destroyed, but that in the red and white pulp was preserved, Figure 4. Consequently, in this system, the substance which caused adherence of material to the marginal sinus behaved differently from the antibody found in either the red or the white pulp. In addition, none of the immunofluorescent studies of which I am aware have shown any immunoglobulin in the marginal sinus. These experiments provide evidence

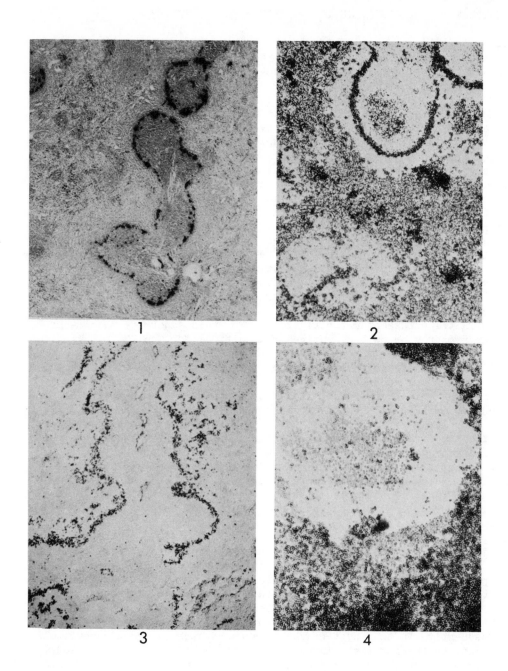

1

2

3

4

Fig. 1. Autoradiograph of isolated perfused rat spleen showing
^{125}I-labeled flagella on the marginal sinus ($\sim$50 X).
Fig. 2-4. Rat spleen frozen sections with adherent sheep red
cells showing the location of receptors for this antigen in an
immunized animal and the effects of 2-mercaptoethanol and heat.
(2 $\sim$60 X, 3 $\sim$50 X, 4 $\sim$100X)

---

that the initial stage of "antigen recognition" for the DRC is due
to some substance present in the marginal sinus which is quite
different from any of the antibody demonstrable in spleen sections.

REFERENCES

1. L. Pringle and R. L. Hunter, J. Reticuloendothelial Soc.,
    5:9, 1968.

2. R. Stejskal and F. W. Fitch, J. Reticuloendothelial Soc.,
    7:121, 1970.

3. F. W. Fitch, R. Stejskal, and D. A. Rowley, in: L. Fiore-Donati
    and M. G. Hanna, Jr, Eds., Lymphatic Tissue and Germinal Centers
    in Immune Response, p. 223. New York: Plenum Press, 1969.

P. Alexander: Dr. Ada, how long does the tolerance persist which
you get under your various regimes, and in terms of persistence,
can you differentiate the various types of tolerance which you
have discovered?

G. L. Ada: High zone tolerance persists for at least two months
after the last injection of antigen. Low zone tolerance and ultra
low zone tolerance do not persist for very long at all.

M. W. Hess: Dr. Ada, did you ever find antigen within lymphoid
cells in tolerant animals?

G. L. Ada: No.

M. Feldman: Most studies on tolerance to flagella have been
performed with rats; mice are apparently much less capable of
evincing tolerance to this antigen. Could you comment on the
differences in antigen localization between rats and mice?

G. L. Ada: There certainly are species differences. It is much
more difficult to make mice tolerant, particularly the CBA mice
that Diener uses. I would hazard a guess that in the rat species
we use, follicular localization is demonstrated much more readily
than in the CBA mouse.

G. J. Thorbecke: Have you ever investigated if the response to fragment A is as thymus dependent as is the response to flagellin? We probably should differentiate between tolerance induction in the T or the B cells, especially when we try to reconcile *in vitro* and *in vivo* data.

G. L. Ada: The tolerance which you get in the adult rat, by using the fragments, extends to the polymerized materials. I think Dr. Lind has shown that the production of antibody to flagella in the rat is thymus dependent.

J. F. A. P. Miller: My question is related to what Dr. Thorbecke just asked. Have you tried to break tolerance in any of your low zone systems with T cells, and if not what would you predict?

G. L. Ada: I will let you know in a few months' time.

V. Anderson: I would just like to put forward the view that any antigenic stimulus which induces antibody production may at the same time induce tolerance in cells that are immunologically immature. There is no time to give the evidence for this, but I think it would fit in with the possibility of the germinal centers may be concerned both with tolerance in the B system and with antibody production. My question is this: Does anybody know if induction of tolerance to thymic independent antigens is associated with germinal center production?

(Editor's Note: no answer)

W. H. Hildeman: Dr. Laissue, given the well established fact that IgG antibody alone will often interfere with, rather than potentiate immune responses, as in tumor enhancement, the Rhesus story or prolonged organ graft survival, one might predict that immune complexes in antibody excess, particularly if IgG antibodies were used, would in fact diminish rather than potentiate the immune response. Do you have any evidence on this? Also, what happens to germinal center development if you should get antibody excess?

M. W. Hess: Primary tetanus antitoxin responses in mice following stimulation with antigen-antibody complexes, prepared in the region of equivalence, antigen excess, or antibody excess, have been compared in a series of experiments performed in collaboration with Drs. Stoner and Terres. Enhancement of primary antitoxin production was invariably observed in mice stimulated with complexes at equivalence and in antigen excess. Animals stimulated with complexes prepared in antibody excess produced less antibody than controls immunized with antigen only.

(Editor's Note: Nobody answered Dr. Hildeman's second question, but it has been shown in at least two systems that excess antibody can suppress germinal center proliferation.)

M. A. B. de Sousa: The experiments we presented were based on the
assumption that lymphocytes would indeed go through germinal centers,
and therefore, fulfill Dr. Ada's hypothesis about the induction of
tolerance. However, we failed to find cells, even previously
sensitized cells, going to germinal centers. I would, therefore,
like to ask Dr. Balfour and Dr. Ada if they would like to comment
on how to conciliate one's results with the other's hypothesis?

G. L. Ada: Dr. Austin and Dr. Nossal in Melbourne have shown traffic
of lymphocytes through primary follicles. The technique essentially
was to pass cells, labelled in one rat, to rats joined by parabiosis.

B. M. Balfour: It is clear that there is a population of cells which
visits the antigen depot and returns to the draining node via the
afferent lymphatic. Following injection of diphtheria toxoid or heat
aggregated HGG which provoke germinal center responses, the number
of blast cells in the afferent lymph rises quite significantly and
a high proportion of these cells do localize in germinal centers of
the node. After injection of antigens such as bovine red cells
the afferent lymph coming from the depot does not contain increased
number of blast cells, but only lymphocytes and these cells do not
localize in germinal centers.

J. E. Veldman: I think the experiments presented by Professor
Keuning and Dr. Bos at the first germinal center conference in Bern
are pertinent. When a peripheral lymph node is locally irradiated
with 750 rads all lymphocytes in it are killed in interphase. Within
12 to 24 hours two sites of influx of lymphoid cells - from the blood -
present themselves. One population of lymphocytes home into the
paracortical areas and another population of lymphoid cells into
outer cortical areas, which present themselves within a very short
time as primary follicles. This last category of lymphoid cells
belongs to the non-thymus derived cell population, presumably the
B-cells. This experiment shows that lymphoid cells can migrate into
primary follicles very rapidly and in large numbers.

A. Cruchaud: I would like to make a hypothesis as to the role of
complement in endocytosis and ask Dr. Phillips-Quagliata if she does
agree with it. Endocytosis by macrophages follows a multiple hit
phenomenon: in other words, a molecule of antigen which hits the
plasma membrane of a macrophage in only one place has little chance
to be endocytosed. Also, macrophages have separate binding sites
for IgG, complement and presumably IgM. When you introduce complement,
increased endocytosis may not be consequent to a modification in the
structure of the antigen-antibody complex, but may be due to a
further increase in the number of hits.

J. M. Phillips-Quagliata: I think that is a reasonable explanation,
but I don't know if there is any real proof of it.

N. L. Warner: In relation to the question of whether the energy of binding of antigen and antibody produces a change in the Fc part of the immunoglobulin that is of importance to the cell, Dr. Ovary and I studied an IgG_{2a} myeloma protein which has the potential for mast cell binding since it gives an RPCA reaction. This myeloma has antidinitrophenol binding activity but will not fix complement or elicit a PCA reaction. It has an extremely low affinity of binding. This raises the possibility that there may be a certain minimum energy of binding, which is necessary to activate the Fc biologically active sites. I therefore wondered if you have studied macrophage immunoglobulin binding with antibodies of differing affinities?

J. M. Phillips-Quagliata: No, I have only used this one purified rabbit antihapten antibody in this system. Also the receptors on the surfaces of macrophages may be entirely different from the receptors on the surfaces of mast cells since an entirely different IgG type molecule is involved. I cannot say anything at all about an allosteric change in the IgA or IgE molecule.

S. Cohen: Dr. Phillips-Quagliata has mentioned the possibilities of allosteric change and summation of binding energies as explanations of the enhancement of antibody binding to macrophages when multi-valent antigens were present at equivalence. There is a third possibility. In analogy with complement fixation, it is possible that each antibody molecule possesses a functionally incomplete binding site. The formation of immune complexes would then serve to link adjacent antibody molecules to form multiple complement sites. This possibility is operationally distinct from that in which multiple complete sites summate their binding energies, and is subject to experimental test.

C. N. Muller-Berat: Dr. Bianco, in your data you mention a population of lymphocytes which is not thymus dependent and which makes rosettes together with complement and antibody and migrates in a particular zone of a BSA gradient. Have you further tested the thymus indepen-dence of these cells by determining their sensitivity to antilympho-cyte serum or to Imuran as described by Drs. Bach and Dormont.

C. Bianco: No, we never tried the antilymphocyte serum.

E. Möller: Is the C'3 receptor present on all B cells? Do you get a 100% cytoxic effect with anti-theta serum after removal of your C'3 receptor bearing cells?

C. Bianco: I cannot answer that. However, the cells that have the receptors for complement are B cells but not all B cells have receptors. For instance in PFC's we do not find the receptor for complement.

E. Möller: But that might be a very small proportion. You mentioned in your talk that there was an inverse relationship between theta sensitivity and the presence of the C'3 receptor. Later you mentioned that the C'3 receptor was present in part of the B cells. It would be difficult to use the C'3 receptor as a marker for B cells, if it is not present on all those cells.

C. Bianco: We are not sure of the percentage of bone marrow derived cells which have these receptors. I think the presence of the receptor may be related to the stage of development of the cells.

M. Raff: I think that there is reasonable evidence in mice that the lymphocytes with receptors for C'3 are the same cells that have readily demonstrable Ig on their surface and that these cells form a subpopulation of thymus-independent B lymphocytes. I say that because in any given population of lymphocytes, spleen or lymph node for example, the percentage of cells that can be killed with anti-MBLA, which we think is the total population of B cells, is greater than the percentage of cells with receptors for C'3 or with readily detectable surface Ig. Thus there would appear to be at least this degree of heterogeneity within the B cell population.

L. Fiore-Donati: Do they also react to phytohemagglutinin *in vitro*? This we believe can show the competence of lymphoid cells engaged in cell mediated responses. This could distinguish the two populations.

C. Bianco: Yes, but we have not tried it.

ROLE OF INDUCTIVE MICROENVIRONMENTS ON HEMOPOIETIC (AND LYMPHOID ?) DIFFERENTIATION, AND ROLE OF THYMIC CELLS IN THE EOSINOPHILIC GRANULOCYTE RESPONSE TO ANTIGEN

J. J. Trentin, M. P. McGarry, V. K. Jenkins, M. T. Gallagher,

R. S. Speirs, and N. S. Wolf

Baylor College of Medicine, Houston, Texas 77025

Hemopoietic spleen colonies arising in lethally irradiated mice repopulated with limited numbers of bone marrow cells have been shown to be clonal in origin (1,2), each arising from a single stem cell or colony forming unit (CFU).

Most if not all hemopoietic spleen colonies and bone marrow colonies arise not from committed but from pluripotent stem cells that are directed (induced) along any one of four lines of hemopoietic differentiation (erythroid, neutrophilic granuloid, eosinophilic granuloid or megakaryocytic) by interaction with their respective microenvironmental area of splenic or marrow stroma (2,3). We have designated these stromal areas as hemopoietic inductive microenvironments (HIM). As judged by the proportion of colonies of each type, erythroid HIM (E HIM) predominate in the spleen stroma, whereas granuloid HIM (G HIM) predominate in the marrow stroma (3).

The progeny of induced CFU are limited to the one line of differentiation for a period of approximately 10 days. That such colonies also continue to replicate pluripotent CFU is indicated by the facts that (a) beyond 10 days they develop a second line of hemopoietic differentiation, of endogenous (intraclonal) origin (2), presumably by overgrowth of the original microenvironment and interaction with an adjacent different HIM; (b) if transplanted earlier than 10 days, colonies of single line of differentiation give rise in secondary irradiated mice to spleen colonies of each of the four lines of differentiation, each again limited initially to a single line of differentiation, and each type of colony occurring in the same proportion as in the case of primary spleen colonies; (c) if growing in a spleen containing a transplanted piece of marrow stroma,

289

single colonies that straddle the border between marrow and spleen stroma are invariably erythroid in the spleen stroma, and granuloid in the marrow stroma (3).

The E HIM is presumed to act by converting pluripotent, erythropoietin insensitive stem cells (CFU) to a state of erythropoietin sensitivity (4).

The present studies were designed (a) to elucidate the possible role of the E HIM in the genetic macrocytic anemia of Sl/Sl^d mice; (b) to search for a hypothetical lymphoid inducing microenvironment (LIM); (c) to study the possible role of the eosinophilic HIM (Eo HIM) in the eosinophilic granulocyte response to certain antigens. In the latter response, an unexpected role of thymic mononuclear cells was discovered.

Role of Erythroid HIM in the Genetic Anemia of Sl/Sl^d Mice

Both the W/W^v and the Sl/Sl^d "genetic" anemias, which occur in congenic stocks of mice, are macrocytic anemias unresponsive to erythropoietin. Both are associated with normal levels of leukocytes, and normal or elevated levels of erythropoietin, depending on the severity of the anemia (5). They are phenotypically indistinguishable, except for a greater severity of the Sl/Sl^d anemia. The W/W^v anemia has been shown to be caused by a deficiency of the stem cell to undergo erythroid differentiation or respond to erythropoietin. Their anemia can be cured by transplantation of congenic non-anemic (+/+) or even Sl/Sl^d (anemic) marrow. The Sl/Sl^d anemia, however, cannot be cured by transplantation of congenic non-anemic (+/+ or Sl/+) marrow or spleen cell suspensions (5). Since the Sl/Sl^d anemic mice have normal stem cells and normal or elevated erythropoietin levels their genetic defect must relate to some other host factor. We have postulated that it may be a deficit of the E HIM (2,6). Such a defect should be correctable by transplantation of splenic stroma, but not splenic CFU.

We have previously shown that subcutaneously transplanted spleens retain functionally normal HIM, in reduced numbers, and yield an erythroid to granuloid (E:G) colony ratio typical of normal spleen in situ (3). Bernstein (7) has recently reported that whereas non-anemic (+/+) spleen cell suspensions do not alter the anemia of Sl/Sl^d mice, intact spleen transplants elevated the hematocrit from 30 to 40, in from 60 to 90 days. We here confirm and extend that observation.

Non-anemic (+/+ or Sl/+) intact spleens were transplanted subcutaneously into weanling or older Sl/Sl^d anemic mice. Hematocrits were determined at weekly intervals. Whereas a single spleen transplant produced no improvement, 2, 3, and 6 intact spleen transplants per anemic mouse produced progressively

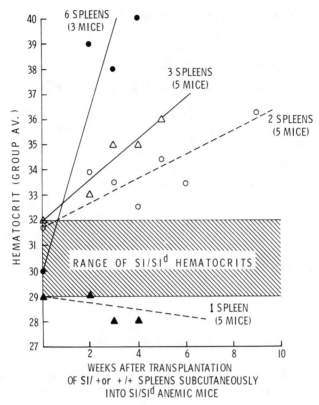

Fig. 1. Hematocrit response of Sl/Sl^d anemic mice to subcutaneous transplantation of one or more intact non-anemic (+/+ or Sl/+) spleens.

greater and more rapid increases in hematocrit. Six intact spleen transplants
increased the hematocrit from 30 to 39 within two weeks (Fig. 1).

In order to determine the number and types of HIM in the Sl anemic and
non-anemic spleens, 1×10^5 Sl/+ (non-anemic) bone marrow cells were injected
intravenously into 1100 R X-irradiated anemic (Sl/Sl^d) and non-anemic (Sl/+)
mice, and spleen colonies harvested 8 days later. While the numbers of spleens
examined histologically to date are small, and the data must be considered
preliminary, they support our theory. Three Sl/+ (non-anemic) spleens each
yielded an average of 12.3 colonies, of which 6.3 were erythroid and 4.3
granuloid, for an E:G colony ratio of 1.46. Four Sl/Sl^d (anemic) spleens
yielded an average of only 3.8 colonies, of which only 1 was erythroid and
2.8 were granuloid, for a very low E:G colony ratio of only 0.36 (Table I).

TABLE I. Spleen colony number and types in irradiated (1100 R) steel anemic (Sl/Sl^d) and non-anemic (Sl/+) mice given 1 x 10^5 Sl/+ bone marrow cells.

| | No. of Mice | No. of Spleen Colonies per Mouse | | | | | | E:G Colony Ratio |
		Total	Ery-throid	Granu-loid	Mega-karyo-cytic	Mixed	Undif-feren-tiated	
Non-Anemic (Sl/+) Mice	3	12.3	6.3	4.3	0.7	1	0	1.46
Anemic (Sl/Sl^d) Mice	4	3.8	1.0	2.8	0	0	0	0.36

Search for the Hypothetical Lymphoid Inducing Microenvironments (LIM)

The spleen and marrow stroma appear not to contain LIM, for none of the spleen or marrow colonies are lymphoid in nature (8). Yet irradiated mice repopulated with chromosomally marked spleen colonies regenerate a lymphoid system bearing the marker of the cells of the hemopoietic spleen colony (9). This and other data suggest that the CFU is pluripotent also for lymphoid differentiation. Since the thymus is one of the first lymphoid organs to regenerate in lethally irradiated, marrow-infused mice, and the regenerated thymocytes contain the markers of the marrow donor, we theorized that the thymus might contain LIM that act on pluripotent CFU, converting them to lymphoid differentiation. If so, CFU should migrate to and be recoverable from the thymus. However, attempts to recover CFU from thymus at intervals after lethal irradiation and marrow cell transfusion yielded no CFU after 1 to 15 days, only .3 to 1.2 CFU per thymus after 1 to 5 hours, and 1.7 and 2.8 CFU after 30 and 15 minutes respectively (Table II). This was comparable to the numbers of CFU recovered from one mesenteric lymph node or from .5cc of blood, but low as compared to the numbers recovered from one femur or from the spleen, in which latter two organs the number of CFU increase with time, rather than decrease. The observed low and only early recovery of CFU from thymus might, of course, be compatible with a rapid interaction of CFU with hypothetical thymic LIM, resulting in loss of hemopoietic differentiating capacity of the CFU. Numerous attempts were made to demonstrate such an interaction by incubation of marrow

TABLE II. Recoverability of CFU from various organs of irradiated mice at intervals after injection.

Harvest Time Post Injection of 5 x 10⁶ Marrow Cells into 1100 R Irradiated (C57 x A) Mice	NUMBER OF CFU RECOVERED FROM				
	One Thymus	One Mesenteric Lymph Node	0.5cc Blood	One Femur	One Spleen
	( ) = No. of Mice				
15 Minutes	2.8 (5)	1.2 (5)	3.3 (6)		18.2 (5)
30 "	1.7 (7)	1.3 (10)	3.5 (11)	8.8 (9)	46.8 (7)
1 Hour(s)	.4 (10)	.5 (11)	.8 (12)		10.9 (12)
2 "	.8 (12)	.3 (12)	.8 (12)		14.9 (12)
3 "	1.2 (11)	.1 (11)	.2 (6)		
4 "	.7 (10)	.5 (12)	.3 (11)		12.3 (12)
5 "	.3 (6)	.6 (5)	0 (6)		16.8 (6)
1 Day(s)	0 (7)	1.0 (4)		9.0 (11)	36.0 (11)
4 "	0 (6)	0 (6)			
6 "	0 (6)	0 (6)			
9 "	0 (6)	.2 (6)			23,000 (6)
11 "	0 (4)	1.2 (6)			4,000 (3)
15 "	0 (6)	.8 (5)		confluent (6)	20,000 (6)
Unirradiated Controls			2.5 (11)		

CFU with minced thymus in vitro before injection of the mixture. No significant loss (or increase) of CFU could be detected, after either 30 minutes interaction at 4° C, or 1 hour at room temperature, or 1 hour at 37° C. Either the thymus does not contain LIM, or the CFU is not the cell of interaction, or a third cell or factor is involved.

Role of Eosinophilic HIM in the Eosinophil Response to Antigen

Eosinophilic granulopoietic colonies constitute only a small proportion of spleen colonies, approximating 1 or 2 percent. Parasitic infections, allergies, and certain other antigenic stimuli evoke a considerable increase in circulating and localized eosinophilic granulocytes (10). Attempts were made to determine whether an eosinophil-evoking antigenic stimulus increased the number of eosinophilic granuloid hemopoietic colonies in the spleen and marrow (it did) and whether this effect of antigen was mediated on the stem cell, or by "turning on" more Eo HIM. In the former case the effect might be expected to be obtained by antigen treatment of the marrow donor only, whereas in the latter case, the effect might be expected to be obtained after antigen treatment of the marrow recipient only.

(C57 x A)F$_1$ mice were irradiated (1000 or 1100 R, ^{137}Cs) and injected intravenously with 5×10^4 or 1×10^5 isologous bone marrow cells. The marrow donors or recipients or both were pretreated with antigen. For the primary antigenic stimulation, mice were injected subcutaneously with 0.2 ml of alum precipitated tetanus toxoid (APTT) mixed with 0.2 ml of a pertussis vaccine, 28 or 45 days before irradiation and bone marrow injection or before sacrifice and use as bone marrow cell donors. In addition, some of the "primed" animals were challenged with one, two, or three secondary and booster injections of 0.2 ml APTT alone, administered intraperitoneally 0–7 days before irradiation and bone marrow treatment or sacrifice for bone marrow cell preparation. Some nonprimed mice of both donor and recipient groups received a single intraperitoneal injection of 0.2 ml APTT alone 0, 1, or 3 days before they were used as donors or recipients. Control animals were not injected with the antigen.

In general, antigen treatment of the marrow recipient, or of both recipient and donor, but not of the marrow donor alone, was found to increase the number of eosinophils in the peritoneal cavity and the femur (Table III), and to increase the percentage of eosinophilic granulopoietic colonies in the spleen and marrow (Table IV). The effect of antigen thus appeared to be mediated more via the Eo HIM than directly on the stem cell. However, in some experiments pretreatment of both the marrow donor and recipient produced a greater increase than treatment of the recipient only. This effect might possibly be related to a role of lymphoid cells, including splenic and thymic cells, in the mediation of antigen-induced eosinophilic granulocyte response, described in the next section.

TABLE III. Effect of antigen treatment of marrow donor and/or recipient on number of eosinophils in peritoneal cavity and femur of 1000 R irradiated mice given 1×10^5 marrow cells.

Antigen To		No. of Mice	No. of Eosinophils in Peritoneal Cavity x 10^3	No. of Mice	No. of Eosinophils in Femoral Marrow x 10^3
Marrow Donor	Marrow Recipient				
−	−	2	0	6	2.1
+	−	8	3.8	24	4.6
−	+	12	278.0	12	24.6
+	+	6	1217.0	6	26.7

TABLE IV.   Effect of antigen treatment of marrow donor and/or recipient on percent of eosinophilic granulopoietic colonies in the spleen and marrow of 1000 R irradiated mice given 1×10^5 marrow cells.

Antigen to		No. of Mice	No. of Colonies In Spleen	% of Colonies Containing Eosinophils			P.
Marrow Donor	Marrow Recipient			Pure	Mixed	All	
−	−	22	264	1.9	1.5	3	.001
+	−	32	422	2	0.2	2	
−	+	46	669	7	5	12	.001
+	+	28	481	6	3	9	
			In Marrow				
−	−	16	125	15	3	18	.1 − .25
+	−	32	189	19	5	24	
−	+	46	313	19	4	23	.01 − .02
+	+	29	200	25	8	33	

Role of Splenic and Thymic Cells in Mediation of the Eosinophil Response to Antigen

The prolonged accumulation of eosinophils in the inflammatory peritoneal exudate after a challenging injection of antigen was earlier shown to be associated with chemotaxis to specific mononuclear cells present in the exudate (11). In the present study quantitative determinations were made of the capacity of large doses of bone marrow cells and/or spleen or thymic cells from primed and unprimed mice to permit an eosinophilic inflammatory and eosinophilic granulopoietic response to challenge with specific antigen (tetanus toxoid) in heavily irradiated recipients.

"Priming" of donor mice consisted of a single subcutaneous injection of APTT with pertussis vaccine 28–45 days prior to use. Unprimed recipient mice were irradiated with 1000–1100 R (^{137}Cs), injected with 10^7 bone marrow cells intravenously from either primed or unprimed donors, and/or 10^7 spleen or thymic cells intraperitoneally from either primed or unprimed donors. One half hour later a challenge dose of APTT was given intraperitoneally. Groups of six mice were sacrificed at 5, 10, and 18 days post irradiation. Total and differential cell counts were made of the peritoneal fluid and of the femoral marrow. Tetanus antitoxin titers of the serum were performed.

Spleen cells from primed mice but not from normal mice had the capacity to adoptively transfer an anamnestic antitoxin response in irradiated animals in the absence of transplanted bone marrow cells, and during retarded myeloid regeneration.

Spleen cells alone or bone marrow cells alone produced an insignificant and a moderate peritoneal eosinophil response, respectively, to antigen.

In the presence of bone marrow cells, normal spleen cells augmented the capacity of recipient animals to mount an eosinophil response to antigen. A much greater augmentation occurred in animals reconstituted with splenic or thymic cells from primed animals (Fig. 2).

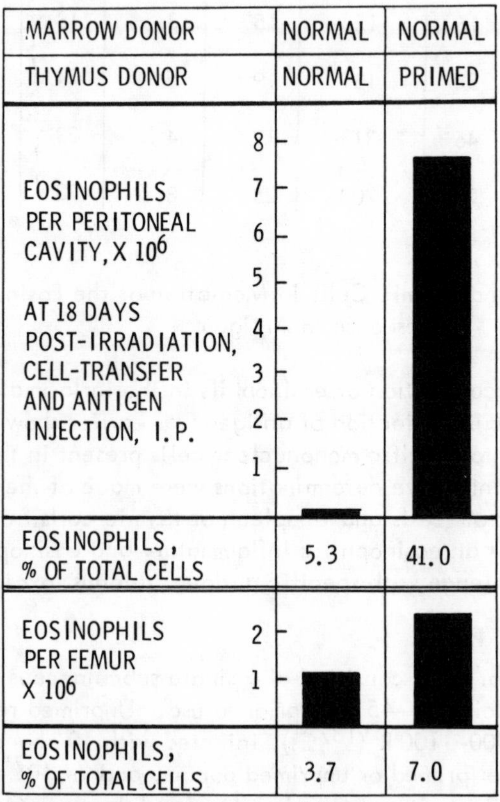

MARROW DONOR	NORMAL	NORMAL
THYMUS DONOR	NORMAL	PRIMED

EOSINOPHILS PER PERITONEAL CAVITY, X 10^6 AT 18 DAYS POST-IRRADIATION, CELL-TRANSFER AND ANTIGEN INJECTION, I.P.

EOSINOPHILS, % OF TOTAL CELLS	5.3	41.0

EOSINOPHILS PER FEMUR X 10^6

EOSINOPHILS, % OF TOTAL CELLS	3.7	7.0

Fig. 2. Effect of antigen treatment of thymus cell donor on 18-day eosinophil response to antigen in heavily irradiated mice receiving 10^7 marrow cells I.V., 10^7 thymus cells I.P., and antigen I.P.

The increase in antitoxin titers appeared to be independent of the response of eosinophils since: (a) marked accumulation of eosinophils occurred in animals with no measurable humoral antitoxin; (b) high antitoxin titers occurred in animals which did not have prior or concurrent eosinophil response.

It is suggested that a thymic derived mononuclear cell population is necessary for optimal eosinophil response to antigen. The neutrophil and mononuclear cell responses to antigen are determined by different mechanisms from those which determine the eosinophil responses.

These experiments are in agreement with the results reported recently by Basten et al. (12) who demonstrated a role of large lymphocytes in the mediation of eosinophilia in response to Trichinella infection. In their experiments, irradiated rats exposed to live parasitic challenge did not develop an eosinophilia unless reconstituted with lymphocytes as well as bone marrow cells. When lymphocytes from sensitized donors were used together with normal marrow cells, a "secondary" type of eosinophil response was obtained. Transfer of the capacity to mount an early eosinophilia was obtained adoptively in normal rats by thoracic duct large lymphocytes collected 3 to 5 days after infection of the donors with Trichinella.

ACKNOWLEDGMENTS

This research was supported by U.S.P.H.S. grants CA 03367, CA 05021, and K6 CA 14,219.

The authors are indebted to Mr. Larry Brown, Mr. Dewaine Edwards, and Mrs. Betsy Priest for their fine technical assistance, and to Mrs. Helen Thomas for manuscript preparation.

REFERENCES

1. A. J. Becker, E. A. McCulloch, and J. E. Till, Nature, 197:452, 1963.

2. J. J. Trentin, in: Albert S. Gordon, Ed., Regulation of Hematopoiesis, Sec. V, Ch. 8. New York: Appleton-Century-Crofts, 1970.

3. N. S. Wolf and J. J. Trentin, J. Exper. Med., 127:205, 1968.

4. J. L. Curry, J. J. Trentin, and N. Wolf, J. Exper. Med., 125:703, 1967.

5. S. E. Bernstein, E. S. Russell, and G. Keighley, Annals N. Y. Acad. Sci., 149:475, 1968.

6.   J. J. Trentin, J. L. Curry, N. Wolf, and V. Cheng, in: The
     Proliferation and Spread of Neoplastic Cells, p. 713, Baltimore:
     The Williams and Wilkins Company, 1968.

7.   S. E. Bernstein, Amer. J. Surgery, 119:448, 1970.

8.   J. L. Curry, J. J. Trentin, and V. Cheng, J. Immunology, 99:907,
     1967.

9.   J. Trentin, N. Wolf, V. Cheng, W. Fahlberg, D. Weiss, and R. Bonhag,
     J. Immunology, 98:1326, 1967.

10. R. S. Speirs and M. X. Turner, Blood, 34:320, 1969.

11. R. S. Speirs and Y. Osada, Proc. Soc. Exper. Biol. Med., 109:929,
     1962.

12. A. Basten and P. B. Beeson, J. Exper. Med., 131:1288, 1970.

DISCUSSION OF DR. TRENTIN'S PAPER

S. Cohen: I just want to mention very briefly some experiments by
Dr. Peter Ward and myself which might shed some light on the inter-
relationship that Dr. Trentin has observed between lymphocytes and
eosinophils. As you all know, when previously sensitized lymphocytes are activated by antigen, they generate a variety of soluble
factors such as migration inhibitory factors, blastogenic factor,
and chemotactic factors for macrophages and neutrophils. We have
recently found that they also make a substance which in itself is
devoid of biological activity, but which can react with preformed
immune complexes to generate an eosinophil chemotactic factor. This
material is unique in that it requires both a non-antibody lymphocyte product and antigen-antibody complexes; chemotactic factors
for other cell types which have been described require one or the
other, but not both. It is unclear whether the eosinophil chemotactic factor plays a role in eosinophilia exudation. Very small
amounts are highly effective in causing the accumulation of eosinophils in normal guinea pig skin. I might add that we had no idea
as to what acronym to associate with this factor. However, in honor
of Dr. Trentin's "HIM" we might call it hyperactive eosinophilic
reactant, or "HER", and suggest that HER leads to HIM or vice versa.

SESSION 6. IMMUNOLOGICALLY ACTIVE CELL KINETICS (MODELS)
CHAIRMAN, J. STERZL, CO-CHAIRMAN, J. F. ALBRIGHT

AN IN VITRO MODEL SYSTEM FOR THE STUDY OF THE INDUCTION OF

CELLULAR IMMUNITY

T. Simmons and L. A. Manson

The Wistar Institute, Philadelphia, Pennsylvania

U. S. A.

The mixed lymphocyte interaction (MLI) observed when allogeneic lymphocytes are cultured together has been interpreted as an
in vitro model system in which to study the alloimmune response.
This interaction has been characterized by cell proliferation and
transformation which are believed to be early events in the response.
The demonstration of the development of specific effector cells in
the MLI has been described (1).

We have previously reported a one-way response by mouse lymphocytes, as measured by enhanced thymidine uptake (2,3), to a particulate microsomal lipoprotein (MLP) prepared from allogeneic tissue.
Such preparations are potent sources of H-2 and non-H-2 transplantation antigens (4). The stimulation of ^{3}H-thymidine uptake was found
to be dose and strain specific. In addition, using a plaque-forming
cell reduction assay (2), it was possible to demonstrate the
induction of specific effector cells in MLP-treated cultures. This
report will be concerned with further studies of the development of
effector cells in the response to cell-free transplantation antigen
preparations.

MATERIALS AND METHODS

Animals. C57BL/10SnJ, B10.D2, DBA/2J, and C3H/HeJ mice were
purchased from Jackson Memorial Laboratories, Bar Harbor, Maine.

Antigens. Microsomal lipoproteins (MLP) were prepared according
to Manson et al. (4) under aseptic conditions from the L-5178Y
murine lymphoblast cell line and from mouse spleens.

299

Lymphocyte cultures. Mice were sacrificed by cervical dislo-
cation and either their spleens or axillary, brachial, inquinal,
superficial cervical, mesenteric, and caudal lymph nodes were removed,
pooled, and placed in cold culture medium. Spleen cell suspensions
were made by teasing while lymph node cell suspensions were made by
pressing the nodes through a #60 sterile, stainless steel mesh screen
into fresh medium. Viable cell counts were made with 1% eosin or
0.5% trypan blue. Spleen cell cultures were initiated at 15 X 10^6
viable cells per ml in a medium adapted from that described by Main
and Jones (5) omitting mouse serum and substituting MOPS for TRIS
buffer (pH 7.4). Lymph node cell cultures were initiated at 1 X 10^6
viable cells per ml in the same medium. Large-scale cultures were
carried out in 8 to 20 ml volumes in 50 ml glass conical centrifuge
tubes or in 30 ml volumes in 125 ml Ehrlenmeyer flasks. Vessels were
foil-capped and incubated in an atmosphere of 5% CO_2, 8% O_2, and
87% N_2 at 37°C. For studies involving enhanced ^3H-thymidine incorporation, 1 uCi/ml (6Ci/mmole) was added for 4 hours to a suitable
aliquot and the acid precipitable radioactivity determined by
liquid scintillation techniques.

Plaque-reduction assay. The details of the assay have been
previously described (2).

Tumor target assay. Washed lymphocytes (killers) resuspended
in target cell growth medium were incubated overnight in various
ratios (1:1, 2:1, 5:1, or 10:1 ratio of killers:targets) with
5 X 10^4 viable L-5178Y lymphoblast targets. Incubations were performed in stoppered, 12-ml glass conical centrifuge tubes in a
slowly revolving roller drum at 37°C. Cultures were then pulsed for
$\frac{1}{2}$-1 hour with 1 uCi/ml of ^3H-thymidine, and the acid precipitable
radioactivity was determined. Controls for the experimental mixes
were killers and targets incubated separately and pulsed in a similar
manner. A value of 100% was assigned to the sum of the two controls
and the incorporation seen in the mixes compared to this theoretical
sum.

Antigen binding assay. The binding of ^{125}I-MLP by washed
lymphocytes was perfomed by a method similar to Byrt and Ada (6).
Cells were incubated at 1-2 X 10^6 viable cells per ml in Eisen's
balanced salt solution with fetal calf serum for 30 minutes at 0°C
with 1-100 ng of ^{125}I-MLP (7). Cells were washed 3 times in medium
and then smears were made and processed for autoradiography using
Kodak NTB3 liquid emulsion film. Autoradiographs were developed
and stained after 4-5 days of exposure in the dark at 0°C. Differential grain counts of at least 500 cells per slide were made.

RESULTS

Lymphocyte stimulation. The details of the MLP-induced stimu-

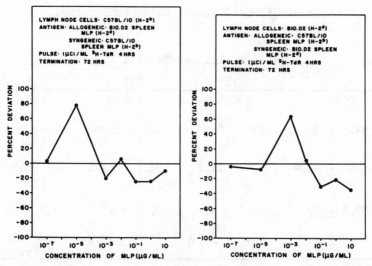

Fig. 1. Cells from each strain were incubated in parallel cultures
with allogeneic or syngeneic spleen MLP. For each concentration of
MLP, for each strain, the average incorporation (sample size of 4) in
cultures containing syngeneic MLP was subtracted from that for cultures containing allogeneic MLP. This difference was then plotted as
the per cent deviation from controls (cells cultured without MLP)
versus antigen concentration.

lation of ^{3}H-thymidine incorporation have been presented elsewhere
(2,3). Low levels of lymphoblast MLP (0.01-0.00001 ug/ml) did induce an enhanced thymidine uptake in lymphoid populations, whereas
high levels of allogeneic L-5178Y lymphoblast MLP (1-10 ug/ml) did
not. Experiments with the congenic-resistant pair C57BL/10 and
B10.D2 demonstrated the immunologic specificity of the low dose
stimulation (Figure 1). Each strain served as a source of spleen
MLP and responding lymphocytes. The figures give the data as the
difference of incorporation in parallel cultures containing corresponding amounts of allogeneic and syngeneic MLP. The genetic differences in these experiments were confined to the antigenic specificities determined by the H-2 locus. Net stimulations of allogeneic
MLP were observed only at low concentrations of MLP. Similar results
were found in the response of C57BL/10 lymph node cells to allogeneic
lymphoblast MLP and syngeneic spleen MLP.

Plaque-reduction assay. The results are reported in detail

Table 1: Ability of C57BL/10 Spleen Cells to Suppress
[3]H-Thymidine Incorporation by L-5178Y Targets

| | | Ratio of Killers:Targets | | |
MLP (ug/ml)	10:1	5:1	2:1	1:1
-	100.0	100.0	100.0	100.0
10	94.5 ± 14.8 (7)	115 ± 8.98 (7)	107 ± 9.06 (5)	110 ± 9.34 (5)
0.1	80.8 ± 4.94 (7)	100 ± 11.1 (7)	82.7 ± 17.0 (5)	105 ± 12.0 (5)
0.01[1]	87.2 ± 27	85.5 ± 27	37.2 ± 12	73.7 ± 19
0.001	64.4 ± 5.97 (7)	86.8 ± 9.90 (7)	90.9 ± 17.1 (5)	95.2 ± 10.8 (5)
Cells from Immune Mice[1]	51.0 ± 3.5	67.0 ± 25	113 ± 25	88.6 ± 22

[1]
The data for cells cultured with 0.01 ug MLP and for cells from
immune mice are from single experiments. The values tabulated
represent the means of 4 replicate incubations for each condition.
In all other cases, the data represent the means of a given number
(in parenthesis) of replicate experiments.

Table 1: C57BL/10 spleen cells (H-2[b]) were cultured for 2 days
with or without L-5178Y MLP (H-2[d]) and then tested against L-5178Y
targets in a 20-hour tumor target assay. The effect of control cells
(cells cultured without MLP) was assigned 100% at each ratio of
killers:targers. The effect of MLP-treated cells is expressed as the
per cent of control. The difference observed at the 10:1 ratio for
cells sensitized in vitro with 0.1 and 0.001 ug/ml and for cells
from immune animals are significantly lower than controls (p values
< 0.01).

elsewhere (3). C57BL/10 (H-2[b]) lymphocytes incubated 3 days with
0.001 ug allogeneic MLP per ml were found to have an enhanced ability,
relative to cells cultured without MLP, to interfere with plaque-
forming cells of the same strain (H-2[d]) as the MLP, but not with a
different strain (H-2[k]) of plaque-forming cells. Cells treated with
the high dose of MLP demonstrated no such enhanced suppressive ability
with respect to either strain of targets.

    Tumor target assay. With C57BL/10 spleen cells, the maximum
differences between control populations (cells cultured without MLP)
and lymphoblast MLP-treated populations were observed for cells that

Table 2: Ability of Cultured C57BL/10 Spleen Cells to
Inhibit L-5178Y Targets [1]

MLP (ug/ml)	Spleen Cells (Killers)	Ratio of Killers:Targets 10:1	Ratio of Killers:Targets 5:1
-	317 ± 57	2350 ± 525	1970 ± 424
10	189 ± 26	1950 ± 150	1890 ± 440
0.01	470 ± 111	2050 ± 100	1520 ± 244
0.001	523 ± 38	2775 ± 255	2275 ± 163

[1]
Targets alone incorporated ^{3}H-thymidine to a level of 3675 ± 165 cpm for 6 incubations

Table 2: C57BL/10 spleen cells (H-2^b) were cultured for 2 days with or without C57BL/10 spleen MLP (H-2^b) and then tested in a 20-hour assay against L-5178Y targets (H-2^d). Incubations of killers alone and killer-target cell mixtures were carried out in quadruplicate. The data is given as the mean cpm for the replicates of each incubation condition. Cultures were pulsed 1 hour with 2 uc/ml ^{3}H-thymidine (3 c/mmole).

were cultured 2 days with low doses of MLP and then incubated approximately 20 hours with lymphoblast targes as described in Table 1. The data have been normalized for each mixture so that the effect of cells unexposed to MLP is 100% in each case. The depression seen with cells treated with low doses of MLP is statistically significant. Specificity tests in this assay were performed by culturing C57BL/10 lymphocytes with and without syngeneic spleen MLP and then testing for their ability to inhibit the growth of L-5178Y tumor target cells. No significant difference was observed between cells cultured with and without syngeneic MLP on allogeneic tumor targets (Table 2).

Antigen binding assay. In neither target cell assay was it possible to quantitate the numbers of sensitized cells that developed in cultures. The technique of autoradiography was applied in order to estimate this number. C57BL/10 spleen cells were cultured 3 days without MLP or with 0.001 ug/ml of lymphoblast MLP and then tested for their ability to bind the homologous iodinated antigen. It appears that the lymphoid population cultured with the low level of MLP contains more cells that bind ^{125}I-lymphoblast MLP as do cells from unimmunized animals (Figure 2). The binding capacities of cells cultured with the low dose of lymphoblast MLP compared very well to cells from immunized mice. The range in binding

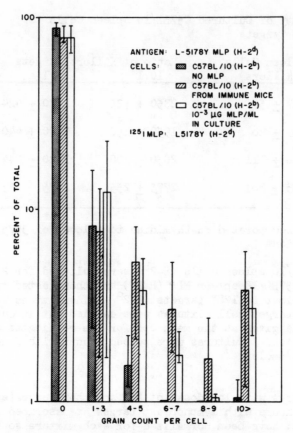

Fig. 2. C57BL/10 spleen cells (H-2^b) were assayed for their capacity to bind iodinated L-5178Y MLP (H-2^d) which was the antigen used in in vivo and in vitro sensitizations. The number of cells with the indicated grain counts is expressed as the per cent of total cells plotted. The figure represents the pooled data from 4 experiments.

capacities observed in replicate experiments is indicated by the vertical bar. The number of cells showing greater than 10 grains per cell in non-immune populations is low, whereas that number in in vitro sensitized populations approaches that found with cells from immune animals.

The data were pooled to compare the binding by normal and sensitized cell populations, with the specificity of the binding also indicated, i.e., the capacity to bind labelled syngeneic (H-2^b) MLP

Table 3: Specificity of Antigen Binding

Treatment	Fewer than 5 grains/cell		More than 5 grains/cell	
	Allo. MLP	Syn. MLP	Allo. MLP	Syn. MLP
--	97.8	99.0	2.2	1.05
in vivo immunized	91.4	96.7	8.5	3.30
in vitro immunized	93.9	98.1	6.0	1.85

Table 3: C57BL/10 spleen cells ($H-2^b$) were assayed in parallel
for their capacity to bind allogeneic iodinated lymphoblast MLP
($H-2^d$) and syngeneic iodinated spleen MLP. The antigen used in sensitization was L-5178Y lymphoblast MLP ($H-2^d$). In the table the
number of cells with fewer than or more than 5 grains is given as
the percentage of the total number counted.

(Table 3). As much as 8.5% of the lymphoid population from immune
mice had the capacity to bind allogeneic antigen, versus a 3.3%
binding of syngeneic antigen. This difference was also seen with
the in vitro sensitized population, but the percentage binding more
than five grains per cell was not as great. The high background of
syngeneic binders observed may reflect the fact that spleen cell
populations can carry out phagocytosis at 0^oC, the temperature at
which the binding assay was performed (Byrt and Ada, 1969). Even
if the degree of binding found with syngeneic MLP is subtracted from
that observed for allogeneic MLP, it appears that the three-day culture in the presence of a low level of MLP led to a rapid increase
in the number of effector cells. This increase also appeared to be
specific.

DISCUSSION

Lymphocytes from adult, untreated mice have been shown to acquire a specific state of immunity due to treatment in vitro with a
variety of immunogens. Specific plaque-forming cells develop during
culture with red blood cells (8,9) and specific effectors of cell-
mediated immunity are induced in mixed cultures of allogeneic lymphocytes (1). Diener and Armstrong (10,11) have shown that low
levels of polymerized Salmonella flagellin (0.02 ug/ml) induced a
specific immune response in culture while higher levels (2-20 ug/ml)
induced immunologic unresponsiveness. This data parallels our observations with the particulate lipoprotein transplantation antigens
with respect to the sensitizing dose of immunogen and the kinetics
of the in vitro response.

The phenomenon of low dose stimulation of lymphocytes in vitro is not surprising when one compares the _in vitro_ and _in vivo_ sensitizing capacities of MLP preparations. In a congenic-resistant pair, 5 ug of MLP per mouse will sensitize for a statistically significant accelerated rejection of a skin allograft (12,13). The immunologically effective dose of MLP is probably less than the 5 ug administered intraperitoneally. Considering the relatively small numbers of lymphocytes used in initiating the cultures, and considering the uniform exposure of all cells to MLP antigens, it is not unreasonable that sensitization in tissue culture should be observed with only a small fraction of the amount of antigens needed to sensitize _in vivo_.

SUMMARY

Lipoprotein transplantation antigens have been shown to induce an immune response in tissue cultures of spleen or lymph node cell populations from untreated mice. Low levels of allogeneic antigens (0.00001-0.01 ug/ml) induced a proliferative response (an enhanced uptake of thymidine) and the development of specific effector cells as demonstrated in the plaque-reduction and tumor target assays. The number of specific effector cells induced in culture was estimated by the binding of iodinated antigen and was found to approach the levels observed in lymphoid cell populations from immunized mice. High levels of antigens in culture appeared to lead to a state of immunologic unresponsiveness in the various tests. It was concluded that this system could be useful as a model for the study of alloimmunity in vitro.

ACKNOWLEDGMENTS

Supported, in part, by Public Health Service Research Grants R01-CA 07973, P01-CA 10815, and R01-CA 10028, from the National Cancer Institute

REFERENCES

1. Häyry, P. and Defendi, V., Science 168:133, 1970.

2. Manson, L. A. and Simmons, T. Transplant. Proc. 1:498, 1969.

3. Manson, L. A., Simmons, T., Mills, L., and Friedman, H., in D. R. McIntyre, Ed., Proc. 4th Leukocyte Culture Conf., New York Appleton-Century-Crofts, 1970.

4. Manson, L. A., Foschi, G. V., and Palm, J., J. Cell. Comp. Physiol. 61:109, 1963.

5. Main, R. K., and Jones, M. J., Nature, Lond. 218:1251, 1968.

6. Byrt, P. and Ada, G. L., Immunology, Lond. 17:503, 1969.

7. Foschi, G. V. and Manson, L. A., Nature, Lond. 225:853, 1970.

8. Mishell, R. I. and Dutton, R. W.; Science 153:1004, 1966.

9. Marbrook, J., Lancet 2:1279, 1967.

10. Diener, E. and Armstrong, W. D., Lancet 2:1281, 1967.

11. Diener, E. and Armstrong, W. D., J. exp. Med. 129:591, 1969.

12. Manson, L. A., Hickey, C. A., and Palm, J., in L. A. Manson,
    Ed., Biological Properties of the Mammalian Surface Membrane,
    Philadelphia, Wistar Institute Press, 1968.

13. Hickey, C. A., Doctoral Thesis, University of Pennsylvania,
    1968.

PRIMARY IMMUNE REACTION OF ALLOGENEIC LYMPH NODE CELLS

AGAINST TISSUE ANTIGENS OF LETHALLY IRRADIATED HOSTS

I. Bašić, D. Dekaris, M. Matošić, V. Silobrčić,
Vesna Tomažić and B. Vitale

Institute "R. Bošković" and Institute of Immunology
Zagreb, Yugoslavia

The precise mechanism of the disease that develops after successful grafting of immunologically competent cells into allogeneic
hosts ("allogeneic disease") is still obscure. We have studied it
using as a model an "acute allogeneic disease" caused by a mixture
of bone marrow and lymph node cells injected into lethally irradiated
allogeneic mice. From serially killed animals we have obtained a
number of very reproducible patterns of the disease (1).

Among these, proliferation of the injected cells within the
recipient's spleen, as a manifestation of the "graft-against-host"
reaction, was very interesting. Namely, we believed that the reaction may be a suitable model for investigating a primary immunological
reaction against tissue antigens.

To further define the reaction, we injected only lymph node cells
into lethally irradiated allogeneic mice. Then we followed the lodging
of the cells and the sequence of cellular events in the spleen.

MATERIALS AND METHODS

Mice. We used 3 highly inbred strains: CBA/H, C57BL/H and A/H.
Donors and recipients of cells were of the same sex, 3-5 months of
age, weighing 18-26 grams. They were kept under conventional
conditions.

Suspensions of cells. We prepared them from subcutaneous lymph
nodes (inguinal, axillary, brachial, cervical) or from the spleen, as
already described (2). There were regularly about 30% of lymph node
and 10-15% of spleen cells stained (tripan blue).

Labeling with ^{51}Cr. A suspension of lymph node cells (2 X 10^8 viable cells/ml) was incubated at room temperature with 120 µC of ^{51}Cr (Sodium chromate, B.P., specific activity: 300 C/g) per ml. After 60 minutes we washed the suspension twice and determined again the number of nucleated and stained cells. Ten million viable cells were injected into the tail vein of irradiated recipients. The activity of the total body and that of the spleen were determined with well type scintillation counters. The percentage values of the actual counts in the spleen were calculated from the amount of label found in the whole body.

Cellularity of the spleen. We prepared a suspension of cells from 10 mg of splenic tissue. From the number of cells in the fragment the number of nucleated cells in the whole organ was calculated.

Histology, large pyroninophilic cells and mitotic figures in the spleen. Four micron sections of the spleen were prepared and stained with methyl green-pyronin. In these we counted large pyroninophilic cells (LPC), as characterized by Gowans (3), and mitotic figures. For each section a total of 1000 cells were scored and the percentage of LPC and mitoses calculated.

Foot-pad test. The test is basically similar to the direct transfer reaction of Brent, Brown and Medawar (4). We prepared a suspension of the spleen cells from the recipients of allogeneic lymph node cells. Five million viable spleen cells suspended in 0.05 ml were injected into the right foot-pad of normal mice, while the same amount of physiological saline served as control injection into the left foot-pad. Four, 24 and 48 hours after the injection we measured the diameter of both foot-pads with a precise dial gauge. The difference in diameter of the right and left foot-pads was statistically evaluated with the Student's t-test.

Peripheral blood. Blood specimens were taken from the tail. We counted leukocytes and differentiated blood smears stained with May-Grünwald Giemsa.

Irradiation. Animals were X-irradiated under standard conditions (1).

Experimental design. We irradiated with 950 R groups of CBA recipients. The irradiated mice were divided into 3 groups: a. injected with physiological saline, b. injected with 1 X 10^7 viable syngeneic (CBA) and c. injected with the same dose of allogeneic (C57BL) lymph node cells shortly after irradiation.

RESULTS

The CBA mice irradiated with 950 R died regularly between 7 and

12 days after irradiation. The same holds true for irradiated CBA recipients of syngeneic lymph node cells. On the other hand, those injected with C57BL cells all died during the 6th day after the injection.

From groups of mice injected with syngeneic or allogeneic lymph node cells 2 animals were used every 24 hours to measure the amount of ^{51}Cr in the whole body. We killed additional 2 mice from each group at 12 hour intervals for determining the activity in the spleen. Twelve hours after the injection of allogeneic cells the spleen contained 16% of the activity, which declined rather slowly for 72 hours. Then followed a statistically significant (P$\angle$0.001) fall and another gradual diminution (bottom third, Fig. 1). There was no conspicuous fall at 84 hours after injection in the spleen of mice injected with labeled syngeneic cells.

The curves for weight and cellularity of the spleen are parallel (middle third, Fig. 1). Cellularity, however, never reached normal values. Therefore, the spleen weight depends on the number of cells within the organ, but a part of it is probably due to noncellular material (oedema, haemorrhage). Weight and cellularity of the spleen in irradiated mice and those receiving syngeneic lymph node cells remains constantly very low.

We killed 2 recipients of allogeneic and 2 or syngeneic lymph node cells every 4 hours after the injection and prepared sections of their spleen. A detailed account of the histology has already been published (1). Mice injected with syngeneic lymph node cells had very few LPC and mitoses in their spleen (5). On the contrary, in mice injected with allogeneic cells the percentage of LPC steadily rose to 68%, declining rapidly soon afterwards. Concomitantly, the number of mitoses increased to nearly 4%, but it remained relatively high even after an almost complete disappearance of LPC (top third, Fig. 1).

Irradiated controls and recipients of syngeneic cells constantly had very few WBC. The same was true for recipients of allogeneic lymph node cells during the first 92 hours. Later WBC rose towards normal numbers, and almost all of them were lymphocytes (bottom third, Fig. 1).

We killed groups of 5 to 10 CBA recipients 1, 2, 3, 4, 5 and 6 days after injection of C57BL cells, harvested their spleens and prepared a single suspension of cells each day. That was injected into the right foot-pad of 10 CBA, 5 C57BL and 5 normal A hosts. The C57BL and A mice were controls for specificity of the reaction and the test was always negative. When the spleen was taken 1, 2 or 3 days after injection of lymph node cells and the suspension inoculated into CBA mice, the foot-pad test was negative. Cells from the

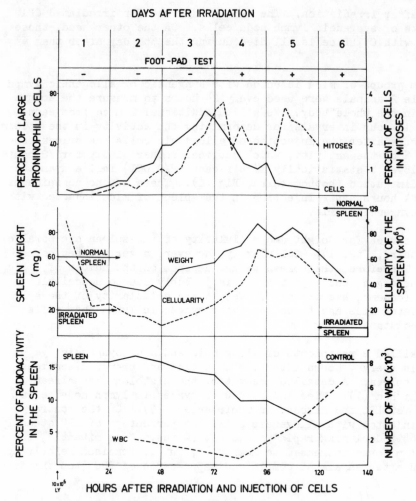

Fig. 1. A composite drawing of the findings in the spleen and
peripheral blood of 950 R irradiated CBA mice injected with
1 X 10⁷ lymph node cells.

spleen harvested on subsequent days, however, caused a positive
foot-pad test, i.e., the right foot-pad was significantly larger
(P/0.01) than the left one, when measured 24 and 48 hours after
the injection.

DISCUSSION

Of the 1 X 10^7 C57BL lymph node cells intravenously injected to irradiated CBA mice 16% lodged in the spleen. For the first 72 hours after injection the amount of the label in the spleen diminished very slowly. There was no evidence of a considerable outflow of labeled cells from the spleen. Gowans has reported that small lymphocytes reacting against their host are quickly fixed in lymphoid tissues (3). Considering also the detailed analysis of labeling with ^{51}Cr by Bainbridge *et al.* (6), we may conclude that the cells found in the spleen at 12 hours remain there. After the first 16 hours we noticed increasing numbers of LPC, which, as there is now ample evidence, are transformed lymphocytes. The transformation was most likely a result of the stimulation of injected lymphocytes by antigens of the host, since it was absent when the cells were syngeneic to the host. The number of LPC increased concomitantly with the number of mitoses. Thus, we may conclude that they originated from lymphocytes, but multiplied by self-replication. The generation time was estimated to be 8 or 9 hours (5). Because of the accumulation of LPC the weight and cellularity of the spleen increased. These cells were unable to cause a positive foot-pad test upon transfer to normal CBA recipients.

At 68 hours after the injection, 68% of the cells in the spleen were LPC. This indicates that CBA antigens powerfully stimulated the transformation of C57BL lymphocytes. After the peak, the number of LPC declined abruptly and more mature forms of lymphocytes appeared. They most probably differentiated from LPC, but also themselves divided, since the number of mitoses remained high even when LPC were few and the mature forms prevailed. The accumulation of lymphocytes further increased the weight and cellularity of the spleen. Simultaneously, however, some of the cells left the spleen, as evidenced by histology and the significant decrease of the label at 84 hours. In addition, concomitantly with the decline of the label, there were more lymphocytes in peripheral blood. The lymphocytes found in the CBA spleen 4, 5 and 6 days after injection of C57BL cells caused a positive foot-pad test in normal CBA hosts.

The replication of lymphocytes kept the weight and cellularity of the spleen at a high level until 108 hours after the injection. Afterwards, the outflow of the cells from the spleen prevailed: there was a constant decline of the label, weight and cellularity. We found at least some of these cells in the peripheral blood, where values for WBC approach normal and almost all of them were lymphocytes.

We could not follow the events in the spleen any further, since all the CBA recipients suddenly died during the 6th day. The cause of such a sudden death remains obscure.

On the basis of our observations, we may conclude that the cellular events in the spleen are stages of a primary immune reaction of the delayed type, in which C57BL lymph node cells react against tissue antigens of their CBA hosts.

ACKNOWLEDGMENT

We are grateful indeed to Mrs. Adela Lechpammer, Mrs. Mila Hršak, Mrs. Lidija Oršanić and Mr. A. Savić for their expert help during experimentation and preparation of the manuscript.

REFERENCES

1. B. Vitale, V. Silobrčić, M. Jurin, M. Matošić and Vesna Tomažić, Effects of Radiation on Cellular Proliferation and Differentiation, IAEA, Vienna, 1968, p. 395.

2. V. Silobrčić, Br. J. Exp. Path., 46:583, 1965.

3. J. L. Gowans, Ann. N. Y. Acad. Sci., 99:432, 1962.

4. L. Brent, J. Brown, P. B. Medawar, Lancet, II, 561, 1958.

5. M. Matošić, Vesna Tomažić, I. Bašić, M. Jurin, V. Silobrčić and B. Vitale, IVth International Congress of Radiation Research, Evian, 1970, Abstr. 540.

6. D. R. Bainbridge, L. Brent, and G. Gowland, Transplantation, 4:138, 1966.

AN ALTERNATIVE MODEL OF ANTIBODY FORMING CELL DIFFERENTIATION

Jan Cerny, Robert F. McAlack and H. Friedman

Depts. of Microbiology, Albert Einstein Med. Ctr. and

Temple University Medical School, Phila., Pa., U.S.A.

Introduction

The recently described model system of specific immune vibriolysis by lymphoid cells of mice immunized with Vibrio cholerae permits some observations impossible in other systems (1). First, there is an absence of "natural" background of lytic antibodies and plaque forming cells (PFC) against the major cell wall antigens of the bacteria. Second, each bacterial cell possess two distinguishable non-crossreacting antigens, A and B (strain Ogawa) or A and C (strain Inaba), respectively. Therefore, we can study the specific PFC response separately against two antigens carried on one particle and "handled" together by the lymphoid cells of the RES. The method allows both enumeration and localization in tissue of anti-A, anti-B and anti-C PFC, as described elsewhere (1,2). The major observations with the present model for this report deal with the early accumulation pattern of PFC and with restricted specificity of antigen reactive cells and their localization in splenic tissue.

Experimental observations

1) After immunization with Vibrio cholerae Ogawa vaccine (A and B antigens) the first PFC appeared in the spleen between 42 and 46 hours. This latent period was the same for both anti-A and anti-B PFC (Fig. 1). Also, the absolute number of the first PFCs were almost the same - 4 anti-A and 6 anti-B PFC per spleen, respectively. However, the further increase was different so that

Supported in part by research grants from the U.S. National Science Foundation (GB 6251X) and the National Institute of Arthritis and Metabolic Diseases (1 RO1 AM/AI 13964-01 ALY).

the accumulation of PFC was not the result of multiplication of
their initial number. This point was substantiated further when
an analysis of the increase in number of PFC at 2 hour intervals
revealed a "staircase" rather than linear type of accumulation
(Fig. 1 and 2). Each plateau was about 4-5 times higher than the

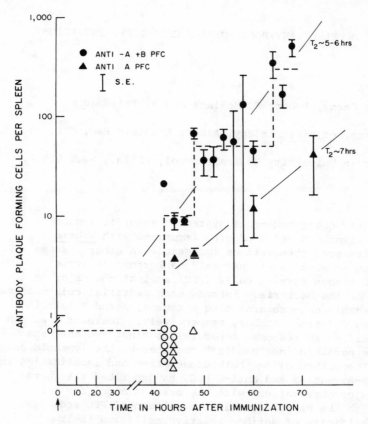

Fig. 1 - Accumulation of PFC in the spleen of mice immunized i.v.
with 5 ug of V. cholerae strain Ogawa vaccine (antigens A + B). The
entire spleen was assayed either against the Ogawa strain (sum of
anti-A and anti-B PFC) or with the Inaba strain (anti-A PFC only).
Subtraction of values give the number of anti-B PFC. (For example,
for 10 PFC found at 42 and 44 hours, 4 were anti-A and 6 anti-B).
Each point (or) represent the average number of PFC (±s.e.) in
the spleen of 6 to 15 mice. Individual mice without any detectable
PFC were not included in the average values, but indicated by open
symbol (or) at zero line. No PFCs detected before immunization
and between 12 and 40 hours thereafter (arrow). (T_2 = approximate
doubling time).

previous one and there were at least 5 such steps from the latent period through the period of rapid accumulation - to the 4th day. This pattern is similar to that described recently by Perkins et al for anti-S-RBC PFC (3). The early PFCs appear to be a homogenous population of IgM producing cells and circulating antibodies do not seem to have a regulatory effect in the stepwise appearance of PFC, since they are not detectable during the first four days after immunization. The stepwise pattern does not change after subtraction of anti-A PFC numbers, suggesting that it represents a periodic process within a population of cells with one specificity.

Studies with cytosine arabinoside - a specific inhibitor of DNA synthesis - showed that cellular proliferation was essential in the differentiation of the first PFC, as well as during their further accumulation (Table 1). However, injection of the drug during the first day of the two-day latent period did not suppress PFC differentiation substantially.

2) As we have shown before, over 95% of the PFC are located within or close to small splenic foci detectable as tiny sharp zones of bacteriolysis under cryostat-prepared sections from immunized spleen. This phenomenon has also been described previously with S-RBC (4). A possible role of circulating antibodies in foci production was ruled out by passive immunization experiments (2).

Table 1 - Suppressive effect of cytosine-beta-D-arabinofuranoside HCl (CA) on appearance of vibriolytic PFC in mouse spleen.

Time of drug injection (hours after immunization)*	Number of PFC per spleen**	
	48 hours	96 hours
	Control mice	
-	60	2,972
	Drug treated mice	
6, 12, 24	34	- (n.d.)
24, 30, 36	2	-
48, 64, 72, 80	-	0

* Groups of mice injected repeatedly i.p. with 100 ug CA per injection at indicated time.

** Average of the number of PFC from 6-8 spleens tested at time indicated after i.v. immunization with 5 ug V. cholerae Ogawa vaccine (assayed against homologous strain).

Individual foci are not distributed randomly but are assembled
closely together in certain areas of the spleen (Fig.2a).   The

Section no.

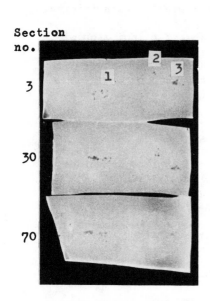

Fig. 2a

Section no.   Assay against

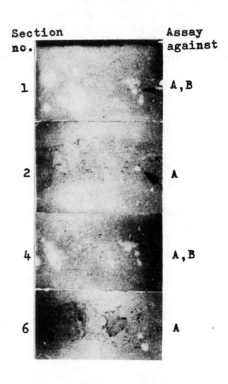

Fig. 2b

Fig. 2a - Consecutive sections from a spleen on the 5th day after
immunization with 5 ug Ogawa vaccine and assayed against homologous
bacteria.   The foci appear in the same positions, i.e., in tri-
dimensional areas of spleen.   Area 1 contains about 10 foci, some
of which are confluent.   Areas no. 2 (3-4 foci) and no. 3 (4 foci)
occupy only part of the spleen proper (Negative image obtained with
indirect light).

Fig. 2b - Adjacent sections from spleen of Ogawa (A + B) immunized
mouse assayed against either Ogawa (A + B foci) or Inaba (A foci),
respectively.   Two foci from area indicated by arrow have anti-A
specificity, whereas others have anti-B specificity.   All other
areas, mostly with confluent lysis, were of anti-B specificity only.
(Comparison of homologous section, 1 and 4, shows good reproducibility of the method) (Positive image with direct light).

number of areas in the spleen does not increase during the immune
response, varying from 1 to 7 (Fig. 3). On the other hand the
average number of foci per area doubled from 4 to 9 between 60 hours
(when they first become detectable) and 5 days after immunization
(Fig. 3).

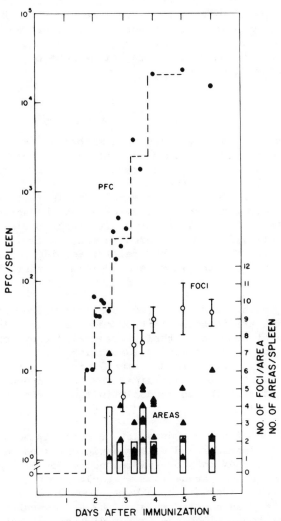

Fig. 3 - Kinetics of areas, foci and PFC in the spleen after 5 ug
of Ogawa vaccine (homologous assay). Average figures of areas are
indicated by columns and their number, in spleens of individual
mice, by triangles. Number of foci in areas are given as average
(± s.e.)(o). PFCs were enumerated per whole spleen in separate
experiment (6-15 mice per point).

Immunological specificity of the foci and the areas was tested by assay of adjacent sections from mice immunized with A + B antigens, either for anti-AB or anti-A specificity (Fig. 2b). Only some of the foci detectable in the anti-A+B assay appeared again in the same position and size in the anti-A assay. Thus, even though both antigens are "processed" together as one bacterial cell, each focus is immunologically specific. On the other hand, one area may contain foci of both specificities, as illustrated in Fig. 2b. Analysis of 31 areas from eight mice showed the ratio between anti-B specific, anti-A specific and mixed areas to be 2:1.4:1, respectively. However, in individual mice, either one or the other type of specificity prevailed.

Conclusions and Discussion

The areas defined here as a portion of a spleen where accumulated antigen reactive cells (ARC) form foci of PFC are considered to be the same as the "areas" described previously as PFC-rich portions of a spleen (5). Their fixed number suggest that they existed before the immunization. One area may contain foci and PFC of different immunological specificity, provided the antigens are part of one complex. However, when two different complexes, unrelated red blood cells, are administered in mixture the areas appear monospecific (5). Therefore, the cell(s) forming an area seems to be immunologically specific to some determinant of the complex antigen.

The foci arising within areas are immunologically specific even when both antigens are integral part of one particle. They appear also after immunization of lethally irradiated recipients of limited numbers of donor spleen cells (unpublished). It follows that antigen reactive cells are already immunologically predestined to one antigen. If so, it must be explained why they accumulate in a few areas, instead of distributed randomly in the spleen as one would expect.

Uniform specificity of a focus does not necessarily mean that each represents a real clone derived by symmetric division on one ARC. The long latent period, the low initial number of PFC and their non-linear accumulation, argue against a clonal origin. Similar evidence has been presented by others, too (3, 6-8). The stepwise increase of PFC can not be explained by a consecutive activation of areas or foci, since the number of areas do not increase with time and the number of foci in a spleen (between 28 and 70) is much higher than the 5-6 steps observed. Therefore, there may be another mechanism for the origin of PFC besides cell proliferation, such as mutual transfer of specific information (9).

The long latent period, a portion of which does not even involve cell proliferation, also indicates that a process of new differentiation is induced by an antigen. A similar latent period was found with other antigens, also, provided there was no pre-immune background (10, 11).

The Model System

With a few additional points the results may be readily explained according to the cooperation of immunocompetent cells in response to a carrier-hapten complex. The concept elaborated by many authors was summarized recently by Plescia (12). Presumably, the help requiring "haptenic determinant," which may be a chemical hapten as well as a natural antigen (13), is directed to an antigen with which the organism did not have any previous immunological experience. On the other hand, the "carrier determinant" of the complex, inducing the helper effect, is to an antigen against which the organism has already been sensitized. The virgin anti-hapten ARC are not capable of reaction without a differentiation step occurring under the influence of a helper effect from anti-carrier ARC.

The A and B cholera antigen (which may not be single determinants) are considered as the haptenic determinants in terms of this hypothesis, since there is no detectable background even after nonspecific stimulation of RES with various stimulators or Gram negative bacteria. Furthermore, a prolonged process of differentiation occurs before PFC appear after cholera immunization.

On the other hand, the cholera bacteria must possess many other antigens and it is likely that a presensitization had occurred against at least one - a carrier determinant X. The anti-X ARC reacts with the determinant and "captures" the whole bacterium and, as a side effect of this interaction, a soluble factor is produced locally in the tissue. The substance has the property of activating other ARC non-specifically so that they migrate into the area (probably against the gradient of the factor concentration) and differentiate. All activated ARC which encounter the appropriate antigen in the area can now react so that foci of PFC of different specificities appear within the same area. A possible candidate for the factor is a polynucleotide. A substance of similar chemistry and with non-specific immuno-enhancing properties is released during an interaction of pre-sensitized cells with the antigen (14).

The suggested model is consistant with the concept of predestined antigen reactive cells. The introduction of the factor is a simplifying rather than complicating point. It explains the non-random distribution of ARC in the spleen and may also explain

the phenomena of antigenic competition and of the non-specific
changes in RES during immunization.

References

1. R. McAlack, J. Cerny, J. Allen and H. Friedman, Science, 168:
   141, 1970.
2. J. Cerny, R. McAlack, M.A. Sajid and H. Friedman, Fed. Proc.,
   29: 769, 1970 (abstract).
3. E.H. Perkins, T. Sado and T. Makinodan, J. Immunol., 103: 668,
   1969.
4. I. Young and H. Friedman, in: H. Cottier, N. Odartchenko, R.
   Schindler and C. Congdon, eds., Germinal Centers in Immune
   Responses, p. 102, New York, Springer-Verlag, 1967.
5. Nakano, M. and W. Braun, Science, 151: 338, 1966.
6. R.W. Dutton and R.I. Mischell, Cold Spring Harbor Symp. Quant.
   Biol., 32: 407, 1967.
7. W.J.K. Tannenberg and A.N. Malaviya, J. Exptl. Med., 128: 895,
   1968.
8. J. Sterzl, J. Vesely, M. Jilek and L. Mandel, in: J. Sterzl and
   co-workers, eds., Molecular and Cellular Basis of Antibody
   Formation, p. 463, Prague, 1965.
9. M. Fishman, J. Exptl. Med., 114: 837, 1961.
10. J. Sterzl, Cold Spring Harbor Symp. Quant. Biol., 32: 493, 1967.
11. Y.B. Kim and D.W. Watson, Fed. Proc., 27: 493, 1968 (abstract).
12. O.J. Plescia, Current Topics in Microbiology and Immunology,
    50: 78, 1969.
13. R.M. McBride and L.W. Schierman, J. Exptl. Med., 131: 377, 1970.
14. M. Nakano and W. Braun, J. Immunol., 99: 570, 1967.

A QUANTITATIVE MODEL FOR THE MECHANISM OF ANTIBODY FORMATION AND TOLERANCE

Stanley Cohen

Department of Pathology, State University of New York

at Buffalo, Buffalo, New York, U.S.A.

INTRODUCTION

Following immunization, an animal can produce a variety of immunoglobulins of different classes, various degrees of specificity, and heterogeneity with respect to affinity for antigen (1). Also, it is primed to respond to a subsequent challenge with an enhanced response (immunologic memory). In addition, under certain conditions exposure to antigen may result in non-reactivity (tolerance) rather than immunity. This was first observed following the administration of massive doses of antigen. Subsequently, however, it was shown that very small doses of antigen, when given in an appropriate manner, may produce unresponsiveness as well. These states are known as "high zone" and "low zone" paralysis. The immunologic phenomena involved are the result of interactions between a variety of different cell types, under the control of poorly understood regulatory mechanisms. The events are ultimately dependent upon the interaction of antigen with some component, presumably on the surface, of one or more of the reacting cells. Because of the specificity of the immune response, this component, or "receptor" must have a stereospecific configuration which complements that of the antigen, and in this sense it is antibody-like. Many otherwise puzzling observations are explainable in terms of receptor theory. Siskind and Benacerraf (2) have presented an elegant model based on these considerations which provides an explanation for the observed changes in antibody affinity during the course of an immune response. The situation with respect to tolerance, however, is more complex. Basically, there are 3 ways in which a cell can "decide" whether to engage in an immune response or become tolerant: (1) the cell may exist in a number of time-dependent states; it is only when it is in an appropriate state that antigen can activate it. At other times,

323

tolerance results. (2) the kind of antigen which contacts the cell
determines the response. If antigen must be processed in order to
become immunogenic, then unprocessed antigen may be tolerogenic.
(3) the way in which antigen contacts the cell determines the response; i.e. the geometric distribution of antigen-bound receptors
on the cell may represent the critical signal for activation or
suppression. In this presentation, we will address ourselves to the
latter possibility. It will be shown that elementary quantitative
considerations lead to some interesting predictions with respect to
antibody induction, memory, tolerance, and the escape from tolerance.

CELL-CELL INTERACTIONS

Although there is much evidence that multiple cell types may
be involved in the induction of an immune response (3), this may
not be an absolute requirement. Thus, although the interaction of
thymic- and marrow-derived lymphocytes is important for the response
to some antigens, it does not appear to be a requirement for all
antigens. Indeed, the "thymic-dependency" of some antigens is dose
dependent; with high doses, marrow-derived cells alone are sufficient
for antibody induction (4). This suggests that the role of the thymic-
derived lymphocyte might be non-specific, perhaps in analogy with
the non-specifically enhancing role of "peritoneal attached cells"
(5). It is known that thymic-derived lymphocytes participate in
reactions of cellular immunity, and do so by means of the elabor-
ation of various effector molecules which are not immunoglobulins.
Many of these substances are chemotactic for various cells. It is
therefore attractive to suggest that antigen-activated, thymic-
derived lymphocytes produce a variety of chemotactic factors, or
"tactins" which help to accumulate both specifically competent
marrow-derived cells capable of antibody production, and ancillary
cell types such as macrophages, in regions of high local antigen
concentration.

Even if it should turn out that both thymic- and marrow-
derived lymphocytes are specific participants in manufacturing
antibody, it is reasonable to consider that there is a crucial
or rate-limiting step which involves the interaction of antigen
with a single critical cell. I will assume the existence of
antibody-like receptors on a cell involved in that critical stage
of the immune reaction. I will also assume that tolerance is based
upon the presence of tolerant cells rather than the selective
destruction of precommitted cells. Evidence for this latter
assumption is the fact that a population of small lymphocytes from
a tolerant donor may lose tolerance after as little as 8 hr of in
vitro incubation. Rapid reversibility of the tolerant state in vitro
argues against cell destruction as the mechanism of tolerance. A
final assumption is that events in the same cell may be responsible
for either tolerance or activation.

INTERACTION OF RECEPTOR AND ANTIGEN

The most general model for antibody induction, based upon cell receptors which can combine with antigen, is one in which certain kinds of antigen-receptor binding lead to cellular activation and other kinds of binding lead to suppression. Whether a given cell is activated or made tolerant is determined by the additive effect of these kinds of binding. In order to account for both high and low zone suppression of the immune response, one would like to find an equation relating activation to atigen binding which is convex, and has a maximum within the range of binding. When activation rises above a critical threshold value, antibody induction, with cellular proliferation and antibody synthesis will occur. For both lower and higher doses of antigen, the threshold is not attained, and tolerance results instead. The simplest case of such a model is the situation where all the receptor sites on a given cell are identical, and there is only one kind of antigen molecule. In this situation, one can derive an activation curve based upon associative pairing of either antigen molecules or occupied receptors on the cell surface. The situation which lends itself best to analysis is the case in which the signal for cellular suppression is a binding of two distinct antigen molecules to two adjacent receptors to form "doublets". The signal for activation is the binding of one antigen molecule to a single receptor to form an unpaired bound site, or "singlet". This is analogous to the mechanism of substrate inhibition in certain kinds of enzyme reactions (7), but is exactly the reverse of that proposed by Bretscher and Cohn (8). They did not explore the quantitative consequences of their assumption, which was that a single antigen-receptor hit leads to paralysis, while doublet hits lead to activation. It is, however, impossible to generate suitable activating curves based upon this assumption, and indeed, the authors required the postulate of a pre-existing "natural" extracellular antibody to serve as carrier for antigen in order to account for both low and high zone tolerance.

The mathematical treatment of the model proposed here has been presented in detail (9). It is based upon simple probability considerations, in order to avoid assumptions about thermodynamic equilibrium and association constants. The general approach is to consider a uniform linear array of receptor sites, each of which has the same probability of combining with antigen. If a fraction "α" of these sites have bound antigen, then one can derive an equation which expresses the fraction "δ" of these bound sites which participate in doublet formation as a function of "α". In a two-dimensional array, which corresponds to the case in which the receptors are distributed on the cell surface, δ is made up of contributions from both dimensions. In any case, it is easy to calculate a value of δ for all values of α, from 0 to 100%. Next, since singlet binding, by assumption, is activating, and doublet formation is suppressive, then activation for antibody formation is proportional

to the difference ($\alpha - \delta$). The theoretical activation curve
which results from these considerations is shown in Fig. 1,

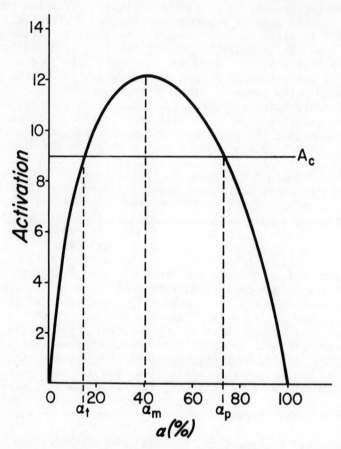

Fig. 1. Immunologic activation (A) of a cell as a function of the
per cent of receptor sites which have bound antigen (α). An arbitrary
activation threshold is illustrated as A_c, which defines threshold
(α_t) and plateau (α_p) values of α. Maximal activation is at α_m=41%.

where activation is plotted as a function of the per cent of the
receptor sites which have bound antigen. For illustration, an
arbitrary activation threshold is represented by the line A_c. This
is taken as the critical level which must be exceeded for antibody
induction to occur. This line defines a threshold and plateau value
of α, which separate the regions of low and high zone paralysis
from the region of antibody induction. Note that even though there

are very few doublets in the former region, the total amount of antigen on the cell is insufficient to bring it to activation, and the cell is therefore suppressed. This assumes that suppression is an active process, and not merely a failure of activation, which is consistent with the nature of tolerance in both zones. It can be seen that maximal cellular activation in this model would occur when 41% of the receptor sites are occupied by antigen. This is a rather quantitative prediction in search of a suitable experiment. It is also of interest that the curve is not symmetric, but is skewed to the right.

ANTIBODY AFFINITY

With the above as background, we can easily account for the variations in affinity with antigen dose which have been observed experimentally (1), by postulating that the number of receptor sites per cell varies from cell to cell. The number of available receptor sites on a cell bears a relationship to the affinity of the antibody which is produced by that cell or its descendants. Cells with only a few receptor sites make high affinity antibody. Please note that this is arbitrary, and does not assume a relationship between receptor affinity and antibody affinity. It is an alternate assumption to that of Siskind that the cell receptor affinity is identical to the affinity of the antibody produced by that cell. It has been shown (9) that this alternate approach is plausible in that very reasonable conclusions about cell receptor affinity follow as a consequence of the assumption.

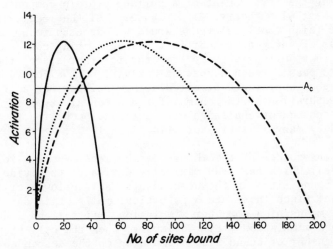

Fig. 2. Activation as a function of number of sites bound, for three hypothetical cells, with 50, 150, and 200 sites.

Fig. 2 shows the activation curve plotted as a function of number of sites bound, rather than per cent of sites bound, for 3 different cells. It is clear that high doses of antigen will tend to saturate the cells with low site numbers first and leave them in their tolerant state. As the dose of antigen descreases, we fall below the activation threshold of the low affinity cells first (higher site numbers) and begin to pick up activity of the high affinity cells. This causes the average affinity of the antibodies produced by the animal to increase. This model predicts that when an animal escapes from high zone tolerance, or when it is in a partially tolerant state, the antibody produced will be of low affinity. This has been found to be the case (1). Interestingly, the model predicts that in escape from low zone tolerance, the antibody first made should be of high affinity. There is no experimental data on this point as yet.

FURTHER PREDICTIONS

Since tolerance, in the above model, is a consequence of the association and distribution of antigen on a cell surface, and is dependent only upon the number of particles involved, the doses required of various antigens to induce tolerance in a given experimental setting should fall within a narrow range. This has been shown to be the case by Mitchison (10). The theory suggests also that induction of tolerance should be a fairly rapid event, since no intervening modification or processing of antigen is required. Recent studies have shown that the time involved may be as little as two hours, and that partial tolerance could be achieved after a 15 minute exposure to antigen (11,12,13). It was shown also that cells lost their ability to become tolerant after trypsinization (11), suggesting the involvement of a surface protein component, again in agreement with theory. Also, in terms of the model, the termination of (high zone) tolerance would be expected to be associated with loss of antigen present in the inactivating configuration. This suggests that during recovery from the tolerant state, the cells involved should pass through a zone of activation, manifested either as the spontaneous appearance of circulating antibody, or as the spontaneous preparation of the animal for a secondary type of response upon subsequent challenge with antigen. Such effects have been described by many investigators (14,15,16,17).

A final consequence of the theory can be seen if one allows a hypothetical cell which has been maximally activated to divide until the number of bound sites on the descendants falls below a critical threshold value. Since these are hypothetical cells, this can only be achieved by means of a computer simulation. Milgrom and I have performed such a simulation (18). Obviously, when the cell stops dividing, the number of bound sites remaining on the descendants can range from zero to the critical value chosen. Fig. 3 shows the frequency distribution of progeny cells as a function of number of

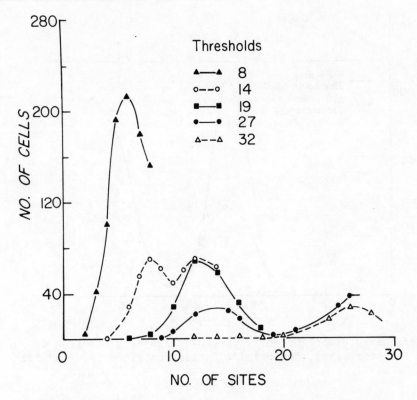

Fig. 3. Frequency distribution of progeny cells as a function of number of receptor sites which retain bound antigen. The original cell contained 128 sites, 41% of which were occupied by antigen.

bound sites, for a variety of such thresholds. It can be seen that at certain thresholds, the frequency distribution becomes biphasic, suggesting that two functionally distinct populations have been formed. These populations have been found to differ in the number of divisions required to reach the critical value. The curves of Fig. 3 have been generated from precursor cells with 128 receptor sites, and each represents the average of 100 computer trials. The effect is quite general; Fig. 4 shows biphasic curves generated from cells with 1024 as well as 128 sites. These curves are based on 1000 trials, which leads to better definition than that seen in Fig. 3.

Since the antigen-bound sites on the original cell were randomly distributed, some descendants fall below threshold after only a few divisions, whereas others progress to a more terminal

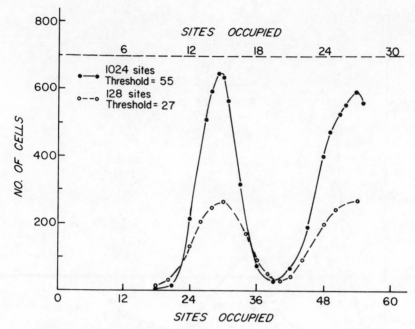

Fig. 4. Frequency distribution of progeny cells as a function of occupied receptor sites. The original cells contained 1024 and 128 sites respectively.

state. It is tempting to equate these two populations with, respectively, memory cells and antibody-forming cells. Further studies will allow us to make predictions as to the relative sizes of these populations as a function of various experimental manipulations of the size and pattern of administration of immunizing dose of antigen.

SUMMARY

Most of the models for antibody formation or tolerance which have been suggested in the literature are based upon the requirement for interaction between antigen and an antibody-like receptor on the surface of an immunocompetent cell as a critical step for either induction or suppression of the immune response. In the simplest situation, where interaction is between identical antigenic fragments and identical receptor units, the nature of the immune response must be dependent upon the geometric distribution of bound receptors on the cell. In this paper, the consequences of doublet suppression and singlet activation have been explored. Analysis of this situation leads to an activation curve which predicts maximal activation of immunocompetent cells when 41% of their receptor sites are bound by antigen. The consequences of this pattern of activation for tolerance and for the affinity characteristics of antibodies as a function of antigen dose have been presented in detail. The behavior of such activated cells under conditions of cellular proliferation have been explored by computer simulation. If maximally activated cells are allowed to divide until the number of antigen-bound receptors falls below certain critical threshold values, the frequency distribution curve for progeny cells is biphasic, suggesting that two functionally distinct populations have been formed. It is suggested that these populations, which differ in the average number of divisions their constituent cells have undergone, represent (1) a pool of end-stage antibody producing cells, and (2) a pool of intermediate cells which remain as a source of immunologic memory.

ACKNOWLEDGEMENTS

This work was supported, in part, by NIH grant AI-09114, and funds from a Dr. Henry C. and Bertha H. Buswell Fellowship.

REFERENCES

1. G. W. Siskind, in: S. Cohen, G. Cudkowicz and R. T. McCluskey, Eds. Cellular Interactions in the Immune Response. Basel: S. Karger, in press.
2. G. W. Siskind and B. Benacerraf, Adv. Immunol., 10: 1, 1969.
3. J. F. A. P. Miller, in: S. Cohen, G. Cudkowicz and R. T. McClusley, Eds. Cellular Interactions in the Immune Response. Basel: S. Karger, in press.
4. J. H. L. Playfair and E. C. Purves, ibid.
5. R. W. Dutton, P. Campbell, E. Chan, J. Hirst, M. Hoffman, J. Kettman, J. Lesley, M. McCarthy, R. I. Mishell, D. J. Raidt and D. Vann, ibid.
6. P. J. McCullagh and J. L. Gowans, in: J. M. Yoffey, Ed. The Lymphocyte in Immunology and Hematopoiesis. London: E. Arnold,1967.
7. J. M. Van Rossum, Molec. Pharm., 2: 201, 1964.
8. P. A. Bretscher and M. Cohn, Nature, 220: 444, 1968.
9. S. Cohen, J. Theor. Biol., 27: 19, 1970.
10. N. A. Mitchison, Immunol.,15: 509, 1968.
11. S. Britton, J. Exptl. Med., 129: 469, 1969.
12. E. Diener and W. D. Armstrong, J. Exptl. Med., 129: 591, 1969.
13. N. A. Mitchison, Immunol.,15: 531, 1968.
14. N. A. Mitchison, Immunol.,9: 129, 1965.
15. G. W. Siskind, P. Y. Patterson and L. Thomas. J. Immunol.,90: 929, 1963.
16. G. Terres and W. L. Hughes, J. Immunol., 83: 459, 1959.
17. J. G. Thorbecke, G. W. Siskind, and N. Goldberger, J. Immunol., 87: 147, 1961.
18. S. Cohen and M. Milgrom, in preparation.

MODELLING OF THE IMMUNE PROCESSES

M. Jílek and J. Šterzl

Department of Immunology, Institute of
Microbiology, Czechoslovak Academy of
Sciences, Prague 4, Czechoslovakia

Extensive immunological studies allow to consider the sequential events between experimental conditions and the results obtained. For this region, not yet covered with enough facts, the biologists are working out hypotheses and models. Such models could be expressed verbally, drawn as figures or formulated mathematically.

To elaborate a mathematical model of biological phenomena, at first the conclusions, based on experimental results, are formulated. These formulated axioms determine the significance of our models: "...If the axioms are true, then the theorems are also true, because the theorems are statements to which the axioms commit us or which follow from them. This procedure compels us to be much more careful than we commonly are in the use of language in biology. It compels us to put all our cards on the table: to say what we mean and to mean what we say. It deprives us of the smoke screens of obscurity that can so bedevil matter when we rely exclusively on natural language." (1).

The set of axioms formulate the theory which was originally expressed by words or pictures. Including different constants resembling experimental conditions allows to compare whether models are in good fit with experimental data. On the basis of such comparisons, this theory (model) is acceptable as a possible explanation or is rejected being unadequate to experimental findings. Using the model, experimental projects could

be proposed: conclusions based on the hypotheses, con-
fronted with experimental results, challenge the fit-
ness of the model.

Models suggested recently do not differ as substantially as the hypotheses on antibody formation proposed
some decades ago (e.g. the theory of Haurowitz,compared
with Burnet´s) because enormous quantities of facts accumulated and conclusions resulting from them are continuously discussed at meetings and in papers. In the
most models, as by Dixon et al. (2), Sercarz and Coons
(3), Šterzl (4), Makinodan and Albright (5), Nossal (6),
and Papermaster (7), at least two stages are assumed:
the phase of adaptation (activation), and the conversion
into antibody forming stage. Only some authors are expressing certain parts of the immune response by mathematical formulae, as e.g. Hege and Cole (8), Marchalonis
and Gledhill (9), Groves et al. (10), Cohen (11).

Data are accumulating which would allow to construct
the models covering and expressing mathematically essential steps of the immune response. Let us consider the
facts which the model should comprise.

Immunocompetent Cell (ICC)

By this term are denoted the cells which possess
the potentiality to respond specifically to an antigen,
but which have not been stimulated yet by the specific
antigenic contact. The capability to react with a certain antigen is being acquired during the differentiation of the lymphoid tissue, by a synthesis of a certain
number of immunoglobulin molecules, or at least of their
variable part containing combining site. The expression
of the genome of the immunocompetent cell is probably
already restricted, i.e. one cell forms only one antibody specificity. That is assumed from the fact that
only very small portion of cells - approximately one
from among 10^6 lymphoid cells - may be stimulated by a
given antigen. Immunocompetent cells do not proliferate
more actively than other cells of lymphoid tissues in
average. It was estimated that relative increase (immunocompetent cells/lymphoid cells) does not occur without specific antigenic stimulus (12, 13).

Stimulation of ICC by Antigen

It is assumed that antigenic molecules in an appropriate, solubilized form (e.g. after processing of particulate antigen by enzymes of phagocytes) are directly reacting with receptors of the immunocompetent cell, with or without need of helper cells. It was demonstrated that only a certain threshold level of anti-gen is effective for such a stimulation in vivo, as well as in closed cultivation system, for stimulation of cells in vitro. Probably a saturation of a certain critical number of receptors on the surface of the im-munocompetent cell is required, and this occurs as a random process. Experimental data suggest that number of receptors on the surface of the ICC is very low. Larger quantity of antigen is needed for stimulation of ICC, compared to immunologically activated cells (IAC). The excess of antigen is not inhibiting ICC directly, but all antigenic doses put them on the differentiation way toward antibody formation (14).

Immunologically Activated Cell (IAC)

Activated cells develop by action of antigen on ICC. These cells actively proliferate. It is not settled whether higher thymidine-labelling of cells involved in antibody formation (compared with other lymphoid cells) is due to their selective activation by the antigen, or due to their shorter generation cycle. Data have been accumulated, suggesting qualitative difference between the ICC and the immunologically activated cell. IAC are not only increased in number 10-100 times compared with ICC but their binding of antigen signifies an increased number of Ig receptors. Activation of the specific Ig gene region is suggested also by the finding that in the same precursor line (producing the same idiotype) IgM and IgG precursors occur subsequently. A second contact with a specific antigen is needed for the terminal differentiation of IAC, i.e. for development of antibody producing cell. IAC are detectable for many months by their ability to respond to a new antigenic dose (memory cells) and to produce characteristic quantitative and qualitative secondary response (14).

The Effect of Different Amounts of
Antigen of the Primary Response

The effect of easily metabolizable protein antigen is considered. This is the case if mice are immunized with sheep erythrocytes (SRBC): the Forssman antigen is not immunogenic in mice, only the labile protein isoantigen of red cell stromas.

1. A threshold quantity of antigen administered is sufficient for activation of ICC. However, during the period of activation, a portion of antigen is metabolized and activated cells are thus deprived of a further antigenic stimulus. The result is the preparation for a secondary response without a detectable antibody production (Fig. 1).

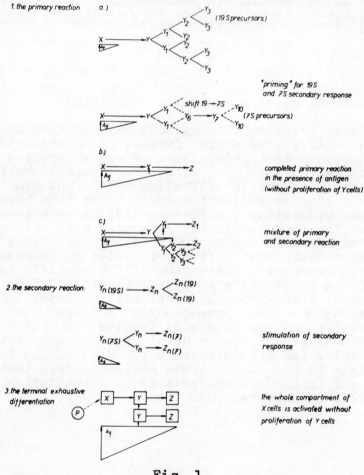

Fig. 1.

   2. An alternate situation occurs if an excessive
amount of antigen is administered, sufficient not only
for activation of most of ICC but also for stimulation
of activated cells. The time of differentiation shortens
and a significant antibody response is detected. The
immediate contact of IAC with the antigen prevents, however, their proliferation. A high dose of antigen, by
forced terminal differentiation, decreases or eliminates
a secondary reaction and establishes the tolerance.

   3. In the organism, due to local concentrations of
antigen, usually both situations occur. With small doses
of antigen, the prevailing part of cells are prepared
for a secondary response, but some of them differentiate
into antibody forming cells (AbFC). On the contrary,
with high doses of antigen, most of cells are transformed into AbFC but some escape from the second antigenic
contact and remain as memory cells (13).

   The half-life of the production period of AbFC is
limited to 2 - 3 days. After finishing their function,
only the cells prepared for a secondary response (IAC,
memory cells) remain in the organism.

The Effect of Different Amounts of Antigen
on the Secondary Response

   1. IAC, stimulated with a minimum amount of antigen (lower than that necessary for ICC), are inactivated
without appearance of AbFC. Therefore the term "abortive
differentiation" is used for that phenomenon: it results
in a low-dose tolerance.

   2. An optimum dose of antigen induces an optimum
secondary response, resulting in a significant antibody
formation, as expansion or maintenance of the immunological capacity, prepared for further antigenic stimuli.

   3. The administration of an excessive dose of antigen leads to a secondary response with, however, a limited proliferation. Thus, if another dose of antigen,e.g.
a third one, is administered the response is much lower
or is completely inhibited by exhaustion of memory cells.

   The effect of various amounts of easily metabolizable protein antigen (sheep erythrocytes - mouse) has
been discussed until now. Another course of the immune
response is observed if sheep erythrocytes are administered in Forssman-negative rabbits. The lipopolysaccharide antigen evokes non-specific irritation, the anti-

body response increases also after administration of
high antigenic doses, similarly as if the protein antigen is administered in Freund s adjuvant. Other is the
course of immunization if pneumococcal polysaccharide
antigen is used: this non-metabolizable antigen remains
in an organism for many months or years, without side
irritation effect. Since this antigen is available for
cells steadily during a very long period it limits the
proliferation of IAC and even in low doses it evokes
the tolerance.

Assumptions for a Mathematical Model

a) The existence of three differentiation stages,
as described above: ICC,IAC, AbFc.

b) A certain time interval (the latent phase) is
required for transformation of ICC into IAC and of IAC
into AbFC.

c) The dynamics of the immune reaction is affected
by the amount of the active antigen, which varies in the
course of the immune reaction (by phagocytosis, binding
on antibody, metabolic decay, etc.). Probably a certain
type of a random process is involved; for simplicity, it
is assumed for the present that the antigen disappears
as negative exponential function. Some results (15) suggest that one may consider the exponential decrease, at
least for kinds of easily metabolizable antigens; we
have accepted such an assumption.

d) Decisive for the fate of the cell is its first
contact with an antigen. We accept the assumption (probably the nearest to reality) that a certain threshold
amount of antigen is required for the activation of ICC,
which the cell meets randomly. Number of critical contacts in the time interval between immunization and the
time t is denoted by the symbol $N(t)$. The following
starting assumptions (axioms) on the $N(t)$ process are
assumed as follows:

1. Until the time of the first immunization (t=0)
the cell has not yet met the given antigen.

Axiom 1: $N(0) = 0$.

2. Although the first contact of the cell with an
antigen is decisive for activation of the ICC it is assumed that further contacts of the cell with an antigen
are as random as the first contact.

Axiom 2: N(t) is a random process with independent increments.

3. The first contact of the ICC with an antigen may (or might not) occur at any moment after immunization.

Axiom 3: $0 < \Pr\left\{N(t) > 0\right\} < 1$ for all $t > 0$.

4. Because of randomness of a contact, two contacts do not occur in absolute synchronization.

Axiom 4: $\lim_{h \to 0} \dfrac{\Pr\left\{N(t + h) - N(t) \geq 2\right\}}{\Pr\left\{N(t + h) - N(t) = 1\right\}} = 0.$

5. The random binding of antigen is dependent on quantity of the antigen present, i.e. on the amount of the antigen injected and on the rate of elimination etc.

Axiom 5: $\lim_{h \to 0} \dfrac{\Pr\left\{N(t + h) - N(t) \geq 1\right\}}{h} = \alpha(t)$

The function $\alpha(t)$ expresses the elimination rate of antigen.

Modelling by Monte Carlo Method

The process corresponding to the above assumptions is termed non-homogeneous Poisson process (16). The simplest method to obtain a model of such a process is the simulation of the natural process by a computer, to which a programme is given respecting the existing relations between individual compartments of the immune response, as well as the randomness involved in the natural process (e.g. randomness of the time of the contact of antigen with the ICC, etc.). This Monte Carlo method has the advantage approaching the variability obtained by the experimental results; for reliable conclusions by this method, however, a large number of individual computations are generally required to obtain the sum of random distributed values.

The computer's simulation of the fate of one ICC after immunization consists of the following steps (Fig. 2):

At first the assumptions (axioms) presented are included in the programme of the computer. The computer starts to analyze one immunocompetent cell. By means of a generator of random numbers, it indicates the time in

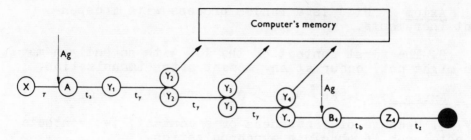

Fig. 2.

which the cell meets the antigen. Randomness of contact
depends on the actual quantity of antigen, and the computer knows that the quantity of antigen available decreases exponentially. The cell starts to proliferate
under this antigenic stimulus: we assume that a symmetric division of IAC (Y) is involved, and that both cells,
formed by division from the original cell, do not differ
in their qualities but in the randomness to realize further differentiation steps. Not all dividing cells can
be simultaneously processed by the computer. In the moment when new IAC (Y) arise by mitotic division, they
are stored in the memory of the computer and the fate
of only one activated cell is followed. The computer
selects one IAC and follows its division; the computer
has in its programme to arrange the second contact of
antigen with the activated and multiplying cell on the
basis of randomness; the available quantity of the antigen at this moment is considerably smaller. As soon as
the second contact of an IAC with antigen takes place,
a terminal differentiation occurs, and an AbFC develops.
In our hypothesis it is assumed that antibody forming
cells, originating from early generations of IAC (Y)
cells, form antibodies of the 19S type, while cells
from later generations (starting about from the 7th generation) form precursors for antibodies of the 7S type.
When the computer is through with differentiation history of that cell it selects another IAC from the memory
and follows similar random events, as described. Certain
constant parameters are selected, based on data obtained
by experimental results: The generation time of proliferating cells is considered as constant (8 hr) and not more
than a given number (eleven) of generations are expected.

    The computer modelates the changes occurring during
differentiation every hour after administration of

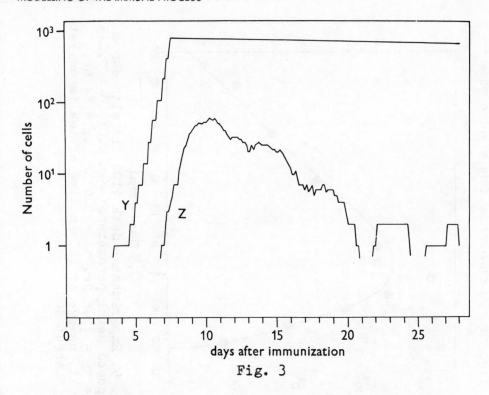

Fig. 3

antigen over 28 days. The results for some individual
cells (dynamics of number of IAC and/or AbFC) are shown
in Fig. 3. The first contact of ICC with antigen occurred in this case relatively late - at 83 hr.

Modelling by Mathematical Analytical Method

When using a computer which should record the random fate of at least one hundred cells, in order to si-
mulate the immune response of one animal it proved that
the requirements for time work of computer are impracti-
cable (a simulation of the fate of one ICC would last in
average one hour of the work of the computer). Therefore
it proved necessary to proceed to a more complicated analytical method. Formulae were obtained for the probability of a random contact of the cell with an antigen (17),

$$P_+ = 1 - \exp(-\alpha/\lambda),$$

and for a probability distribution of the epoch at which
this first contact takes place, conditioned with the
density of probability (18)

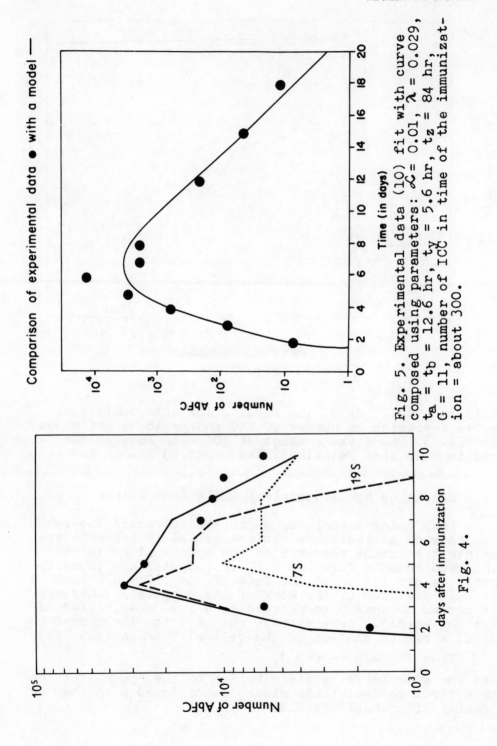

Fig. 5. Experimental data (10) fit with curve composed using parameters: $\alpha = 0.01$, $\lambda = 0.029$, $t_a = t_b = 12.6$ hr, $t_y = 5.6$ hr, $t_z = 84$ hr, $G = 11$, number of ICC in time of the immunization = about 300.

Fig. 4.

Influence of the amount of antigen on the course
of the primary reaction

Amount of antigen : A – 0.001   D – 0.02
B – 0.005   E – 0.05
C – 0.01   F – 0.1

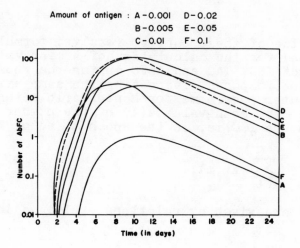

Fig. 6

Immunological capacity (relative amount of memory cells y)
after several antigenic doses (k)

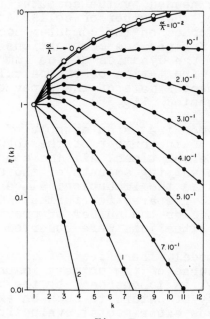

Fig. 7

$$f_+(t) = \frac{\lambda M}{\exp(M)-1} \exp(-\lambda t) \exp\left\{M \exp(-\lambda t)\right\}$$

with $M = \alpha/\lambda$.

In virtue of these partial results, formulae were then obtained for the calculation of a mean value of the number of ICC, IAC and AbFC during the whole course of the immune response, respecting the same axioms as in the computer programme for Monte Carlo method (19). For example, the mean value $z(t)$ of the number of AbFC formed from one ICC is, in the epoch t, equal to the sum of

$$z(t) = \sum_{g=1}^{G} z_g(t);$$

where $z_g(t)$ are given by relations explained in the Appendix.

Preliminary verification was done by a table calculating machine only for a certain combination of the initial values and the curve obtained was compared with experimental data (20)(Fig. 4).

Analytical mathematical work substantially decreased the time needed by the computer to calculate the mean value of the number of cells. At present, calculation is performed on the computer according to obtained formulae for various combinations determining the character of the dynamics of the immune response. As example, a confrontation of the calculated curve with the experimental data of the paper of Groves et al. (10) is presented (Fig. 5).

Figure 6 demonstrates an example of curves showing the mean values of the number of the AbFC in the primary response in different times. All the conditions are the same, except the varying amounts of the antigen injected. Fig. 7 demonstrates the immunological capacity (relative amount of the IAC prepared for further antigenic stimulus) in dependence on the number of previous immunizations (21). Both situations were observed in experiments.

Using the model, the effect of changed initial values on the course of the primary immune response is studied. The goal is to approach by the mathematical model the reality of nature to such an extent that instead of laborious experimental evaluations the course of immunity, e.g. the preparation of optimum secondary response or tolerance by certain type of antigens and different doses, will be predicted by the computer.

REFERENCES

1. J. H. Woodger, Ann. N. Y. Acad. Sci., 96:1093,
    1962.

2. F. J. Dixon, D. W. Talmage, and P. H. Maurer,
    J. Immunol., 68:693, 1952.

3. E. Sercarz and A. H. Coons, in: Mechanisms of Immu-
    nological Tolerance, p. 73. Prague: Czechoslovak
    Academy of Sciences, 1962.

4. J. Šterzl, in: Advances in Biological Sciences,
    p. 149. Prague: Czechoslovak Academy of Sciences,
    1962.

5. T. Makinodan and J. F. Albright, in: P. Grabar and
    P. A. Miescher, Eds., Immunopathology, 3rd Int.Symp.,
    p. 99. Basel: Schwabe, 1963.

6. G. J. V. Nossal, K. D. Shortman, J. F. A. P. Miller,
    G. F. Mitchell, and J. S. Haskill, Cold Spring Har-
    bor Symp.Quant. Biol.,32:369, 1967.

7. B. W. Papermaster, Cold Spring Harbor Symp. Quant.
    Biol., 32:447, 1967.

8. J. S. Hege and L. J. Cole, J. Immunol., 97:34, 1966.

9. J. J. Marchalonis and V. X. Gledhill, Nature, 220:
    608, 1968.

10. D. L. Groves, W. E. Lever, and T. Makinodan, J. Im-
    munol., 104:148, 1970.

11. S. Cohen, J. Theor. Biol., 27:19, 1970.

12. J. Šterzl and A. M. Silverstein, Adv. Immunol. 6:
    337, 1967.

13. J. Šterzl, Cold Spring Harbor Symp. Quant. Biol.
    32:493, 1967.

14. J. Šterzl, P. Šíma, J. Medlín, H. Tlaskalová, L. Man-
    del, and A. A. Nordin, in: Developmental Aspects of
    Antibody Formation and Structure. Prague: Academia,
    1970.

15. R. Franzl and J. Morello, Information Exchange Group
    No. 5., Scientific Memorandum No. 59, 1965.

16. E. Parzen, Stochastic Processes. San Francisco:
    Holden Day Inc., 1964.

17. M. Jílek and Z. Ursínyová, Folia Microbiol., 15:
    294, 1970.

18. M. Jílek and Z. Ursínyová, Folia Microbiol., 15,
    Nr. 6, 1970 (in press).

19. M. Jílek and J. Šterzl, in: Developmental Aspects
    of Antibody Formation and Structure. Prague:
    Academia, 1970.

20. J. Šterzl, J. Veselý, M. Jílek, and L. Mandel, in:
    Molecular and Cellular Basis of Antibody Formation,
    p. 463. Prague: Czechoslovak Academy of Sciences,
    1965.

21. M. Jílek, Folia Microbiol., 16, Nr. 1, 1971 (in
    press).

APPENDIX

Notation

This notation is used throughout the formulae given:

α ... a constant proportional to the amount of antigen injected

λ ... rate of elimination of antigen

t_a ... length of the latent phase for transition ICC→IAC

t_b ... length of the latent phase for transition IAC→AbFC

t_z ... length of the production of antibodies by an AbFC

t_y ... generation time of IAC

G ... maximum number of generations of IAC.

Mean value of the number of antibody forming cells Z_g at the time t is

$$(5) \quad z_g(t) = \begin{cases} 0, \quad t < t_a + t_b + (g-1)t_y, \\[2mm] 2^{g-1} e^{-\frac{\alpha}{\lambda}} \left\{ \dfrac{e^{\frac{\alpha}{\lambda}[1-e^{-\lambda t_a}(1-e^{-\lambda(g-1)t_y})]}}{1-e^{-\lambda t_a}(1-e^{-\lambda(g-1)t_y})} + \right. \\[4mm] \left. + \dfrac{1}{1-e^{-\lambda t_a}}\left[\dfrac{e^{\frac{\alpha}{\lambda}[1+e^{\lambda(g-1)t_y}(e^{\lambda t_a}-1)]}e^{-\lambda(t-t_b)}}{1+e^{\lambda(g-1)t_y}(e^{\lambda t_a}-1)} - \right.\right. \\[4mm] \left.\left. - e^{\frac{\alpha}{\lambda}[1-e^{-\lambda t_a}+e^{-\lambda(t-t_b)}]}\right]\right\}, \\[4mm] \qquad\qquad t_a+t_b+(g-1)t_y \leqslant t < t_a+t_b+gt_y, \\[2mm] 2^{g-1} e^{-\frac{\alpha}{\lambda}}\left\{ \dfrac{e^{\frac{\alpha}{\lambda}[1-e^{-\lambda t_a}(1-e^{-\lambda(g-1)t_y})]}}{1-e^{-\lambda t_a}(1-e^{-\lambda(g-1)t_y})} - \right. \\[4mm] - \dfrac{e^{\frac{\alpha}{\lambda}[1-e^{-\lambda t_a}(1-e^{-\lambda gt_y})]}}{1-e^{-\lambda t_a}(1-e^{-\lambda gt_y})} + \\[4mm] + \dfrac{1}{1-e^{-\lambda t_a}}\left[\dfrac{e^{\frac{\alpha}{\lambda}[1+e^{\lambda(g-1)t_y}(e^{\lambda t_a}-1)]}e^{-\lambda(t-t_b)}}{1+e^{\lambda(g-1)t_y}(e^{\lambda t_a}-1)} - \right. \\[4mm] \left.\left. - \dfrac{e^{\frac{\alpha}{\lambda}[1+e^{\lambda gt_y}(e^{\lambda t_a}-1)]}e^{-\lambda(t-t_b)}}{1+e^{\lambda gt_y}(e^{\lambda t_a}-1)}\right]\right\}, \\[4mm] \qquad\qquad t_a+t_b+gt_y \leqslant t < t_a+t_b+t_z+(g-1)t_y, \\[4mm] \text{(contin.)} \end{cases}$$

$$
\text{(5 cont.)} \quad z_g(t) = \begin{cases}
\begin{aligned}
& \text{(contin.)} \\
& 2^{g-1} e^{-\frac{\alpha}{\lambda}} \left\{ \frac{1}{1-e^{-\lambda t_a}} \left[\frac{1}{1+e^{\lambda(g-1)t_y}(e^{\lambda t_a}-1)} \times \right. \right. \\
& \quad \times \left(e^{\frac{\alpha}{\lambda}[1+e^{\lambda(g-1)t_y}(e^{\lambda t_a}-1)]e^{-\lambda(t-t_b)}} \right. \\
& \quad \left. - e^{\frac{\alpha}{\lambda}[1+e^{\lambda(g-1)t_y}(e^{\lambda t_a}-1)]e^{-\lambda(t-t_b-t_z)}} \right) + \\
& \quad + e^{\frac{\alpha}{\lambda}[1-e^{-\lambda t_a}+e^{-\lambda(t-t_b-t_z)}]} - \\
& \quad \left. - \frac{e^{\frac{\alpha}{\lambda}[1+e^{\lambda g t_y}(e^{\lambda t_a}-1)]e^{-\lambda(t-t_b)}}}{1+e^{\lambda g t_y}(e^{\lambda t_a}-1)} \right] - \\
& \quad \left. - \frac{e^{\frac{\alpha}{\lambda}[1-e^{-\lambda t_a}(1-e^{-\lambda g t_y})]}}{1-e^{-\lambda t_a}(1-e^{-\lambda g t_y})} \right\}, \\
& \quad\quad t_a+t_b+t_z+(g-1)t_y \leqslant t < t_a+t_b+t_z+g t_y,
\end{aligned} \\[2em]
\begin{aligned}
& \frac{2^{g-1}e^{-\frac{\alpha}{\lambda}}}{1-e^{-\lambda t_a}} \left\{ \frac{1}{1+e^{\lambda(g-1)t_y}(e^{\lambda t_a}-1)} \times \right. \\
& \quad \times \left(e^{\frac{\alpha}{\lambda}[1+e^{\lambda(g-1)t_y}(e^{\lambda t_a}-1)]e^{-\lambda(t-t_b)}} \right. \\
& \quad \left. - e^{\frac{\alpha}{\lambda}[1+e^{\lambda(g-1)t_y}(e^{\lambda t_a}-1)]e^{-\lambda(t-t_b-t_z)}} \right) - \\
& \quad - \frac{1}{1+e^{\lambda g t_y}(e^{\lambda t_a}-1)} \times \\
& \quad \times \left(e^{\frac{\alpha}{\lambda}[1+e^{\lambda g t_y}(e^{\lambda t_a}-1)]e^{-\lambda(t-t_b)}} \right. \\
& \quad \left. \left. - e^{\frac{\alpha}{\lambda}[1+e^{\lambda g t_y}(e^{\lambda t_a}-1)]e^{-\lambda(t-t_b-t_z)}} \right) \right\}, \\
& \quad\quad t \geqslant t_a+t_b+t_z+g t_y,
\end{aligned}
\end{cases}
$$

$$(6) \quad z_G(t) = \begin{cases} 0 \ , \ t < t_a + t_b + (G-1)\,t_y \ , \\[2mm] 2^{G-1} e^{-\frac{\alpha}{\lambda}} \left\{ \dfrac{e^{\frac{\alpha}{\lambda}}\left[1 - e^{-\lambda t_a}\left(1 - e^{-\lambda(G-1)t_y}\right)\right]}{1 - e^{-\lambda t_a}\left(1 - e^{-\lambda(G-1)t_y}\right)} + \right. \\[4mm] \left. + \dfrac{1}{1 - e^{-\lambda t_a}}\left[\dfrac{e^{\frac{\alpha}{\lambda}}\left[1 + e^{\lambda(G-1)t_y}\left(e^{\lambda t_a}-1\right)\right]e^{-\lambda(t-t_b)}}{1 + e^{\lambda(G-1)t_y}\left(e^{\lambda t_a}-1\right)} - \right. \right. \\[4mm] \left. \left. - e^{\frac{\alpha}{\lambda}}\left[1 - e^{-\lambda t_a} + e^{-\lambda(t-t_b)}\right]\right]\right\} , \\[4mm] \qquad\qquad t_a + t_b + (G-1)t_y \leqslant t < t_a + t_b + t_z + (G-1)t_y \ , \\[4mm] 2^{G-1} e^{-\frac{\alpha}{\lambda}} \left\{ \dfrac{e^{\frac{\alpha}{\lambda}(1 - e^{-\lambda t_a})}}{1 - e^{-\lambda t_a}} \times \right. \\[4mm] \times \left(e^{\frac{\alpha}{\lambda}} e^{-\lambda(t-t_b-t_z)} - e^{\frac{\alpha}{\lambda}} e^{-\lambda(t-t_b)} \right) + \\[4mm] + \dfrac{1}{\left(1 - e^{-\lambda t_a}\right)\left[1 + e^{\lambda(G-1)t_y}\left(e^{\lambda t_a}-1\right)\right]} \times \\[4mm] \left. \times \left(e^{\frac{\alpha}{\lambda}\left[1 + e^{\lambda(G-1)t_y}\left(e^{\lambda t_a}-1\right)e^{-\lambda(t-t_b)}\right]} - e^{\frac{\alpha}{\lambda}\left[1 + e^{\lambda(G-1)t_y}\left(e^{\lambda t_a}-1\right)e^{-\lambda(t-t_b-t_z)}\right]} \right) \right\} , \\[4mm] \qquad\qquad t \geqslant t_a + t_z + t_z + (G-1)t_y \end{cases}$$

Co-chairman's remarks: It has been our feeling that some of the
complexities in the analysis of the cytokinetics of antibody production might be substantially reduced if we were able to perform
analysis of clones of antibody-forming cells. Some of the results
which we hope to be able to provide through this approach are, for
example: a) to estimate homogeneity of the antibody produced by a
given immunologically competent unit, that is, a unit composed
presumably of one antigen reactive cell and one precursor cell;
b) the proliferative capacity of a single precursor cell, presumably
bone marrow-derived; c) the actual composition of the immunocompetent
units, that is, whether or not a unit consists of a single antigen
reactive cell and one or more precursor cells of bone marrow origin;
and d) gain additional information with regard to the mechanism of
antigen competition. Those are just some of the problems that
might be attacked if we were able to perform this particular kind
of analysis. Our approach is a variation of the procedure of transferring donor cells to irradiated recipients wherein the inoculum
transferred is of limited cell number. The spleen of the recipient,
after appropriate length of time, is removed, cut into fragments
(3 pieces). Individual fragments are assayed for their content of
antibody-forming cells using the Jerne hemolytic plaque assay.
Individual pieces of other spleens are cultured *in vitro* and provided
with C^{14}-amino acids; later, the culture fluids are recovered and
antibodies removed with immuno-absorbent. Antibodies are eluted
and analyzed by acrylamide gel electrophoresis followed by autoradiography. Some of the variations one can introduce into the procedure
are, for example, priming the prospective recipients 3 days prior to
irradiation and transfer of cells, thus creating depots of antigen
in the recipient's spleen. The number of depots can be varied by
varying the antigen dose. In addition, donor cells can be introduced
which are derived from an intermediate host that has been irradiated
and repopulated with bone marrow cells. Thus, there is the possibility
to introduce varying numbers of bone marrow-derived spleen cells.

Now I will turn to a brief description of studies on transfer
of a limited number of cells from donors that have been previously
primed with antigen (sheep RBC). A limited number of spleen cells
(about 10^5) was transferred to irradiated recipients together with
more antigen. The spleen of a recipient was removed 7 days later,
cut into 3 fragments, and each fragment assayed for indirect PFC's.
In other experiments the fragments were cultured for 48 hours in the
presence of C^{14}-amino acids and the specific antibody produced was
analyzed. We have not yet completed analysis of the specific eluates.
I will briefly talk about the behavior of the eluates in sucrose
density gradients. Figure 1 shows that the eluate is specific antibody.

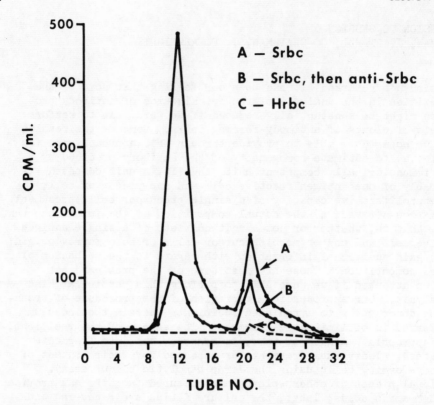

Fig. 1.   Incorporation of ^{14}C-amino acids into specific antibody
against Srbc during 24 hour culture, *in vitro*, of spleens from mice
injected as follows: (A) with Srbc 5 days prior to spleen culture;
(B) with Srbc, followed 2 days later by high-titered anti-Srbc serum,
and 3 days later spleen was cultures; (C) with horse rbc 5 days
prior to spleen culture.   Antibody absorbed on Srbc stroma, eluted
and resolved by centrifugation in a linear sucrose density gradient.

Eluate obtained after stimulus with SRBC is shown in curve A.   The
second curve G is the eluate obtained by the same procedure except
that 3 days after injecting the SRBC into the culture animal a high
titered SRBC antiserum was introduced.   Far less antibody was obtained in the eluate.   In C the cells were stimulated with HRBC
(horse erythrocytes).   Table I shows the analysis of spleens from
the group of recipients that were injected with 10^5 primed donor
spleen cells.   A, B, C refer to the three fragments, cut from the
spleen of a single recipient.   The table records the analysis of
the PFCs directed against SRBC in these fragments.   In addition, the
counts incorporated into specific antibody during *in vitro* culture
and absorbed on erythrocyte stroma are recorded.   The counts eluted,

Table I.

PFC AND Ab FORMATION IN SEPARATE SPLEEN FRAGMENTS

NO. DONOR CELLS	RECIP. SERUM TITER (DAY 7-8)	SPLEEN FRAGMENT	CULTURE FLUID TITER	NO. PFC (IN VITRO) ((48 HR.)	CPM/ml CULTURE FLUID (CORRECTED FOR CONTROLS)			PERCENT ELUTED
					ELUATE	STROMA	TOTAL	
0	0	—	0	8	2,820	6,459	9,280	30
1 X 10^5	0	a	0	84	3,040	2,645	5,685	53
		b		10	0	0	0	—
		c		22	200	0	200	100
	0	a		6	480	0	480	100
		b		10	520	1,093	1,613	32
		c		112	2,840	2,277	5,117	56
	1	a		0	180	0	180	100
		b		2	0	0	0	—
		c		198	1,300	343	1,643	79
	2	a		152	3,880	4,709	8,589	45
		b		26	2,840	2,001	4,841	57
		c	↓	16	2,220	2,537	4,757	47

the counts remaining attached to stroma and the percentage of counts eluted are shown. A key point is that, in the case of small cell inocula, we found good correspondence between the number of PFC's in a given piece and the amount of radioactivity incorporated into antibody. Table II shows the analysis of PFC's in the spleen pieces as a function of donor cell dose. In this table we tabulated the three spleen fragments according to highest, middle and lowest number of PFC's. At the lowest donor spleen cell dose we expected to obtain one focus, presumably clone, per recipient spleen.

When the donor spleen cell dose was doubled we found some spleens that showed additional clones in other pieces. A point that I wish to make is that on the average the number of PFC's obtained in a given piece, derived presumably from a single clone, was twice as great with a donor inoculum of 2.5 X 10^5 cells as was the number of PFC's found when the inoculum was only 10^5 cells. This finding suggests that two precursor cells were present in the immunocompetent unit resulting from inoculation of 2.5 X 10^6 donor cells whereas only one precursor cell occurred in the unit established from inoculation of half as many donor cells. Analysis of the relative homogeneity of the specific antibody formed by such units may verify this conclusion.

Table II.

PFC IN RECIPIENTS' SPLEENS

NO. DONOR CELLS	PFC/SPLEEN FRAGMENT			TOTAL PFC PER SPLEEN
	HIGH	MEDIUM	LOW	
1×10^5	78	16	4	98
	106	4	0	110
	192	0	0	192
	146	20	10	176
	58	32	0	90
$\bar{X}$	116	14	3	133
2.5×10^5	181	9	5	195
	353	73	61	487
	393	73	65	531
	381	145	113	639
	89	69	13	171
	877	93	1	971
	65	33	21	119
	333	37	0	370
	65	61	0	126
	153	41	1	195
$\bar{X}$	289	63	28	376

R. Paque: Dr. Simmons, I am impressed with the quantities of antigen employed in your model of cellular immunity. The reason I say this is that in our laboratory where we use the cell-migration-inhibition technique assay for cellular immunity, and in Dr. Baram's laboratory, who also uses thymidine incorporation as an assay, both of us routinely use various antigens such as PPD, histoplasmin, KLH, and BGG in quantities of at least 10 to 30 μg/ml of culture. Other investigators use similar amounts. I have two questions: 1) Do you consider the very low quantity of your MLP antigen needed to stimulate mouse cells as a reflection of the cell system, or perhaps the nature of your antigen? 2) Can you tell us anything about the details of preparation and the nature of this evidently highly potent MLP antigen? Is it similar to Reisfeld's soluble transplantation antigens which he prepares from guinea pig cells?

T. Simmons: We believe these results reflect the nature of the antigens employed. Our antigens are particulate lipoproteins extracted from the microsomes of cells disrupted by nitrogen decompression and isolated by differential centrifugation through sucrose. We don't think the MLP is directly comparable to the Reisfeld antigen and believe the response observed is more in line with that obtained with flagellin antigens. The low dose response is possibly a function of the particulate nature of the lipoproteins.

L. A. Manson: The sensitizing activity of the microsomal lipoproteins when assayed *in vivo* is quite high. We find that the minimal sensitizing dose for allograft rejection, when antigen is given to a whole animal as a single injection, is 5 micrograms of the lipoprotein when assayed in the congenic resistent pair $C57B4_{10} - B_{10} D2$. Therefore, in the *in vitro* system we think we are using roughly the same physiological level of antigen scaled down to the number of cells that are being sensitized.

W. L. Ford: I wish to suggest to Dr. Silobričić an alternative interpretation of his data on the distribution of ^{51}Cr-labeled lymph node cells in irradiated, allogeneic recipients. This is based on the following assumptions: 1) Only a minority of cells, say less than 10%, react against recipient antigen. The majority are distributed in the recirculating pool as syngeneic lymphocytes would be. 2) The great majority of lymph node cell lymphocytes enter the recirculating pool and all of these are capable of migrating from the blood into the spleen. However, there are alternative sites of migration from the blood, especially the lymph nodes. Moreover, the lymphocytes which have migrated into the spleen begin to leave it again for the blood in 3-6 hours. Therefore the amount of label which you detect in the spleen after 12 h or 24 h represents an approach to a steady state at which the rate of lymphocytes leaving the spleen balances the rate at which lymphocytes enter the organ.

D. R. Bainbridge: I would tend to agree with Dr. Ford - I don't think the evidence from the chromium labeling technique can distinguish a static state from a dynamic steady state when the amount of label remains the same. Some preliminary work I have been doing with another label suggests very strongly that there is a rapid turnover of cells in the mouse spleen, as distinct from mouse lymph nodes. This would support Dr. Ford's suggestion that there may well be a rapid traffic of cells through the spleen, and what one is observing with a constant level of about 16% is in fact a steady state.

V. Silobrčić: I did not mean to say that your data suggest that the cells remain in the spleen, although we have taken those published by Gowans to suggest that. We have studied other organs, blood, lung, liver, kidney, lymph nodes, and found no evidence of increased labeling in the liver, for example. So, on the basis of this and the evidence of Dr. Gowans, we have concluded that the cells remained in the spleen.

L. J. Cole: I was interested in your observations that the irradiated mice which had received allogeneic cells died early, say around
6 days, in contrast to the controls injected with saline and syngeneic cells. We have made similar observations some years ago (P. C.
Nowell and L. J. Cole, Transplantation Bull., 27:94, 1961) from
experiments in which we had injected similar allogeneic lymphocytic
cells into heavily X-irradiated mice. We found that the animals
that died early under these conditions exhibited inhibition of
intestinal epithelium regeneration, suffering from a form of intestinal radiation death. Since you mentioned that the cause of the
early deaths was obscure, I wonder whether you have looked at histological changes in the gut in these mice which died early.

V. Silobrčić: Not systematically. The death is so sudden that it
seems like some sort of intoxication. The animals appear quite well
until the 5th day and the next day you find all of them dead. But
we did not study the gut systematically.

C. N. Muller-Berat: D. W. van Bekkum and L. M. van Putten and I used
a similar system as yours, i.e., acute allogeneic disease in the
irradiated F_1 mice injected with parental spleen cells. We also
found that there was a very critical period between days 0 and 4
after transplantation that was related to cellular kinetics of lymphoid cells. In order to prolong the life of these animals which
all died of secondary disease between day 8 and day 9, we had to
treat the recipient within a narrow period after the transplantation.
We postulated that owing to the immense quantity of host antigen, the
stimulated lymphoid cells of the inoculum had an exponential growth
and that at day 4 they might already have an irreversible killing
effect on the tissues. Thus, in order to prevent death, we had to
adapt a regimen of chemotherapy to these speculated kinetics. We
found out two things: a) Cytostatic agents had to be used before
day 4; b) methotrexate, which is known now to block cells in S-phase,
was active only at day $3\frac{1}{2}$ to day 4, after transplantation, never at
day 1, 2, or 3. When we used an alkylating agent like cytoxan,
which is known to exert its action on a much broader lag time of
the cell cycle, we could inhibit the secondary disease as early as
day 1. By using both agents we could prolong life in a very significant fashion. I think that it is very important to map the cellular
events during graft vs. host reactions, because this model is very
similar to what is observed in bone marrow transplantation in primates,
including man. If we hope to treat this disease in humans, it will
surely be necessary to use a cell cycle phase adapted chemotherapy.

V. Silobrčić: We have started these studies for exactly the same
purpose, and we have done experiments very similar to yours. With
cyclophosphamide we saw that we can eliminate completely proliferation of cells in the spleen and save the animals for more than
double the time that they would otherwise live.

M. Feldman: I want to add one piece of information to support an important point made by Dr. Černy and to suggest an alternative model to your alternative model regarding antigens of cholera. Now I do so, not because cholera became a public issue during the last couple of weeks in the Middle East, but rather in response to one point that was made, namely that an increase in antibody-forming cells cannot be attributed just to an exponential replication of antibody-forming cells. I think that this is a very important point and we have also arrived at that conclusion using the DNP as an antigen.

In studies made by Dr. Segal, Dr. Globerson and myself, we found that if DNA synthesis in our organ cultures is inhibited at time zero, that is if cytosine arabinoside is applied with the antigen, no antibody is formed. If, however, cytosine arabinoside is applied 24 hrs after the antigen, just to allow one cycle of replication, antibodies are formed. Hence, one and only one, cycle of replication is necessary for antibody production. Now in studying the kinetics of antibody-forming cells, in collaboration with Dr. Nakamura, we found that in fact you get an increase in antibody-forming cells when no further cell replication takes place. So you do get recruitment, which was the point you have made. Yet I think an alternative model can be suggested to your notion of cellular cooperation. In order to save your time looking for an unknown carrier in your cholera system, let me suggest the following: Indeed you have a system of cell corporation, but the cell corporation is based on the fact that the T cells differ with regard to the degree of specificity of their receptors. The receptors of the T cells might have a much wider range of cross reactivity than the receptors of the B cells. Therefore they may recognize more determinants of the cholera complex than the B cells.

J. Černy: I don't want to comment on that. I do find it very stimulating. Thank you very much.

A. T. Cunningham: I wonder if you have any direct evidence that the foci you describe do represent antibody-forming cells? I bring this up because in a comparison we made of the distribution in spleens of hemolytic foci and of plaque-forming cells to SRBC, we found, to our surprise, a rather poor correlation. Some foci contained very few plaque-forming cells, while other areas of the spleen which were negative in the focus test contained many plaque-forming cells. This point would be crucial to your model.

J. Černy: I cannot explain your finding, but I can give the indirect evidence upon which we based our conclusion. First, the number of foci found in one half of a spleen was plotted against the number of PFC found in the other half of the same spleen. With a high number of mice assayed at different times after immunization we obtained a straight line relationship. Second, we cut a spleen into two sagittal parts along the long axis, expecting the areas of foci to occur in both splenic parts. One part of the spleen was further cut transversally into pieces and each one was assayed separately for PFC content. The other part of the spleen was assayed for foci. Over 95% of all PFC was found in the pieces corresponding topographically to the foci.

H. Cottier: I was interested in your demonstration of a partially synchronized population of proliferating cells. This phenomenon may give more insight into the problem concerning the number of divisions involved, the generation time and the number of cells produced in a single focus. I have two questions: 1) How does the final number of cells per focus compare with the number of steps you found in your plot of cell numbers against time, and 2) can the shape of the curve indicating a stepwise increase in cell numbers be changed by varying the antigen dose?

J. Černy: I will start with the last question. The "staircase" pattern of the PFC curve can be changed completely by increasing the antigen dose. In fact, the "stairs" may even be replaced by "waves" with increasingly higher peaks. However, a systematic study after several different doses is still to be done.

Concerning the first question: there is no correlation in number and rate of increase between foci and single "steps" of the PFC curve. We conclude that one "step" does not correspond to one activated focus.

J. Šterzl: I would like to discuss the suggestion of Dr. Cerny that the focus is developing around one multipotential cell, and a similar one of Dr. Feldman that such a cell could be thymus-derived, bearing immunoglobulins of broader specificity. In the past two days we have learned that transferred cells are randomly distributed in many organs and there in different tissue spaces. At least for several days they do not leave their new homes. It was established also that increasing the number of transferred cells in linear relation increases the number of antibody-forming foci. It would mean, according to the suggested function of the thymus cells, that these T cells are limited in number and surrounded by precursors of antibody-forming cells. Such a hypothesis seems to me improbable: at the meeting on cell interaction in Helsinki (edited by Dr. Mäkelä) we presented a statistical estimation that unreasonably high amounts of specific immunocompetent cells (B) should be available in the suspension of transferred cells so that each may meet an antigen-reacting cell (T), in order to preserve the linear increase of foci.

M. Feldman: You are absolutely right, but we try to do the experiment in a slightly different way. An indication that the degree of diversity among T cells might be more limited than among the B cells can be derived from the experiment of Simonsen. Simonsen showed that

random samples of 50 cells could cause a graft vs. host response in
chickens. If the effector cells are T cells - as I believe they
are - then the diversity seems more limited here than among B cells.

   I think that a way to test it directly is the following: Take
carriers which are synthetic polyaminoacids. Take a variation of
polyaminoacids which, althoughly closely related structurally, will
elicit different types of antibodies. Now test whether such carriers,
that are slightly different from each other, will still be "homogenous" with regard to the "carrier effect." Since the carrier
sensitivity is the function of T cells, this might indicate cross-
recognition, i.e., a more limited diversity.

J. Šterzl: In respect of two-cell cooperation (B + T), to establish
it as a generally valid hypothesis, the exceptions have similar or
greater value than data supporting it. From that standpoint, there
are very important experiments proving that some antigens do not
need T-cell helper effect (e.g., in Dr. Thorbecke's presentation)
and, on the same line, that the carrier effect, which is explained
by two-cell cooperation, is not observed in hyperimmunized animals
in which the response to hapten is not carrier-dependent (Eisen,
H. N. et al., J. Israel Med. Sci., 5:338, 1969).

J. Černy: Let me pour some oil on the water. Dr. Šterzl may be
right and the chance of cells' encounter may be low, under certain
circumstances. This may be reflected in the experimental fact that,
in adoptive transfer, increasing of cell inoculum may result in an
unproportional increase of the immune response as shown by Celada,
for example. However, within certain optimal limits of cell number
the "functional encounter" of cooperating elements seems to be
ensured. This is one reason why we have suggested the existence of
a soluble factor attracting one cell to another during the latent
period of antibody formation.

J. R. Anderson: Dr. Cohen, you postulated three mechanisms which
might determine whether the antigen directs a cell towards an antibody
response or towards tolerance. I am interested in why you chose the
third possible mechanism (namely, the pattern of binding of antigen
on the cell surface) as the basis of your analysis. In particular,
did your calculations (which I didn't altogether understand) depend
on the exclusive operation of the third possible mechanism, or would
they be equally applicable if all three mechanisms were involved?

S. Cohen: A partial explanation is laziness; it turns out to be the
easiest situation model in mathematical terms. One can do a computer
stimulation of the other two possibilities, but it seems fairly difficult at the present stage of knowledge. As Dr. Šterzl has pointed
out, the computer tends to take as long a time as the animal does,
if not longer, and this negates some of the advantages of modelling.

D. Nachtigal: Dr. Cohen, your model for tolerance fits very nicely
the findings in the mouse. In the mouse low level and high level
tolerance are 100% reproducible phenomena. However, to my mind
too many generalizations are made from experiments performed in
the mouse and this is a somewhat unfortunate practice. Now, if we
try to correlate your model with the findings in the rabbit, we
encounter immediately some difficulties. In the rabbit, to be
sure, low level tolerance has been demonstrated, but it is far from
being 100% reproducible. Actually, only a few animals in an experiment will respond that way. On the other hand, high level tolerance
in the rabbit has never been demonstrated. Overloading with antigen
will give temporary specific suppression, but as soon as the overloading is stopped an immune response will ensue. Therefore, I have
some doubts about the universal applicability of this model.

S. Cohen: I think the fact that one can at least reproduce the
immunological behavior of one species by suitable experimental
manipulation in others gives some hope that there is at least a
little universality to the immune response in different species.
I suspect the underlying patterns will probably turn out to be the
same, but that there are a whole set of species-specific complica-
tions superimposed in these patterns. If different species really
operate through different mechanisms, then obviously the situation
is terrible, if not hopeless. I can't believe nature designed
things that badly.

G. Wick: I would like you to comment a little bit more on the singlet
and doublet theory as far as low dose tolerance is concerned. It
seems hard to me to understand how low dose tolerance can be explained
by the theory.

S. Cohen: It is not really an explanation, it is a description based
upon an opinion, again as Dr. Šterzl has pointed out in another context. Basically what one assumes is the following: the cell begins
life as a virgin. Then it comes in contact with antigen. Whether
this is a good union or a bad union determines its response. The
assumption here is that there are two different kinds of signals,
one of which is a vote for cellular suppression, the other for activation. It's only when the sum of these votes is in favor of activation that the cell becomes activated. Obviously at the beginning
stage (low zone) there are very few signals for activation. The
difference falls below the threshold. I drew one such threshold
line which was obviously arbitrary. From the shape of the curve,
no matter where we draw such an activation line, certain doses of
antigen exist where the cell will be below this line. This happens
for both low and high doses of antigen. A difference in these two
states is that in recovery from high zone tolerance, one should find
antibodies of rather low affinity. This is what in fact happens.
When you come up the curve the other way you are first activating
the cells that are high affinity cells, and coming back from low

zone tolerance one should immediately produce very high affinity
antibody in small amounts. This prediction is different than what
my intuition would have suggested. Luckily (or unluckily) no one
has done this latter experiment.

D. R. Bainbridge: Could you tell us if in your model the apparently
skewed nature of the curve to the left is actually an intrinsic
feature? It is my impression that in some of the experimental data
the dose response curve tends to be skewed to the right rather than
to the left.

S. Cohen: You mean that they are flatter at the left border?

D. R. Bainbridge: Your curves are flatter to the right.

S. Cohen: Correct, they slope off more to the right. This is an
intrinsic feature. It follows the assumptions.

D. R. Bainbridge: I may be wrong, but I think that data, for
instance the BSA induction of tolerance, tend to be the other way,
skewed in the other way.

S. Cohen: This doesn't reflect the dose. You see, there you are
looking at some experimental measure of tolerance. Here you are
looking at what is allegedly happening, or at least a mathematical
analogue of what's happening in a single cell in terms of what the
activation curve itself looks like. I don't see why the experimental measure that you're looking at need be a linear function of
this activation curve. There is no reason to make this assumption.
This is one class of predictions that cannot be made from this
model.

D. R. Bainbridge: Sure, but the model is only the simplest hypothesis
and since we are talking in terms of simplest hypotheses, the simplest
hypothesis would be that there is a linear relationship between your
activation curve and the observed experimental results. Would you
like to try and reconcile them?

S. Cohen: Not really, since they are measures of different events.
What happens in the animal is not only the result of the individual
cell activations, but also many of complex events relating to
distribution of antigen, etc.

J. Černy: Dr. Šterzl, it is very impressive to see that you put
certain premises into a computer and you can get a curve fitting
your experimental data back. However, are you sure that you would
not obtain the same curve using different premises? I have been
playing with this approach, too, and let us say I would give a
certain experimentally obtained curve to a mathematician and ask
him: "Are you able to create one and only one theoretical model

fitting this curve?" And he would say: "Of course not! There will be several such models, quite different."

J. Šterzl: You are quite right; for the experimental data you can construct various models, especially if you are using only words. Starting with the computer and giving to it certain initial information (axioms) you wait only what the result will be. When you obtain from the computer data and curves which completely differ from the experimental results you can exclude many of the premises you started with. If the computed results are near the reality it does not mean yet that the model is true. Are we able to judge at all whether the model approaches the complexity of nature? I think that we could trust the model more if on its basis some crucial experiments are suggested and confirmed experimentally. The most convincing, of course, would be if the computer working with the model and starting from different initial conditions (which can be changed so quickly) produced some unexpected data, "discovered" facts which will later on be confirmed experimentally on this basis.

S. Cohen: I just wish to add something to Dr. Šterzl's comment. The situation is obviously very complex. In addition to a given immunocompetent cell existing in a set of different states, clearly there are many cell types involved. For at least some antigens there is an interaction between thymus-dependent and marrow-dependent lymphocytes. The macrophage is also involved somehow, and so are various factors, chemotactic and otherwise, elaborated by cells as a consequence of antigen contact with a sensitized cell. The location where these things happen may also be crucial. Things are almost certainly quite different when contact occurs in a germinal center than when it occurs elsewhere. It is clear that as a result of this complexity one can construct a whole set of "iso-paradigms" in which you assume that one or more of these events is crucial, or rate-limiting. You therefore get a whole set of different basic assumptions which, as is true in many sciences, will lead to models which are very much like each other. Luckily, however, they are not entirely like each other. There are areas where the predictions are distinct. It is only in those areas where the predictions are distinct that we can hope to decide which of our opinions are best. The only purpose for playing this fantasy game is that it often makes reality a bit clearer. We essentially do the pilot experiment in our heads, or in a machine.

H. Ginsburg: I want to contribute to the studies of models of cellular immunity by discussing our *in vitro* system in which we produce stimulation of lymphocytes by two means and get complete graft rejections *in vitro*. We have stimulated lymphocytes with living embryo fibroblast monolayers of allogeneic or xenogeneic origin. By incubating the lymphocytes for 5 days large pyroninophilic blast cells accumulate. Now we can collect these cells and plate them on any

other monolayer and we find several interesting things. Rat lymphocytes were collected after 5 days of incubation and plated on a mouse
monolayer, then incubated for 24 hours on this target monolayer. At
a dilution of 2 X 10^6 pyroninophilic cells complete lysis occurred
after 24 hours; with half the dose, 10^6 cells, there was still some
lysis. The reaction is specific for the sensitizing monolayer.
Cells derived from other sources are not lysed. The same number of
lymphocytes but incubated with L-asparaginase had no effect. We can
do a similar thing with pokeweed mitogen. Instead of incubating the
lymphocytes initially on monolayer we incubated with pokeweed mitogen,
and got the same kind of blast cells. We collected these cells after
3, 4 or 5 days and plated them on a syngeneic monolayer which was
coated with pokeweed conjugated to the monolayer. After incubation
for 24 hrs lysis was obtained at different dilutions of blast cells
but not in controls with pokeweed by itself. This effect is specific
to the pokeweed because, if you incubate it with PHA, no effect is
obtained except the one caused by the phytohaemoglutinin itself.
The interesting results seem to imply that by incubating the cells
with pokeweed, we heterogenize the lymphocytes. The heterogenization produces blast cells, which specifically destroy the coated
monolayer.

ATTEMPT TO SEPARATE ANTIBODY-FORMING CLONES OF DIFFERENT AFFINITY

FOR ONE ANTIGENIC DETERMINANT ON A MACROMOLECULE

A.J.L. Macario, E. Conway de Macario, C. Franceschi
and F. Celada
Department of Tumor Biology, Karolinska Institutet

Stockholm, Sweden

Circulating antibodies directed against a given antigen show
an evolution of their binding characteristics from low to high
affinity during both the primary and the secondary response. This
may be interpreted as progressive selection for the most affine
clones of antibody-forming cells forced by antigen limitation. To
test this hypothesis one would like to be able to follow the quality
of the antibody produced by single clones of cells during long
periods of time under chosen antigen pressure. We did experiments
in this direction on the assumption that the heterogeneity of the
antibodies against a single determinant may be limited, i.e. that
they may be synthesized by a discrete number of clones (1). The
results - still preliminary in nature - indicate that the clonal
level can be reached in in vitro culture of lymph node cells.

We combined a) A lymph node fragment culture method by which
a long lasting secondary response can be obtained with b) The use
of an antigen, E. Coli β-galactosidase having characteristics specially favorable for our purpose, namely: 1) Immunization of animals
with this antigen causes the production of antibodies, titrable by
precipitation, directed against up to 10-20 determinants; 2) In
contrast only antibodies directed against a particular site of the
molecule have the property of activating a point mutant β-galactosidase (AMEF (2, 3, 4)). Thanks to the size of the factor of activation ($\sim$1000 times) both activating titer and binding energy can be
determined on very small quantities of antibody.

To approach the level of discontinuity of the response in
vitro two means have been employed, namely: reduction of the size
of the fragments cultured (down to 5×10^4 cells) and graded antigen
pressure in vitro. The results were judged according to the follow-

ing criteria: 1) - The frequency of fragments from a given node
producing activating antibodies should be low. 2) - The ratio
Activating titer/Precipitating titer should show a wider variation
than that observed in randomly assembled sera from immune rabbits.
3) - The affinity study should reveal homogeneity (index of heterogeneity tending to unity).

MATERIALS AND METHODS

Tissue culture technique. A modification of the lymph node
fragment culture method (5, 6) was applied. Lymph nodes were
aseptically removed and cut into fragments (54,400 $\pm$ 14,700 cells/
fragment). They were distributed into Leighton Tubes (1 to 20/
Tube) and 1.0 ml of Medium 199 + 20% normal rabbit serum was added.
The in vitro challenge with antigen was done by incubating the
fragments with different β-galactosidase doses (0.5 to 500 μg/ml)
for different periods of time (1 to 6 hours). After incubation
the fragments were carefully washed and placed in position. Samples
were collected every 3-5 days by pouring the used Medium into small
sterile tubes.

Immunization of the donor rabbits. Different doses (1-3-5
mg) of β-D-galactosidase in complete Freund's adjuvant were injected in one footpad of 2-4 kg rabbits. Sera obtained sterily
were stored at -30°C.

Enzyme activation assay. Activating antibodies were detected
by incubating (2 h at 37°C) 0.05 ml of the Sample (or serum)
dilution with 0.02 ml of AMEF. The mixture was then assayed for
enzymatic activity in the presence of 2 ml of ONPG (o-nitrophenyl-
β-D-galactopyranoside). The OD per minute was measured and then
converted to concentration of o-nitrophenol liberated using a
molar extinction coefficient of 4,700. One enzyme unit (EU) is
defined as the amount of β-galactosidase which hydrolyzes 10^{-9}
Moles of substrate in one minute. The activating antibody titer
of samples were determined by confronting several dilutions with
an excess of AMEF and utilizing the value of the tube situated
two steps above the background (controls were Medium or normal
rabbit serum). The titer was expressed as EU produced by one μl
of undiluted sample using the formula $\frac{EU/ml}{1,000}$ x dilution factor.

Quantitative precipitation assay. 0.1 ml of β-D-galactosidase was added to a series of tubes containing 0.1 ml of progressive dilutions of the Sample or serum. The mixture was incubated 30 min at 37°C and 30 min at 4°C. The tubes were then
centrifugated at 15,000 rpm for 5 min. The enzyme remaining in
the supernatant was determined as described above. The μl of

sample or serum needed to precipitate 50% of the enzyme was calculated by plotting the data on probability paper, then the titer
- expressed in EU precipitated by 1 μl sample - was calculated.

Determination of binding affinity of activating antibodies.
The method employed to determine affinity of activating antibodies
is based on the measurement of the binding capacity of a given
amount of serum in the presence of varying concentrations of
antigen in the mixture, in analogy with the determination of
enzyme constants. Since the binding of activating antibodies can
be detected by a specific signal, there is no need to purify either
antigen or antibodies. The affinity is expressed as K_m, in M^{-1}
(the [AMEF] at which one half of the antibodies are bound). This
constant is determined from double reciprocal plots 1/EU vs. 1/
[AMEF]. Linearity of this function indicates homogeneity of the
antibodies.

RESULTS

1) Frequency and titer of tubes showing activating antibodies.
A drastic reduction in the frequency of the response (from 100%
to 50%) is seen when fragments from non regional lymph nodes are
used; in this case the number of responder tubes is independent
of the number of fragments (1 or 2) they contain. Both frequency
and titer of responder tubes are lower when fragments from non
regional lymph nodes are used specially when the antigen stimulation is diminished (see Fig. 1).

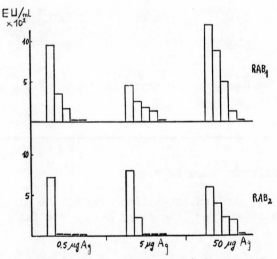

Each bar represents a culture tube containing one fragment either
from a draining lymph node (upper part, RAB_1) or from a non
regional lymph node (bottom, RAB_2).

Table I.

Culture tube	Period of Ab production(d)	Titer (EU/ml)	Binding constant M^{-1}
22 (1 frag.)	3-7	85	3×10^6 (het)**
5 µg Ag*	11-15	220	1.2×10^7 (het)
	15-19	125	2×10^7 (het)
17 (2 frag.)	3-7	97	10^6 (het)
0.5 µg Ag	15-19	1700	10^7 (het)
	26-30	1200	8×10^6 (het)
31 (1 frag.)	3-7	83	1.2×10^6 (het)
50 µg Ag	11-15	414	3×10^7 ($\sim$hom)
	15-19	210	3.2×10^7 ($\sim$hom)
42 (2 frag.)	15-19	304	1.4×10^7 ($\sim$hom)
500 µg Ag	23-26	206	1.5×10^7 ($\sim$hom)
	35-38	89	1.5×10^7 ($\sim$hom)
16 (2 frag.)	7-11	850	3×10^7 (hom)
0.5 µg Ag	15-19	850	4×10^7 (hom)
38 (2 frag.)	7-11	2900	3.8×10^7 (hom)
50 µg Ag	15-19	2900	4.7×10^7 (hom)
	23-26	900	5×10^7 (hom)
Donor rabbit (serum)	1 month	35430	10^7 (het)
	9 months (after priming)	3021	3.5×10^7 ($\sim$hom)

*Antigen stimulatory dose *in vitro*.

**In parentheses, hom indicates linearity of the plot; $\sim$hom, limited deviation from linearity; het, curve function (heterogeneity).

2) Ratio activating titer/precipitating titer in samples and
sera. The ratio activating titer/precipitating titer was determined in 51 samples belonging to 8 different tubes. They varied
from 0.01 to 1.28, and at the peak of the activating response those
8 tubes had ratios between 0.09 and 1.28. In contrast, rabbit sera
had ratios between 0.24 and 0.60. At the peak of the activating
response the 8 culture tubes had ratios between 0.09 to 1.28, while
for the rabbits the ratios varied from 0.42 and 0.60.

3) Maturation of activating antibody response in terms of
affinity. The analysis of a number of cultures at different times
(a sample of which is shown in Table 1) indicates a) as a rule
there is increase of affinity with time only in cultures showing
antibody heterogeneity. b) The "homogeneous" cultures tend to
have high titers and high affinity, and are not necessarily those
with smaller initial inoculum.

Taken together the present results show that it is possible
to reach conditions resulting in homogeneity (of clonal type) in
the immune response in vitro. However, the correlation between
antigen dose, titer and degree of affinity suggest that the expression of a single clone is made possible by functional factors -
possibly by the same operating in vivo - rather than by mere dissection out of the organ.

ACKNOWLEDGEMENTS

This work was supported by the International Union Against
Cancer - American Cancer Society, the Swedish Cancer Society and
the Sir Samuel Scott of Yews Trust.

REFERENCES

1. D. Pressman, O.A. Roholt and A.L. Grossberg, Ann. N.Y. Acad. Sci.,
   169:65, 1970.

2. M.B. Rotman, and F. Celada, Proc. Nat. Acad. Sci. USA, 60:660,
   1968.

3. F. Celada, J. Ellis, K. Bodlund and M.B. Rotman, in manuscript.

4. F. Celada, R. Strom and K. Bodlund, Proc. Lac Operon Meeting,
   Cold Spring Harbor, 1969, pp. 67-79.

5. M.C. Michaelides and A.H. Coons, J. Exp. Med. 117:1035, 1963.

6. M. Richter, A. Juhasz, B. Drechsler and J. Myers, Nature (Lond.),
   210:645, 1966.

CELLULAR IMMUNITY IN VITRO: SPECIFIC ANTIGEN INDUCES SENSITIZATION AND ACTIVATES A NONSPECIFIC CYTOLYTIC EFFECT[1]

I.R. Cohen and M. Feldman

Department of Cell Biology

The Weizmann Institute of Science, Rehovot, Israel

In order to learn which processes of a cellular immune reaction depend upon an immunospecific interaction between lymphocytes and antigens, we studied a system in which both primary sensitization of lymphocytes against sensitizing fibroblasts and cytolysis of target fibroblasts can be observed in vitro (1-4).

MATERIALS AND METHODS

Animals. Inbred Wistar or Lewis rats or C3H/eb mice were used as cell donors.

Fibroblasts. Sensitizing and target fibroblasts were obtained and prepared as described previously (1-4). Sensitizing monolayers contained 3×10^6 fibroblasts in 60-mm plastic Petri dishes and target monolayers contained 0.7×10^6 fibroblasts in 35-mm dishes. Labeling of target fibroblasts with radioactive 51-chromate was done according to the method of Berke et al. (2).

Antiserum. Normal rat serum or rat anti-C3H antiserum (raised by multiple i.p. injections of 10^8 C3H spleen cells in complete Freund's adjuvant or PBS) was used in preincubation experiments. Target fibroblasts received 0.1 ml and sensitizing fibroblasts 0.5 ml for 30-40 min at 37°C

---

[1] This work was supported by a postdoctoral fellowship awarded to I.R. Cohen by the Arthritis Foundation, New York; by a grant from the Freudenberg Foundation for Research on Multiple Sclerosis, Weinheim, Germany, and by the Max and Ida Hillson Foundation, New York.

before lymphocytes or 0.5 ml fresh adsorbed guinea pig complement was added.

Sensitization and effector phase in vitro. Primary sensitization in vitro was done using minor modifications (3, 4) of the method developed by Ginsburg et al. (1, 2). Rat lymph node cells were dispersed in Eagle's medium containing 20% horse serum and 20 x 10^6 were incubated for 5 days in sensitizing cultures with foreign rat or mouse fibroblasts. Sensitization of lymphocytes was evidenced by the appearance of large, transformed cells and by the ability to lyse target fibroblasts after transfer to target cultures. Lysis was measured by the release of ^{51}Cr from target fibroblasts during 20 hrs of incubation (2, 3). The recorded values have been corrected for spontaneous release of ^{51}Cr measured in control cultures.

RESULTS

Immunospecificity of sensitization phase. We used antibodies to block the antigenic sites of sensitizing fibroblasts in order to test whether sensitization of lymphocytes in vitro was dependent upon contact with specific antigens. Figure 1 shows that preincubating C3H fibroblasts with anti-C3H antiserum inhibited sensitization of Lewis rat lymphocytes. Both the number of recovered lymphocytes and their cytolytic capacity were progressively inhibited by increasing concentrations of rat anti-C3H antiserum compared to normal rat serum. This suggests that immunospecific contact with fibroblast antigens is necessary to initiate the sensitization phase of the in vitro cellular reaction.

Immunospecificity of cytolytic effector phase. The immunospecificity of the effector phase was tested by sensitizing lymphocytes against fibroblasts of a specific genotype and measuring their cytolytic effects against target fibroblasts of the specific or an unrelated type. We found (Table I) that cytolysis of unrelated fibroblasts consistently occurred although cytolysis of the specific sensitizing fibroblasts was usually 4-fold greater. There was no difference in the numbers of lymphocytes recovered after the lytic phase in target cultures containing antigen-specific or unrelated fibroblasts (Table II). Hence, the greater lysis of antigen-specific target fibroblasts was not due to a greater proliferation of lymphocytes. These findings suggest that the cytolytic mechanism of sensitized lymphocytes may be stimulated or activated by contact between lymphocytes and specific antigens.

Augmented cytolysis of unrelated fibroblasts in presence of specific sensitizing fibroblasts. Mixed target cultures containing equal numbers of two different types of fibroblasts were prepared to study the effect of the presence of specific antigen-bearing fibroblasts on lymphocyte-mediated cytolysis of unrelated fibroblasts. Lysis of selected fibroblasts in a mixed culture can be measured by labeling them with ^{51}Cr before mixing the cell

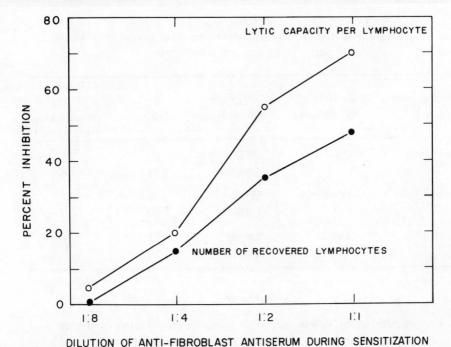

Fig. 1. Inhibition of lymphocyte sensitization by anti-fibroblast antiserum. Sensitizing cultures of C3H fibroblasts were preincubated with normal rat serum or dilutions of rat anti-C3H antiserum. Lewis lymphocytes were counted and their cytolytic capacity against C3H target fibroblasts was measured after 5 days. Percent inhibition was computed by comparison to sensitizing cultures which were preincubated with normal rat serum.

types together. Such mixed target cultures were incubated with sensitized lymphocytes or antibody and complement. We found (Table III) that anti-C3H antibody and complement produced cytolytic release of ^{51}Cr from labeled C3H fibroblasts, but not from labeled Lewis fibroblasts which were mixed with either unlabeled C3H or Lewis fibroblasts. This indicates that there was no transfer of ^{51}Cr from labeled Lewis to Unlabeled C3H fibroblasts, and that lysis of unlabeled C3H fibroblasts did not by itself cause the release of ^{51}Cr from adjacent Lewis fibroblasts. However, in contrast to antibody and complement, the lysis of ^{51}Cr-labeled Lewis fibroblasts by syngeneic Lewis anti-C3H lymphocytes was significantly augmented by the presence of antigen-specific C3H fibroblasts. These findings suggest that activation of the lymphocyte cytolytic effector mechanism is immunospecific, but that the effector mechanism itself does not discriminate between antigens once it is activated.

Table I

Cytolytic effects of sensitized lymphocytes against target fibroblasts of sensitizing or unrelated type

Lymphocytes (2.4 x 10^6)	Sensitizing fibroblasts	Target fibroblasts	% lysis	Ratio of % lysis sensitizing: unrelated
Lewis	C3H	C3H	56	4
		Lewis	14	
Lewis	Wistar	Wistar	35	4
		C3H	9	
Wistar	Lewis	Lewis	51	4
		Wistar	12	

Table II

Changes in number of Lewis anti-C3H lymphocytes during cytolysis of target fibroblasts of sensitizing or unrelated type

Cell type	No. sown	Number recovered post lysis Target fibroblasts		% lysis	
		C3H	Wistar	C3H	Wistar
Total	3.0	3.2	3.5	86	21
Large	0.9	1.8	2.0		

Inhibition of cytolysis by antibodies. It was shown above (Fig. 1) that antibodies to fibroblast antigens inhibited primary induction of lymphocyte sensitization probably by blocking antigenic sites. Hence, lysis too should be inhibited by antibodies to fibroblasts if the cytolytic effector phase is dependent upon a second immunospecific activation by antigens. We therefore studied the effects of preincubating Wistar or C3H target fibroblasts with anti-C3H antiserum. The target fibroblasts were then incubated with Lewis lymphocytes which had been sensitized against Wistar or C3H fibroblasts. We found (Table IV) that anti-C3H antiserum had no inhibitory effects on lysis of Wistar fibroblasts. However, anti-C3H antiserum inhibited lysis of C3H fibroblasts caused by either anti-C3H or anti-Wistar lymphocytes. The latter effect cannot be explained by inhibition of immunospecific activation since the anti-Wistar lymphocytes were activated by Wistar antigens.

Table III

Augmented cytolysis of Wistar fibroblasts in the presence of C3H fibroblasts. Comparison of effects produced by anti-C3H lymphocytes and
anti-C3H antiserum + complement

Lewis anti-C3H preparation	Mixed target fibroblasts		% lysis of ^{51}Cr-labeled cells
	^{51}Cr-labeled cells	Unlabeled cells	
Antiserum + complement	C3H	Lewis	53
	Lewis	Lewis	2
	Lewis	C3H	1
Lymphocytes (2 x 10^6)	C3H	Lewis	31
	Lewis	Lewis	10
	Lewis	C3H	21
			(P 0.01)

Table IV

Effect of anti-C3H antiserum on cytolysis of C3H or Wistar
target fibroblasts

Lymphocytes (2.5 x 10^6)	Target fibroblasts	% reduction of lysis by anti-C3H compared to normal serum	
Lewis anti-C3H	C3H	63	(P 0.01)
	Wistar	0	
Lewis anti-Wistar	Wistar	0	
	C3H	67	(P 0.01)

It is therefore likely that the antibodies coating the C3H target fibroblasts
inhibited lymphocyte-mediated cytolysis by acting as a physical barrier to
cell contact. It remained, therefore, to demonstrate that antibodies could
inhibit immunospecific activation of sensitized lymphocytes without being
bound to the target fibroblasts.

Figure 2 shows the results of an experiment in which Lewis anti-C3H
lymphocytes were incubated with ^{51}Cr-labeled C3H or Wistar target fibroblasts, or ^{51}Cr-labeled Wistar in the presence of unlabeled C3H fibroblasts.
The target cultures were preincubated with normal rat serum or with rat
anti-C3H antiserum before the lymphocytes were added. Normal rat serum
had no effect on the augmented cytolysis of nonspecific Wistar fibroblasts
which occurred in the presence of antigen-specific C3H fibroblasts. How-

ever, anti-C3H antiserum significantly reduced both the cytolysis of specific C3H fibroblasts and the augmented cytolysis of ^{51}Cr-labeled Wistar in
the presence of unlabeled C3H fibroblasts. Thus, the augmented lysis of
the nonspecific Wistar fibroblasts was apparently inhibited by antibodies
binding to C3H fibroblasts which blocked specific C3H antigenic activation
of the anti-C3H lymphocytes. These findings indicate that antibodies can
inhibit the effector phase of the reaction by blocking immunospecific activation of sensitized lymphocytes, as well as by acting as a physical barrier
to contact between lymphocytes and target fibroblasts.

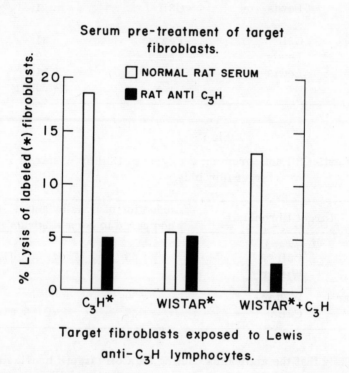

Fig.2 Effect of anti-C3H antiserum on C3H-augmented lysis of nonspecific
Wistar fibroblasts mediated by 2.4×10^{6} Lewis anti-C3H lymphocytes.
^{51}Cr-label is indicated by (*).

DISCUSSION AND SUMMARY

The results presented in this report indicate that contact with fibroblast antigens is necessary to induce sensitization of rat lymphocytes in
vitro. The sensitized lymphocytes must then interact with antigen a second time to activate their cytolytic effector mechanism. The effector

mechanism itself, however, does not appear to discriminate between antigens and any target fibroblasts, including syngeneic, with which close contact is made can be injured by antigen-activated lymphocytes (3).

Thus, the induction of the sensitization phase of this in vitro cellular immune reaction appears to be immunospecific. Sensitized large lymphocytes are able to increase in number even when they are cultured with fibroblasts unrelated to those against which they have been originally sensitized (Table II). Preliminary evidence (I.R. Cohen and M. Feldman, unpublished) indicates that less than 72 hrs of contact with foreign fibroblasts can be sufficient to induce sensitization. After 72 hrs of induction, large lymphocytes can proliferate on unrelated or syngeneic fibroblasts and maintain the immunospecificity of their cytolytic effects when transferred to target fibroblasts. Hence, the sensitization phase can be divided into a first stage of antigen-dependent induction, and a second stage of proliferation which appears to occur even in the absence of specific sensitizing antigen.

The effector phase of the reaction can also be divided into two stages. The first is immunospecific activation by the sensitizing antigens. The second is the mediation of injury to target cells which is not immunospecific, but which appears to depend upon close contact between lymphocytes and target cells (3). Results obtained from studies of the cytolytic effects of lymphoid cells sensitized in vivo also have indicated the importance of cell contact, and suggested that the cytolytic effect occurs as a two-stage process, only one stage of which appears to be immunospecific (5, 6). We consistently observed a degree of cytolysis of unrelated target fibroblasts which occurred in the absence of added antigen-specific fibroblasts (Tables I—III). This can be explained by the possibility that some sensitizing antigen was transferred to target cultures with sensitized lymphocytes, and/or that some of the transferred lymphocytes were already activated in the sensitizing culture.

It has recently been shown (7) that lymphocytes taken from rats with delayed hypersensitivity to protein antigens secrete a nonspecific cytotoxic substance when incubated with specific antigens in vitro. However, we were unable to demonstrate the existence of extracellular cytotoxic substances in our system (3). Perhaps delayed hypersensitivity to soluble antigens is mediated by a different effector mechanism than that which operates in cellular immunity to fibroblast antigens.

Antibodies to fibroblast antigens inhibited the sensitization phase of the cellular immune reaction, probably by binding to antigens and blocking immunospecific contact between lymphocytes and fibroblasts. Antibodies appeared to inhibit the cytolytic effector phase in two distinct ways: they prevented immunospecific activation of lymphocytes by binding to fibroblast antigens, and they acted as a physical barrier to contact between activated lymphocytes and target fibroblasts.

REFERENCES

1. H. Ginsburg, Immunology 14:621, 1968
2. G. Berke, W. Ax, H. Ginsburg and M. Feldman, Immunology 16:643, 1969
3. I. R. Cohen and M. Feldman, Cellul. Immunol., in press
4. I. R. Cohen, L. Stavy and M. Feldman, J. Exptl. Med., in press
5. D. B. Wilson, Transplantation 5:986, 1967
6. W. Rosenau, Fed. Proc. 27:34, 1968
7. N. H. Ruddle and B. H. Waksman, J. Exptl. Med. 128:1267, 1968

CONTROL OF LYMPHOCYTE GROWTH IN RESPONSE TO PHYTOHEMAGGLUTININ STIMULATION[1]

Arnold D. Rubin[2]

Department of Medicine (Hematology), The Mount Sinai

School of Medicine, New York, New York USA

Circulating lymphocytes under appropriate stimulation transform into large proliferating blast cells in a predictable fashion. When compared to resting lymphocytes, the proliferating blast cells can be distinguished morphologically by their large size, open, finely textured nuclear chromatin, prominent nucleoli and copious cytoplasm abounding with ribosomes clusters (1). These characteristics reflect heightened metabolic activities such as increased RNA and protein synthesis (2). We have previously demonstrated that phytohemagglutinin (PHA) induced enlargement of resting lymphocytes into proliferating blast cells is accompanied by an early increase in the synthesis and utilization of ribosomal RNA (rRNA) (3). Presumably this new rRNA provides for the delivery of additional cytoplasmic ribosomes and secondarily increased protein synthesis which ultimately culminates in lymphocyte growth and the morphologic appearance of a blast.

The present study will describe certain descrete metabolic processes which govern the synthesis of lymphocyte rRNA and the possible role of these processes regulating the growth process.

---

[1]Supported in part by USPHS Grant CA 10478 from the National Cancer Institute and Contract AT(30-1)3833 from the Atomic Energy Commission and by the Albert A. List, Frederick Machlin and Anna Ruth Lowenberg funds.

[2]Leukemia Society of America Scholar

MATERIALS AND METHODS

Suspensions of lymphocytes isolated (3) in 96-99% purity from the blood of normal volunteers were suspended in medium (50x10^6 cells/ml in Eagles Minimal Essential Medium containing 2mM glutamine and 15% human serum) and incubated for specified intervals in tightly stoppered bottles at 37°C. PHA-P (Difco, 19 µg/culture) was employed as the mitogen. At specified times before harvest the cells in each culture were resuspended in methionine fr-e medium containing sodium formate (20mM) and exposed to tritiated methyl methionine (3HMe, 4C/mM, 20 µc/ml). The cultures were harvested over a frozen slurry of Earle's balanced salt solution and washed. RNA was extracted from each culture by previously described methods (3) and the final extract was layered on a 5-20% sucrose gradient for ultracentrifugation (37,000 rpm for 180 min.) in an SW65 rotor of a Spinco Model L-2. Gradients were divided into approximately 30 equal fractions on filter paper discs which were then processed for liquid scintillation counting of acid precipitable RNA. Unlabeled rat liver rRNA served as sedimentation rate markers at 28S and 18S.

Quantitation of the various nacent RNA species was accompanied by planimetry measurements to determine the area under descretely sedimenting peaks of radioactive RNA (3).

RESULTS

In mammalian cells, rRNA is transcribed in the nucleolus as a single 45S molecule which becomes immediately methylated and then is incorporated into a ribonucleoprotein particle (4). As part of the nucleoprotein particle still in the nucleolus, the 45S rRNA precursor molecule cleaves to 32S and 18S subunits. The 18S subunit proceeds into the cytoplasm while the 32S subunit further cleaves to a 28S subunit. Thus, a 60S particle containing a 28S rRNA and a 40S particle containing an 18S rRNA combine to form a mature ribosome. During the cleavage processes, methylated segments of the 45S rRNA precursor are quantitatively retained and expressed in the mature 28S and 18S rRNA products (5). All segments not representing potential rRNA precursor are not methylated. Therefore, radioactive methylated RNA provided a convenient means of identifying the new rRNA moieties and of following the kinetics of rRNA precursor transcription and processing to mature 28S and 18S rRNA.

Independent studies of 3HMe incorporation into an intracellular acid soluble nucleotide pool demonstrated saturation of the pool with label within 1 hour after exposing resting lymphocytes to 3HMe. Prior treatment of the lymphocytes with PHA did not affect the rate of pool saturation nor did PHA treatment alter the size of the acid soluble methyl pool. Thus, quantitative assessment of labeled methylated RNA (Me RNA) could be utilized as a direct measurement

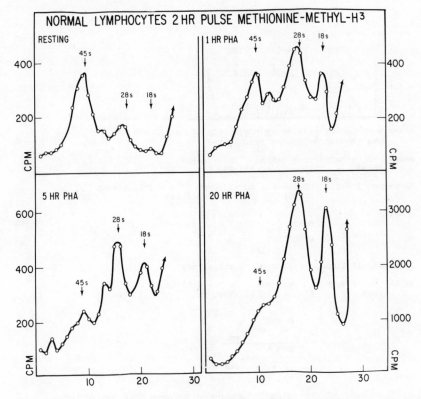

Fig. 1.   Sedimentation patterns of methylated RNA (3).

of 45S rRNA precursor transcription both in resting and in PHA-treated
cultures.

During a 2 hour exposure of resting lymphocytes to [3]HMe, radioactive rRNA remained as precursor with only a minor proportion being
processed to 32S-28S rRNA during the interval. Note the barely
detectable 18S peak (Fig. 1, upper left). After a 1 hour incubation
with PHA, more rRNA was labeled during the exposure to [3]HMe (Fig. 1,
upper right) and the prominent peaks at 28S and 18S reflect to the
more rapid processing of the precursor molecules. Longer incubations
with PHA resulted in a progressive increase in the rate of 45S
transcription and processing to 28S and 18S rRNA (Fig. 1, bottom
left and right).

In the PHA-treated cultures, the 18S peak relative to the
32S-28S peak was clearly defined while in the resting culture the
32S-28S peak predominated over a barely detectable peak at 18S.

CALCULATIONS

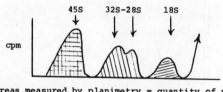

Areas measured by planimetry = quantity of methylated
   rRNA (MeRNA) molecules synthesized

$MeRNA_{total} = MeRNA_{45S} + MeRNA_{32S-28S} + MeRNA_{18S}$

Assuming: 1 mole. $rRNA_{45S} \longrightarrow$ 1 mole. $rRNA_{32S-28S}$ + 1 mole. $rRNA_{18S}$

Then:

$$\text{ratio } r = \frac{MeRNA_{18S}}{MeRNA_{32S-28S}} = 0.67$$

Thus, at all times, total MeRNA synthesized:

$MeRNA_{total} = MeRNA_{45S} + MeRNA_{32S-28S} + 0.67\ MeRNA_{32S-28S}$

$$R = \frac{MeRNA_{total\ PHA}}{MeRNA_{total\ resting}}$$

Fig. 2. Method for quantitating ribosome RNA moieties.

Considering that 32S-28S RNA and 18S RNA represent equimolar products
of one 45S precursor molecule (6), some 18S RNA must have been wasted
by resting cells and PHA treatment rapidly reduced the wastage of
these subunits (3,7).

The complex metabolic processes reflected in these sedimentation
profiles could be dissected into several components utilizing calcu-
tions based on availability knowledge regarding the chemistry of the
various rRNA moieties. Thus, total 45S transcription was estimated
from the sum of the measured areas under the 45S peak plus the
32S-28S peak plus a calculated value for 18S Me RNA (Fig. 2). The
calculation for 18S RNA was necessitated by the apparent wastage of
these subunits in resting cultures. For this calculation equimolar
products of the 45S precursor molecule and complete conservation of
methylated segments were assumed. From the known molecular weights
and concentration of methyl groups on the 32S-28S and 18S moieties

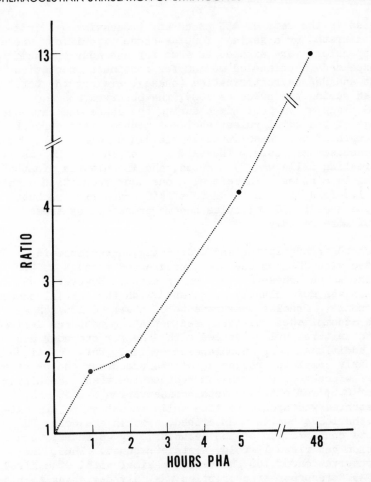

Fig. 3. Effect of PHA treatment on ribosomal RNA transcription. Ratio ("R" in Fig. 2) expresses the change in total rRNA transcription produced by incubation with PHA for specified intervals.

an ideal ratio (7) of 18S/28S Me RNA with complete conservation of 18S subunit would be 0.67. Any value less than 0.67 indicated 18S RNA wastage (3,7). The total 18S RNA originally transcribed was calculated according to Figure 2. The final sum Me total RNA yielded an estimate of the total 45S RNA transcribed and included the observed rRNA 45S precursor peak plus all of the 45S rRNA processed to mature rRNA during the exposure to radioactive precursor. Figure 3 demonstrates a 1.8-fold rise in 1 hour progressing to a 13-fold rise by 48 hours incubation with PHA.

An increase in the rate of 45S precursor processing was independently demonstrated by a series of pulse-chase experiments where lymphocyte suspensions were exposed to ^{3}HMe for one hour (pulse) and then resuspended in unlabeled medium for continued incubation before harvest and RNA characterization (chase). Taking the total 45S transcribed during the pulse as 100%, the observed 28S and calculated 18S peaks at various times during the chase was expressed as a percentage of the total pulse label. A plot of this percentage against the length of the chase interval yielded a half life (50%) for the 45S precursor molecule. The half life of the 45S Me RNA precursor in resting cells was 24 minutes, and in cultures treated with PHA it was 14 minutes. Therefore, a one hour incubation with PHA induced a 1.8-fold rise in the rate of 45S transcription but, in addition, the nacent 45S molecules became processed by these lymphocytes 70% more rapidly.

The increased transcription and processing, detectable in cultures treated with PHA for one hour, progressed through to 48 hours during the actual phase of cell enlargement. However, 18S RNA conservation was more closely associated with the initial phases of the PHA response. Precise measurements of observed 18S/28S Me RNA ratios was accomplished utilizing sedimentation patterns derived from lymphocyte cultures pulse-labeled with ^{3}HMe for one hour and chased for an additional hour in unlabeled medium. This technique allowed for nearly complete processing of 45S precursor and provided the most descrete peaks of sedimenting radioactive rRNA. Recalling that a ratio of 0.67 reflects the total conservation of 18S RNA, Table I demonstrates wastage in resting cells amounting to approximately 50% of the 18S subunits transcribed. Within one hour, PHA induced complete conservation of 18S subunits. By 48 hours, when 45S transcription had risen 13-fold, wastage resumed. Thus, the PHA-induced conservation of 18S RNA became maximal within the first 5 hours while 45S precursor transcription was only beginning to rise.

Table I.

Normal Lymphocytes	$\dfrac{\text{Me RNA } 18S}{\text{Me RNA } 28S}$
Hours Incubation with PHA	r ± 1SD
0	0.38 ± 0.04
2	0.63 ± 0.06
6	0.64 ± 0.03
48	0.55 ± 0.010

PHA-induced 18S RNA conservation took on added significance
from the following experiment: 45S precursor was labeled in a pair
of resting cultures after which the cells of both cultures were
resuspended in unlabeled medium. After one culture received PHA,
both were incubated for an additional 2 hours. While the ratio of
0.32 reflected the anticipated 50% wastage in the untreated culture,
complete conservation of 18S RNA (r = 0.67) resulted when PHA was
introduced. Therefore, rRNA which had been transcribed by resting
cells was efficiently conserved under the subsequent influence of
PHA.

DISCUSSION AND CONCLUSIONS

The small lymphocyte must maintain its resting condition for an
indefinite period, yet it must retain the ability to enlarge and
proliferate in response to antigenic stimulation (8). The intracellular mechanisms for controlling growth must provide stability as
well as adaptability for rapid change. Cell growth depends ultimately
on protein synthesis. In theory, protein synthesis could be regulated
at the level of messenger RNA transcription or perhaps during trans-
lation on the cytoplasmic ribosome. However, the marked contrast
between the sparsely populated ribosomes in the resting lymphocyte
and the dense clusters of these organelles observed in transformed
blast cells (9) suggests that the concentration of ribosomes might
limit the protein synthetic rate in these cells. During the initial
phase of the PHA response, the ribosome concentration in small lymphocytes could be substantially augmented by a rapidly increasing
rate of new ribosome delivery. The present data demonstrated at
least two independent processes regulating the synthesis of rRNA.
Resting lymphocytes transcribed 45S rRNA precursor at relatively
low rates. But even at this slow rate of rRNA precursor transcription, actual delivery of mature 28S and 18S subunits was even further
restricted by limited 45S RNA cleavage and by a pronounced wastage
of 18S RNA subunits. Since unpaired 28S RNA subunits cannot be found
in the cytoplasm and since rRNA does not accumulate in resting cells
(10), at least 50% of the nacent 45S precursor molecules transcribed
by resting cells become degraded without ever being utilized for
ribosome assembly. Thus, stability is maintained in resting lymphocytes by an active metabolic process.

Within one hour after an initial introduction to PHA, the effect
of increased RNA precursor transcription is greatly augmented by more
rapid cleavage of the 45S molecules and by conservation of 18S subunits resulting in efficient utilization of the nacent precursor
molecules for ribosome assembly. The demonstrations that maximal
conservation of 18S subunits appeared only during the first 5 hours
in PHA stimulated cultures and that this phenomenon was independent
of the PHA effect on precursor transcription suggest that 18S conservation plays a critical role in regulating the initial phases of the

PHA-induced growth response. Thus, removal of an active process restricting ribosome assembly could provide for a 4-6-fold increase in the rate of new ribosome delivery with less than a 2-fold change in the rate of nucleolar RNA transcription.

Conceivably, the rapid induction of efficient ribosome assembly can raise the rate of new ribosome delivery above a certain critical level. Above this level, protein synthesis could increase sufficiently to support progressively heightened nucleolar RNA transcription as was observed in the blase cells at 48 hours. Therefore, a self-reinforced, upwards scaling of cellular metabolism, perhaps initiated by a rapid change in the efficiency of rRNA precursor utilization, offers an intriguing model to study the mechanisms governing antigen stimulated lymphocyte growth — one of the key reactions in the immune response.

REFERENCES

1. S. D. Douglas, J. Borjeson, and L. N. Chessin, J. Immunol., 99:340, 1967.

2. L. I. Johnson and A. D. Rubin, in: A. S. Gordon, Ed., Regulation of Hematopoiesis. Appleton-Century-Crofts, 1970.

3. A. D. Rubin, Blood, 35:708, 1970.

4. R. P. Penman, J. Mol. Biol., 17:117, 1966.

5. U. E. Loening, in: H. P. Charles and B. C. J. G. Knight, Ed., Organization and Control in Prokaryotic Cells, p. 77. Cambridge Press, 1970.

6. B. Maden, Nature, 219:685, 1968.

7. H. L. Cooper, J. Biol. Chem., 244:5590, 1969.

8. J. L. Gowans and D. D. McGregor, Progr. Allergy, 9:1, 1965.

9. D. R. Inman and E. H. Cooper, J. Cell Biol., 19:441, 1963.

10. H. L. Cooper, J. Biol. Chem., 244:1946, 1969.

STUDIES OF THE MECHANISM OF PREVENTION OF IMMUNOLOGIC DEFICIENCY IN SUCKLING DWARF MICE[1]

René J. Duquesnoy

Department of Microbiology, Medical College of Wisconsin

Milwaukee, Wisconsin 53233

The pituitary dwarf mouse has been used as a model of study of immunologic deficiency disease. Endocrinological studies (1) of dwarf mice of the Snell-Bagg strain have demonstrated absence of pituitary acidophils, lack of growth hormone and decreased thyrotropic hormone and prolactin. Although the autosomal recessive dwarf mutant is infertile the gonadotrophins appear to be within normal ranges. Baroni first demonstrated immunologic deficiency of the Snell-Bagg dwarf mouse with decreased antibody response to sheep erythrocytes, lymphopenia, and early death with symptoms of wasting and extensive involution of lymphoid tissue (2, 3). We have confirmed his observations and it appears that the immune deficiency of the dwarf is rather limited to the thymus-dependent system (4). Fabris, Pierpaoli and Sorkin showed delayed allogeneic skin graft rejection of these mice (5). Immunoglobulins IgG_1, IgG_2a, IgG_2b, IgM and IgA were in the normal range as compared to normal littermates (4); and these observations were confirmed by Wilkinson, Singh and Sorkin (6). Pierpaoli, Baroni, Fabris and Sorkin (7) demonstrated immunological reconstitution in dwarf mice following injections of preparations of bovine growth hormone in combination with thyroxine.

We have also studied another dwarf mouse, the Ames dwarf, which was originally discovered in 1961 by Schaible and Gowen (8) in the offspring of irradiated C57Bl mice. The immunologic deficiency of the Ames dwarf is similar to that of the Snell-Bagg

[1] Continuation of a study begun at the University of Minnesota during the author's post-doctoral fellowship with Dr. Robert A. Good, Regent's Professor of Microbiology and Pediatrics.

dwarf mouse. We have studied the effect of prolonged nursing with
foster mothers on the lymphoid system of dwarf mice. Three-week
old dwarf mice continued to have a strong suckling instinct for
several weeks and consequently it was possible to foster-nurse
them for a prolonged period beyond the usual time of weaning.

Continued nursing prevented the drop in peripheral lymphocyte
counts in dwarf mice which otherwise occurred soon after weaning
(Fig. 1). The hemagglutinating antibody response to sheep erythrocytes was similar in nursed dwarfs and normal littermate
controls, and markedly decreased in weaned dwarfs. Although the
body weight was not different in nursed and weaned dwarfs, the
relative spleen weight of nursed dwarfs was significantly greater
and approached the values of normal littermates. The results of
nursing experiments on Snell-Bagg dwarf mice have been published
(9). All nursed dwarfs were alive at the end of these experiments
while a great number of weaned dwarfs died before 6 weeks of age
with symptoms of wasting.

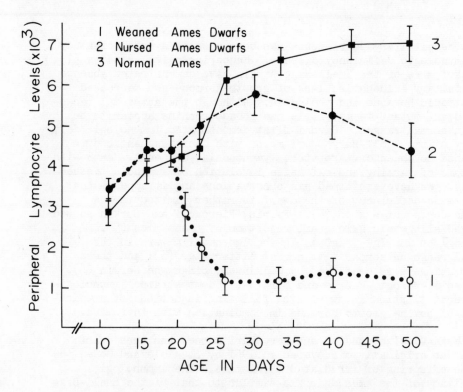

Fig. 1: Effect of prolonged nursing on peripheral lymphocyte
         levels of Ames dwarf mice.

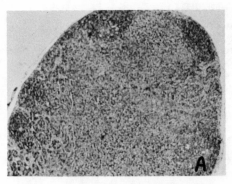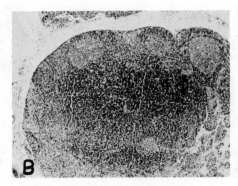

Fig. 2:   Mesenteric lymph nodes of Ames dwarf mice following
          antigenic stimulation with sheep erythrocytes (x40).
          A: Weaned dwarf lymph node with lymphocyte depleted
          paracortical areas and no germinal centers.   B: Nursed
          dwarf lymph node with abundant presence of lymphocytes in
          paracortical regions and well-developed germinal centers.

Histologically, the lymphoid tissue of nursed dwarf mice had a
normal appearance in contrast to the involution of the lymphoid
tissues of weaned dwarfs. Fig. 2A is a micrograph of a stimulated
mesenteric lymph node of a weaned Ames dwarf after sheep erythrocyte immunization. The lack of germinal center formation and
the depleted paracortical areas were typical. Fig. 2B shows a
stimulated mesenteric lymph node of a nursed Ames dwarf with
normal germinal center formation and the presence of lymphocytes
in the thymus-dependent paracortical areas.

     It is evident from these observations that continued nursing
of dwarf mice prevented, to a large degree, the immunologic deficiency which otherwise progressively occurred in these mice after
weaning. We have two possible explanations for this observation.
First we may deal with a specific effect. Because the lymphoid
system appears to be so distinctively affected it could be that
mouse milk or specific factor(s) (hormones) in mouse milk acted
in some way on the lymphoid system of the dwarf mouse. Thus far,
no reports have appeared in the literature that have indicated
presence of pituitary hormones in mouse milk.

     Non-specific factors related to nutrition and stress could
also explain the occurrence of immunologic deficiency in weaned
dwarf mice and its prevention when nursing is prolonged. Change
of diet (from milk to mouse chow) at weaning may result in stress
with subsequent involution of lymphoid tissue and deficient immune
function. In stress, the pituitary-adrenal axis is activated in
normal animals and corticosteroid levels are increased. Unfortu-

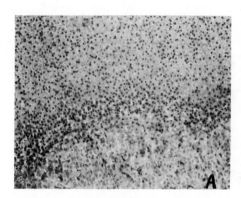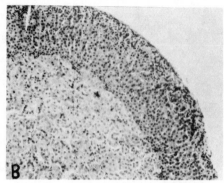

Fig. 3: Adrenal glands of a normal and a dwarf Snell-Bagg mouse
         (x100). A: Normal adrenal. The adrenal cortex which is
         in the upper half contains clear foamy cells. Note the
         so-called X-zone of degeneration between cortex and
         medulla. The physiological significance of the X-zone
         is unknown. B: Dwarf adrenal with thin cortex consisting
         of eosinophilic cells. The X-zone of degeneration is
         absent.

ately with the present methodology it is not feasible to measure
corticosteroid levels in dwarf mice. The dwarf is apparently
incapable of producing sufficient quantities of ACTH as judged by
the atypical appearance of the very small adrenal glands (1). The
adrenal cortex is reduced in thickness and the eosinophilic cells
of the zona fasciculata compared with the clear foamy cells of
zona fasciculata in the normal adrenal cortex, suggested a lower
metabolic activity of the dwarf adrenal cortex (Fig. 3).

     These observations suggest that the activity of adrenal-
pituitary axis in the dwarf is rather low and cannot be included
as an important mediator of stress-induced lymphoid involution in
the dwarf mouse. However, other factors related to stress cannot
be ruled out as causes for the immune deficiency. The endocrinological deficiencies of the dwarf affect many metabolic processes to various extents. Alteration of the nutritional status at
weaning (milk→mouse chow) must result in an adaptation by the
mouse of the nutrient metabolism, in particular the digestive
processes in the gut. We have studied some aspects of carbohydrate metabolism in the dwarf mouse. The major carbohydrate in
the food changes at weaning from lactose to sucrose. Since carbohydrate is transported through the intestinal mucosa mainly in the
form of monosaccharide (glucose), adequate quantities of disac-
charide digestive enzymes in the intestinal tract are necessary
for sufficient carbohydrate uptake. We have measured jejunal and
ileal lactase and sucrase levels in 14-day old and 25-day old
dwarf and normal Snell-Bagg mice. In normal mice during the

suckling stage, the activity of lactase is high and the sucrase
activity is low. Normal adult mice have increased sucrase and
decreasing lactase activities. Hedberg, Reiser and Reilly (10)
have studied these enzymes in 10-day old immunologically runted
mice. They found a marked deficit in intestinal lactase which led
to a malabsorption of lactose, which they suggested contributed to
the pathogenesis of runting in these mice.

Our results (Figure 4) have shown that 14-day old dwarfs
have the same lactase and sucrase activities as compared to normal
littermate controls. In the weaned 25-day old dwarf the lactase
activity is somewhat increased, and the sucrase activity was
threefold higher as compared to normal 25-day old Snell-Bagg mice.

These observations indicate that dietary carbohydrate digestion is at the least sufficient and probably does not contribute
to the wasting of dwarf mice. At the present time we are studying
the effects of dietary lipids in dwarf mice. We have no sufficient
data to report now. Our impression is that high and low fat diets
have no different effect on the lymphoid system of dwarf mice.

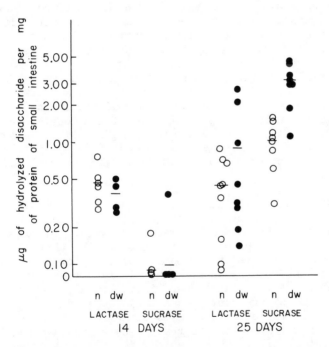

Fig. 4. Lactase and sucrase activities of small intestine homo-
         genates from normal and dwarf Snell-Bagg mice measured by
         the methods of Dahlquist (12).

Although we have not completely ruled out non-specific factors related to stress which significantly contribute to the immune deficiency of dwarf mice, specific lymphopoietic factors present in milk which prevented the immune deficiency in these mice should be considered. In other words, the nursed dwarf mouse may get specific factors through the milk which help to maintain his immune system thereby preventing the immunologic deficiency which appears to be limited to the thymus-dependent system. This would indicate that at least in the dwarf mouse specific factors in milk influence cellular immune function. Previous investigations of the immunologic influence of milk have only dealt with immuno-globulins and humoral immunity. Thus far immunological analysis has not concerned an association between milk and cellular immune function, even though cellular immunity in the newborn seems to play a most important role in host defense against many infectious agents and in immunological surveillance.

A logical sequence of our nursing experiments was to inject mouse milk into weaned dwarf mice and to study their immune system. However, one should not exclude the possibility that a better route of administration of milk is through the intestinal tract, where even some kind of activation of milk factor may take place. Mouse milk was obtained from nursing Snell-Bagg mice with 10-18 days old litters. We used a milking device designed by Feller and Boretos (11) which was applied to the mammary nipples 5 minutes after intraperitoneal injection of oxytocin. With this method it was possible to obtain almost 1 cc of milk every day. Twenty-five day old dwarf mice were injected with 0.4 ml milk. To our disappointment we observed an adverse reaction in the dwarfs as demonstrated with a drop of peripheral lymphocyte counts from about 2,500 to a few hundred and symptoms of wasting. A few days later about 25% of the injected dwarfs had died. Surprisingly, the remaining dwarfs recovered and are still lively and well at six months of age.

Our hypothesis that prevention of immune deficiency in dwarf mice by prolonged nursing is mediated by specific lymphopoietic factors, has been strengthened. It seems unlikely that the pitui-tary-adrenal axis and also changes in nutrition at the time of weaning play an essential role in the pathogenesis of immune de-ficiency disease of the weaned dwarf. We would rather suggest that the immune deficiency of the weaned dwarf is the result of a de-fective thymotropic pituitary control and the discontinuation in the supply of specific thymotropic or lymphopoietic factors through the milk. Experiments are now in progress to determine a specific lymphopoietic effect of milk, which possibly depends on the mode of administration of milk.

ACKNOWLEDGEMENT

This research was supported by USPHS General Research Support Grant 5 SO1 FR- 434 and by grants from American Cancer Society (Minnesota Division) and Minnesota Heart Association.

REFERENCES

1. U. J. Lewis, Mem. Soc. Endocr., 15:179, 1967.

2. C. Baroni, Experientia, 23:282, 1967.

3. C. Baroni, N. Fabris, and G. Bertoli, Exp. Haemat., 17:33, 1968.

4. R. J. Duquesnoy, P. K. Kalpaktosoglou, and R. A. Good, Proc. Soc. Exp. Biol. Med., 133:201, 1970.

5. N. Fabris, W. Pierpaoli, and E. Sorkin, In Developmental Aspects of Antibody Formation and Structure (Czechoslovak Academy of Science) in press.

6. P. C. Wilkinson, H. Singh, and E. Sorkin, Immunology, 18:437, 1970.

7. W. Pierpaoli, C. Baroni, N. Fabris, and E. Sorkin, Immunology, 16:217, 1969.

8. R. Schaible, and J. W. Gowen, Genetics, 46:896, 1961.

9. R. J. Duquesnoy, and R. A. Good, J. Immunol., 104:1553, 1970.

10. C. A. Hedberg, S. Reiser, and R. W. Reilly, Transplantation, 6:104, 1968.

11. W. F. Feller, and J. Boretos, J. Natl. Cancer Inst., 38:11, 1967.

12. A. Dahlquist, Anal. Biochem., 7:18, 1964.

CHAIRMAN'S INTRODUCTION TO THE DISCUSSION

THE REGULATION OF ANTIBODY FORMATION

Jonathan W. Uhr, Jean-Claude Bystryn, and Martin W. Graf

Irvington House Institute and Department of Medicine, New

York University School of Medicine, New York, N.Y. USA

The immune response is regulated by the complex interaction of many processes, most of which are not antigen-specific. In this presentation, however, I want to discuss antigen-specific mechanisms only, because these influence the immune response in an exquisitely selective manner and because their manipulation offers the best opportunities of modifying the immune response in a directed manner to achieve therapeutic goals.

It is well known that the nature of an immunogen and its metabolism by the host are critical features in determining the type of immune response (1-4). Thus, the dose and physico-chemical characteristics of an antigen, the way it is distributed between and within organs, and the rate it is catabolized are decisive factors in determining whether tolerance or immunity results, and, if the latter, when antibodies appear, their persistence, the classes of antibody, the binding affinity and the change in affinity with time after immunization.

Evidence is accumulating that continued antibody formation implies continued immunogenic stimulation. The persistence of antigen long after immunization has been well documented by Campbell and Garvey (5). The most decisive evidence for this conclusion, however, comes from experiments in which passive antibody administered to immunized animals inhibited the immune response (6). Particularly impressive in this regard is the experiment by Wigzell (7) in which antiserum was administered as late as one month after conventional immunization with heterologous red blood cells without adjuvants. Even at this late stage, there was a marked inhibition of continued antibody formation. These experiments imply that the

395

small number of immunogenic molecules which persist long after a
conventional primary immunization are constantly stimulating new
cells that synthesize antibody and/or carry immunologic memory for
the specific antigens. Thus, when passive antibody combines with
persisting immunogen, the driving force for the immune response is
diminished and antibody synthesis decreases.

Although this type of "addition" experiment with passive antibody indicates a critical role for the persistence of immunogenic
stimulation, the question arises as to whether antibody formed in
response to immunization can control its own synthesis. The
simplest answer is that antibody actively produced in an animal
behaves like the passively administered antibody, however, serum
antibody levels are raised to unphysiological levels in the addition
experiments casting doubt on this explanation. I think the first
evidence for a physiological role of antibody as a regulatory
mechanism is the observation of Britton and Möller that immunization
of mice with E. coli lipopolysaccharide results in a cyclical
appearance of plaque-forming cells and serum antibody levels (8). I
believe they correctly interpreted this experiment as suggesting
that serum antibody regulates the immune response to this non-
metabolizable antigen.

Other evidence along these lines comes from experiments of
Dr. Martin Graf and myself in which we removed antibody from immunized animals by exposing their plasma to an immunoadsorbent containing the specific antigen, and returned the adsorbed plasma back
to the animals (9). We observed that after the removal of 50-80%
of a specific serum antibody by this method, the titers of that
antibody eventually rose to the levels that would have existed if
it had not been removed. We thought it likely that the removal of
antibody had stimulated an increased rate of antibody formation.
In these experiments we obtained considerable data showing that
antigen had not leaked back from the immunoadsorbent into the animals.
This was a critical point because it represented the difference
between a conventional immune response due to exogenous antigen and
a new type of "secondary" antibody response not stimulated by exogenous antigen but rather the removal of antibody and the increased
immunogenicity of endogenous antigen.

We have now performed further experiments in which antibody
has been removed from immunized animals under conditions in which
re-exposure to exogenous antigen was not possible (10). The plan
of these experiments was as follows. Groups of four rabbits were
immunized with one antigen. One of these rabbits, the prospective
recipient, was also immunized with a second antigen. Two and one
half weeks to two months later, antibody levels were determined in
all four animals on the same day. The next day, the two rabbits
whose antibody levels were closest to that of the recipient were

exsanguinated. This blood was then exchanged with that of the recipient animal, thereby maintaining the level of the shared "control" antibody, but decreasing the level of the other antibody. In addition, serum antibody to a third unrelated antigen was administered passively to some of the recipient animals 4 to 10 days before the exchange transfusion, to investigate the effect of re-equilibration of antibody from extravascular spaces upon serum antibody levels after removal.

Serum antibody levels of four representative rabbits are shown in the Figure and the results with these animals and four

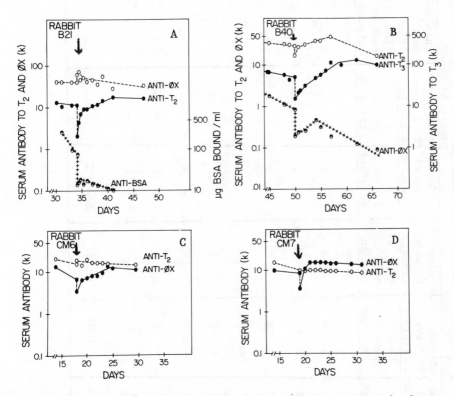

Fig. Serum antibody levels in immunized rabbits before and after exchange transfusion. Four individual rabbits each immunized to two antigens are shown. Exchange transfusion with blood from rabbits immunized to one antigen only was performed on the day designated by the arrow. Rabbits B21 and B40, also passively received antibody to a third antigen 4-7 days before exchange. ●——● antibody removed by exchange transfusion; o----o control antibody; ●xxxxxx● passive antibody. (10)

TABLE (10)

Changes in Serum Antibody Levels Resulting from Exchange Transfusion

Animal no.	Test Antibody			Passive Antibody			Control Antibody	
	Serum antibody level (% of pre-exchange titer)		Interval between transfusion and peak of rebound	Serum antibody level (% of pre-exchange titer)		Interval between transfusion and peak of rebound	Serum antibody level (% of pre-exchange titer)	
	Post-exchange	Peak post-exchange	days	Post-exchange	Peak post-exchange	days	Post-exchange	Peak post-exchange
CM 6	− 50	+ 100	6	−	−	−	+ 20	0
CM 7	− 58	+ 80	2	−	−	−	− 8	− 6
CM 8	− 68	+ 54	3	−	−	−	+ 5	− 5
B 17	− 84	+ 82	7	−	−	−	+ 23	− 60
B 21	− 83	+ 48	7	− 82	− 76	1	+ 48	− 33
B 25	− 75	+ 222	19	− 79	− 67	1.5	− 32	− 20
B 36	− 50	+ 75	7	− 71	− 54	1	− 19	− 11
B 40	− 70	+ 130	12	− 77	− 59	4	− 41	+ 42
Average	− 67%	+ 100%	8	− 77%	− 64%	2	− .5%	− 22%

− = not done

additional ones are summarized in the Table. As can be seen in the
Table, serum levels of the antibody to be depleted were lowered
50-85%, whereas on the average, levels of a control antibody were
unchanged. Following this procedure, there was a rapid rise, or
"rebound" in the levels of the depleted antibody (see Figure) so
that approximately 8 days later, serum levels of the depleted
antibody were 54-222% above the pre-exchange levels, whereas at
that time the levels of the control antibody were an average of
22% below pre-exchange levels. Passive antibody which was depleted
as efficiently as antibody appearing after active immunization,
showed a rebound after depletion whose peak was on the average
60% below the pre-exchange level.

    We considered several possible explanations for these results:
(i) Ig concentration had changed non-specifically due to hemo-
concentration, reaction to stress, etc. This explanation could be
excluded because the control antibody levels did not increase. (ii)
The possibility that the rebound was due to redistribution of
antibody from the extravascular space into the serum was excluded
by the finding that passively administered antibody showed only a
small rebound. (iii) We considered the possibility that the class
or average binding affinity of serum antibody had changed and
accounted for the increase in antibody activity in the serum. It
is known that IgM antibody to bacteriophage can decrease the neutralizing capacity of IgG antibody (11). Therefore, we looked at
the class of antibody appearing during the rebound phase in these
animals. Sucrose density gradient analysis showed that almost all
the antibody was 7S immunoglobulin both before and after exchange.
Furthermore, the rebound was still evident when IgM activity was
inhibited by 2-mercaptoethanol in pre- and post-exchange serum.
The possibility that the average binding affinity of serum antibody
had changed could not be excluded, however. Changes in the average
avidity of antibody to bacteriophage have been described by ourselves
and others (12-14). However, a marked change over a one-week
period as late as two months after immunization would not be expected. We therefore consider the likely explanation to be that
the rate of antibody formation has increased after the removal of
antibody. We emphasize that we do not have proof of this tentative
conclusion. Proof would require evidence that the rate of incorporation of radioactive precursor into specific antibody had increased or that the number of antibody-forming cells in these
animals had increased.

    Assuming for the moment, however, that this tentative inter-
pretation is the correct one, I would like to discuss a provocative
problem which this interpretation raises. Two months after injection of a microgram of bacteriophage, there are very few antigenic
molecules left in the host. Phages such as T_2 and ϕX have a very
short half life in the circulation (15,16). We can detect them in

the lysosome-rich fraction of liver and spleen within one hour and
we can demonstrate rapid catabolism of these phages within these
fractions (17). In other words, they are catabolized like other
antigenic proteins. Clearly, 2 months later, the number of intact
antigen fragments in the whole animal is very small, perhaps in the
nanogram or picogram range. At this time, even after depletion of
antibody from these well-immunized animals, there remains high
levels of antibody in the serum, perhaps 10-100 ug of antibody
nitrogen per ml. Thus, considering the animal a test tube, the
ratio of antibody to antigen is at least 10^7. Yet these handful
of immunogenic molecules apparently can detect the difference
between a ratio of 10^8 to 10^7 and stimulate antibody synthesis.

If this appears to be fanciful, it is to be remembered that
the same type of problem exists in the secondary challenge. The
host is a rabbit immunized 6 months previously which now has 100 ug
of antibody protein per ml and also has primed cells tucked away
in various lymphoid organs. One ug of T2 phage is introduced into
the circulation. Immediately, the antigen is bound by antibody
under conditions of extreme antibody excess and complexes are formed
that are rapidly removed and destroyed by reticuloendothelial cells
of the liver and spleen. It is amazing that this puny amount of
antigen is able to fight its way through a sea of antibody molecules,
reach the appropriate sites, and make effective contact with the
corresponding subpopulations of lymphocytes. Clearly, antigen can
do the job in the secondary response under conditions which superficially appear unfavorable and are analogous to the problem of
stimulation by endogenous antigen.

We have previously discussed several explanations for this
phenomenon (9) none of which can be excluded. We favor the
possibility, however, that the binding of antigen to antigen-
reactive cells (ARC) is favored energetically over the binding of
antigen to circulating antibody. It has been shown by Hornick and
Karush (18) that the association constant of antibody bound to
polyvalent hapten can be 10^4 fold higher than the same antibody
bound to monovalent hapten. They attribute this enormous increase
in binding energy when polyvalent hapten is used to the simultaneous
interaction of both combining sites of the antibody molecule with
two hapten groups on a single carrier. Present information suggests
that an ARC has a large number of antibody-receptor molecules on its
surface (19,20). Our working hypothesis is that multiple interactions between these receptors on the ARC and repeating similar
antigenic determinants on the immunogen (e.g., virus, antigenic
fragments bound to the surface of a macrophage, etc.) may also lead
to an energetic advantage when compared to the interaction of antigen and the same number of antibody molecules free in solution.
Apart from these energetic considerations, it should be noted that
antigen-ARC interaction may lead to an irreversible biological

event, i.e., differentiation to an antibody-secreting cell in
contrast to antigen-circulating antibody interaction. On the biological level, therefore, there may be amplification of the effect
of antigen-ARC interaction.

We would like to finish by stating that we believe the manipulation of the immune system by alteration of antigen and serum
antibody levels will be interesting not only from the point of
view of revealing mechanisms of regulation of the immune response,
but also because these maneuvers offer the possibility of manipu-
lating the immune response in a therapeutic manner.

This work was done under the sponsorship of the Commission on
Immunization of the Armed Forces Epidemiological Board, and was
supported in part by the United States Army Medical Research
Development Command, Department of the Army, under research contract
DADA 17-69-C 9177, in part by USPHS Grant no. AI-0834, and by the
National Science Foundation Grant no. GB-7473-X.

One of the authors (J.-C. B.) is the recipient of the USPHS
Fellowship Dermatology Training Grant no. TI-AM-5326.

REFERENCES

1. J. W. Uhr, and M. S. Finkelstein, Prog.Allergy, 10:37, 1967.
2. B. Benacerraf, IN: Textbook of Immunopathology (P.A. Miescher
        and H.J. Muller-Eberhard, eds.), Grune and Stratton, N.Y.,
        p. 3, 1968.
3. G. W. Siskind, P. Dunn, and J.G. Walker, J. Exp. Med., 127:55,
        1968.
4. D. W. Dresser, and N. A. Mitchison, Adv. Immunol., 8:129, 1968.
5. D. H. Campbell, and J. S. Garvey, Adv. Immunol., 3:261, 1963.
6. J. W. Uhr, and G. Möller, Adv. Immunol., 8:81, 1968.
7. H. Wigzell, J. Exp. Med., 124:953, 1966.
8. S. Britton, and G. Möller, J. Immunol., 100:1326, 1968.
9. M. W. Graf, and J. W. Uhr, J. Exp. Med., 130:1175, 1969.
10. J.-C. Bystryn, M. W. Graf, and J. W. Uhr, J. Exp. Med.,132:
        Dec. 1970, in press.
11. K. J. Turner, and V. Krishnapillai, Immunochemistry, 5:9, 1968.
12. M. S. Finkelstein, and J. W. Uhr, J. Immunol., 97:565, 1966.
13. N. K. Jerne, and P. J. Avegno, J. Immunol., 76:200, 1956.
14. S. E. Svehag, Acta Path. et Microbiol. Scandinav., 64:103, 1965.
15. J. W. Uhr, M. S. Finkelstein, and J. B. Baumann, J. Exp. Med.,
        115:655, 1962.
16. N. K. Jerne, IN: Mechanisms of Antibody Formation (M. Holub
        and L. Jarošková, eds.), Czechoslovak Academy of Science,
        Prague, p. 60, 1960.
17. J. W. Uhr, and G. Weissmann, J. Immunol., 94:544, 1965.

402 J. W. UHR, J.-C. BYSTRYN, AND M. W. GRAF

18. C. L. Hornick, and F. Karush, Israel J. Med. Sci., 5:163, 1969.
19. D. Naor, and D. Sulitzneau, Nature (Lond.), 214:687, 1967.
20. G. L. Ada, and Pauline Byrt, Nature (Lond.), 222:1291, 1969.

DISCUSSION TO SESSION 7
CHAIRMAN, J. W. UHR, CO-CHAIRMAN, G. MÖLLER

J.W. Uhr: Firstly, Dr. Macario, what does your "affinity index" mean? This is important to the theme of the paper. Secondly, at the conclusion of the experiment when you looked at the lymph node fragments histologically to see if your affinity did not change, you might have had only one clone of antibody secreting cells. Were there any clones visible histologically? Do you have anything like a plaque method by which you could investigate that important aspect?

A. Macario: The index of affinity is determined by testing a critical dilution of the sample (capable of activating less than 1% of the AMEF molecules) in the presence of decreasing concentration of AMEF. Data are plotted in a log-log paper and the slope of the straight lines obtained is calculated. The index of affinity is 1 - slope. This is because earlier in our laboratory another test for affinity has been developed to make use of data obtained by the Farr's technique. In this previous test the index of affinity correlates directly with the slope. So now we can compare both tests in which highest affinity has an index of one. In the present system using β-galactosidase as antigen, we can also measure the binding constant, using the Lineweaver-Burk type of plot. Now the second question: we have not analyzed the fragments histologically. We know the number of cells we set in culture because we count the cells contained in fragments that can be considered "twins" of those placed into the culture. Concerning the meaning of the changes of affinity with time, we consider this an open question at the present time.

S. Segal: The molecular structure responsible for enzyme activity probably includes more than one immunogenic determinant. There-fore, antibodies may bind to different antigenic loci with the same degree of affinity and yet produce different degrees of inactiva-tion of the enzyme. Hence, there may not be a direct relationship between affinities of antibodies to the enzyme and their influence on enzyme kinetics. This question could better be studied by using chemically defined immuno-dominant determinants.

A. Macario: For the theoretical approach to this test I would like to call on Dr. Celanda who has developed the method and studied these things.

F. Celanda: We have several lines of evidence which convinced us completely that a single site of the defective enzyme has to be covered for the activation to occur. This stems from the analysis of the kinetics of activation with different concentrations of antibody, and also by single molecule studies done recently by Boris Rotman, using Fab from anti-Z serum. That not all antibodies binding

403

to the enzyme activate, but only a "specific" one, is shown by the
fact (obtained by injecting the point mutant in question) that
antisera exist, which are indistinguishable for precipitating
capacity of the enzyme, but fail to activate. Summing up the data
I think we can say that we are looking at a single site and, since
every hit gives a signal, we can study the affinity of the antibodies by following their efficiency in the presence of various
antigen concentrations. If you were questioning the use of the
term affinity and would prefer avidity because we are looking at
a definite site on a macromolecule and not at a free hapten binding the antibody, we would probably go along with you.

D. Pressman: I think that even if you have a single region against
which the antibody is formed, that there can be antibodies of different nature and of different specificity still interacting with
the one particular region. Although they would be different antibodies and probably with different affinities, they would still
cause the change in enzyme activity which is observed.

N.L. Warner: Do you have any evidence as to whether these clones
are making IgM or IgG? Are there any that switch from IgM to IgG,
and, if so, have you studied whether there is a change in affinity?

A. Macario: No, we haven't studied that.

R. Hard: A question for both Dr. Cohen and perhaps Dr. Möller.
You have often shown that lymphocytes attack and destroy allogeneic cells. Could you reconcile this work with the results in vivo
that indicate that two allogeneic lymphocytes interact with re-
sultant death of innocent bystanders? In vivo it seems that an
allogeneic cells is not capable of attacking directly target cells.
such as allogeneic kidney cells in the local host versus graft
system described by Elkins.

J. Cohen: I do not think that findings obtained in immune systems
in vitro can fully explain immune effects observed in vivo. Our
present work merely emphasizes that the effector phase of a cellular reaction can be divided into two separate stages. The first
stage appears to be immunospecific activation of sensitized lymphoid cells, and the second stage seems to be the cytolytic effect
itself. Cytolysis does not appear, however, to discriminate between antigens. The results which we have presented today do not
really bear upon the nature of the cytolytic effector mechanism.
It would be hazardous, therefore, to expand our findings to interpret immune effects in vivo. However, preliminary studies have
been made in which we compared immune effects in vitro and in vivo
of mouse spleen cells allosensitized in vitro. We found that sensitized mouse cells, which are highly effective in producing the
rejection of tumor allografts in vivo, may not necessarily cause
cytolytic effects in vitro. This also suggests that lymphocyte

recognition and effector functions are distinguishable, and emphasizes the danger of comparing immune effects in vitro and in vivo.

H. Ginsburg: In relation to Dr. Cohen's presentation I would like to
comment on a very interesting result concerning this kind of cultures.
When we obtain blastoid cells after stimulation of lymphocytes we
find that if they are continuously associated with the stimulant,
e.g. poke weed mitogen, they remain large and divide. They specifically lyse target cells that are conjugated with the mitogen.
The blastoid cells die a few days later. But if we dissociate the
cells from the stimulant by plating them on a fibroblast monolayer
free of the stimulant, they transform back to lymphocytes. If we
expose these lymphocytes again to the stimulant in the presence of
the fibroblast monolayer, toxic effects appear and the whole culture degenerates, while the transformation starts. This effect is
not a specific one and can be transferred to another culture with
the cell-free medium.

     Now, if we expose the newly developed lymphocytes in the ab-
sence of the fibroblast monolayer, we obtain complete transformation and large pyroninophilic cells appear. If we plate these
large cells on the cell monolayer that was conjugated with the
pokeweed mitogen they lyse, by contact, the target cells. This lytic
reaction is specific to the presence of the mitogen on the target
cell surface. In certain cultures both the specific and non-specific effects may occur in the same culture. Fortunately, in many
cases, we can separate entirely the one from the other.

H. Oerkerman: We have tried to inhibit the cytoaggressive reaction
of phytohaemagglutinin-stimulated human lymphocytes upon HeLa cells
by coating the HeLa cells with rabbit anti-HeLa cell antibodies,
and we could not inhibit the cytoaggressive effect at all. The
lymphocytes destroyed the target cells as usual. Do you have any
explanation for these results in comparison with the results of
your experiments?

J. Cohen: It seems to be a completely different system. The activating substance, the effector cells, and the target cells are all
different. I think therefore, that one is free to make any reasonable interpretation one wants to explain the difference in results.

N.R. Sinclair: Does binding of antibody to the bystander fibroblast
affect the specific attack on homologous fibroblasts?

J. Cohen: This experiment is certainly called for, but has not yet
been done.

K. Schumacher: You have shown that a non-specific lysis occurred in
your experiments. My question is: can you exclude that there are
identical antigenic sites on your different fibroblasts? If this

is not the case, have you any idea upon the nature of the receptor
which allows the unspecific binding of the lymphocytes?

J. Cohen: There are three findings which offer circumstantial evidence against the possibility that cross-reactivity between fibroblast antigens could explain non-specificity of the cytolytic effect.
First of all, among the non-specific fibroblasts which were attacked
were included those which were syngeneic with the sensitized cells.
It is quite possible that there may be an aspect of autoimmunity in
the system and this is open to further investigation. Secondly,
the anti-fibroblast antibodies did not show any cross-reactivity
between the two types of fibroblasts. And thirdly, antigen-specific
fibroblasts were able to augment the cytolysis of unrelated fibroblasts. It is most difficult to explain this finding on the basis
of cross-reactive antigens. Therefore, I believe that specific
antigens activated the cytolytic effector mechanism against unrelated fibroblasts.

M. Feldman: I was impressed by the data presented by Dr. Rubin,
particularly with regard to the wastage of the 18S component. I
would like to direct a question regarding a phenomenon which appears
to me to be a wasteage of the whole ribosomal population of the
transformed cells. Let me explain what I mean. On an a priori
basis one could have assumed that a transformation of lymphocytes
might be associated with the activation of new genes, or the suppression of new genes, of the small lymphocyte. And yet all the
experiments using hybridization competition techniques, whereby
the old RNA was allowed to compete with the new RNA, have demonstrated that in fact one cannot indicate within the limitations of
these methods the formation of new RNA in the transformed cells.
This was done on human lymphocytes in our laboratory. Dr. Berke
did it for rat lymphocytes both following transformation by PHA and
in the experiments of the in vitro sensitization by antigen. So
one could have assumed, perhaps there is just a magnification of
the different type of transcriptional events which might be eventually manifested in the magnification of the rate of protein synthesis. Now you have a cell full of ribosomes, full of polyribosomes, the transformed cell. According to the population of these
ribosomes one could have assumed that these cells manifested dramatic raise of protein turnover, but in effect, if you measure the
increase in protein turnover in the transformed cells you find a
maximum of 2 fold to 4 fold increase in protein turnover. Why the
hell do we need that huge amount of ribosomes and polyribosomes?
Is it not a tremendous functional wastage? I am looking for a
teleological answer.

A.D. Rubin: Well, thank you, Dr. Feldman. I do not have any clear
insight in this particular sort of problem. I would comment that
the utilization of transcribed RNA moieties may represent an important control of cellular metabolism. These cells turn over RNA

at a rapid rate and such a phenomenon is poorly understood.

J. Cerny: I should like to answer Dr. Feldman's question. Is it
not possible that a biological system appears as tremendous wastage
due to our ignorance, only? For example, most of RNA synthesized
does not even leave nucleus and we do not know what function it
has.

J.W. Uhr: What happens to the 28 S particles which do not have a
partner? Have you studied the half-life of these?

A.D. Rubin: Yes, this was included in the paragraph that I would
have gone into, if time had not run out. We know that there is no
net increase in ribosomal RNA in the resting cells. Therefore,
unpaired 28 S RNA units are eventually degraded but at a much slower
rate than 18 S subunits. It seems that the final degradation of the
transcribed 45 S unit depends upon this independent mechanism
working on 18 S RNA.

K. Borum: I would like to ask you, Dr. Duquesnoy, if you have considered the possibility of a thymic humoral factor being transferred
from the mother through the milk? This possibility could be tested
by performing neonatal thymectomy upon the mice to become mothers
and fostermothers and see whether the milk would still have the
beneficial effect upon the young ones.

R.J. Duquesnoy: I have thought about this. Before I do these experiments I want to determine with certainty whether or not our
observations are non-specifically related to stress. I have looked
at neonatally thymeotomized dwarf mice and they behave quite similar
to unoperated dwarf mice.

M.W. Hess: Have any attempts been made to raise these animals under
germ-free conditions?

W. Pierpaoli: Yes, it has been done. In germ-free condition they
show slightly prolonged life span, but they are still dwarfed and
the immune response is deficient.

C.D. Baroni: My first comment to Dr. Duquesnoy's paper is related
to the MMF factor. You reported that prolonged nursing of dwarf
mice prevents the decrease of their immune functions and that this
interesting finding can be due to a specific maternal milk factor.
Don't you think that this finding can be explained considering that
in the maternal milk are present those hormones necessary for the
development of the immune system?

We have reconstituted dwarf animals immediately after weaning
with growth hormone and thyroxin, and after 21 days of hormonal
treatment we got a perfectly normal primary immune response. For

this reason we do not think that MMF could be considered as a specific factor.

My second comment is about the thymus-dependency of the immune defect of the dwarf mouse. We do not agree with this interpretation. In fact, we have evidence that the primary site of action of growth hormone and thyroxin, and consequently the defect of the dwarf animal, is mainly located in the bone marrow and in the B-cells. During intrauterine life and the nursing period the dwarf animals receive their supply of growth hormone and thyroxin from the mother via the placenta and the milk. Thus, the maternal hormones are able to compensate for the hormonal lack and to exert their actions on the lymphoid system. After weaning the dwarfism syndrome clearly develops. But at this time T-cells have already migrated from the thymus into the thoracic duct and peripheral lymphoid tissues. In fact, peripheral lymphoid tissues of untreated dwarfs show striking evidence of cellular depletion in the bursa-dependent areas and in bone marrow, but not in the thymus-dependent areas. After hormonal treatment we always observed evidence of repopulation of bone marrow and bursa-dependent areas, together with a reconstitution of the immune capacity.

R.J. Duquesnoy: First I would like to comment on Dr. Baroni's remark that the immunologic defect of the dwarf mouse is located in the bone marrow. I agree that in particular in the wasting phase the bone marrow is depleted but not so much before wasting. We have transplanted bone marrow cells from normal mice into dwarfs and there was no effect on the immune deficiency. Apparently the microenvironment of the dwarf thymus did not allow the induction of immunological competence of normal bone marrow cells. My main criticism of the hormonal experiments is that heterologous bovine growth hormone preparations were used which may be contaminated with other hormonal substances, perhaps a specific thymotropic hormone. We have administered monkey antiserum to purified rat growth hormone into newborn rats for up to four weeks of age and found no effect on the lymphoid system, although a considerable impairment of body growth was observed.

As for Dr. Baroni's remark on MMF (which I have said is a speculative concept) I do not think that such a factor is a known pituitary hormone. Also no reports in the literature have appeared which indicate the presence of pituitary hormones in milk. As for the deficiency of the thymus-dependent system of the dwarf, I want to say again that immunological deficiency of the dwarf is relatively limited to cellular immune function. We have ample evidence for this. We must consider that in general the metabolism of the dwarf is abnormal and this may play an important role in the immune deficiency. But we really do not know to what extent. This makes the dwarf mouse a less ideal model of study of immunologic deficiency disease. The immunologic deficiency of the dwarf mouse resembles in many aspects early thymectomy of the mouse.

W. Pierpaoli: I cannot agree with the preliminary remarks of Dr.
Uhr on the possible function of some non-specific factors on the
lymphoid tissues when he includes hormones among them. We cannot
consider the hormones only as general activators or amplifiers of
cellular processes simply because we are ignorant of their mechanism of action. I would like to remind you of the aphorism of Sir
Peter Medawar: "It is not hormones that have changed in evolution
but the use to which they are put." This use includes certainly
the sophisticated lymphoid system of mammals. Therefore the central
point to consider is that if one wants to say that hormones act
non-specifically on cells, at least one has to accept that some
target cells are very specifically reacting to some hormones and
this sensitivity determines the future function of these cells.
Isn't it specificity? Some of these cells are the lymphocytes
which are exceedingly sensitive to hormones. Therefore to go on
discussing what germinal centers are and how they are formed, for-
getting the hormones, is for me a source of great astonishment and
concern.

C.D. Baroni: Previous reports from our group have indicated that
primary haemolysin response to sheep red blood cells (SRBC) is
markedly impaired in hereditary pituitary dwarf mice as compared to
normal litter mates. These results have been confirmed by Duquesnoy
and coworkers in 1969. We have recently suggested that hormonal
deficiency in pituitary dwarfism acts primarily on the cellular
precursors in the bone marrow, perhaps through this pathway, 19S
antibody-producing cells.

The present report describes a comparison of morphology of
secondary lymphoid tissues and of haemagglutinin titres during
primary and secondary response to SRBC in pituitary dwarf mice.

Histological studies of the peripheral lymphoid tissues have
shown patterns of cellular depletion in bursa-dependent areas in
dwarfs killed during primary response, while these areas appeared
markedly cellular after a second antigenic stimulation.

It has also been found that 19S primary haemagglutinin response
was suppressed to a great extent, while 7S secondary response has
reached practically normal levels.

The possible explanation of these apparently contrasting results could be based on the suggestion that 19S and 7S immunoglobulins are formed by two different lymphoid lines with distinct
specificities, one for the production of 7S antibodies. Accordingly, we may explain the markedly depressed 19S primary response in
the dwarf mouse considering that this animal is particularly defi-

cient in the bone-marrow-derived lymphoid cells, and that separate
functions have been defined for thymus-derived and non-thymus-
derived lymphocytes only in the primary 19S haemolysin response of
mice to SRBC (J.F.A.P. Miller and G.F. Mitchell, J. Exptl. Med.,
131:675, 1969). Therefore in dwarf mice thymus-derived lymphocytes
are able to respond to a primary immunization with SRBC, but they
can subsequently interact only with a limited number of non-thymus-
derived precursors of 19S antibody-forming cells.

The interpretation of a practically normal 7S haemolysin
response in pituitary dwarf mice could be based on the assumption
that some 19S producers interact directly with SRBC at low concentrations, whereas other 19S and almost all 7S producers require
cooperation by thymus-derived cells, whose numbers and/or function
seem to be only moderately impaired in dwarf mice.

In conclusion, our findings seem to reasonably support the
implication that the lymphoid cell systems involved in antibody
production during primary and secondary responses to sheep erythrocytes, may be separate and with distinct immunological specificity.
If so, such observations would also explain why the hormonal deficiency of the dwarfs can affect the primary response without
manifesting itself in the secondary response. It is not known at
this time whether this difference is attributable to qualitative
or quantitative factors.

W. Pierpaoli: I would like here to mention some relevant experiments which we have done in the course of the last two years. The
dwarf mouse is simply one of the many experimental models which
have been used or developed to study the interrelationship between
some developmental hormones and the function of the immune system.
The findings obtained by Dr. Fabris, Prof. Sorkin and myself are
now in course of publication and can be summarized as follows:
1) The white cell number in peripheral blood in dwarf mice is significantly lower than in normal litter mates during the first 90
days of life. This deficiency can be prevented by 20 daily injections of somatotropic hormone and thyroxine, beginning at 30 days
of age. Two points are of additional interest: a) the reconstitution obtained with such a hormonal treatment lasts many months
beyond the hormone injections and b) this reconstitution can also
be achieved by beginning the hormone treatment at 60 days of age
(Fig. 1). 2) The immune response to sheep erythrocytes is only
slightly deficient in dwarf mice in comparison with normal litter
mates. The main conclusion on this point is that the primary
immune response is delayed rather than quantitatively defective
and that such a delay is due to a deficient formation of 19S plaque
forming cells, while the production of 7S plaque forming cells both
during primary and secondary response is completely normal (Fig. 2).
3) Cellular immunity, evaluated by skin graft survival, is clearly
deficient in dwarf mice. They show a delay of rejection of about

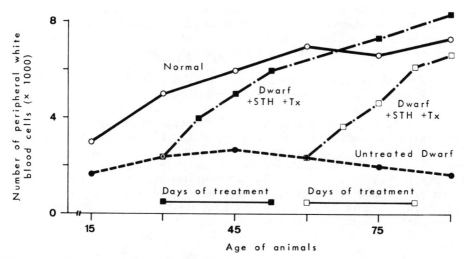

Fig. 1.   Hormone-dependent deficiency of number of peripheral blood white cells in Snell-Bagg dwarf mice.   Reconstitution after 20 daily injections of 250 µg somatotropic hormone (STH) and 1 µg thyroxine. The treatment was begun at day 30 or 60 of age.

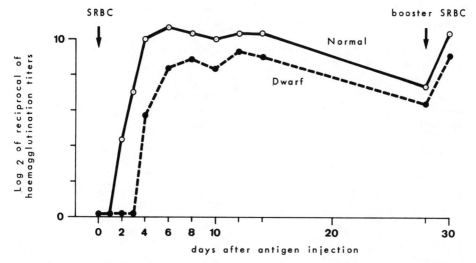

Fig. 2.   Delayed primary haemagglutinins formation against sheep erythrocytes (SRBC) in Snell-Bagg dwarf mice.   Dose of antigen: 4×10^8 SRBC.

15-20 days with respect to normal litter mates. Such a delay can
be overcome by injection of somatotropic hormone. It should be
noted that reconstitution of immunocompetence following hormonal
treatment is long-lasting, and that it can be obtained beginning
the hormone treatment of the dwarf mice at any age.

    Taken together these and other findings obtained in our labo-
ratory allow us to conclude that a) dwarf mice show a block of
maturation of the immune system and mainly of the thymus and thymus-
dependent system, which begins about at the time of weaning; b)
the immunological maturation and the normalization of number of
peripheral blood white cells, of humoral immune response and of
cellular immunity can be achieved by 20 daily injections of somatotropic hormone; c) reconstitution of the immunological maturation can be induced at any age of the dwarf mouse and d) once such
a maturation is achieved it lasts for many months even in the absence of further hormonal treatments.

SESSION 8.   MODIFICATION OF IMMUNE RESPONSE BY EXTERNAL AGENTS
WITH SPECIAL REFERENCE TO GERMINAL CENTERS
CHAIRMAN, M. HESS, CO-CHAIRMAN, G. W. SANTOS

A QUANTITATIVE ASSESSMENT OF CELLULAR RECOVERY IN LYMPHOID TISSUE

Cornelius Rosse, Ruth W. Tyler and N. B. Everett

Department of Biological Structure, University of

Washington, Seattle, Washington 98105 U.S.A.

INTRODUCTION

Measurement of cellular responses in quantitative terms is an
essential requisite for elucidating the basic processes of hemopoiesis under normal physiological conditions as well as under conditions of specific stimulation or suppression. In man, the lymphomyeloid complex does not lend itself readily for direct cell
quantitation and inferences have to be drawn from qualitative observations on the hemopoietic tissues, the possibility of cell
quantitation for practical purposes being confined to the peripheral blood. Even in experimental animals, quantitative studies of
lymphomyeloid tissues are virtually confined to portions of the
lymphoid tissue and bone marrow of the rat (1,2) and to the bone
marrow of the guinea pig (3).

In experimental hematology, the regeneration of lymphoid tissue following radiation injury is frequently used to investigate
cellular interrelationships within the lymphomyeloid complex. Thus
far, our knowledge of this regenerative process is based on topographically limited sampling of this complex, on changes in organ
weights, and on qualitative histological observations. In the present study, the train of events following sublethal irradiation was
investigated with the following objectives in mind: (1) to establish the events of post-irradiation recovery quantitatively in terms
of cell numbers in different parts of the lymphoid tissue complex;
(2) to identify the cells participating in the regenerative process
localizing them topographically within the tissues.

413

MATERIALS AND METHODS

Animals and Procedure

Male guinea pigs of the Hartley strain were used. The animals weighed approximately 400 g at the time of sacrifice. Eighty guinea pigs received 150 r total body irradiation from a Co^{60} teletherapy unit. This dose is somewhat less than the LD-50 for guinea pigs (4). After irradiation, the animals were sacrificed in groups of eight on alternate days over a period of 20 days. Ten normal unirradiated guinea pigs served as controls. Thirty minutes before exsanguination, all animals were injected intracardially with H^3-thymidine (1 μ Ci/g body weight, specific activity 6.5 Ci/m mole).

Tissues

The two lobes of the thymus, the glandula mesenteria magna, and an anatomically constant deep cervical lymph node from each side of the neck were excised. The popliteal and the largest axillary node of the subscapular group (constant in position) were rendered visible by injection of trypan blue into the footpads before they were removed from each side. All tissues were immediately weighed on a torsion balance and a portion of each was fixed for histological study while the remaining part was used for cell quantitation.

Cell Quantitation

The total amount of DNA was determined in weighed tissue samples by the indole-colorimetric method of Ceriotti (5) after extraction with 5% trichloracetic acid (6). The DNA content of a single cell was measured by the same method on thoracic duct lymph in which the cells were counted in a hemocytometer. The number of cells per mg tissue and per organ could thus be calculated.

Radioactivity

The trichloracetic acid extract of tissues was also used for measuring the radioactivity in a scintillation counter. Values were computed for the entire organs. Localization of the isotope within the tissues was determined on radioautographs of sections.

RESULTS

Thymus

<u>Radioactivity (Fig. 1)</u>. The rate of H^3-thymidine incorporation declined from the normal value after irradiation, the lowest point being reached on the 4th day. By the 8th day, however, the level of specific activity increased more than fivefold. A marked secondary decline was followed by steady recovery to values twice above the normal on the 18th day.

<u>Cellularity (Fig. 1)</u>. Changes in the number of cells paralleled the changes in H^3-thymidine incorporation. Cell depletion was maximal on the 4th day. Two days later, the number of cells per mg of tissue recovered to the normal level which was maintained thereafter. The total number of cells in the thymus recovered to the range of normal by the 8th day. A secondary depletion on the 10th day was followed by an increase in cellularity to a level twice above the control by the 20th day.

<u>Cells in DNA Synthesis</u>. During the first peak of H^3-thymidine incorporation (6th and 8th days post-irradiation), the labeled cells were localized predominantly in two distinct areas of the thymus: one band of labeled cells at the corticomedullary junction and another band of labeled cells subjacent to the trabeculae or septa. During the second phase of regeneration, these two zones became confluent and, by the 20th day, the cortex of the thymus was thicker than in the controls.

Lymph Nodes

<u>Radioactivity (Figs. 1,2)</u>. Although there was an over-all similarity in the pattern of H^3-thymidine incorporation, lymph nodes of different topographical locations showed different rates of recovery in cellularity. Furthermore, in the lymph nodes changes in the number of cells did not consistently reflect those of H^3-thymidine uptake as they did in the thymus. The number of cells per mg and per organ continued to decline during the conspicuous peak of increased H^3-thymidine uptake observed on the 2nd day. Cell depletion was maximal on day 4.

The cervical lymph node showed the earliest signs of recovery in cellularity. By the 8th day, the number of cells per mg of tissue and per organ reached the range of the control. Recovery did not occur to this extent in organ cellularity until day 16 in the axillary and until day 20 in the popliteal nodes. In the mesenteric node, the number of cells per mg recovered to the normal level by the 10th day but the total number of cells in the node remained be-

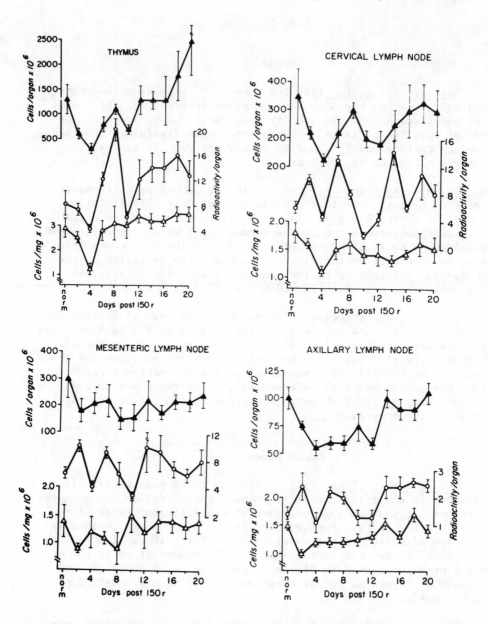

Fig. 1. Comparison of changes in cells per mg (△), cells per organ (▲) and radioactivity per organ (O) in the thymus, cervical, mesenteric and axillary lymph nodes following 150 r total body irradiation of guinea pigs (means ± standard deviation). Note same scale but different range of values along ordinates in various tissues.

low the control throughout the experiment.

Cells in DNA Synthesis. The histological findings were similar in the cervical, mesenteric and axillary nodes. On the 2nd day post-irradiation, at the time of the first peak in specific activity, heavily labeled cells were scattered throughout the markedly depleted node. On the 4th day, all nodes consisted predominantly of reticulum cells, plasma cells and a few lymphocytes.

The second peak in radioactivity on the 6th and 8th days was associated with the appearance of heavily labeled cells, particularly in the region of the corticomedullary junction.

The third peak in H^3-thymidine incorporation marked the regeneration of germinal centers. Germinal centers never completely disappeared from the nodes, but their reappearance in large numbers was conspicuous at this stage.

Germinal centers did not appear in the popliteal node. It is significant that the peak in H^3-thymidine incorporation coinciding with the phase of regeneration of germinal centers was absent in this node (Fig. 2).

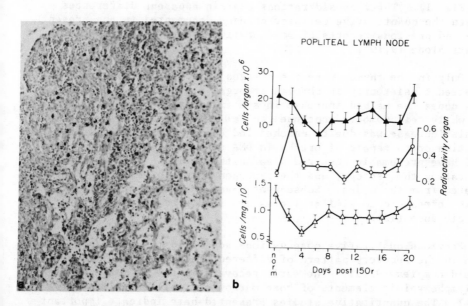

Fig. 2. Radioautograph of a 5 μ thick section of the popliteal node on the 18th day after irradiation shows the absence of germinal centers (a-X 150). Cellular recovery and changes in rate of H^3-thymidine incorporation are shown in b.

DISCUSSION

The limitations of observations based on histology and organ weights were recognized by some of the first investigators of radiation effects upon tissues of hemopoiesis (9). The present work reflects these limitations in the variation of cell numbers per mg tissue. An increased amount of extracellular fluid and the relative predominance of cytoplasmic mass over nuclei accounted for as much as 60% of thymic weight and more than 30% of weight in the lymph nodes at the time of greatest cell depression (Fig. 1). Later, at the commencement of regeneration, the medullary sinusoids contained considerable quantities of blood.

The number of cells per mg of tissue in the normal unirradiated control has not been exceeded significantly in any of the organs during post-irradiation recovery. As a rule, cellularity per mg was recovered relatively early and considerably before the normal level of cellularity per organ was reached. Only in the thymus did organ cellularity rise above control. This occurred through an increase in the volume of the organ. The data suggest that the maximum cellularity per unit weight of each lymphoid organ is relatively constant around the value in the normal. Variation does occur, however, from tissue to tissue, in the same animal (Fig. 1). These considerations explain apparent differences between the quantitative cellular changes documented in the present study and previous reports of regenerative events based on organ weights alone (9,10).

Only in the thymus were the changes in H^3-thymidine uptake reflected consistently in changes of organ cellularity. In the lymph nodes the marked increase in specific activity on the 2nd day, while cell numbers continued to fall, is difficult to explain. If this increase was due to unscheduled DNA synthesis, repair replication or to repair of breaks in DNA strands (11), an increase would have presumably occurred also in the thymus. The cells incorporating the isotope, and their progeny, must have perished or migrated from the nodes. Subsequent waves of increased H^3-thymidine uptake correspond to similar increases of labeled cells in the thoracic duct (12).

Previous qualitative observations suggested topographic variation in the recovery pattern of different members of the lymphomyeloid complex (9,13). The early recovery of the thymus and of the lymphomyeloid elements of bone marrow are well established (9, 10,14). The quantitative studies presented here indicate important differences between lymph nodes of various locations. Recovery in the cervical node showed some similarities to the thymus which may be related to the fact that lymph from the thymus drains predominantly to these nodes (15). The delayed cellular recovery of the glandula mesenterica magna is particularly notable. The more sharply defined changes in the cervical node make it probably the most suitable lymph node for sampling the lymphoid tissue.

All the lymph nodes studied reached a near normal level of organ cellularity by the 20th day post-irradiation. From these observations it is not clear why the thoracic duct output of lymphocytes should remain markedly below the normal level for a much longer period (16,17,18).

The findings relating to the distribution and identity of cells in DNA synthesis in the thymus and lymph nodes are in accord with previous reports (7,19). The phase of reappearance of germinal centers in increased numbers coincided with the period of recovery of competence in cell-mediated immune responses by lymphocytes as detected by the mixed lymphocyte reaction and the lymphocyte transfer reaction (18). Although the production of long-lived lymphocytes, known to participate in these reactions, have not yet been investigated after sublethal irradiation, the findings suggest that germinal centers are necessary to enable lymphocytes to partake actively in these reactions.

SUMMARY

After sublethal irradiation of guinea pigs, changes in absolute cell numbers correlated with H^3-thymidine incorporation show a differential response in thymus and lymph nodes of various topographical location. Cellularity per mg tissue recovered to the normal level considerably before normal organ cellularity was reached. Normal cell numbers were exceeded only in the thymus. In lymph nodes regeneration was best defined in the cervical node while cellular recovery of the mesenteric node was delayed in comparison. In the thymus the first increase in H^3-thymidine incorporation was associated with the appearance of labeled cells subjacent to the trabeculae and at the corticomedullary junction, whereas in lymph nodes, the first increase occurred while cell numbers were declining. In lymph nodes commencement of regeneration was marked by the appearance of labeled cells at the corticomedullary junction leading later to accelerated germinal centers formation.

ACKNOWLEDGEMENTS

This work was supported by grants from the National Institutes of Health (AM 13145) and from the Atomic Energy Commission (AT[45-1]-1377).

REFERENCES

1. Kindred, J. E. Amer. J. Anat. 62, 453, 1938.
2. Everett, N. B., Caffrey, R. W. and Rieke, W. O. Ann. New York Acad. Sci. 113, 887, 1964.
3. Yoffey, J. M. Bone Marrow Reactions. Edward Arnold Ltd., London, 1966.
4. Ellinger, F. Radiology 44, 125, 1945.
5. Ceriotti, G. J. Bio. Chem. 198, 297, 1952.
6. Schneider, W. C. J. Biol. Chem. 161, 293, 1945.
7. Everett, N. B., Rieke, W. O., Reinhardt, W. O. and Yoffey, J. M. In: CIBA Foundation Symposium on Haemopoiesis, Churchill, London, 1960.
8. Everett, N. B. and Tyler, R. W. Cell and Tissue Kinetics 2, 347, 1969.
9. Brecher, G., Endicott, K. M., Gump, H., and Brawner, H. P. Blood 3, 1259, 1948.
10. Harris, P. F. Brit. J. Exptl. Path. 39, 557, 1958.
11. Spiegler, P. and Norman, A. Rad. Res. 39, 400, 1969.
12. Osmond, D. G. Personal communication.
13. Laissue, J., Hess, M. W., Stoner, R. D., Riedwyl, H., and Cottier, H. In: Lymphatic Tissue and Germinal Centers in Immune Response. (Ed.: Fiore-Donati, L. and Hanna, Jr., M.G.) Plenum Press, New York, 1969.
14. Hulse, E. V. Brit. J. Haematol. 9, 365, 1963.
15. Harris, P. F. and Templeton, W. R. Acta Anat. 69, 366, 1968.
16. Schreck, R. In: The Lymphocyte and Lymphocytic Tissue (Ed.: Rebuck, J. W.) Hoeber, New York, 1960.
17. Ross, M. H., Furth, J., Bigelow, R. R. Blood 7, 417, 1952.
18. Lamberg, J. D. and Schwarz, M. R. In: Proceedings of 4th Leucocyte Culture Conference (Ed.: MacIntyre, R. O.) Appleton-Century-Croft. In Press.
19. Yoffey, J. M., Reinhardt, W. O., and Everett, N. B. J. Anat. 95, 293, 1961.

A STUDY OF THE PROPERTIES AND EFFECTS OF ANTI-MACROPHAGE SERA

Ruth Gallily

Department of Immunology

The Hebrew University-Hadassah Medical
School, Jerusalem, Israel

Several studies in the last ten years have indicated that macrophages are essential in the induction of antibody production
(1-4). Heterologous antisera which are specific against macrophages
can provide an important tool for further study and elucidation of
the participation of macrophages in the immune response.

This paper describes the preparation of anti-macrophage serum
(AMS) and its assay, and reports its effect regarding phagocytosis,
antibody production and allograft survival. The effect of AMS on
DNA synthesis in macrophages is also shown.

Antisera were prepared by giving a group of rabbits two IP
injections of 10^9 peritoneal macrophages fourteen days apart (the
peritoneal cells were withdrawn from C57BL or BALB/c mice four days
after thioglycollate injection, when 80 to 85% of the cells were
macrophages). A second group of rabbits were given three injections of 10^8 cells of a cultured macrophage preparation once a week
(in which about 98% of the cells were macrophages). The rabbits
were bled seven days after the last injection. The sera were inactivated and stored at -20°C.

Before studying the properties of AMS a method was devised for
defining the cytotoxic activity of different anti-macrophage sera.
Essentially, the method consisted of growing peritoneal macrophages
in small disposable Petri dishes in media consisting of 10% fetal
calf serum (FCS) and 90% Hank's salt solution. After twenty-four
hours *in vitro* the media were replaced by AMS of various dilutions.
The cells were incubated with these antisera for an hour, after
which 5% commercial guinea pig complement was added. Three hours

Table 1. Cytotoxicity of pre-immunization sera and
anti-macrophage sera (AMS)[1] against macrophages

Rabbit No.	pre-immunization sera		AMS	
	Dilution	% of dead cells	Dilution	% of dead cells
79	1:10	0	1:5000	66
119	1:100	0	1:5000	73
239	1:10	0	1:1000	72
242	1:10	0	1:1000	73
1	1:10	0	1:1000	52
2	1:10	0	1:1000	88
5	1:10	0	1:1000	55

[1]The sera were inactivated for 30 minutes at 56°C and adsorbed
with sheep erythrocytes. 5% guinea pig complement was added to
the media.

later, the viable cells were scored by exposing them to 0.4% Ery-
throsin B. Only the dead cells were stained red by this test. The
assay proved to be sensitive as well as repeatable.

The cytotoxicity of seven anti-macrophage sera was assayed.
It was found (Table 1) that the antisera killed 52-88% of the macrophages in 1000 to 5000 fold dilutions. In order to determine
if the specificity of these antisera were limited to macrophages,
cytotoxicity of AMS against other two types of cells, lymphocytes
and granulocytes,was tested. Spleen lymphocytes were incubated in
tubes with different dilutions of AMS to which 5% complement was
added. The viability of the cells was scored (Table 2). It can
be seen that the four AMS tested were cytotoxic to lymphocytes in a
1:1000 dilution (two of the antisera had the same cytotoxic titers
against lymphocytes as against macrophages and two had somewhat
lower titers).

Likewise, these four AMS were found to be cytotoxic to granulocytes in a similar *in vitro* assay; AMS in 100 - 1000 fold dilution killed 50-96% of the granulocytes.

It is apparent that this cross reactivity of AMS with lymphocytes excludes its use for elimination of macrophages from a mixed
population of macrophages and lymphocytes *in vitro*. Moreover, injection of AMS into animals might affect cell types other than macrophages. It could be postulated that adsorption experiments with

Table 2. Cytocoxicity of AMS against lymphocytes and granulocytes

Serum	Cytotoxicity against Lymphocytes		Cytotoxicity against Granulocytes	
	Dilution	% of dead cells	Dilution	% of dead cells
AMS 79	1:1000	96	1:100	96
AMS 119	1:1000	97	1:1000	50
AMS 239	1:1000	82	1:1000	60
AMS 242	1:1000	55	1:100	82

the right concentration of other cell types might leave some specific residue activity against macrophages. Indeed, if such a specific antisera were available, it might provide an important tool for studying the role of macrophages in the immune response (experiments along these lines are now being carried out in our laboratory).

In the next set of experiments the effects of AMS on phagocytosis and antibody production, as well as on allograft survival, were studied. In the phagocytosis experiments we added AMS as well as anti-thymocytic serum (ATS) or normal rabbit serum (NRS) to macrophages growing *in vitro*. One hour after the addition of the sera *Bacillus subtilis* was added and the percentage of phagocytosis was scored one hour later (Table 3). It was found that the phagocytosis of the bacilli by the macrophages was almost completely inhibited by the AMS. It is interesting to note that phagocytosis was not completely inhibited, although it was significantly reduced by the ATS. This difference between ATS and AMS regarding phagocytosis of *Bacillus subtilis* revealed an apparent difference in their modes of action.

The unique effect of AMS on the phagocytosis of macrophages *in vitro* was not manifested when we studied the effect of AMS on humoral antibody production and allograft survival. In the *in vivo* experiments C57BL mice were injected intraperitoneally with AMS (adsorbed with SE (5) and ME) two hours before *Shigella para-*

Table 3.   Effect of AMS, ATS and NRS on phagocytosis
of Bacillus subtilis by macrophages in vitro

Medium	No. of sera samples	percentage of phagocytosis
Hanks		49
Hanks + 10% NCS	2	67
Hanks + 10% NRS	2	33
Hanks + 10% ATS	2	20
Hanks + 10% AMS	5	3

dysenteriae inoculation and subsequently three or four additional
injections of AMS were given (Table 4).   No decrease of anti-
Shigella antibody production in AMS treated mice was found.   Like-

Table 4.   Effect of AMS injections on anti-shigella antibody
production by C57BL mice

Treatment of recipients	No. of mice	Agglutinin titer	
		5 days $\log_2$ of titer (mean)	8 days $\log_2$ of titer (mean)
Shigella	5	5.6	9.4
AMS[1] + Shigella	5	7.4	9.8
AMS[2] + Shigella	5	–	10.0

[1] Recipients were treated with a total dose of 0.1 ml AMS given
on days 0,1,2,3.

[2] Recipients were treated with a total dose of 0.8 ml AMS given
on days 0,1,2,4,6.

Table 5.   Effect of NRS, AMS and ATS injections on skin allograft
          survival

| Serum[1] | Balb/c graft on C57BL mice | | C57BL graft on Balb/c mice | |
	No. of mice	Mean survival ± S.D. (days)	No. of mice	Mean survival ± S.D. (days)
–	(5)	13.5 ± 1.3	(8)	12.6 ± 0.4
NRS	(4)	17.3 ± 1.7	(6)	19 ± 2.1
AMS	(9)	16.8 ± 2.1	(7)	21 ± 2.7
ATS	(6)	23.1 ± 5.8	(5)	23.2 ± 3.1

[1] Recipients were treated with a total dose of 0.25 ml given in 6 or 7
injections.

wise, (Table 5) five or six IP injections of AMS did not increase
significantly the survival times of skin allografts above the
times found after treatment with NRS. On the other hand, injections of ATS prolonged the survival of the skin grafts, as was
known from experiments done by other investigators. The allograft
transfer was performed reciprocally between C57BL and BALB/c mice.

From these two sets of experiments one can conclude that application of AMS in the amounts and schedules used did not affect
either anti-Shigella antibody production or skin allograft survival.
Since AMS diminished phagocytosis *in vitro*, we treated macrophages
in vitro with AMS before adding Shigella. After incubation, the
washed macrophages were transferred to 550r X-irradiated mice
(Table 6). To our great surprise, we did not find any decrease in
antibody production by the animals which received AMS-treated macrophages. Apparently, the macrophages could recover from the
effect of the AMS, and the small amount of Shigella which was phago-
cytised or stuck to the macrophages was sufficient to trigger antibody production.

In the last experiment the effect of AMS on DNA synthesis of
macrophages was studied. It was found (Figure 1) that in cultured
macrophages incubated with 10% AMS for twenty-four hours, the DNA
content per plate increased 50 to 100% (as was determined by indole
colorimetric estimation of DNA). The DNA content of similar cultured macrophages was not affected when NRS was added.

<u>Table 6</u>.   The effect of macrophages treated in-vitro with
                 AMS on the induction of antibody by irradiated mice

Treatment of recipients	No. of mice	Agglutimin titer on day 7 $(\log_2)$
15×10^6 macrophages incubated with shigella	13	6.7
15×10^6 macrophages incubated with AMS and shigella	11	6.8
Shigella	15	1.8

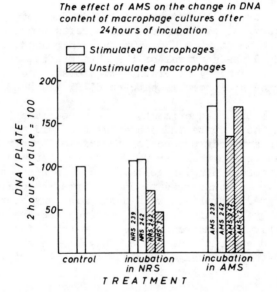

Legend to Figure 1: The experiment began two hours after the
macrophages had been cultured. The value 100 represents the DNA
content per plate at the beginning of the experiment. The macrophages were withdrawn from the peritoneum of thioglycollate injected mice (blank bars), as well as taken from unstimulated mice
(lined bars).

In summary, anti-macrophage sera (AMS) showed high cytotoxic activity against macophages in culture. Likewise, the AMS showed cross reactivity to lymphocytes and granulocytes.

Injection of AMS into mice did not affect anti-Shigella antibody production, nor did it prolong skin allograft survival. Furthermore, AMS treated macrophages did not lose their ability to induce anti-Shigella antibody production in irradiated mice.

On the other hand, AMS inhibited phagocytosis of *Bacillus subtilis* by macrophages and likewise increased the synthesis of DNA in cultural macrophages.

REFERENCES

1. Fishman, M. *J. Exp. Med.*, 114:837, 1961.

2. Askonas, B.A. and Rhodes, J.M. *Nature*, 205:471, 1965.

3. Gallily, R. and Feldman, M. *Immunology*, 12:197, 1967.

4. Moiser, D.E. *Science*, 158:1573, 1967.

5. Tanaka, N. and Leduce, E.H. *J. Immunol.*, 77:198, 1956.

EFFECT OF L-ASPARAGINASE ON THYMUS-DEPENDENT IMMUNE REACTIVITY*

Marc E. Weksler and Babette B. Weksler

Department of Medicine, The New York Hospital-Cornell

Medical Center, New York, N.Y. 10021, U.S.A.

Asparaginase is the second enzyme reported to have immuno-suppressive properties. Ribonuclease was shown to depress the transfer reaction (1) and Mowbray and Scholand (2) suggested that mice pretreated with ribonuclease complexes did not produce normal titers of anti-sheep erythrocyte antibody. Recently asparaginase has been reported to inhibit a number of "thymic dependent" immune reactions: the rejection of skin grafts (3), the production of anti-sheep erythrocyte antibody (4), the transformation of lympho-cytes in response to phytohemagglutinin (PHA) (5), and the development of graft-versus-host-disease (6).

We have examined the immunosuppressive properties of aspara-ginase and suggest that the action of this enzyme is mediated by depletion of asparagine which in turn appears to impair the function of thymus-derived lymphocytes.

METHODS

Balb/c mice were the subjects of all animal studies. Hemag-glutinating antibody activity was determined 6 days after the injection of 0.2 ml of a 10% suspension of sheep erythrocytes. Grafts of C57Bl/6J ear skin on Balb/c mice were performed by standard techniques. Grafts were covered with vaseline gauze and secured by a plaster cast. Casts were removed on day 9 and the grafts inspected daily for rejection. Dissociated lymph node cells were incubated with chromium-51 for 30 minutes at 37°C. The cells were washed three times and 10 million cells were injected intravenously into syngeneic recipients. These mice were sacrificed 24 hours

*Supported in part by the American Cancer Society Grant CI 28.

later and the radioactivity in pooled lymph nodes, in spleen and
in liver was determined. Graft-versus-host reaction was assayed
in 7 week old F_1 mice (C57Bl/6J x DBA/2J) given 30 million spleen
cells from either untreated or asparaginase-treated C57Bl/6J mice.
Spleen index at 7 days was used to quantitate the reaction. Anti-
mouse thymocyte serum was made by immunizing rabbits intravenously
with 1 billion thymocytes on day 0 and 14. On day 21 the rabbits
were exsanguinated, the serum collected, decomplemented and
sterilized.

Human lymphocyte transformation was measured in culture in the
presence of PHA. The standard culture consisted of 1.6 ml of TC
199 (containing Penicillin 100 U and Streptomycin 100 micrograms),
0.4 ml of plasma containing 0.4 million lymphocytes and 0.025 ml
of PHA-M (Difco).

E. coli L-asparaginase from a single lot: C-7938 (Merck,
Sharp and Dohme) was used throughout the study.

RESULTS

The peripheral lymphocyte count falls following a single
intraperitoneal injection of 1000 U of asparaginase. The number
of lymphocytes was reduced after 3 hours and remained significantly
reduced for 24 hours. Lymphocytopenia was not produced by heat-
inactivated asparaginase but did occur in adrenalectomized animals
(Table I). Asparaginase-treated mice showed marked atrophy of
their lymphoid organs. Normal mice treated daily for 6 days with
1000 U of asparaginase showed a marked reduction in weight of lymph
nodes (45%), spleen (50%) and thymus (80%) after correction for
body weight. Adrenalectomized animals which received only 10 U

Table I

Effect of a Single Dose of L-Asparaginase on Blood Lymphocytes#

Animals	Asparaginase	Hours after Asparaginase			
		0	3	8	24
Normal (4)	0	6800	6450	6850	9850
Normal (4)	inactivated	6750	--	6920	8600
Normal (4)	1000 U	7100	4250	3700*	4240*
Adrenalectomized (4)	1000 U	13600	--	10100*	8250*

#mean tail blood lymphocyte count/mm^3
*values significantly different from initial values. (p < .01)

Table II

Effect of Asparaginase Treatment on Hemagglutination Titer

Animals	Asparaginase Dose=	Mean Titer (log$_2$)
Normal (10)	1000 U inactivated	9.1
Normal (7)	50 U	6.3*
Normal (7)	100 U	4.7*
Normal (7)	1000 U	4.5*
Normal preimmunized with Asparaginase (5)	1000 U	4.6*
Adrenalectomized (8)	100 U inactivated	6.6
Adrenalectomized (7)	100 U	4.2*

= Asparaginase given daily by intraperitoneal route from day-2 to +5
*Values significantly different from controls

of Asparaginase daily for 6 days also showed marked reduction in lymphoid mass.

A significant reduction in antibody to sheep erythrocytes was found in normal and adrenalectomized animals treated with asparaginase (Table II). Mice were given asparaginase daily beginning 2 days before immunization with sheep erythrocytes and continuing until the day of sacrifice 6 days after immunization.

The survival of C57B1/6J skin on Balb/c mice treated with inactivated asparaginase, active asparaginase, ATS and ATS combined with asparaginase was studied. Not only was a prolongation

Table III

The Survival of Skin Grafts on Mice Treated with Asparaginase and/or Anti-Thymocyte Serum (ATS)

Treatment+	Mean Survival and Standard Deviation
1000 U inactivated	11.0 ± 1.1 days
500 U	13.5 ± 1.5 days
1000 U	15.8 ± 1.8 days
2000 U	17.5 ± 2.1 days
ATS	16.8 ± 1.6 days
ATS + 500 U	25.6 ± 2.9 days

+Asparaginase given daily via intraperitoneal route. ATS given as 1/2 ml subcutaneous injection on day 2 and 5.

Table IV

Effect of Asparaginase on Lymphocyte Migration in Syngeneic Mice

Donor	Recipient	Percent Labeled Lymphocytes		
		Lymph Node	Spleen	Liver
Normal	Normal (5)	6.3	12.4	30.2
Normal incubated in vitro with Asparaginase	Normal (5)	5.9	13.1	27.6
Asparaginase treated	Normal (5)	2.8	7.2	34.6

of graft survival seen with asparaginase treatment but a very marked synergism was seen with the combination of ATS and asparaginase (Table III).

These studies indicate that asparaginase alters the number and function of lymphocytes. These effects were further studied by investigating the "homing" of lymphocytes to lymphoid organs. Lymphocyte labeled with chromium-51 and incubated in vitro with asparaginase (500 U/ml) did not release their label and migrated normally to lymph nodes and spleen of syngeneic recipients demonstrating the lack of a direct cytotoxic action of asparaginase on lymphocytes. In contrast lymphocytes obtained from animals treated for 6 days with asparaginase did not migrate normally to the lymph nodes and a higher percent were retained in the liver (Table IV).

We have also assayed the function of lymphocytes by measuring the capacity of spleen cells to induce graft-versus-host disease in adult F_1 mice. Thirty million spleen cells taken from parental mice treated for 5 days with 1000 U/day of asparaginase produced significantly less splenomegaly than did equal numbers of cells taken from untreated animals.

DISCUSSION

The present studies show that asparaginase produces lymphocytopenia and atrophy of the lymph nodes, spleen and thymus. Repeated injection of asparaginase inhibits the rejection of skin grafts and the formation of antibody by treated mice. Lymph node cells from asparaginase-treated mice do not migrate normally in syngeneic mice. Similarly, spleen cells from treated mice do not elicit graft-versus-host disease in F_1 mice. While it is most likely that the immunosuppressive activity of asparaginase is attributable to its enzymatic activity, the possible roles of antigenic competition, endotoxin contaminating the E. coli asparaginase preparation and the release of adrenal steroids in the intact animal need be discussed.

Although it is difficult to exclude antigenic competition, two aspects of the study militate against this phenomenon explaining the immunosuppressive activity of asparaginase: (I) Control animals received heat-inactivated enzyme yet showed no depression in their antibody response and (II) animals pretreated with asparaginase showed no enhancement of immunosuppression whereas immunosuppression by antigenic competition is augmented by pretreatment with competing antigen (7). Endotoxin has been found to potentiate antibody formation (8) and stimulate lymphocyte transformation (9) and therefore would not explain the immunosuppression observed. The activity of asparaginase in adrenalectomized animals indicates that endogenous adrenal steroid release is not the main mechanism of immunosuppression by this enzyme.

We therefore conclude that asparaginase is immunosuppressive by virtue of its capacity to convert asparagine to aspartic acid. This has been the mechanism defined by in vitro studies of lymphocyte transformation (5). The administration of asparaginase to mice produces a rapid and profound fall in the serum asparagine level. That this deficiency of asparagine underlies the immunosuppressive activity of the enzyme is supported by the reversal of asparaginase inhibition of antibody formation by the administration of asparagine to asparaginase-treated mice. How asparagine depletion results in immunosuppression is not clear. One of the few known metabolic requirements for asparagine involves the synthesis of glycoprotein where N-acetyl-glucosamine is linked through the beta amide of asparagine to the polypeptide chain. Asparaginase is known to inhibit glycoprotein synthesis by mouse leukemia cells (10). Gessner and Ginsberg (11) have demonstrated that lymphocytes treated with glycosidase do not migrate normally presumably because of an alteration in surface glycoprotein. The alteration in lymphocyte migration we have observed after asparaginase treatment of animals may reflect a similar alteration in surface components produced by asparaginase inhibition of lymphocyte glycoprotein synthesis. Normal surface glycoprotein may be required for the emigration of the lymphocyte through the post-capillary venule into the lymph node. It is also possible that surface glycoproteins may play a role in the normal response of lymphocytes to antigen.

The primary subpopulation of lymphocytes affected by asparaginase may be the thymus-derived lymphocytes because: (I) Asparaginase produces a striking depletion of thymocytes in vivo. (II) Direct toxicity studies performed in vitro suggest that asparaginase may be more cytotoxic to thymocytes than to lymphocytes (12). (III) The thymus of mice contains 30% more asparagine than the spleen, 300% more asparagine than the kidney and 500% more asparagine than the liver (13). (IV) The immune reactions observed to be inhibited -- skin graft rejection, the antibody response of mice to sheep erythrocytes and the induction of graft-versus-host-disease -- are all "highly thymic dependent" phenomena (14). (V) Impairment of PHA-

induced lymphocyte transformation can be related to a reduction
in the number of thymus-derived lymphocytes (15) and (VI) Asparaginase appears predominantly to affect the primary and not the
secondary response to sheep erythrocytes (3) as does thymectomy
(16).

Thus the inhibition of skin graft rejection, the suppression
of antibody formation to sheep erythrocytes and the inhibition of
graft-versus-host reactions observed in our studies may reflect
an alteration in the function of thymus-derived lymphocytes.

REFERENCES

1-Jankovic, B.D. and H.F. Dworak J. Immunol. 89:571 (1962)
2-Mowbray, J.F. and J. Scholand Immunol. 11:421 (1966)
3-Nelson, S.D., M.B. Lee and J.B. Bridges Transplant 9:566 (1970)
4-Charkrabarty, A.K. and H. Friedman Science 167:869 (1970)
5-Ohno, R. and E.M. Hersh Blood 35:250 (1970)
6-Hobik, H.P. Naturwissenschaft 56:279 (1969)
7-Brody, N.I. and G. Siskind Fed. Proc. 29:770 (1970)
8-Langevoort, H.L., R.M. Asofsky, E.B. Jacobson, T. DeVries
   and G.J. Thorbecke J. Immunol. 90:60 (1963)
9-Oppenheim, J.J. and S. Perry Proc. Soc. Exp. Biol. Med.
   118:1014 (1965)
10-Bosman, H.B. and D. Kessel Nature 226:850 (1970
11-Gessner, B.M. and V. Ginsburg Proc. Nat. Acad. Sci. 52:750 (1964)
12-Dolowy, W.C., L.M. Elrod, R.N. Ammeraal and R. Schrek.
   Proc. Soc. Exp. Biol. Med. 125:598 (1967)
13-Broome, J.D. J. Exp. Med. 127:1055 (1968)
14-Miller, J.F.A.O. and G.F. Mitchell Transplant Rev. 1:1 (1969)
15-Rodney, G.E. and R.A. Good Int. Arch. Allergy 36:399 (1969)
16-Sinclair, N.R.S.C. and E.V. Elliot J. Immunol. 101:251 (1968)

THE ULTRASTRUCTURE OF ANTIBODY-FORMING SPLEEN CELLS IN IMMUNOLOGICALLY SUPPRESSED LEUKEMIC MICE [1]

W. S. Ceglowski, G. Koo, and H. Friedman

Temple University School of Medicine, Philadelphia,

Pennsylvania, USA

Previous studies in our laboratory and studies by others have demonstrated that infection with the murine leukemia viruses results in a significant depression in immunologic responsiveness (1,2). The extent of this suppression is dependent upon the dose of virus administered and the time interval between infection and immunization. These and other observations have been used to support the concept that there may be a competition between the leukemia virus and antigen for a limited number of precursor cells.

The present study was an attempt to correlate morphologic aspects of leukemia virus-induced immunosuppression with immunologic events. The first part of the study was devoted toward the study of the cell types involved in leukemia virus infection and the immune response. The second part of the study concerned the ultrastructural study of individual antibody plaque forming cells in order to gain some insight into the possible interaction of a leukemia virus with a committed antibody forming cell.

MATERIALS, METHODS AND EXPERIMENTAL DESIGN

Inbred BALB/c strain mice were used in this study. They were infected with a preparation of Friend Leukemia Virus (FLV) which

---

[1] Research currently supported by grants from the American Cancer Society, Inc. (T-382E), the National Science Foundation (GM-25996), and the Damon Runyon Memorial Fund for Cancer Research Inc. (DRG-1037).

had been stored at -60 C. The mice were inoculated intraperitoneally
with 0.5cc of an appropriate dilution of the virus. Splenomegaly
was used as the indicator of infection. Sheep red blood cells were
used as the antigen. They were washed and standardized to a 10%
concentration prior to inoculation. The direct hemolytic assay
technique in agar gel was used to determine the number of antibody
plaque-forming cells (PFC), as described previously (1).

On the 4th day after immunization mice were sacrificed and
spleens excised. Segments were cut from each spleen and immersed
in 3% cold glutaraldehyde in 0.1 M phosphate buffer, pH 7.4 (3).
The pieces were then cut with a razor blade and transferred to
small vials containing the same glutaraldehyde solution. After
2-3 hours the tissue pieces were washed in phosphate buffer containing 10% sucrose. The spleen pieces were then fixed in 1%
osmium in phosphate buffer. The fixed sections were dehydrated,
using graded concentrations of cold ethanol and embedded with
Epon (4). After the blocks had hardened, they were sectioned with
a Reichert ultramicrotome. Sections approximately 0.5 μ thick were
cut and stained with pyronin Y and toluidine blue (5). Fixed blocks
with well-defined lymphoid follicles and white pulp were selected
for further study. These portions of the spleen contained mainly
lymphoid cells surrounding an arteriole and were readily distinguishable from the red pulp. When a suitable block was obtained,
silver-gray sections were cut with the microtome and stained with
6% uranyl acetate and Reynold's lead citrate (6). The sections
were then examined with a Siemens Elmiskop 1A, with magnification
ranging from x4000 to x30,000.

For the electron microscopic studies of single cells agar
plates containing approximately 5 to 10 x 10^6 viable leukocytes
were used. Immediately after plaque development, the agar plates
were treated with cold 3% glutaraldehyde in 0.1 M cacodylate
buffer, pH 7.4 (3). Individual antibody plaques were punched out
with a small-bore Pasteur pipette. The plaques were fixed and then
washed in the same buffer with 10% sucrose. The plaques were placed
in 1% osmium in 0.1 M s-collidine buffer, pH 7.4 (7). Then were
dehydrated with graded concentrations of ethanol and then infiltrated
with Epon (4). Plaques containing only a single cell in the center
were selected and used for embedding. Flat embedding was used to
facilitate orientation of the plaque. Sections approximately
600 Å thick were cut and placed on 75 x 300 mesh Formvar and carbon-
coated grids. They were stained with 4% aqueous uranyl acetate
and lead citrate (6). The sections were examined with a Siemen's
Elmiskop 1A electron microscope. Three to 12 sections were examined
for each cell. A total of 25 PFC's were studied from 9 control
animals and 20 cells from 9 FLV-infected mice.

For studies of the ultrastructure of spleen sections, groups
of mice were infected either 3 or 8 days before, the same day, or

2 days after antigenic stimulation. On the fourth day following
immunization the immune response was assayed by means of the plaque
assay and sections of spleen were prepared for electron microscopy
as described. For the study of individual plaque forming cells,
groups of mice were infected 8 days prior to immunization with
sheep erythrocytes. Four days after immunization, the mice were
sacrificed, their spleens excised and plaque assays performed. The
plaque forming cells were then selected, processed and studied.

RESULTS

The suppressive effects of infection with FLV are demonstrated
in Table I. These results are similar to those previously reported
(8) and demonstrate that infection prior to immunization has a
marked immunosuppressive effect while infection simultaneously with
or following immunization has little or no immunosuppressive effect.

Ultrastructural observations of spleen sections from animals
exhibiting the immune response presented in Table I can be characterized in the following manner. Study of spleen sections of the
white pulp of normal non-immunized mice revealed that small to
medium lymphocytes were the predominant type of nucleated cells.
The other major type of nucleated cell observed was the macrophage.
The organization of these cells and the reticulum cells was unre-
markable and similar to that reported by Reynolds (6) and Movat
and Fernando (9). Representative spleen sections from animals
immunized 4 days previously revealed abundant lymphoid cells and
macrophages, with the appearance of the various cell types of the
plasmacytic series. Among these were plasmablasts, proplasmocytes
and mature plasma cells. Plasmablasts were usually observed 1 to
2 days after immunization, while proplasmacytes and plasmacytes

TABLE I.   Effect of Infection with FLV on the Immune
           Response to Sheep Erythrocytes

Experimental Group	PFC per Spleen*	Percent of Control
Control	7.8×10^4	---
Infected 2 days after immunization	4.5×10^4	58
Infected same day as immunization	1.4×10^5	173
Infected 3 days prior to immunization	1.3×10^4	17
Infected 8 days prior to immunization	4.9×10^2	1

*Results 4 days after immunization.

appeared on the 3rd and 4th day after immunization. Spleen sections
prepared from mice infected with virus 2 days after immunization
were essentially identical to those of control immunized mice. No
virus particles were observed in any of the more than 1000 sections
studied.

Examination of spleens of mice infected on the same day as
immunization and sacrificed 4 days later revealed the presence of
undifferentiated blast cells. These cells constituted approximately
10% of the cells observed in a typical section. Careful search of
more than 1000 sections failed to reveal the presence of FLV
particles. Study of spleen sections from mice infected 3 days prior
to immunization revealed an infiltration of immature neoplastic
cells. These neoplastic cells constituted 40 to 50% of the cells
observed in a section. Many virus particles were observed budding
from the plasma membranes of these neoplastic cells. There appeared to be a paucity of plasma cells in these sections. There
was approximately one identifiable plasma cell per 10,000 nucleated
cells. There was an extensive infiltration of leukemic cells in
spleen sections from mice infected 8 days prior to immunization.
These leukemic cells constituted 80 to 90% of the cells observed.
Virus particles were numerous and were observed to be budding from
the plasma membranes of undifferentiated cells. No mature plasma
cells were observed in the more than 1000 sections examined.

The above observations prompted the studies on the ultrastructure of antibody forming cells from control immunized and
FLV-infected immunized mice. Study of individual plaque forming
cells would give information regarding the morphologic types of
cells involved in antibody production in nofmal and FLV-infected
mice and would also give information regarding the interaction
between a committed antibody forming cell and the virus. Figure 1
shows an electron micrograph of a single antibody forming cell
from a mouse 4 days after immunization. The morphology is that of
a mature plasmocyte. It contains dense chromatin material, has a
well-developed golgi apparatus and exhibits a continuous and distended endoplasmic reticulum. Figure 2A shows an electron micrograph from a mouse immunized 8 days after infection with FLV. This
cell is also a mature plasmocyte, however there are C type virus
particles at the plasma membrane. Figure 2B is a higher magnification
of the same cell in which there appears to be continuity of the
virus particle with the cell membrane, suggesting active virus
proliferation.

The summary of the morphologic type distribution of the 25
cells from control-immunized and the 20 cells from infected-
immunized mice is presented in Table 2. All the antibody forming
cells from the control immunized mice were of the plasmacytic
series. In the infected immunized group 90% of the antibody forming cells were of the plasmacytic series while 2 out of 20 or 10%

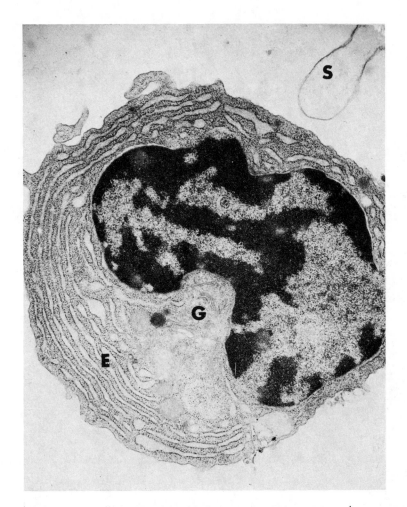

Fig. 1. A single PFC from an immunized control mouse 4 days after immunization. A mature plasmacyte with dense chromatin material, well-developed golgi apparatus (G) and continuous and distended endoplasmic reticulum (E). (S) is a remnant of a lysed sheep erythrocyte. 16,200x.

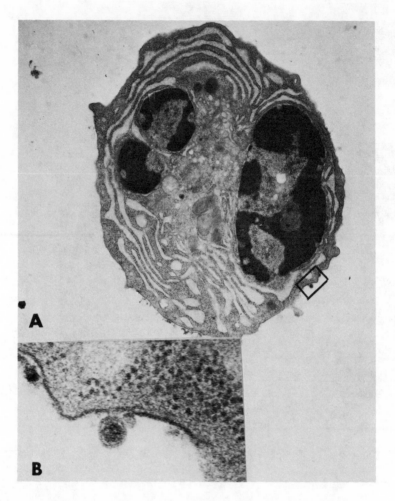

Fig. 2. A single PFC from an FLV-infected and immunized mouse
which contains C-type particles. (A) is a mature plasmacyte with
C-type particles at the plasma membrane. 13,600x. (B) is a
higher magnification showing continuity of virus particle with
cellular membrane. 100,200x.

Table 2. Distribution of Morphologic Types of Single
Antibody Forming Cells from Normal-Immunized
and Infected-Immunized Mice.*

	Group			
	Normal		FLV-Infected**	
Cell Type	Frequency	Percent	Frequency	Percent
Lymphocyte	0/25	(0)	2/20	(10)
Plasmablast	0/25	(0)	0/20	(0)
Proplasmacytes	6/25	(24)	2/20	(10)
Plasmacytes	14/25	(56)	12/20	(60)
Degenerated	5/25	(20)	4/20	(20)

*All animals were killed and assayed 4 days after immunization.

**Mice were infected with FLV 8 days before immunization.

were lymphocytic. This appeared to be the only difference in the
distribution of cell types between the two groups.

Ultrastructural observation of individual antibody plaque
forming cells revealed the presence of virus-like intracisternal
A type particles in cells from both control and virus-infected
mice. The intracisternal A type particles could be differentiated
from C type particles by 1, the fact that the intracisternal A
type particles were found only in the intracisternal spaces, 2. they
were electron-lucent with 2 electron-dense shells, and 3. their
diameter averaged 70-8 mμ. The incidence and distribution of A type
and C type particles is presented in Table 3. A type particles
were observed at a rather high frequency in cells from both control
and infected mice. C type virus particles were observed only in
the cells from virus infected animals. The percentage of cells,
in which neither A nor C type particles were observed, was essentially similar for both groups.

TABLE 3. Frequency of Observation of Intracisternal A Type
Particles and C Type Particles in Single Anti-
body Plaque Forming Cells from Normal and FLV
Infected Mice.

Virus Particles Observed	Mouse Group	
	Control	FLV-Infected
Intracisternal A type only	16/25	3/20
C type only	0/25	4/20
Both A and C type	0/25	7/20
None	9/25	6/20

DISCUSSION

By the 4th day after immunization with sheep erythrocytes, lymphoid follicles of spleens of BALB/c mice contained many plasmacytes at different stages of maturity. As shown in this study, morphologic changes evident in intact spleens after immunization are reflected by the ultrastructural morphology of individual antibody-forming cells. The majority of the plaque-forming cells from spleens of both infected and control micr consisted of typical plasmacytic cells - both proplasmacytes (10 and 24% respectively) and typical mature plasma cells (60 and 56% respectively). Degenerated cells comprised about 20% of the PFC's observed. Two large lymphocytes were observed among the 45 PFC's examined; these cells were derived from infected mice. Harris et al. (10) had previously reported that PFC's are comprised of either lymphocytic or plasmacytic cells.

The virus-like particles (intracisternal A particles) were observed in PFC's from both control and infected mice. There have been reports that similar particles appear in the tissues of normal and germ-free mice (11,12). These particles are generally regarded as noninfectious and their exact role is not clear (13).

Previous studies concerning the immune response in leukemic animals have suggested a competition between virus and antigen for functional stem or antigen-sensitive cells as the mechanism of immunosuppression. The ultrastructural studies of intact spleen sections, from infected and immunized mice, have further supported this postulate, indicating that a marked decrease in plasmacytic cells occurred in the spleens of FLV-infected mice. This decrease paralleled the decrease in immune responsiveness, as assessed on both the cellular and humoral level. Furthermore, typical FLV particles were observed mainly in blast cells. Such observations were consistent with the concept that stem cells are the target cells of the leukemic virus. The induced deficiency in the number of PFC's in spleens of infected mice seemed due to depletion of precursor cells, rather than to infection and/or destruction of immunocompetent cells. However, the single cell studies indicate that a leukemia virus may be intimately associated with active antibody-secreting cells.

Recent studies with Rauscher virus in sarcoma tissue cultures have shown that lymphoblasts infected with the leukemia virus particles could produce a specific anti-virus antibody demonstrable by fluorescent antibody microscopy (14). Such results complement the findings reported in this study. However, it should be pointed out that Siegel et al. (15) recently reported the absence of Rauscher virus in antibody plaque-forming cells studied by electron microscopy.

Competition between leukemia virus and antigen may still be the most adequate explanation for the mechanism of virus-induced immunosuppression. Although virus might infect antibody-forming cells at all stages of differentiation and maturation, it may be that only those cells infected at an early stage are arrested in their function and proliferation, resulting in a significant decrease in the number of potential antibody-forming cells and their progenitors. Those cells infected at a later stage of differentiation, or after "commitment" to antibody formation, may maintain their function despite the presence of virus. Regardless of the actual mechanism, it seems apparent from this study that virus infection and antibody synthesis are not mutually exclusive events for individual cells.

ACKNOWLEDGEMENTS

The excellent technical assistance of Mrs. Vivian Simmons is acknowledged.

SUMMARY

The effect of infection of mice with Friend leukemia virus on single antibody-forming cells was studied. Individual plaque-forming cells from normal immunized mice were examined and found to consist almost exclusively of cells of the plasmacytic series. Virus-like intracisternal A particles were found in many of these cells. Many cells (55%) from the center of plaques derived from spleens of mice infected with FLV contained typical murine leukemia virus particles. The ultrastructure of these spleen cells was similar to that of the control animals. The results of this study indicate that leukemia virus infection and antibody formation are not mutually exclusive processes at the single cell level.

REFERENCES

1. Ceglowski, W.S. and Friedman, H. J. Nat. Cancer Inst. 40: 985. 1968.
2. Salaman, M.H. Antibiot. Chemotherapia 15:393. 1969.
3. Gomori, G. Methods in Enzymology, Edited by S.P. Colowick and N.O. Kaplan, P. 142. Academic Press, Inc. New York. 1955.
4. Luft, J.H. J. Biophys. Biochem. Cytol. 9:409. 1961.
5. Trump, G.F., Smuckler, E.A. and Benditt, E.P. J. Ultrastruc. Res. 5:343. 1961.
6. Reynolds, E.S. J. Cell. Biol. 17:208. 1963.
7. Bennett, H.S. and Luft, J.H. J. Biophys. Biochem. Cytol. 6: 113. 1959.
8. Ceglowski, W.S. and Friedman, H. Proc. Soc. Exp. Biol. Med. 126:662. 1967.
9. Movat, H.Z. and Fernando, V.P. Exptl. Mol. Path. 3:546. 1964.

10. Harris, T. N., Huemmeler, K. and Harris, S. J. J. Exp. Med. 123:161. 1966.
11. DeHarven, E. J. Exp. Med. 120:857. 1964.
12. Feldman, D. G. and Gross, L. Cancer Res. 24:1760. 1964.
13. Kindig, D. A. and Kirsten, W. H. Science 155:1543. 1967.
14. Trujillo, J. N., Hearn, M. J., Pienta, R. J., Gott, C. and Sinkovics, G. Cancer Res. 30:540. 1970.
15. Siegel, B. V., Neher, G. H. and Morton, J. Lab. Investigation 20:347. 1969.

EFFECTS OF ANTILYMPHOCYTE SERUM ON THE LOCALIZATION OF ^{125}I-LABELED FLAGELLA, COLLOIDAL CARBON, AND TITANIUM DIOXIDE IN SPLENIC LYMPHOID FOLLICLES

Rolf F. Barth[1], Robert L. Hunter[2], and John N. Sheagren[3]

[1]Department of Pathology and Oncology, University of Kansas Medical Center, Kansas City, Kansas; [2]Department of Pathology, University of Chicago, Chicago, Illinois; and the [3]Laboratory of Clinical Investigation, National Institute of Allergy and Infectious Diseases, Bethesda, Md.

Studies were undertaken in order to further define the effects of antilymphocyte serum (ALS) on the localization of antigen and colloidal particles in splenic lymphoid follicles.

Rabbit and burro anti-mouse lymphocyte sera were prepared as previously described, and were shown to markedly suppress the cellular and humoral antibody response of mice to sheep erythrocytes (1). _Salmonella_ _typhi_ (Ty 2w) flagella were prepared and iodinated with ^{125}I to a specific activity of 2.5 μc ^{125}I/μg flagella (2). BALB/c mice were injected intraperitoneally (i.p.) with 0.25 cc of ALS on days -1, -1 and 0, 0 and +1, or -1, 0, and +1 relative to the day of intravenous (i.v.) injection with 5 μg of ^{125}I labeled flagella. Mice treated with ALS had a significant decrease in the amount of labeled antigen retained by the spleen 6 days later. The effect was greatest in mice injected with ALS on days -1 and 0, with a mean splenic count of 3,150 dpm compared to 9,500 dpm for normal serum treated controls. In contrast to this, no differences were noted in the hepatic localization of antigen. Autoradiographs showed decreased follicular retention of ^{125}I flagella in ALS treated animals at 6 days, but by 43 days no significant differences were observed either in the amount of labeled antigen retained by dendritic macrophages (follicle reticular cells) or the total splenic radioactivity when compared to normal serum treated mice. The anti-flagella

Table I.   Effects of Antilymphocyte Serum on the Antibody Response
to <u>Salmonella typhi</u> Flagella

Serum Treatment	Anti-Flagella Agglutinin Titer[1] (Reciprocal Log_2)	
	ALS	Normal Serum
Day		
-1	7.3	9.3
-1, 0	8.0	9.6
0, +1	8.3	9.3
-1, 0, +1	9.0	8.2

[1]Determined 6 weeks following immunization with 5 µg of
<u>S</u>. <u>typhi</u> flagella.

agglutinin titers were only slightly depressed in ALS treated mice
at the time of peak response 6 weeks following immunization
(Table I).   These findings correlate with the observation that
there were no significant differences in the follicular localization of antigen at this time, since otherwise a more significant
depression of the IgG response might have been expected (3).   Although ALS initially affects the follicular localization of antigen
(4), this appears to be transient.

The effects of ALS on the follicular localization of colloidal
carbon and titanium dioxide (TiO_2) were also studied.   Intravenous
administration of 0.25 cc of ALS produced an immediate acceleration
in the clearance of simultaneously administered colloidal carbon
given in a dose of 0.01 ml/g weight of mouse (5).   The clearance
rate slowed to normal by about 4 hr, and impairment was demonstrated from 8 hours on.   Histologic sections taken during either
phase of clearance revealed a virtual absence of colloid in the
marginal zones of splenic lymphoid follicles in ALS treated mice
(Fig. 2) when compared to normal serum injected controls (Fig. 1).
This was evident as early as 2 hours following injection (Fig. 1
and 2), and became even more pronounced by 24 hours (Fig. 3 and 4).
In contrast to this, only slight differences were noted in the
amount of carbon localized in hepatic sinusoids.

Mice given a single dose of ALS, followed immediately by an
i.v. injection of TiO_2 (Dupont TiPure R 900), had normal follicular
localization 4 hours later.   If ALS was injected on day -1, however,

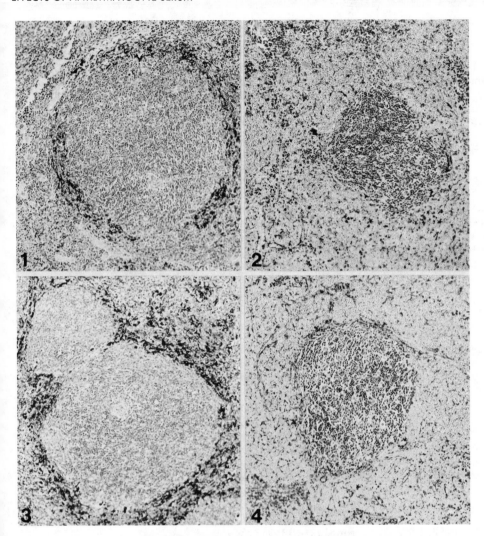

Fig. 1-4.   BALB/c mice were injected intravenously with 0.25 cc of
either burro anti-mouse lymphocyte serum (ALS) or normal burro
serum (NBS), and immediately thereafter with colloidal carbon in a
dose of 0.01 cc/g weight.   Two hours following injection of the
colloid significant amounts of carbon were seen in the marginal
zones of splenic lymphoid follicles of NBS treated mice (Fig. 1),
while in contrast virtually none was seen in ALS treated animals
(Fig. 2).   These findings were even more prominent at 24 hours
(Fig. 3 and 4).   Congestion of the splenic red pulp was noted in
ALS treated mice at both times (Fig. 2 and 4).   Formalin fixation
and stained with hematoxylin and eosin.   125 X

there was increased uptake of TiO_2 by dendritic macrophages.

The data indicate that ALS has complex effects on the follicular localization of antigens and colloids, which may result in either decreased or increased uptake and retention by dendritic macrophages. ALS may stimulate the dendritic macrophage system and be carried into the follicle, thereby reducing the amount of flagella which is transported. Decreased follicular localization may simply be a result of this competition for transport sites. It is known that TiO_2 can displace flagella (2), and if it could also displace ALS then this might explain the increased uptake which was observed in mice pretreated with serum on day -1. The effects of ALS on the clearance of colloidal carbon might be due to a reduction in the rate of perfusion of the lymphoreticular system, so as to physically prevent the interaction between colloidal particles and phagocytizing cells (5). The observed congestion of the splenic red pulp (Fig. 2 and 4) supports this hypothesis. In addition, ALS has been shown to contain opsonizing antibodies for lymphocytes (6-8), and it is possible that opsonized cells may compete with colloid thereby producing an apparent RES blockade.

In summary, the degree, duration and probably even the basic mechanisms by which ALS affects the localization of antigen and colloidal particles in splenic lymphoid follicles seems to be dependent upon the test substances used to evaluate RES activity.

Acknowledgments

This work was supported in part by Public Health General Research Grant #5 S01 RRO 5373-09. We thank Mr. J. B. Edelin for his technical assistance, Mr. G. Gsell for his excellent photography, and Mrs. Louise Conaughton for secretarial assistance.

References

1. R. F. Barth, J. Immunol., 103:648, 1969.

2. R. L. Hunter, Jr., New Physician, 15:111, 1966.

3. R. L. Hunter, R. W. Wissler, and F. W. Fitch, in Lymphatic Tissue and Germinal Centers in Immune Response, p. 101, New York: Plenum Press, 1969.

4. R. F. Barth, R. L. Hunter, J. Southworth, and A. S. Rabson, J. Immunol. 102:932, 1969.

5. J. N. Sheagren, R. F. Barth, J. B. Edelin, and R. A. Malmgren, J. Immunol. 105:634, 1970.

6. P. G. Gill, J. Immunol. 102:1329, 1969.

7. M. F. Greaves, A. Tursi, J. H. L. Playfair, G. Torrigiani, R. Zamir, and T. M. Roitt, Lancet 1:68, 1969.

8. N. B. Everett, M. R. Schwarz, R. W. Tyler, and W. D. Perkins, Fed. Proc. 29:212, 1970

ELECTRON MICROSCOPIC OBSERVATIONS IN RAT LYMPH NODES FOLLOWING

INJECTION OF AMS AND ATS

H.K. Müller-Hermelink and W. Müller-Ruchholtz

Depts. of Pathology and Hygiene, University of Kiel
W.-Germany

Studies on the _in vivo_ action of rabbit-anti-rat macrophage sera (AMS), exhaustively absorbed with rat thymocytes, revealed prolongation of allogeneic skin graft survival time in rats (fig. 1).

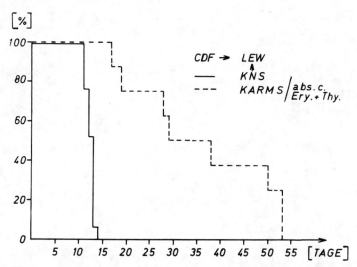

Figure 1: Survival times of allogeneic rat skin, grafted in the CDF → LEW inbred strain system (normal MST = 12.3 days): No prolongation following 2 injections of normal rabbit serum (KNS) on days +1 and +4; significant prolongation following similar application of rabbit-anti-rat macrophage serum (exhaustively absorbed with rat erythrocytes and thymocytes).

        Morphological studies were performed on regional lymph nodes
after s.c. injection to elucidate whether or not such antisera act
differently as compared to macrophage-absorbed antithymocyte sera
(ATS). It has been found that both types of antisera initiates
much faster appearing and quite different alterations than normal
rabbit serum and induce no in vivo damage to that cell type used
for absorption.

        Following the application of AMS three main observations have
been made: (1) Cytoplasmic edema of sinus macrophages followed by
complete cytolysis with appearance of cellular debris are to be
seen (fig. 2).   (2) Macrophages are phagocytosed by other macrophages, which themselves may show signs of cytoplasmic degeneration.   (3) Cortical reticulum cells, especially those localized
in the paracortical zone, show cytoplasmic edema and cytolysis.

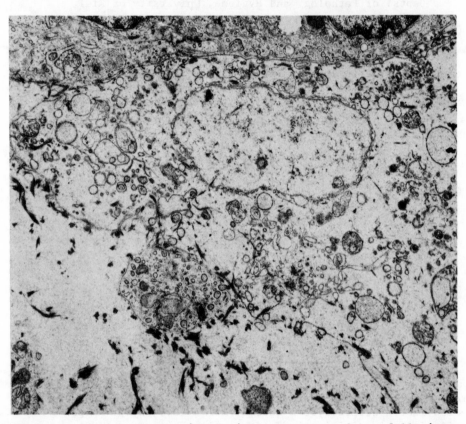

Figure 2: Complete cytolysis of sinus macrophage 2 hrs following
application of AMS: Shadowy structures of nucleus and cytoplasm
with release of cellular debris in the sinus lumen (intact sinus
wall at the bottom, sinus lumen in top of the graph).   x 17,000

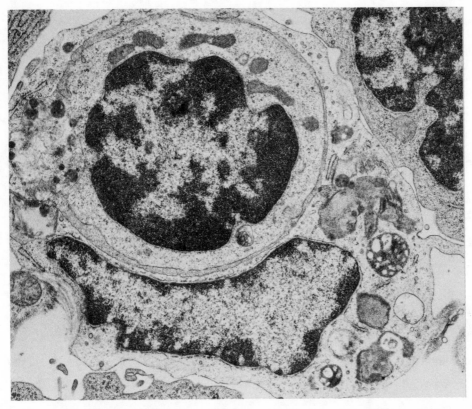

Figure 3: Phagocytosis of a lymphocyte 10 min. following application of ATS: note the almost intact structure of its cytoplasm and
nucleus. x 20,000

Following application of ATS, on the other hand, two main
types of lymphocyte damage were observed: (1) Macrophages of cortex, pulp cords and sinuses phagocytose morphologically intact
lymphocytes shortly after the injection of ATS (fig. 3). Such
cells, subsequently, are digested intracellularly. (2) Extracellular lympyocytolysis occurs in the same lymph node areas.

These morphological data may help to understand the immunosuppressive capacity of AMS.

MODIFICATION OF THE IMMUNE RESPONSE BY EXTERNAL AGENTS.

AN INTRODUCTION TO THE DISCUSSION

M. W. Hess and R. D. Stoner

Department of Pathology, University of Bern, Switzerland, and Medical Research Center, Brookhaven National Laboratory, Upton, Long Island, New York 11973 USA

In introducing the following discussion a sketchy catalog of unresolved problems will be presented rather than a review of the whole subject of this session. The problems involved in any attempt at modifying immune responsiveness by external agents may be visualized to center around: 1) the target cell system, 2) the immunosuppressive agent, and 3) the environment in which agent and target interact.

Most target cells in this context belong to the lymphoreticular system, which is composed of at least the following categories of cells: 1) a pool of non-differentiated precursor or "stem" cells; 2) immunologically competent cells; 3) immunologically active cells; and 4) a group of ancillary cells, instrumental in a more general rather than specific sense for the expression of immune responsiveness. This last group includes cells such as macrophages, mast cells, cells of the granulocytic series, and even epithelial cells. Kinetic data indicate that each of these categories of cells not only has its own mode of proliferation and differentiation pathways, but is also governed by different environmental and regulatory influences. In addition, elements belonging to the lymphoreticular system may be found at different sites of the organism, with a constant exchange of cells, however, between organs or between sites within an organ. Needless to say that the migrational behavior of lymphoid cells and of members of the group of ancillary cells again is governed by different mechanisms, many of which are unknown.

As a working hypothesis, let us assume that the following events take place in the course of an immune response: undifferentiated precursor cells, which themselves may be in a restive phase or in

455

proliferation, acquire immunological competence by differentiation.
Immunologically competent cells, a pool maintained by self-renewal
and/or feeding-in from the precursor compartment, in turn, respond
to antigenic stimulation with a wave of proliferation and differentiate into immunologically active cells; i.e., antibody-producing
elements or sensitized cells effective in cell-mediated types of
immune reactions. In addition, a population of "memory" cells is
generated, often long-lived elements largely responsible for rapid
and effective reactions in the course of anamnestic immune responses.
This scheme of events remains theoretical in nature until we know
more about 1) the identity and origin of the cells involved; 2)
pool sizes and kinetic behavior of the different cell populations;
and 3) mechanisms governing both proliferation and differentiation
at any given stage of development.

   A number of factors, called "environmental" in a rather broad
sense, are known to influence the organism's capacity to mount an
immune response. The most important among these is antigenic
stimulation. There is abundant evidence indicating that the development of the lymphoreticular system, with the relative exception
of the thymus, depends on exposure to antigenic material. This
"environmental" stimulation is neither constant with regard to its
specificity nor to its intensity. In any attempt to understand the
regulatory effect of both "environmental" and experimental antigenic
stimulation upon the kinetic behavior of lymphoid cells a number of
factors has to be taken into account, some of which have already
been alluded to in preceding sessions. The type of immune response
developing following contact with antigen is determined to some
extent by each of these factors, such as 1) chemical composition,
physical form, and amount of antigenic material; 2) route of entry;
3) primary or secondary contact; 4) antigenic competition; and 5)
cross-reactivity between antigen and preexisting antibody. It is
surprising that despite these variables the healthy organism apparently is able to exert a certain regulatory control over proliferation
and differentiation of cells of the lymphoreticular system. As we
heard from Dr. Uhr, part of this control is exerted by antibody, one
of the end products of the reaction. Other regulatory factors,
hormonal, humoral, cellular, and genetic, may be mentioned in passing.

   Among non-immunological influences on the target system, an
important role is played by the afore-mentioned ancillary cells.
With the exception perhaps of the macrophage system the function of
which has been the subject of a large number of studies, we know
little about the influence such cells, as for instance epithelial
cells, granulocytes or mast cells, may have on the overall immunologic capacity of the organism. And yet, they all participate in
some way in the inflammatory reaction which accompanies an immune
response. Surely, agents causing epithelial damage or destruction
of granulocytes indirectly influence the delicate functional balance

which ensures the integrity of the organism. This balance further
is known to be in jeopardy with advancing age: in the older organism
involution of lymphoid tissue is a common finding. It is largely
unknown whether the concomitant decline of immune functions is due
to 1) decreased numbers of immunologically competent cells or their
precursors, in the sense of an exhaustion of the "stem cell" pool;
2) a summation of somatic mutations; 3) a genetically fixed limitation of the number of successive mitoses possible within a given
cell line; 4) a functional insufficiency of immunologically active
cells; or a combination of these or other factors.

This short description of the target of immunosuppression or
immunological enhancement most certainly is incomplete. It served
only to reemphasize the discrepancy between the complexity of the
very system to be influenced and our ignorance with respect to
many mechanisms governing its functional integrity.

Turning now to the agent, a series of questions arises. Although
the problems raised are pertinent both to measures aimed at immunosuppression and to those resulting in enhanced immune responsiveness,
emphasis is placed on immunosuppressive agents. The first question,
then, may be: Does the agent reach the target? Theoretically, an
affirmative answer may be given only for whole-body radiation.
Evidence for immunosuppressive substances to reach the entire target
system are based on more or less empirical findings. It may also
be recalled in this context that none of the immunosuppressive
measures currently available act exclusively on the target system.

We can look at the problem from another angle by asking: For
what period of time and in what local dose does the agent act on
target cells? For all immunosuppressive agents, except for radiation,
this depends obviously on factors such as vascularization, diffusion,
metabolism, antigenicity, to mention just a few. Our knowledge of
the pharmacodynamics of immunosuppressive drugs, however, is frag-
mentary at present, and studies on the antigenicity of ALS and
microbial or viral agents yielded controversial results.

The next question we have to ask ourselves is: How well can the
action of the agent be timed? In view of cellular events taking
place in the course of an immune response, the administration of an
agent will result in immunosuppression only when the timing is right
with regard to antigenic stimulation. To give an example, the
effects of whole-body irradiation may be considered, the one immunosuppressive measure that can be accurately timed. It may be recalled
that the repression of both primary and secondary antibody formation
following whole-body irradiation is dose-dependent, on the one hand,
primary responses being significantly more radiosensitive than
secondary responses. On the other hand, dose-dependency varies
with the time interval between irradiation and antigenic stimulation.
In other words, relative repression of antibody formation induced

with a given radiation dose varies with the time interval between irradiation and antigenic stimulation. This time relationship directly reflects the rate of functional recovery of the lymphoreticular tissues. The cellular kinetics of recovery following a well-timed and accurate dose of whole-body radiation are highly complex. Even more experimentation is necessary to better understand the events taking place after the administration of substances we know little about with regard to their fate in the organism, their effective tissue dose, and the types of cells they affect.

A final question, at the same time the most difficult to answer: At what stage of the proliferation, differentiation and migration pathway of immunologically competent or active cells does an immunosuppressive agent or measure have to intervene in order to be effective?

Removal of a major source of non-committed lymphoid cells theoretically represents the most clear-cut possibility of achieving absolute immunosuppression. Studies on immunological deficiency states in man and results obtained in animal experiments point to the thymus and possibly to the hemopoietic system as such a source. In practice, however, immune responsiveness has never been completely abolished by experimental thymectomy, probably because absolute sterilization of the pool of precursor or stem cells is incompatible with life. Removal of lymphoid organs other than the thymus is effectively compensated for by the remainder of the lymphoreticular system. Functional compensation is facilitated by circulation and recirculation of lymphocytes. A gradual depletion of this mobilizable pool of lymphoid cells may be brought about by removal of cells from blood or lymph, for instance with the aid of extracorporeal irradiation of blood or lymph, or thoracic duct drainage. The more sessile pool of lymphocytes, such as the one in the outer cortex of lymph nodes, however, contains members of both committed and non-committed elements. Since complete depletion of this sessile population of cells is not achieved with the techniques mentioned above neither primary or secondary antibody formation nor skin homograft rejection are drastically altered even after prolonged removal of circulating lymphocytes. In contrast, removal of specifically sensitized lymphocytes by draining the lymphatics of either a regional lymph node following antigenic stimulation or the bed of a skin transplant prevents in the first case the generalization of anamnestic responsiveness, and in the second, fast graft rejection. With the use of antilymphocytic sera or immunoglobulin fractions (ALS, ALG) circulating and recirculating lymphocytes are more readily destroyed than the more sessile ones. Immunosuppressive effects of ALS or ALG, therefore, are similar to some extent to those obtained by the removal of part of the mobilizable pool of lymphocytes. Additional effects of ALS or ALG may be due in part to the consequences of an interaction with non-lymphoid cells. Morphological

and functional effects of ionizing whole-body irradiation have been
studied extensively. Radiation not only affects proliferating cells
but also those that are in a resting stage. As a general rule,
radiosensitivity decreases with increasing differentiation of the
target cell. Accordingly, most small lymphocytes and lymphoblasts
are much more sensitive to ionizing radiation than plasma cells.
Since with the aid of whole-body irradiation cells of the entire
organism are affected, information obtained in studies on radiation
induced depression of immune responsiveness may help to understand
or even predict to some extent the effects of immunosuppressive
drugs. The most effective among these interfere with DNA synthesis
or replication of cells. With better knowledge of the action and
pharmacodynamics of these agents on the one hand, and of the kinetics
of the cell system to be influenced on the other hand, we should be
in a position to monitor the proliferation and differentiation of
cells of the lymphoreticular system in a differential manner, i.e.,
without the sometimes life-threatening interference with the function
of other vital organ systems.

DISCUSSION TO SESSION 8

CHAIRMAN, M. HESS, CO-CHAIRMAN, G. W. SANTOS

Co-chairman´s remarks: The immunosuppressive drugs have been useful tools for studies of the immune response. A variety of agents (6-mercaptopurine, methotrexate, cyclophosphamide and X-ray) may under certain conditions block 7S antibody synthesis selectively in animals and man. Either 7S producing cells are more sensitive to the various agents than are 19S producing cells or the "switch" mechanism whereby 19S antibody production is converted to 7S antibody production is most sensitive to the action of these agents.

To examine this question further we employed an in vivo tissue culture technique. Mice given 300 mg/kg of cyclophosphamide cannot elicit a serological response to the injection of sheep erythrocytes. If one transfers graded doses of syngeneic spleen cells together with sheep erythrocytes to cyclophosphamide treated mice, the agglutinin titer measured 6-7 days later is directly related to the number of cells injected. If the spleen cells come from unprimed mice, the antibody produced is predominantly 19S. The transfer of spleen cells from mice previously primed with sheep erythrocytes, however, results in 7S antibody production.

In the experiments, cyclophosphamide pretreated mice were given a constant cell number of primed or unprimed syngeneic spleen cells together with sheep erythrocytes. Graded single doses of cyclophosphamide were given immediately after the cell transfer or 2 days later. Agglutinin titers were determined 6-7 days after the cell transfer. The regression lines that resulted when the mean agglutinin titers of the various groups of mice were plotted against the dose of cyclophosphamide measure the sensitivity of 19S and 7S producing cells to the agent. In each case the regression lines for 19S and 7S producing cells were parallel. Similar studies employing methotrexate and 6-mercaptopurine also indicated that 19S and 7S producing cells had equal sensitivities to these agents. These data strongly suggest that the most sensitive phase of the primary immune response to a variety of agents is the "switch" mechanism of conversion of 19S to 7S antibody production.

The germinal centers are known to be very sensitive to these agents and perhaps they function directly or indirectly in the "switch" mechanism.

G.A. Kool: I do have a remark on the work of Dr. Santos concerning the equal sensitivity of the 19S and 7S producing cells to cyclophosphamide.

In our model we used paratyphoid H vaccine as an antigen. We injected a single dose of cyclophosphamide into rats at different times before and during the primary immune response. It is known

461

that cyclophosphamide, administered from two days before until two days after antigen, will prevent an antibody titer to occur. However, cyclophosphamide given on the third day after antigen injection does not completely inhibit the antibody production.

In the secondary response, the results were reversed. A secondary response could be evoked although the primary response was completely inhibited in those animals treated with cyclophosphamide from two days before until two days after the first antigen injection. In the animals which received cyclophosphamide on the third day after primary stimulation, secondary stimulation did result in an antibody titer comparable to a normal primary response.

Now, the third day after stimulation with paratyphod H vaccine, is the day of the de novo formation of germinal centers and furthermore, the first morphological change induced by cyclophosphamide is the destruction of germinal center cells. Perhaps these results suggest a correlation between the formation of germinal centers and the production of memory cells in a cyclophosphamide sensitive phase.

D. Eidinger: We have for several years been studying antigenic competition and should like to present one slide illustrative of data pertaining to one possible underlying mechanism, one which perhaps provides an alternative to account for the work of Dr. Friedman. I should like to say that we believe this to be only one of the mechanisms operative in antigenic competition. In this work, we used a model of antigenic competition employing two antigens administered in sequence, using the first as the suppressing antigen and the second as a test antigen. One of our favorite non-cross-reacting antigen pairs has been goose followed by rat erythrocytes.

One of the questions we have posed in the past was the role of the thymus-derived cell in antigenic competition. As part of the study, we tested the percentage of theta positive cells in spleen following administration of the suppressing antigen, goose red cells. This work has been carried out by Robert Kerbel in my lab.

For those of you who are familiar with antigenic competition the change in the proportion of theta positive cells illustrated in the slide (Fig. 1) is very similar to the curve of suppression generated by varying the time interval between administration of two antigens, in that the proportion of theta positive cells slopes down sharply and is followed by a more gentle slope of recovery. One can see that the proportion of theta positive cells in the spleen following goose erythrocytes falls to a low level at 3 days, which corresponds to the time at which it is maximally suppressive in a competition system (D. Eidinger et al., J. Exp. Med., 128:1183, 1968). However, the total number of theta positive cells did not diminish and, in fact, generally exceeded the numbers contained in

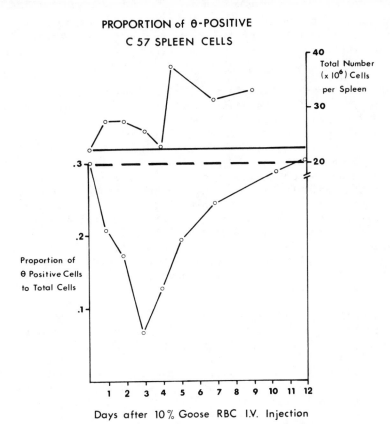

Fig. 1. Total number (upper curve) and proportion of theta positive cells in C57 spleen following immunization with goose erythrocytes.

normal spleen. Therefore, we would like to suggest that immunization with antigen simply creates a relative reduction of thymus-derived cells in the micro-environment. This in effect reduces the potential cellular interaction in which theta bearing thymus-derived cells are an essential part, to account for the immune response to the second antigen. Unfortunately, time does not permit a description of further studies which pertain to this data. Nevertheless, we should like to suggest that the above represents an attractive, simple model to account for antigenic competition compatible with clonal selection and with the data deriving from cell receptor studies.

D.G. Osmond: I would like to add some data which are complementary to the study reported by Dr. Rosse. These experiments were designed to quantitate the numerical changes in newly-formed lympho-

cytes in thoracic duct lymph and blood following 150r whole body
irradiation in Hartley guinea pigs. They are therefore comparable
with, and complementary to, the study just reported by Rosse, Tyler
and Everett.

Thoracic duct lymph was collected through a cervical fistula
in animals sampled 24-26 hours after intraperitoneal administration
of thymidine-H^3 (1 μc/g; spec. act. 1.9 c/mM) and at close intervals of up to 36 days after 150r gamma irradiation.

The total lymphocyte content of thoracic duct lymph was depleted rapidly to values of one third to one half normal by the second
day after irradiation. Thereafter, cell numbers recovered in two
main phases. Fluctuant increases towards low normal values occurred
from 2 to 9 days, but at 11-14 days counts as low as those of the
second day were observed. This secondary fall coincided with a
transient anaemia and reduction in body growth rate. Only subsequently was there a slow rise towards sustained normal values.
The same general pattern of recovery in numbers was shown by the
subpopulation of large and medium-sized lymphocytes.

Thymidine-H^3 labelled lymphocytes fell from normal values
(6.2%) to very low levels (0.22%) at 2 days, followed by approximately twice normal labelling percentages at 3-10 days, a second
minimum at 13-15 days, and finally sustained values. In absolute
numbers the labelled lymphocytes followed the same course but at no
time exceeded normal levels. The proportion of labelled large and
medium lymphocytes to labelled small lymphocytes remained unchanged
throughout, except during the first efflux of labelled cells at
2-5 days when labelled large cells predominated.

In the blood, changes in newly-formed labelled lymphocytes
resembled those in thoracic duct lymph in their timing. However,
both at 2-10 days and after 16 days the absolute numbers of labelled
lymphocytes reached over twice normal values.

Thus, following 150r whole body irradiation in the guinea pig
the reappearance of newly-produced lymphocytes occurs in two main
phases in both thoracic duct lymph and blood, reflecting apparently
abortive waves of proliferation at 2-10 days and sustained lymphocytopoiesis after 15 days. The quantitative differences in number
of labelled lymphocytes between thoracic duct lymph and blood indicate that many newly-formed lymphocytes enter the blood stream
directly in addition to those entering via the lymph.

C.C. Congdon: I would like to mention in connection with the remarks by Dr. Rosse and Dr. Hess some results on germinal centers
in irradiated mice treated with bone marrow. This work was done
with David Brynmor Thomas of Birmingham, England. It is well known
that heavily irradiated mice transfused with syngeneic bone marrow

show essentially complete recovery of the lymphatic tissue. The
number of germinal centers counted in the spleen and mesenteric
lymph node reaches very high levels by the end of one month. However, with allogeneic marrow the lymphatic tissues do not recover
completely after irradiation. The graft versus host reaction is
added on to radiation damage. The variability in recovery can be
quite extreme, however. In the mesenteric lymph node and spleen,
there was poor development of germinal centers. There is also
some evidence, I think, that lymph nodes show poorer recovery after
graft versus host than the spleen.

G.A. Kool: Dr. Rosse, if I understood you well you said the formation of germinal centers was a prerequisite for immunological competence. In your popliteal lymph nodes you did not see any germinal centers. You did see them, however, in your mesenteric lymph
nodes and in these last lymph nodes the probability of antigenic
stimulation is much greater than in the popliteal lymph node. So
I would say the formation of germinal centers is more a result of
immunological stimulation than a prerequisite for immunological
tolerance.

C. Rosse: I will not take issue with you on this. From the data
I presented one can only say that chronologically the reappearance
of germinal centers and the recovery of immunological competence
coincide in these animals.

T. Trentin: I would like to address a comment to Dr. Friedman with
reference to the theory that the Friend virus erythroblastosis
produces a suppression of plaque-forming cells by draining off uncommitted immunocyte precursors. Has it been shown that such animals suffer a serious depletion of the uncommitted CFU pool in the
bone marrow?

H. Friedman: I am really not competent to answer that. I believe
Cudkowitz is doing something like that, but I am not sure. What
we have shown is the depletion of precursor cells capable of responding to antigen after transfer to irradiated animals. On the
immunological side we have shown a depletion of immunological competent cells infected with Friend disease virus using a transfer
assay, the transferred cells were spleen cells.

J.J. Trentin: Before one could conclude that draining off uncommitted CFU is the mechanism, one would have to demonstrate that the
bone marrow pool of CFU is depleted. I would like to propose an
alternate explanation for this phenomenon. This relates to some
of the things I spoke about yesterday, about the spleen being a
house with many "rooms" each designated for different purposes.
Many of the rooms are painted red for erythropoiesis, and these
are the rooms in which the Friend virus leukemogenesis occurs.
Bennett et al. have shown that both the W anemic mouse and the

Steel anemic mouse are resistant to this virus-induced erythroblastosis. The W/W^v anemic mouse lacks the uncommitted stem cell,
but has the erythroid HIM. The Steel anemic mouse has the uncommitted stem cells, but lacks the erythroid HIM. Thus, it would
appear that the target for the virus is neither of these, but is
likely the erythropoietin-sensitive stem cell that results from
the interaction of the two. If so, it would be hard to see how
this would deplete the remaining peripheral CFU pool. As you have
pointed out, there is an explosive proliferation of erythroblasts
such that at 8 days after virus infection 90% of the spleen cells
are malignant erythroblasts. Many of them undoubtedly spill out
of the little red rooms into uncommitted hallways and into other
rooms. We know that in the spleen there are rooms for the proliferation of SRBC hemolytic plaque forming cells resulting from
interaction of thymic and marrow cells. It may simply be a matter
of physical crowding of these rooms with malignant erythroblasts.

H. Friedman: I have a list of six possible mechanisms of which
only one was the stem cell interaction, and I think our electron-
microscopic data puts that on the bottom of the list.

SURFACE ANTIGENS OF IMMUNOCOMPETENT CELLS

G.J. Thorbecke, T. Takahashi and W.P. McArthur

Dept. Pathology, New York University Sch. Med. and

Div. Immunology, Sloan Kettering Institute, New York, N.Y.

INTRODUCTION

It is now well established that in the mouse, at least in the humoral immune response to the "thymus-dependent" antigens, a synergistic cooperation between thymus-derived, "T-cells" and bone marrow, but not thymus-derived, "B-cells" takes place [1,2]. This cooperation can be shown in the primary response to sheep erythrocytes, and in the secondary response to hapten-conjugates, where the T-cells represent the so called "carrier-sensitive" cells, and memory against the two different components of the immunogenic molecule, the hapten and the carrier, appears to be represented in the B-and T-cells respectively [2-6]. Surface antigens peculiar to the T-cells, primarily the theta antigen [7-9], are very useful in the analysis of cooperation between B-and T-cells in primary [10-12] and secondary responses [11,13]. An equally useful marker for the B-cells is still lacking, although it seems reasonable to conclude from a variety of observations [14,18] that a high degree of reactivity of the cell surface with antisera to immunoglobulins characterizes a large proportion of these cells and that many if not all B-cells have a complement receptor on their surface [19]. Evidence accumulated during the last few years in this laboratory has suggested the germinal center as a site for memory cell proliferation [20]. Since germinal centers arise independently of the presence of the thymus and thus belong to the B-cell group [21], it would also be of interest to determine whether B-cell memory exists.

MATERIALS AND METHODS

<u>Animals</u>: Female BALB/c mice were obtained from the colonies

maintained in the Sloan-Kettering Laboratories or from Jackson Lab.
(Bar Harbor, Maine). White leghorn F_1 hybrid chickens (line 96),
homozygous for the major B histocompatibility locus, were obtained
as hatching eggs from the Basic Research Laboratory, Hy-line Poultry
Farms (Johnston, Iowa).

Antigens used were sheep erythrocytes (SE: obtained through
the courtesy of the Public Health Laboratories of the City of New
York) and B. abortus stained ring test antigen (BA: generously
supplied by the US Department of Agriculture, Agricultural Research
Service, Ames, Iowa).

Antisera: Allo-antiserum to θ-C3H (AKR anti-C3Hf/Bi thymocytes)
was prepared as described (22). Antisera to immunoglobulins were
prepared in rabbits, by immunization with ammonium sulfate precipitated normal mouse IgG, or by immunization with chicken γ-
globulin prepared according to Benedict (23). Anti-mouse k-chain
was obtained through the courtesy of Dr. R. Asofsky (National
Institute of Health, Bethesda, Maryland) and a chicken L-chain
preparation was generously donated by Dr. A.A. Benedict, (University
of Hawaii, Honolulu, Hawaii). Prior to use rabbit antisera to
immunoglobulin as well as normal control rabbit sera were always
absorbed with mouse or chicken thymus cells (from agammaglobulinemic bursectomized chickens) in order to remove nonspecific cytotoxicity. Such absorption did not appear to diminish their reactivity with immunoglobulin. Rabbit anti-bursa and anti-thymus sera
were made by subcutaneous immunization with 2×10^8 bursa or thymus
cells (from 4-week old chickens) in complete Freund's adjuvant.
Two weeks later the rabbits were boosted intravenously with 10^8
cells and then bled repeatedly. Antisera were heat-inactivated,
absorbed once with chicken erythrocytes, and 2 or 3 times with
either bursa or thymus cells from 4-week old chickens.

Experimental details are given in the text and in footnotes
to the tables (see also ref. 11). Cell viability was determined
with the trypan blue exclusion test. Spleen cell cultures were
prepared and maintained according to Mishell and Dutton (24) with
minor modifications for chicken spleen cells developed in this
laboratory (25). Tissue culture medium used was RPMI-1640 with 10%
fetal calf serum (Associated Biomedic Systems, Inc., Buffalo, N.Y.).

Murine plaque forming cells (PFC) were detected as described
previously (11) and chicken PFC were developed by exposure to
rabbit anti-chicken IgG followed by guinea pig C'. Results of
transfer experiments are expressed as averages of PFC numbers and
titer values obtained for 3-5 recipients per group.

STUDIES WITH MOUSE SPLEEN CELLS

Cytotoxic tests performed on cells after incubation with antisera and prior to cell transfer confirmed previous observations on

TABLE 1

ABILITY OF MOUSE SPLEEN CELLS TO TRANSFER * PRIMARY OR SECONDARY IMMUNE RESPONSES TO SE REMAINING AFTER INCUBATION WITH ANTI-θ AND C'

Mouse Serum for Pre-Incubation +	Normal Cells Added ‡	Percent of Control PFC per Recipient Spleen			
		PRIMARY	SECONDARY AFTER PRIMING FOR		
			1 WEEK	4 WEEKS	
		19S (day 7)	19S (day 4)	19S (day 6)	19S + 7S (day 6)
Normal	None	100 (40,000)	100 (6,000)	100 (6,200)	100 (74,000)
Anti-θ	None	2	3	4	1
Anti-θ	Thymus	30		16	3
Anti-θ	Spleen	<1	3	39	6
-	Thymus		2	<1	<1
-	Spleen			36	5

*) 650 r irradiated BALB/c recipients received i.v. 2 x 10^7 normal or 10^7 immune syngeneic spleen cells and were challenged with sheep erythrocytes (SE: 0.1 ml 20%). Immunization of donor mice was by i.v. injection of 0.1 ml 20% SE with 10 μg E. coli endotoxin, once (1 week) or twice at a 2-week interval (4 weeks).

+) Pre-incubation for 45 min. at 37°C with 1 ml anti-θ-C3H and 0.7 ml fresh rabbit serum (C') per 2 x 10^8 spleen cells at a final concentration of 6.7 x 10^6 cells per ml. Control cells were incubated with normal BALB/c serum and C'.

‡) For "reconstitution" of the primary response 2 x 10^7 thymus cells were injected separately and for the secondary response 10^7 normal spleen or thymus cells.

TABLE 2

ABILITY OF MOUSE SPLEEN CELLS TO TRANSFER * PRIMARY OR SECONDARY
IMMUNE RESPONSE TO SE REMAINING AFTER INCUBATION WITH ANTI-MOUSE IG AND C'

Rabbit Serum + for Pre-Incubation	PRIMARY		SECONDARY					
	% of Control PFC/recip. spl. 19S	1/log 2 HA titer recip. sera	% of Control PFC/recip. spleen				1/log 2 HA titer recip. sera	
			19S		19S + 7S			
			Exp.1	Exp.2	Exp.1	Exp.2	Exp.1	Exp.2
Normal	100 (12,800)	7.6	100 (6,000)	100 (2,300)	100 (72,800)	100 (30,600)	10.7	9.3
Anti-k	100	7.4	27	-	27	-	10.2	-
Anti-Ig	-	-	9	95	17	50	9.7	9.3

*) 650 r irradiated BALB/c recipients received i.v. 2 x 10^7 normal or 10^7 immune syngeneic spleen cells and were challenged with sheep erythrocytes (SE: 0.1 ml 20%). Immune cells were taken 2 weeks after the last of 2 i.v. injections of 0.1 ml 20% SE with 10 μg E. coli endotoxin at a 2-week interval. Recipient spleens and sera were analyzed on day 7 (primary) and day 6 (secondary) after transfer.

+) Pre-incubation for 45 min at 37°C with 0.8 ml anti-Ig or anti-k and 1.7 ml fresh guinea pig serum (C') per 2 x 10^8 spleen cells at a final concentration of 6.7 x 10^6 cells per ml. Control cells were incubated with normal rabbit serum and C'.

spleen cells. Allo-antiserum against θ-C3H killed 30 to 40% in the presence of C' (22) and rabbit anti-mouse Ig or anti-mouse k-chain killed approximately 40 to 50% (14).

The effect of incubation with anti-θ is illustrated by results of typical experiments in table 1. Several experiments were done with essentially similar results, as was shown elsewhere (11). Anti-θ treatment drastically reduced the ability of 1 to 2 x 10^7 spleen cells to transfer either a primary or a secondary response. Reduction of the numbers of PFC in recipients spleens was more than 95%, while serum hemagglutinin titers of recipients' sera suffered a 5-7 log 2 reduction. Addition of 2 x 10^7 normal thymus cells to the anti-θ treated spleen cells resulted in a reconstitution of the ability of these spleen cells to transfer a primary immune response to about 30% of the level obtained with control (normal mouse serum-treated) spleen cells. Normal thymus cells, by themselves, did not transfer a significant immune response, and were also unable to reconstitute the ability of anti-θ treated immune spleen cells to transfer a secondary response. Normal spleen cells were equally ineffective in reconstituting anti-θ treated immune spleen cells. The results obtained upon transfer of the combination of anti-θ treated long-(4 weeks) or short-term (1 week) immune spleen cells with normal spleen cells was indistinguishable from the results obtained with normal spleen cells alone, both for 19S and for 7S + 19S PFC (Table 1).

Incubation of BALB/c spleen cells with rabbit anti-Ig or anti-k was completely ineffective in reducing the ability of the spleen cells to transfer primary or short-term 19S PFC secondary responses. However, in two experiments performed on transfer of the long-term memory (4 weeks) there was a variable degree of reduction by anti-Ig treatment both for 19S and for 7S + 19S PFC (Table 2). A slight (1 log) reduction of hemagglutinin titers in recipients' sera was seen in only one of these experiments.

When antisera treated short-term (1 week) immune spleen cells were examined for their ability to form a secondary immune response in vitro the results obtained with anti-θ treated cells were exactly comparable to those of transfer experiments. Table 3 gives the results of a typical experiment expressed as averages of PFC numbers in duplicate dishes. Anti-Ig was more effective when the treated cells were tested in vitro than upon transfer to irradiated recipients and caused a 90% reduction in the ability to form a secondary response to SE.

The ability of antisera-treated BALB/c mouse spleen cells to transfer a primary or secondary immune response to BA was also examined (Table 4). The results contrasted sharply with those obtained in the transfer of the response to SE. Anti-θ treated cells were only slightly, if at all, inhibited in their ability to form agglutinins to BA, whereas anti-Ig had a severely inhibitory effect on the transfer of the primary, and a slight to moderate inhibitory effect on the transfer of the secondary response.

These results are in complete agreement with the fact that the response to bacterial antigens such as BA is much less thymus dependent in mice than the response to SE (26). In addition, these results suggest that anti-Ig and C' affect an entirely different cell type from the one killed by anti-θ and C'. Other attempts were made to affect the precursor of PFC by treatment with allo-antiserum to the PC.1 antigen of myeloma cells and PFC recently described by Takahashi, et al. (22). However, it was found that treatment with this antiserum and C' had no detectable effect on the ability of spleen cells to transfer a primary or secondary response to either SE (11) or BA (unpublished observations), and also did not affect to a significant degree the ability of immune spleen cells to form a secondary response in vitro (unpublished observations). It was concluded that the PC.1 antigen is present on differentiated B-cells, but not on their precursors.

TABLE 3

ABILITY OF MOUSE SPLEEN CELLS TO FORM A SECONDARY
IMMUNE RESPONSE TO SE IN VITRO * REMAINING AFTER
PRE-INCUBATION WITH ANTISERA AND C'

Serum for pre-incubation +	Normal cells added	% of control PFC per dish 19S
Normal mouse	-	100 (39,800)
Anti-θ	-	1
Anti-θ	Thymus (5 x 10^6/dish)	3
Normal rabbit	-	108
Rabbit anti-Ig	-	12

*) Immune spleen cells were obtained from BALB/c mice 1 week after i.v. injection of 0.1 ml 1% SE. Rocking duplicate cultures were prepared of all pre-incubated cells, at 10^7 cells per dish, challenged with sheep erythrocytes, and assayed for PFC 4 days later.

+) Conditions for pre-incubation as described in corresponding footnotes of tables 1 and 2.

STUDIES WITH CHICKEN SPLEEN CELLS

The bursa appears to contain precursors of immunoglobulin synthesizing cells in the chicken (27,28), as well as the progenitors of the germinal centers in peripheral lymphoid tissue (29, 30). Since the bursa, particularly in young chickens, is a very discrete lymphoid organ, it seemed appropiate to look for surface antigens specific for B-cells by immunizing with bursa cells. Attempts were therefore made to prepare specific antisera in rabbits to bursa and thymus cells.

The results of cytotoxicity tests performed on thymus, bursa and spleen cells are represented in table 5. These results will be published in greater detail elsewhere (31). The antiserum dilution (1/20) used in these studies was lower than needed to obtain the degree of cytotoxicity shown. It was also noted that at this concentration of antiserum the cell concentration could be varied up to 5×10^7 per ml without diminishing the antiserum effect. Although bursa cell suspensions had a rather high background level of non-viable cells, the relative specificity of the antisera was

TABLE 4

ABILITY OF MOUSE SPLEEN CELLS TO TRANSFER [*]
PRIMARY OR SECONDARY IMMUNE RESPONSES TO <u>BRUCELLA</u>
<u>ABORTUS</u> (BA) REMAINING AFTER INCUBATION WITH ANTISERA AND C'

Serum for pre-incubation [+]	1/log 2 anti-BA titer in recip. sera			
	PRIMARY		SECONDARY	
	Exp. 1	Exp. 2	Exp. 3	Exp. 4
Normal mouse	2.2	2.7	9.5	11.0
Anti-θ	1.8	2.2	8.5	11.5
Normal rabbit	-	4.7	9.5	11.0
Anti-Ig	-	0.8	7.0	10.7

*) 650 r irradiated BALB/c recipients received i.v. 2-4 x 10^7 normal or 10^7 immune syngeneic spleen cells and were challenged with 2×10^8 Brucella organisms. Immunization of donor mice was by a similar i.v. injection of BA 1 week prior to transfer. Agglutinin titers were determined in sera taken from recipients day 7 (primary) or day 5 (secondary) after transfer.

+) Conditions for pre-incubation as described in corresponding footnotes of Tables 1 and 2.

obvious. Anti-Ig showed a higher cytotoxic index for bursa than
for thymus or spleen cells. This is in agreement with results
reported by Cooper (32) who obtained suppression of bursa development by injection of anti-μ chain into chick embryos.

The ability of bursa and spleen cells to transfer a primary
response to BA has been established in previous studies (33). In
these studies it was also shown that spleen but not bursa cells
could transfer a response to SE. Although this would suggest a
similar cooperation between bursa-and thymus-derived cells in the
response to SE in the chicken as is known to occur between B-and
T-cells in the mouse (1,2), attempts to demonstrate synergism between bursa and thymus cells were not convincing (33).

Therefore, the antisera to bursa and thymus are currently
being used in this laboratory to attempt to demonstrate cooperation between lymphoid cells in the chicken. Preliminary results
of transfer experiments are shown in table 6. While the ability
of spleen cells to transfer a primary response to SE was virtually abolished by treatment with anti-thymus serum and C',
the ability to transfer a response to BA was only slightly, if
at all, affected. Anti-bursa serum did not seem to inhibit the
ability to transfer either response, nor did anti-Ig inhibit the
transfer of the response to SE.

TABLE 5

PERCENT CYTOTOXICITY IN CHICKEN LYMPHOID CELLS [*]
AFTER EXPOSURE TO RABBIT ANTISERA AND C'

SERUM	THYMUS	BURSA	SPLEEN
Anti-thymus	>95	40	56
Anti-bursa	<12	>95	38
Anti-L chain (Ig)	26	69	30
Normal	12	22	16

*) Lymphoid cells (10^7/ml from 4 week-old chickens
were incubated for 40 min. at 37° with 1/20
rabbit serum and 1/10 guinea pig serum (C')
final dilutions.

TABLE 6

ABILITY OF CHICKEN SPLEEN CELLS TO TRANSFER [*]
A PRIMARY RESPONSE TO SE AND TO B. ABORTUS (BA)
REMAINING AFTER INCUBATION WITH ANTISERA AND C'

Rabbit serum for pre-incubation [+]	% of control PFC/recip. spleen	1/log 2 anti-BA in recip. sera
Normal	100 (1100-2300)	7.1
Anti-thymus	3	6.4
Anti-bursa	100	8.8
Anti-Ig	105	-

[*) Cells were taken from 4-week old chickens, transferred intraperitoneally to 650 r irradiated, neonatal, partially inbred recipients and challenged with sheep erythrocytes (0.1 ml 20%) and BA (4 x 10^8 organisms). Recipient spleen and sera collected 7 days after transfer.

+) Conditions for pre-incubation as in corresponding footnote of Table 5, except that cells were kept at 5 x 10^7/ml.

TABLE 7

ABILITY OF CHICKEN SPLEEN CELLS [*]
TO FORM A SECONDARY IMMUNE RESPONSE IN VITRO TO SE
REMAINING AFTER PRE-INCUBATION WITH ANTISERA AND C'

Rabbit serum for pre-incubation [+]	% of control PFC per dish
Normal	100 (550-3000)
Anti-thymus	1
Anti-bursa	58
Anti-Ig	3

*) Spleen cells taken from chickens 7-10 days after i.v. injection of 0.2 ml 20% sheep erythrocytes (SE), challenged in vitro with SE, and assayed for plaque forming cells (PFC) 4 days later.

+) Conditions for pre-incubation as in corresponding footnote of Table 5.

Results of in vitro experiments were somewhat different
(Table 7). As was shown in the mouse, the ability of spleen cells
to form a secondary immune response to SE in vitro was abolished
by anti-thymus and C' as well as by anti-L chain, whereas several
anti-bursa sera examined caused a 50% reduction of the response.
Additional results suggested a comparable sensitivity to anti-Ig
of the primary response to SE in vitro confirming results obtained
by others with mouse spleen cells (34,35). Reconstitution of the
ability of antisera-treated spleen cells to form a secondary response in vitro has also been attempted. The results so far suggest
that normal spleen cells cannot reconstitute the ability of anti-
thymus treated immune spleen cells to respond to SE. However,
addition of normal spleen cells appears to restore to full activity
the anti-Ig or anti-bursa treated immune spleen cells.

DISCUSSION AND CONCLUSIONS

These observations suggest a striking similarity in the immune
response of mice and chickens to SE and BA. In both species the
response to BA is relatively unaffected, whereas the response to
SE is severely inhibited by removal of the T-cells. Anti-Ig treatment of spleen cells is much less effective in lowering their
ability to transfer immune responses than in reducing their in
vitro capacity to form a secondary response to SE. In both species
anti-Ig or anti-L chain, in the presence of C', appear to inactivate
primarily the B-cells. This does not of course, rule out the
possibility that T-cells have immunoglobulin determinants on their
surface, but are not killed by exposure to these antisera and C'.
In fact, several recent reports suggest that T-cells exert their
immunological functions by means of some immunoglobulin molecules
on their surface (36,37).

It is clear from the present results that, both in the mouse
and in the chicken, the numbers of T-cells are the limiting factor
in the primary and secondary responses to SE. Lack of reconstitution
of T-cell depleted immune spleen cells by normal spleen cells suggests
the presence of immunological memory in the splenic T-cell population,
although further studies are needed to determine the specificity of
such "memory" cells. The observation that normal spleen cells can
reconstitute the ability of anti-Ig treated immune spleen cells to
form a secondary response in vitro appears in agreement with the
observed difference between the abilities of anti-Ig treated spleen
cells upon transfer in vivo and in vitro. It would seem that, with
respect to the SE antigen, the B-cell population is present in excess
in normal as well as in immune spleen cells, and that removal of a
large percentage of these cells has, therefore, relatively little
effect.

It should be noted that the ratio of 7S + 19S/19S PFC in the
recipients' spleens after transfer of T-cell depleted long-term
immune mouse spleen cells + normal spleen cells was exactly the

same as with normal spleen cells alone, and much lower than the one
seen after transfer of untreated immune spleen cells. Since studies
of   others (38) have suggested that the precursor of the PFC in
the bone marrow determines the type of immunoglobulin to be produced,
the present findings suggest some functional activity of the T-cells
in determining which B-cells will be activated. If, however, B-
cells go from a stage of 19S antibody production to a stage of 7S
antibody production of similar specificity, then the presence of T-
memory cells may accelerate this change in the B-cells.

Since T-cells appear of relatively little importance in the
response to the BA antigen, in both species studied, it follows
that B-cells must be important in the expression of memory for the
response to BA. The inhibitory effect of anti-Ig on the transfer
of the anti-BA response is in agreement with this assumption.

ACKNOWLEDGEMENTS

These studies were supported by United States Public Health
Service grants AI-3076 and CA-08748 and by grant T-524C from the
American Cancer Society. W.P.A. is the recipient of a Stipend from
training grant 711-44-108, and G.J.T. is the recipient of Career
Development Award #2-K3-GM-15,522 from the United States Public
Health Service.

REFERENCES

1. H.N. Claman, E.A. Chaperon and R.F. Triplett, Proc. Soc. Exp.
    Biol. Med., 122:1167, 1966.
2. G.F. Mitchell and J.F.A.P. Miller, J. Exp. Med., 128:821, 1968;
    see also J.F.A.P. Miller, These Proceedings.
3. N.A. Mitchison, in: M. Landy and W. Brown, Eds., Immunological
    Tolerance, p. 149, New York: Academic Press, 1969.
4. D.H. Katz, W.E. Paul, E.A. Goidl and B. Benacerraf, J. Exp. Med.,
    132:261, 1970.
5. M. Feldman, These Proceedings.
6. E.B. Jacobson, J. L'Age-Stehr and L.A. Herzenberg, J. Exp. Med.,
    131:1109, 1970.
7. A.E. Reif and J.M.V. Allen, J. Exp. Med., 120:413, 1964.
8. M.C. Raff, Nature (London), 224:378, 1969.
9. M. Schlesinger and I. Yron, Science (Washington), 164:1412,
    1969.
10. A. Schimpl and E. Wecker, Nature, 226:1258, 1970.
11. T. Takahashi, E.A. Carswell and G.J. Thorbecke, J. Exp. Med.,
    in press.
12. E. Moller and M.F. Greaves, Eur. J. Immunology, in press.
13. M.C. Raff, Nature, 226:1257, 1970.
14. T. Takahashi, L.J. Old, R.K. McIntire and E.A. Boyse, manus-
    cript in preparation.
15. M.C. Raff, M. Sternberg and R.B. Taylor, Nature, 225:553, 1970.

16. F. Daguillard and M. Richter, J. Exp. Med., 131:119, 1970.

17. G.V. Alm and R.D.A. Peterson, J. Exp. Med., 129:1247, 1969.

18. R.E. Kaplan and G.J. Thorbecke, Cellular Immunology, in press.

19. C. Bianco, R. Patrick and V. Nussenzweig, J. Exp. Med., 132: 702, 1970.

20. G.J. Thorbecke, in: L. Fiore-Donati and M.G. Hanna, Jr., Eds., Advances in Exp. Medicine and Biology, p. 83, New York: Plenum Press, 1969.

21. B.H. Waksman, B.G. Arnason and B.D. Jankovic, J. Exp. Med., 116:187, 1962.

22. T. Takahashi, L.J. Old and E.A. Boyse, J. Exp. Med., 131:1325, 1970.

23. A.A. Benedict, in: M.W. Chase and C.A. Williams, Jr., Eds., Methods in Immunology and Immunochemistry, p. 229, New York: Academic Press, 1967.

24. R.I. Mishell and R.W. Dutton, J. Exp. Med., 126:423, 1967.

25. W.P. McArthur, Manuscript in preparation.

26. J.H. Humphrey, D.M.V. Parrott and J. East, Immunology, 7:419, 1964.

27. N.L. Warner, Folia Biol., 13:1, 1967.

28. G.J. Thorbecke, N.L. Warner, G.M. Hochwald and S.H. Ohanian, Immunology, 15:123, 1968.

29. M.D. Cooper, R.D.A. Peterson, M.A. South and R.A. Good, J. Exp. Med., 123:75, 1966.

30. H.G. Durkin, G.A. Theis and G.J. Thorbecke, These Proceedings.

31. W.P. McArthur and G.J. Thorbecke, manuscript in preparation.

32. M.D. Cooper, These Proceedings.

33. D.G. Gilmour, G.A. Theis and G.J. Thorbecke, J. Exp. Med., 132:134, 1970.

34. H. Fuji and N.K. Jerne, Ann. Inst. Pasteur, 117:801, 1969.

35. J. Lesley and R.W. Dutton, Science, 169:487, 1970.

36. M.F. Greaves, G. Torrigiani and I.M. Roitt, Nature, 222:885, 1969.

37. N.L. Warner and P. Byrt, Nature, 226:942, 1970.

38. G. Cudkowicz, G.M. Shearer and R.L. Priore, J. Exp. Med., 130: 481, 1969.

DISCUSSION OF DR. THORBECKE´S PAPER

R.K. Gershon: My question is related to the work of Dr. Thorbecke on memory-cells in the bone marrow. In collaboration with Dr. Paul at NIH, we studied the affinity of antibodies made to haptens in thymus-deprived reconstituted mice. We found that the high affinity antibodies were highly thymus-dependent, i.e. the more thymus cells present when antibodies are being made, the higher the affinity of the antibody produced. Now, since antibody acts as a marker of the bone-marrow-derived cells, this indicates that the emergence of high affinity bone-marrow-derived cells is thymus-dependent. Therefore, in the secondary response, there will be more of these cells than before antigenic stimulation and this could possibly be a form of memory in the bone marrow population.

G.J. Thorbecke: I think the mere fact that you have to immunize with the DNP-conjugate before you can boost with another DNP-conjugate to which the helper cells (T-cells) are sensitized, already shows the same thing: memory in the B-cells to the DNP-determinant.

B.D. Jankovic: Dr. Thorbecke, you have found, using cytotoxic tests, that rabbit anti-bursa serum preferentially kills bursa cells. We have tested the rabbit anti-thymus and anti-bursa sera by means of local agglutination, passive hemagglutination and cytotoxic tests, and we observed that anti-bursa and anti-thymus sera were not capable of discriminating in vitro against thymus and bursa cells (Jankovic et al., Clin. Exp. Immunol. 7:693, 1970). We attribute these results to the presence of a high number of lymphocytes in both thymus and bursa cell suspensions which were employed for immunization. My question is, therefore: Do you have any data on differential counts in suspension of thymus and bursa cells used to inject the rabbits? How do you explain this discrepancy between yours and our results?

G.J. Thorbecke: We indeed have very different results with our anti-sera, also when we tried them in vivo. Even starting administration of the antisera early after hatching in attempts to affect responses to sheep erythrocytes and Brucella abortus, there has been no effect. We have attributed this to the inability of rabbit antisera to fix chicken complement. It could also mean a difference in the type of antigen that the antisera detect on the cell surface. With respect to the specificity, both for our in vitro studies and for our immu-nization of rabbits, we have always taken cells from very young chickens, in which the organs are still relatively pure in cell types. I think that it may make a big difference in trying to get specific antisera and tests. In addition, we always absorb our anti-bursa with thymus and our anti-thymus with bursa cells.

G. Wick: I would like to support the findings in vivo which Dr. Thor-becke just mentioned. In testing antilymphocyte sera against chicken

bursa and thymus cells in goats we could not find any in vivo immunosuppressive effect which exceeded that of normal goat serum. We
also attribute this to the inability of mammalian sera to bind avian
complement. On the other hand, if we prepared our antisera in turkeys there was a very marked immunosuppressive effect. An anti-
bursa serum prepared in turkeys could, for example, completely inhibit thyroiditis which I mentioned above. Anti-thymus serum did
also prevent it to a certain extent, but not as much as anti-bursa
serum. In vitro, no specificity was detected.

SESSION 9.   TOLERANCE AND AUTOSENSITIZATION
CHAIRMAN, W. O. WEIGLE, CO-CHAIRMAN, N. ODARTCHENKO

THE SIDE EFFECTS OF HIGH ZONE TOLERANCE

Maria de Sousa, John H. Humphrey and Brigid M. Balfour

Bacteriology and Immunology Department, Glasgow University

National Institute for Medical Research, London

In the course of experiments designed to investigate the process
of germinal centre formation, it was found that the lymphoid tissues
of mice kept in a high zone tolerance regime to either HSA or lysozyme appeared to be abnormal in many ways (1). The abnormalities
affected in particular the so-called thymus-independent zones of the
lymphoid organs (2,3), namely, the primary nodules and the medulla
in the lymph nodes, the red pulp and the perifollicular area in the
spleen. It was then considered necessary to establish a base line
of the morphology of the lymphoid tissues from mice receiving repeated
injections of either antigen from birth and correlate it with the
animals' immunological capacity beyond their known inability to
respond to the tolerogenic antigen.

Mice from the C3H/Bi and the CBA strains were kept in a high
zone tolerogenic regime (0.25 mg antigen/g body weight/week given
from birth in 2 divided doses each week) to either HSA or lysozyme
and the development of their lymphoid organs followed by the histological examination of samples from groups of 5 to 8 mice killed
when aged 2-3, 5, 11 and 21-23 weeks. Selected mice from the HSA
and control groups were injected with ^{3}H-thymidine 2-3 hrs before
death and their tissues processed for autoradiography. In the older
age groups (21-23 weeks) IgG levels and antibody response to haemocyanin, pneumococcus polysaccharide type III and sheep red blood
cells were also investigated using the methods described by Fahey
and Humphrey (4).

RESULTS

During the observation period a considerable number of animals
in both experimental groups died (HSA: 15/78; LYS: 8/50) in contrast

with the untreated control group where no losses were recorded
(0/30). The highest incidence of deaths occurred when the animals
were about 2½ to 4½ weeks old; within some litters, a proportion of
the mice failed to thrive, lost weight, had ruffled fur, and eventually were either found dead or killed sick. There were no significant differences between the HSA and the lysozyme treated groups,
and within each litter males and females appeared equally vulnerable.
The body weight from mice of all groups was followed for a period of
10 weeks; it was observed that once the mice receiving the antigen
injections had thrived through the apparently critical first 4 weeks
of life, their development was no longer different from that of the
controls.

Microscopy

1) Histology. An arbitrary scale ranging from (-) to (+++) has been
devised so as to allow the plotting of histological findings against
time, because we wished to stress the importance of the overall
resulting picture (or curve) as opposed to the limited value of a
single observation at an isolated time. The meaning attributed to
each division in the scale has been summarized in Table I.

Peripheral lymph nodes (Fig. 1). The perhipheral nodes appeared
well delineated at a slightly earlier age (2 wks) in the tolerant
than in the control groups (3-4 wks). At 5 weeks, however, most
experimental mice killed and particularly those killed sick had very
small peripheral nodes and a very poor histological picture. At 11
weeks, the experimental groups appeared to have recovered and most

Table I. Arbitrary scale for the lymph node histology

-	+	+++
Poorly developed	'Quiescent' node	'Hyper-active' node
Ill-defined primary nodules or ill-defined medullary architecture, normal T. D. A.	Clearly defined primary nodules, well-defined cords and sinuses in medulla, a number of germinal centres (<5), some plasma cells. Normal T. D. A.	High numbers of germinal centres (>5, >10 in some cases), vast sheets of plasma cells in medullary cords, normal T. D. A.

+ and ++ : intermediary values

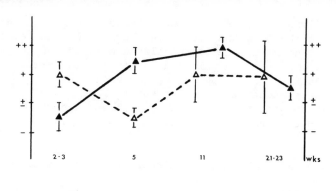

Fig. 1.   Peripheral lymph node development in tolerant and control mice.

peripheral nodes at this time had well developed germinal centres and a considerable number of medullary plasma cells. In the mice killed at later stages (21-23 wks) there was a great variation in the lymph node morphology. Although the majority of lymph nodes studied were hyperactive others had extensive atrophic lesions. These lesions did not occur in the thymus-dependent populations but consisted mainly of loss of definition between medullary cords and sinuses due to either fibrosis or extensive macrophage choking of the sinuses. There was far less variation in the peripheral lymph nodes of the control animals, and although they were not clearly defined until a slightly later age (3 weeks) than the experimental ones, they then evolved steadily without a depression at 5 weeks.

   Mesenteric lymph node. With the exception of those mice killed sick when all lymph nodes showed atrophy of the thymus-independent zones in particular of the primary nodules, the mesenteric node in the tolerant groups was generally more 'active' or responsive than the peripheral nodes. This higher responsiveness consisted of high numbers of plasma cells and germinal centres. In the control group, the mesenteric and peripheral nodes appeared to have kept in step until 11 weeks. In the older control mice, the mesenteric node was also more active than the peripheral nodes.

2) Autoradiography. Examination of the autoradiographs emphasized differences between the control and tolerant mice; the number of

labelled, i.e., dividing cells, was much higher both in the spleen and lymph nodes of the tolerant mice. In the spleen, the labelled cells belonged to the haemopoietic and plasma cell series and were found predominantly in the red pulp and perifollicular area, and in the mesenteric and inguinal lymph nodes they were also predominantly in the non-thymus-dependent zones. The autoradiographs of the spleen were particularly important, since they revealed a hyperactivity which was not deduced from the conventional histology.

IgG Levels in Adult C3H/Bi Mice Tolerant to HSA or Lysozyme

Determinations of the IgG levels in the blood of 10 mice tolerant to HSA and of 8 tolerant to lysozyme were done by the Mancini plate technique. The IgG levels were increased in all animals of both tolerant groups; the average value in the HSA tolerant group was 1.47 mg/ml (range: 0.96-2) and 1.5 mg/ml (range 1.35-1.9) in the lysozyme tolerant group, in contrast with the control value of 1.0 mg/ml.

Antibody Responses in C3H/Bi and CBA
Mice Tolerant to HSA or Lysozyme

The antibody responses were all primary responses to single first intravenous injections of a cocktail of the 3 antigens (haemocyanin, pneumococcus polysaccharide type III and sheep red blood cells). The animals were bled at 5 and 10 days after the immunizing injections. Untreated control mice of the same age were included in each experiment.

The levels of sheep cell haemolysin (not included in Fig. 2) and sheep cell agglutinin (Fig. 2) in the tolerant mice were similar to those of the controls. The antibody responses to the other two antigens, however, were very different in the tolerant and control groups (Fig. 2). Four out of the 5 control mice bled at 5 days had haemagglutination titres less than 1:10, the majority of both HSA and lysozyme tolerant mice, however, had much higher antibody titres than the controls. In the SSSIII immunized animals bled at 10 days the difference between tolerant and control mice was still obvious, though not so striking. Four out of the 7 HSA tolerant, and 3 out of the lysozyme tolerant mice had haemagglutination titres up to 1:160, only 1 out of the 5 controls had similar antibody levels. The anti-haemocyanin levels were also much higher in all HSA and lysozyme tolerant animals than in the controls, both at 5 and 10 days after immunization.

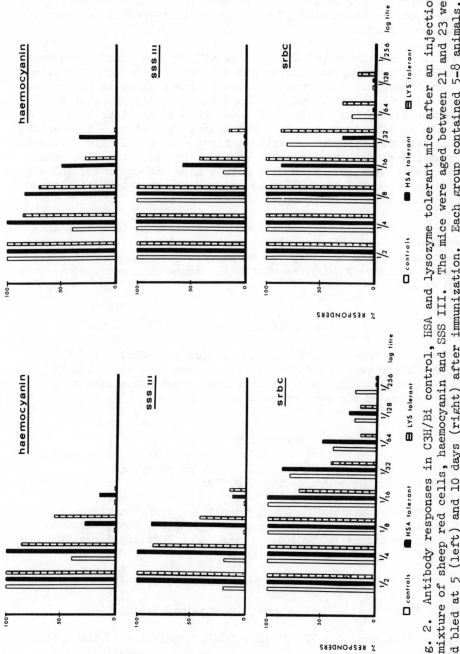

Fig. 2. Antibody responses in C3H/Bi control, HSA and lysozyme tolerant mice after an injection of a mixture of sheep red cells, haemocyanin and SSS III. The mice were aged between 21 and 23 weeks, and bled at 5 (left) and 10 days (right) after immunization. Each group contained 5-8 animals.

CONCLUSIONS

The paralysing effect of the repeated injection of an antigen from birth on the production of antibody to that specific antigen is well documented (5).

We have now investigated the 'side effects' of such a treatment using HSA and lysozyme as tolerogenic antigens on the animal's life span, development of the lymphoid tissues, immunoglobulin and antibody production to other antigens. We found that the life span of a significant number of the tolerant mice was reduced and that this coincided with an atrophy of the thymus-independent system. Those animals that survived the apparently critical first 4 weeks of life developed a 'thymus-independent hyperplasia' of their lymphoid tissues, which was paralleled by higher serum IgG levels than the controls, and also by antibody responses to SSSIII and haemocyanin that were significantly higher than those produced by the controls.

The thymus-dependent population did not seem to be so dramatically affected, and this correlated well with the antibody responses of the tolerant mice to sheep red blood cells (a well known 'thymus-dependent' antigen) which were within the range of those in the control groups.

ACKNOWLEDGEMENTS

We wish to thank Mrs. R. de Rossi, Miss J. McKinlay and Mr. H. Cairns for their valuable technical assistance. We wish also to acknowledge Miss M. Sinclair's and Mrs. E. Hough's assistance on the preparation of the typescript.

REFERENCES

1. D. M. V. Parrott, B. M. Balfour, J. H. Humphrey and M. de Sousa, these Proceedings, p. 235.

2. M. A. B. de Sousa and D. M. V. Parrott, in: H. Cottier, N. Odartchenko, R. Schindler and C. C Congdon, Eds., Germinal Centers in Immune Responses, p. 361. New York: Springer-Verlag, 1967.

3. M. A. B. de Sousa, Adv. exp. Med. Biol., 5:49, 1969.

4. J. L. Fahey and J. H. Humphrey, Immunology, 5:110, 1962.

5. N. A. Mitchison, in: B. Cinader, Ed., Regulation of the Antibody Response, Chapter II, p. 54. C. C. Thomas, Springfield, Ill., 1967.

THE MECHANISM OF BREAKDOWN OF IMMUNE TOLERANCE TO PROTEIN ANTIGEN IN RABBITS[1]

David Nachtigal

Department of Cell Biology

The Weizmann Institute of Science, Rehovot, Israel

Experimental termination of the state of immune tolerance to protein antigens has been extensively studied on the assumption that it could yield information relevant to the mechanism of unresponsiveness in general. One of the main points under discussion concerned the problem whether the abolition of tolerance to an antigen represents an authentic restoration of the previously deleted immune capacities or whether it results from an induction of a new type of antibody which cross-reacts with the tolerogen. Studies conducted on these lines demonstrated that the abolition of tolerance could elicit an antibody which displays the same specificity as that of an antibody formed by normal non-tolerant animals (1). Nevertheless, this observation can by no means serve as a proof of a genuine reversal of tolerance, since the reasoning based on it might be obsolete in the light of recent evidence. According to available reports (2, 3), immune tolerance may result from the functional elimination of specific antigen-reactive cells (ARC) and does not affect the antibody forming cells (AFC). Moreover, evidence is accumulating that the immunogenic determinants of the antigen molecule which are operative on the recognition level to interact with the ARC and those which interact with the AFC, thus presumably determining the specificity of the antibody formed, may be entirely unrelated (4, 5). Consequently, the specificity of the antibody formed as a result of termination of tolerance may have no bearing on the specificity of unresponsiveness on the cellular level which involves, apparently, antigen-reactive cells only. The study reported here presents information relevant to this problem.

[1] This work was supported by a grant from the Freudenberg Foundation for Research on Multiple Sclerosis, Weinheim, Germany .

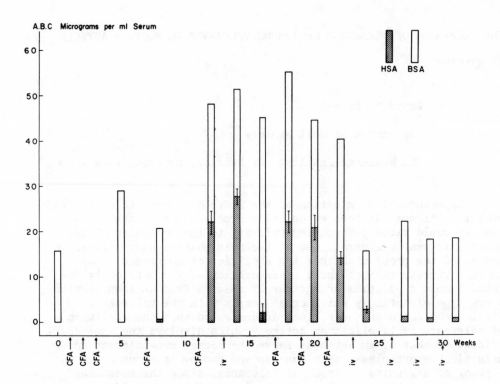

FIGURE 1.   The response of HSA-tolerant rabbits to hyperimmunization
with HSA or BSA in adjuvant.

CFA — 25 mg protein antigen given subcutaneously in complete Freund's
adjuvant; iv — 25 mg protein antigen given intravenously in saline; ABC—
the antigen–binding capacity; micrograms of ^{125}I-labeled antigen bound per
milliliter serum.

Adult rabbits were made tolerant to human serum albumin (HSA) after sublethal x-irradiation (6) and then hyperimmunized with either HSA or bovine serum albumin (BSA) incorporated in complete Freund's adjuvant (CFA). The doses were 25 mg protein per rabbit given subcutaneously at weekly intervals with a rest period between the third and the fourth injections. On the 8th week of immunization and after a total of 4 injections, an antibody to HSA could be demonstrated, irrespective of whether the animals received HSA or BSA (Fig. 1). The antibody bound ^{125}I-labeled HSA but did not precipitate the protein nor agglutinate HSA-coated sheep red blood cells. It fixed complement specifically, although most of the antibody was destroyed at 56°C. An additional feature of this response was its strict dependence on the method of immunization. Thus, when a switch was made, on week 13, from subcutaneous stimulation with antigen in CFA to an intravenous injection of the same amount of protein in saline, the antibody titer dropped to 8% of its previous value (Fig. 1, week 13) while a subsequent return to the former schedule boosted up the antibody response again. Thus, the termination of tolerance in this experiment resulted in an anti-HSA antibody which was non-precipitating (and not agglutinating), representing therefore, in all probability, a response restricted in its range of specificities (7, 8). Furthermore, since it was elicited both by the cross-reacting BSA and by the original tolerogen (HSA), it appears to be a limited response directed towards residual non-tolerized specificities shared by both antigens. Such a response could be stimulated by intensive immunization of otherwise tolerant animals and would obviously be specific for a limited number of minor determinants (9). The characteristics of this limited response remained constant throughout an immunization period lasting for nearly six months, and at about this time, the schedule was changed from antigen-adjuvant stimulation to a series of intravenous injections of antigen in saline. As a result, the anti-HSA titer dropped practically to zero, the animals demonstrated a prolonged retention of HSA in their circulation while at the same time showing a good binding of BSA (Fig. 1, weeks 27-31) and could thus be considered tolerant to HSA again. This relapse into unresponsiveness provided an opportunity to gain insight into the mechanisms operative in tolerance breakdown. Assuming that the initial state of unresponsiveness in this experiment was terminated by the boosting up of residual non-tolerized specificities, then the reinstatement of tolerance represented most probably an additional step in tolerance induction through the elimination of ARC specific for those residual determinants, thus practically exhausting the recognition potential of the animals for HSA. If this interpretation is correct, then by repeating, after tolerance reinstatement, the original schedule of immunization which terminated unresponsiveness in the first phase of the experiment, no anti-HSA response would be reproduced. To test this, the rabbits which backslided into tolerance were divided randomly into two

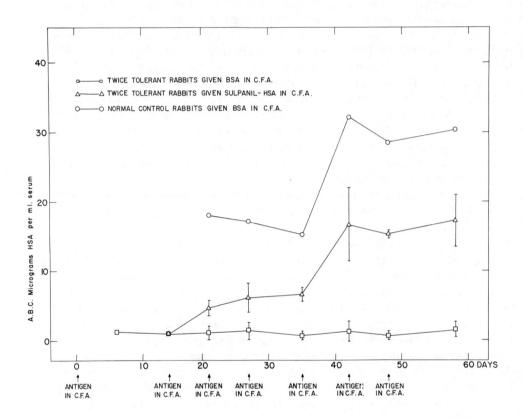

FIGURE 2. The anti-HSA response of rabbits which had been made tolerant to HSA for the second time, as compared with normal controls. Rabbits were immunized either with sulphanil-HSA or with native BSA incorporated in complete Freund's adjuvant (CFA), 25 mg antigen per dose.

ABC—the antigen binding capacity; micrograms of ^{125}I-labeled antigen bound per milliliter serum.

groups. One group received a repeat immunization with BSA in adjuvant while the other was treated identically with sulphanilated
HSA carrying about 10 sulphanilic groups per molecule. The sulphanil-HSA elicited a specific anti-HSA response after 4 weeks of
immunization. The resulting antibody could neither precipitate
HSA nor agglutinate HSA-coated cells, similarly to the anti-HSA
formed during the first phase of the study, suggesting thus also
a restricted range of specificities. It differed, however, from
the other antibody by being stable at 56° C. Contrary to this, the
BSA treated rabbits remained unresponsive to HSA when tested up to
8 weeks from the beginning of repeat immunization (Fig. 2).

In conclusion, these findings are in agreement with the assumption that immune tolerance represents a deficiency on the recognition level. Once the ARC specific for the determinants of an
antigen are completely eliminated, the animal enters a phase of
persistent tolerance. If, however, new determinants are conjugated
to the tolerogen, provided respective specific ARC are available,
the tolerogen will again become 'recognizable' and on its presentation to the AFC antibody to the native (as well as to the conjugated) specificities will be formed.

References

1. D. Nachtigal, R. Eschel-Zussman and M. Feldman, Immunology $\underline{9}$:
    543, 1965.
2. J.F.A.P. Miller and G.F. Mitchell, J. Expl. Med. $\underline{128}$:80, 1968.
3. I.A. Nabih and M. Richter, J. Exptl. Med. $\underline{130}$:165, 1969.
4. K. Rajewsky, V. Schirrmacher, S. Nase and N.K. Jerne, J. Exptl.
    Med. $\underline{129}$:1131, 1969.
5. S. Segal, A. Globerson and M. Feldman, in publication.
6. D. Nachtigal, E. Greenberg and M. Feldman, Immunology $\underline{15}$:343,
    1968.
7. J.H. Humphrey, Immunology $\underline{7}$:462, 1964.
8. C.L. Christian, Immunology $\underline{18}$:457, 1970.
9. C.R. Wyttenbach, Develop. Biol. $\underline{2}$:173, 1960.

PRESENCE OF ANTIGEN BINDING CELLS IN MICE TOLERANT

TO E. COLI POLYSACCHARIDE[1]

Olof Sjöberg

Department of Bacteriology, Karolinska Institutet

Medical School, S-104 01 Stockholm 60, Sweden

The immune response involves the appearance of antibody secreting cells (plaque forming cells, PFC) (1) as well as antigen binding cells (rosette-forming cells, RFC) (2). Howard *et al.* (3) have reported the presence of RFC in animals, which were tolerant to pneumococcal polysaccharide, as judged by the absence of a detectable serum antibody response. They suggested that antibody forming cells existed but that the antibodies produced were neutralized by excess antigen in the serum. To study if this hypothesis was true for another polysaccharide the cellular basis for tolerance towards polysaccharide of E. coli origin was examined in this study.

CBA mice were used. Tolerance was induced by repeated injections of 3 mg of alkali detoxified polysaccharide from E. coli 055:B5 (CPS) (4) and maintained by weekly injections of 3 mg of CPS. Animals tolerant to CPS showed a normal PFC response to sheep red cells (SRC).

For detection of PFC in the local hemolysis in gel assay (1) CPS was absorbed to SRC (5). Since CPS stimulates 19S antibody synthesis exclusively for a prolonged time period, only direct PFC were studied (6). RFC were assayed by the method of McConnel (7). In this test CPS was absorbed to CBA mouse red cells. Treatment with anti-theta serum was performed as described by Greaves and Möller (8).

---

[1]Supported by the Swedish Medical Research Council, the Swedish Cancer Society, Anders Otto Swärds stiftelse, and the Damon Runyon Memorial Fund (DRG-1038).

Spleen cells from normal, immune and tolerant animals were assayed for the presence of RFC and PFC (Table I). The number of RFC increases from 115 to 382 after optimal immunization. In tolerant animals, which gave no PFC response, there still existed RFC; in fact, in the "tolerant mice B" group the number of RFC was significantly higher than in unimmunized mice but was not as high as in optimally immunized animals.

Table I. Cellular immune response in spleens
of mice immunized with E. coli polysaccharide.

	$PFC/10^6$ spleen cells	$RFC/10^6$ spleen cells
Normal mice	-0.23 ± 0.23 (0.6)[1]	2.06 ± 0.07 (115)
Immune mice[2]	2.19 ± 0.08 (154)	2.58 ± 0.06 (382)
Tolerant mice A[3]	-0.23 ± 0.22 (0.6)	2.21 ± 0.14 (164)
Tolerant mice B[4]	0.66 ± 0.25 (4.5)	2.37 ± 0.04 (235)

[1]The figures are given in $_{10}$logs for the mean ± standard error. The corresponding antilogs are given in parenthesis.

[2]Immune animals were tested 5 days after the injection of 0.01 mg of CPS.

[3]Tolerant mice A were tested 5 days after the last tolerance maintaining dose of 3 mg of CPS.

[4]Tolerant mice B were given 0.01 mg of CPS 7 days after the last injection of 3 mg of CPS and assayed 5 days later.

To exclude the possibility that the rosette formation in tolerant mice is due to a binding of mouse erythrocytes to lymphocytes, the number of RFC against CBA erythrocytes was tested in normal and tolerant animals. The mean values were found to be 29 $RFC/10^6$ spleen cells in normal mice and 35 $RFC/10^6$ spleen cells in tolerant mice. CPS tends to stick to cells passively. It would therefore be possible that the RFC in tolerant animals are caused by nonspecific binding of CPS coated red cells to surfaces of lymphocytes. However, the RFC in tolerant animals were found to be inhibitable to 70-92% with rabbit anti-mouse immunoglobulin serum. It therefore seems likely that the RFC detected in tolerant mice represents an immunologically specific reaction although the presence of some nonspecific RFC cannot be excluded.

Treatment of spleen cells from tolerant mice with anti-theta serum caused an inhibition of the RFC against CPS with -16 to +18%. Spleen cells from optimally immunized animals were inhibited with -2 to 8% after the same treatment. In contrast to this RFC against SRC from animals injected 5 days earlier with SRC were inhibited with 20 to 32% (Table II).

Table II. % inhibition of RFC by anti-theta serum treatment of spleen cells.

Mice immunized to CPS[1]	8, -2, 3
Mice tolerant to CPS[2]	-4, 18, -16, -2
Mice immunized to SRC[3]	27, 20, 32, 32, 26

[1]Normal mice were immunized with 0.01 mg of CPS 5 days before the assay.

[2]Tolerant mice were injected with 0.01 mg of CPS 7 days after the last tolerance maintaining dose and their spleens assayed 5 days later.

[3]Normal mice were immunized with 4×10^8 SRC 5 days before the assay.

The present findings cannot be explained on the basis suggested by Howard *et al.* (that the tolerant state is due to neutralization of antibodies by excess antigen. Thus tolerance to polysaccharide seems to inhibit selectively the steps leading to the appearance of antibody secreting cells without affecting those resulting in RFC to a similar extent.

A number of different alternatives seem possible to explain the findings.

1. The receptors on the RFC in tolerant animals may be directed to other antigenic determinants than the antibodies secreted by the PFC in immune animals. These determinants may occur in such a low density on the sensitized SRC that antibodies against them do not cause plaques. This possibility cannot be ruled out, but seems unlikely since Humphrey *et al.* (9) found that one single hit by a 19S antibody can cause lysis of red cells.

2. Tolerant animals may contain cells actually secreting antibodies directed against the same determinants as the antibodies produced in

optimally immunized animals, which cause plaque in the local hemolysis
in gel assay, but of very low affinity (10). It would be possible
that cells producing antibodies of such a low affinity are detected
as RFC but not as PFC. This explanation seems unlikely, however, if
it is considered that the receptors on the RFC must have an affinity
sufficiently high to bind the antigen during the suspension of the
cell pellet. It is assumed in this discussion that the antibodies
produced have the same properties as the receptors on the precursor
cells for antibody production (11).

3. Tolerance induction leads to blockage of antibody secretion without affecting division and differentiation of precursor cells for
antibody production. It can be argued against this possibility that
RFC are fewer in tolerant than in optimally immunized animals.

4. Tolerance may be caused by the inhibition of division and differentiation of precursor cells for antibody production. The RFC in
tolerant animals may in that case be formed by thymus derived lymphocytes (T cells) or by bone marrow derived lymphocytes (B cells),
which do not give rise to PFC. T cells and B cells are known to
cooperate in the antibody response to certain antigens (12). The
lipopolysaccharide is not dependent on T cells in order to induce a
humoral antibody response (13, 14). This does not necessarily imply
that there are no receptors for the antigen among the T cells. The
independence of T cells for an adequate immune response to CPS may
be related to the fact that the structure of this antigen is characterized by repeating units of identical determinants. Such an antigen
may bind well to bone marrow precursor cells with multivalent receptors
and stimulate them to antibody production without the presence of T
cells. It would be possible that T cells are stimulated to respond
in tolerant animals. Such cells would be revealed as RFC but not as
PFC and may therefore be the explanation for the findings of RFC in
tolerant animals. However, as shown above, there was no inhibition
of RFC against CPS after treatment with anti-theta serum. The RFC
against CPS are therefore not likely to be T cells, but rather B cells.

It is possible that a high dose of antigen will only stop division of B cells with receptors for the antigen above a certain level
of affinity. Such cells would give rise to PFC after an optimal
immunization dose. B cells with receptors of lower affinity would
be stimulated to divide but not to produce antibodies after optimal
immunization as the energy of binding is not sufficiently high. In
tolerant animals these cells are not prevented to divide as they
escape tolerance induction due to the low affinity of their receptors.
Such cells with rather low affinity receptors could therefore be the
explanation for the RFC in tolerant animals.

A final possibility is that at least some of the RFC in tolerant
animals are inactivated precursor cells which would normally give
rise to antibodies after an optimally immunizing dose.

The lack of thymus-derived RFC to CPS may explain some features of the immune response to this antigen. The inability of T cells to increase the response is mentioned above. Low dose tolerance has not been possible to obtain to CPS, which is to be expected if low dose tolerance is caused by inactivation of TdL, as suggested by Mitchison (15). Finally, long lasting memory, which generally is attributed to TdL, is poor for CPS.

In conclusion, it was found that mice tolerant to CPS contain antigen binding cells against this antigen. In some cases the number of antigen binding cells was higher in tolerant than in unimmunized animals. It was not possible to inhibit the number of antigen binding cells against CPS, neither in tolerant nor in optimally immunized animals with anti-theta serum treatment.

REFERENCES

1. N. K. Jerne and A. A. Nordin, Science, 140:405, 1963.

2. N. R. Nota, M. Liacopoulos-Briot, C. Stiffel, and G. Biozzi, C. R. Acad. Sci., 259:1277, 1964.

3. J. G. Howard, J. Eisen, G. H. Christie, and R. G. Kinsky, Clin. Exp. Immunol., 16:513, 1969.

4. S. Britton, Immunology 16:513, 1969.

5. G. Möller, Nature (Lond.), 207:1166, 1965.

6. S. Britton and G. Möller, J. Immunol., 100:1326, 1968.

7. I. McConnell, A. Munro, B. W. Gurner, and R. R. A. Coombs, Int. Arch. Allergy 35:209, 1969.

8. M. F. Greaves and E. Möller, Cellular Immunology (in press).

9. J. H. Humphrey and R. R. Dourmashkin, in: Ciba Foundation Symposium on Complement, G. E. W. Wolstenholme and J. Knight, Ed., p. 175. London: Churchill.

10. G. A. Theis and G. W. Siskind, J. Immunol., 100:138, 1968.

11. O. Mäkelä, A. M. Cross, and E. Rouslahti, in: Cellular Recognition, R. T. Smith and R. A. Good, Ed., p. 287. Appleton-Century-Crofts.

12. G. F. Mitchell and J. F. A. P. Miller, Proc. Nat. Acad. Sci., 59:296, 1968.

13. B. Andersson, personal communication.

14. G. Möller, personal communication.

15. N. A. Mitchison, personal communication.

CELLULAR AND HUMORAL ASPECTS OF "HIGH AND LOW DOSE" TOLERANCE TO

SHEEP ERYTHROCYTES IN MICE[1]

Herman Friedman

Departments of Microbiology, Albert Einstein Medical

Center and Temple Univ. Med. School, Phila., Pa.,U.S.A.

The mechanism of specific immunologic tolerance is still poorly understood (1-3). Nevertheless, it is widely recognized that any new information concerning tolerance induction might also have significant bearing on understanding the equally unresolved problem of antibody formation. In this regard, several studies have shown that immunologic tolerance can be induced with sub-immunogenic doses of antigen, either in neonatal or adult animals, thus giving rise to the concept of "high and low zones" of tolerance (4,5). Most studies concerning low zone tolerance were based on work with serum protein antigens. Recent reports, however, indicate that tolerance also can be achieved in two dose ranges to strongly immunogenic bacterial antigens, as assessed by serum antibody titrations (6,7).

Cellular aspects of tolerance have, in general, been limited to the "high dose" range. One of the earliest uses of the immuno-plaque procedure for enumerating antibody forming cells was concerned with hemolysin forming cells in rodents given sheep red blood cells (RBC) as newborns or adults (7-9). For example, repeated injections of the RBCs into adult rats appeared to induce immunologic tolerance, as demonstrated by a marked suppression in appearance of antibody plaque forming cells (PFC) in the spleens of treated animals. However, there was no concommitant decrease in the level of serum antibody. In contrast, similar tolerance-inducing injections of RBCs into newborn rats resulted in a marked decrease of both PFCs and serum antibody. However, no distinction was made between the high efficiency (19S) and low efficiency (7S)

[1] Supported in part by research grants from the U.S. National Science Foundation (GB 6251X).

PFCs. Similar studies in this laboratory showed that repeated injections of sheep erythrocytes into adult mice markedly stimulated appearance of low-efficiency 7S hemolysin-forming cells, with a simultaneous decrease in the number of 19S PFCs. On the other hand, repeated injections of the red cells into newborn mice suppressed both 19S and 7S antibody forming cells, as well as serum antibody (10-12).

Since the mechanism of unresponsiveness induced by repeated injections of RBCs was unclear, it seemed of value to examine the effect of antigen dose on tolerance induction. Thus, a schedule of injections, as well as dosage range, was utilized similar to that employed by others with bacterial antigens (6,7). Newborn mice were given graded doses of erythrocytes and both direct (19S) and indirect (7S) PFCs enumerated. One of the goals of the study was to ascertain if "high" and "low" dose tolerance could be achieved.

METHODS AND MATERIALS

For these experiments litters of newborn NIH albino A mice were injected daily with sheep RBCs for a period of 2-3 weeks, starting on the day of birth. The antigen dose ranged from 10^4 to 10^{10} RBCs per injection. Representative mice from each group were tested for the presence of splenic PFCs, both 19S and 7S, before and after challenge immunization, using the direct and indirect hemolytic plaque assays (13,14). At least 3-5 mice were tested before challenge immunization. For post-challenge studies, groups of mice were injected with 4×10^8 S-RBC at either 14 or 21 days of age and the number of PFCs appearing in their spleens determined 4 days later. Serum antibody titers were also determined, before and after challenge, using the standard microtiter assays for hemagglutinins and hemolysins. 2-mercaptoethenol (2-ME) treatment was used to estimate presence of 7S and 19S hemolysins. The degree of responsiveness was assessed in relation to the responses of normal, non-treated mice challenged at the same age.

RESULTS

Immunization of 2 to 4 week old mice with 10^5 to 10^9 RBCs resulted in rapid appearance of splenic PFCs and humoral antibody (Table 1). Although the magnitude of the response varied among the age groups, the peak of the response occurred on the 4th day, regardless of age or antigen dose. In general, mice given 5×10^7 RBCs responded with the largest number of PFCs. The lower dose (10^5 RBCs) resulted in fewer PFCs, especially in the youngest mice (Table 1).

Table 1 - Cytokinetics of antibody plaque response in spleens of mice immunized with different doses of sheep erythrocytes at several ages.

Age at immunization[a]	Antigen dose (RBC)	Day after immunization[b]				
		2	4	7	10	15
14 days	5×10^5	785	1,930	1,500	1,150	658
	5×10^7	1,200	7,350	5,310	4,250	2,150
	5×10^8	1,350	6,950	6,830	5,700	2,350
21 days	5×10^5	1,250	10,300	5,100	2,300	1,560
	5×10^7	2,350	12,650	6,450	3,150	2,700
	5×10^9	2,850	11,360	10,650	7,310	6,050
28 days	5×10^4	1,650	21,000	12,100	5,300	1,230
	5×10^7	3,500	36,500	19,650	6,350	4,500
	5×10^9	4,650	32,400	31,300	17,500	12,300

[a] Groups of mice immunized at age indicated by i.p. injection of several doses of sheep RBCs.
[b] Average PFC response of 3-5 mice on day indicated.

Mice given daily injections of sheep RBCs during the first 14 days of life had a markedly different response. As seen in Table 2, very few PFCs, either 19S or 7S, were present before challenge immunization in mice given the lowest doses of antigen (10^4 to 10^7 RBCs). However, mice given the 10^8 to 10^{10} doses from birth generally had moderate numbers of PFCs in their spleen prior to challenge at 14 or 21 days. The largest number of pre-challenge 7S PFCs were present in the "high dose" treated mice tested at 21 days of age (7 days after the last injection of RBCs).

Table 2 - Effect of daily injections of neonatal mice with indicated dose of sheep erythrocytes on appearance of splenic PFCs before challenge immunization.

RBC dose for neonatal injections[a]	Number of splenic PFCs before challenge at age indicated			
	14 days		21 days	
	19S	7S	19S	7S
None	< 100	< 100	<100	< 100
10^4	< 100	< 100	<100	<100
10^5	< 100	< 100	<100	< 100
10^6	< 100	<100	<100	< 100
10^7	< 100	<100	< 100	389
10^8	452	265	493	1,120
10^9	321	134	365	963
10^{10}	120	<100	<100	284

[a] 2-3 litters of mice injected i.p. for 14 days, starting on day of birth, with indicated antigen dose.
[b] Average response of 3-5 mice per group at age indicated; 7S PFCs detected by enhancement with anti-gamma globulin serum.

The development of serum antibody before challenge is of particular interest. As can be seen from Fig. 1, mice given the smallest and largest doses (RBCs) had insignificant titers before challenge, either at 14 or 21 days of age. However, the other groups showed considerable serum antibody activity, ranging from 1:8 to 1:64. Except for the mice given 10^{10} RBCs, the highest titers occurred in serum specimens from mice given the largest doses of antigen.

After challenge the different groups responded with varying numbers of PFCs and serum titers. As can be seen in Fig. 1, mice given the largest doses of antigen (10^9 and 10^{10} RBCs) responded with relatively few PFCs when challenged at 14 days of age. Similarly, mice given 10^5 RBCs also had very few PFCs, either 7S or 19S, after challenge. On the other hand, the 10^6 RBC dose stimulated an enhanced response, with large numbers of both 19S and 7S PFCs. The mice given 10^4, 10^7 or 10^8 RBC doses responded relatively similar to the controls as far as 19S PFCs were concerned; these mice also developed moderate numbers of 7S PFCs.

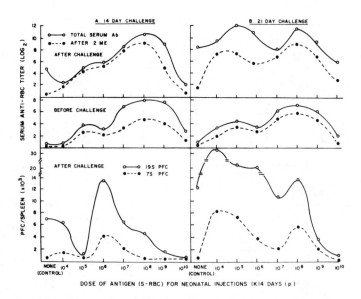

Fig. 1 - Cytokinetics of antibody plaque response (lower panels) and serum antibody (upper panels) to sheep erythrocytes in mice treated as neonates with daily injections of graded doses of RBCs. Each point indicates average response of 3-5 mice treated with indicated dose of antigen and then challenged with 4 x 10^8 RBCs at 14 days of age. PFC responses and serum anti-RBC titers determined 4-5 days after challenge immunization.

The serum antibody response after challenge also was markedly influenced by the dose of antigen used for neonatal injections (Fig. 1). Mice given the 10^8 antigen dose showed the most marked post-challenge response; these animals, however, had not developed the largest number of splenic PFCs.

A different pattern of responsiveness appeared when challenge occurred at 21 rather than 14 days. Control mice of this age responded with nearly twice as many 19S PFCs as compared to the younger mice. Following challenge, mice treated with the two largest antigen doses evinced tolerance, with very few 19S and 7S PFCs in their spleens. Mice given 10^8 RBCs repeatedly responded with the same number of 19S PFCs as the controls, but showed many more 7S PFCs. Mice given one log less RBCs (10^7) responded with fewer PFCs, both 19S and 7S. However, those animals given the three lowest doses of antigen responded with the most PFCs after challenge, exceeding the control level by 10,000 or more PFCs. All of these mice developed relatively large numbers of 7S PFCs, with the largest number in mice given the smallest dosage (10^4 RBCs).

The serum antibody titers after challenge immunization at 21 days paralleled the cellular responses. Before challenge most of the mice had significant titers, with somewhat lower activity in mice given the highest and lowest doses. After challenge most of these mice responded with relatively large amounts of 2-ME resistant antibody, regardless of antigen dose. Even the mice given the 10^{10} RBC dose had a moderate hemolysin titer after challenge.

DISCUSSION AND CONCLUSIONS

The major point which emerges from these studies is that immunologic tolerance, at least on the cellular level, may occur in two zones after neonatal injection of mice with sheep erythrocytes. However, the nature and mechanism of this unresponsiveness is not clear. Earlier work had shown that newborn animals given repeated injections of relatively large doses of sheep RBC developed a marked immunosuppression as manifested by decreased responsiveness to challenge immunization with the red cells (10-12). The present study confirmed and extended those observations. Graded doses of sheep RBCs were used for the neonatal injections. It was anticipated that no "low dose" tolerance could be achieved with a complex particulate antigen such as erythrocytes. Nevertheless, a dose as low as 10^5 RBCs, injected daily starting on the day of birth, induced unresponsiveness as profound as that obtained with a dose 100,000 times greater (10^{10} RBCs). Such "low dose" unresponsiveness was apparent, however, only when mice were challenged immediately. Delay of challenge immunization until day 21 resulted in an anamnestic like response in the low-dose treated mice. In contrast, mice given the largest RBC doses during neonatal life were still unresponsive. Thus, the different levels of responsiveness among the groups appeared to be a function of both time and antigen dose.

The apparent lack of correlation between serum antibody activity and the number of splenic PFCs in the different mouse groups
was noteworthy. Except for mice in the highest antigen dose
groups, most animals showed significant levels of serum antibody
to the RBCs, both before and after challenge immunization. Furthermore, much of the antibody was resistant to 2-ME, suggesting
the presence of 7S IgG. Even those mice which showed depressed
numbers of PFCs after challenge had significant levels of 2-ME
resistant antibody after challenge.

Despite the several inconsistancies discussed above, the
results of this study appear to support the concept of high and
low dose tolerance (4-7), and extend this phenomenon to include
complex particulate antigens. In this regard, several possible
mechanisms may be considered to explain the marked unresponsiveness
occurring in the mouse groups given these differing antigen doses.
Among these obviously is the possibility of an "overloading" or
masking phenomenon in mice given the largest doses of RBCs (1-3).
At the other extreme is the possibility of serum antibody-mediated
"feedback" suppression (15,16). Thus, one of the essential
questions to be answered is the importance of serum antibody, as
well as the low number of PFCs, before challenge immunization.

It is not difficult to reconcile the "high dose" tolerance
results of this study with similar studies by others using various
soluble and particulate antigen. One explanation for high dose
tolerance suggests that large concentrations of antigen, especially
when administered over a prolonged time period, may "drive"
precursor cells into antibody formation, without concommitant
induction of "memory cells" (17,18). Depletion of such cells would
result in failure of a subsequent response due to exhaustion of the
relevant cell types. This hypothesis predicts that antibody forming
cells should develop during tolerance induction. Thus, the PFCs
before challenge in this study may reflect this effect by antigen,
especially with the repeated high doses.

The "low dose" tolerance, on the other hand, may more likely
reflect the "feedback" type suppression. Neither of these explanations, however, take into account the apparently important role of
macrophages and/or other "processing" cells during the initial
stages after antigen administration. Furthermore, it is now
generally recognized that there are various cell-to-cell interactions
during antibody formation. This may also occur during tolerance.
The role of thymus and bone marrow derived cells in the responses
of both the high and low antigen dose treated mice remains to be
elucidated more fully in the sheep RBC system. In addition, it
should be remembered that the sheep erythrocytes offer a mosaic of

antigens to the test animals. The responses to different surface
antigens of the red cells cannot be readily differentiated by the
hemolytic plaque assay, especially since PFCs with specificity to
any one of many RBC determinants should induce similar hemolytic
plaques.

Despite the aforementioned shortcomings, further studies with
this model may provide additional information of direct relevance
to tolerance. The hemolytic plaque assay provides a system for
direct assay of the immune response, as well as its absence, on
both the cell and serum level.

SUMMARY

Neonatal mice were injected daily for 14 days with graded
doses of sheep erythrocytes, ranging in concentration from 10^4 to
10^{10} RBCs, starting on the day of birth. The number of splenic
antibody plaque forming cells and the level of serum antibody to
the erythrocytes were determined before and after challenge immunization with sheep red blood cells at 14 and 21 days of age. Except
for the high and low dose groups, most mice had significant levels
of serum antibody before challenge, although the number of splenic
PFCs was low.

Mice given both the largest and smallest doses of antigen
responded with the fewest immunocytes after challenge at 14 days.
Mice given intermediate doses had an "immunity hump" after
challenge. Both 7S and 19S antibody forming cells were stimulated
in these mice, as was 2-mercaptoethanol resistant serum antibody,
indicative of 7S globulins. Only those mice treated with the
largest doses of antigen showed tolerance when challenged at 21 days
of age. The low dose groups responded with an anamnestic-like
response, with many 7S PFCs.

These results appear to confirm and extend the concept that
two doses of antigen can induce tolerance. However, the incon-
sistency between serum activity and the cell response suggests that
different and possibly opposing mechanisms might be involved. These
differences could be compounded by the heterogeneity of the immune
response to a particulate antigen as complex as xenogeneic
erythrocytes.

ACKNOWLEDGEMENT

The capable assistance of Mrs. Leoney Mills and Mrs. Joyce
Thompson during this study is acknowledged.

REFERENCES

1. R.T. Smith, Adv. Immunol., 1:67, 1961.

2. D.W. Dresser and N.A. Mitchison, Adv. Immunol., 8:129, 1968.

3. T. Hraba, Monographs in Allergy, 3, S. Karger Co., N.Y., 1968.

4. N.A. Mitchison, Proc. Roy. Soc., B., 161:275, 1965.

5. G.J. Thorbecke and B. Benacerraf, Immunol., 13:141, 1967.

6. M. Shellam and G.J.V. Nossal, Immunol., 14:273, 1968.

7. G.J.V. Nossal, K.D. Shortman, J.F.A.P. Miller, G.F. Mitchell and J.S. Haskill, Cold Spring Harbor Symp. Quant. Biol., 23:396, 1967.

8. D.A. Rowley and F.W. Fitch, J. Exp. Med., 121:671, 1965.

9. F.W. Fitch and D.A. Rowley, J. Exp. Med., 121:683, 1965.

10. H. Friedman, in Immunological Tolerance, ed. by M. Landy and W. Braun, Academic Press, p. 32, 1969.

11. H. Friedman, Nature, 205:508, 1965.

12. J.L. Allen and H. Friedman, Fed. Proc. 28:767, 1969.

13. N.R. Jerne and A.A. Nordin, Science, 140:405, 1963.

14. J. Sterzl and I. Riha, Nature, 208:858, 1965.

15. J.W. Uhr and J.B. Baumann, J. Exp. Med., 113:935, 1961.

16. K. Sahier and R.S. Schwartz, Science, 145:395, 1964.

17. E. Sercarz and A.H. Coonis, in Mechanisms of Immunological Tolerance, ed. by M. Hasek, A. Lengerova and M. Vojtiskowa, Academic Press, N.Y., p. 73, 1962.

COMPARATIVE STUDIES OF ANTIGEN INJECTED INTO ADULTS AND NEONATAL RABBITS

Justine S. Garvey

Division of Chemistry and Chemical Engineering

California Institute of Technology; Pasadena, California

Tolerance induced in newborn rabbits (1-4) by an injection of soluble protein antigen resulted in a state of specific unresponsiveness that was dependent in duration upon the amount of antigen injected at birth. Influenced by these findings Medawar (5) modified an earlier definition of tolerance to read: "if an animal is exposed to an antigen before it has developed the capacity to react against it, then the development of that capacity is delayed and, in the continued presence of antigen, can be indefinitely postponed." Within the past decade, additional investigations have confirmed and extended the earlier findings, but the lack of information on antigen handling by the neonate and the questionable persistence of antigen during maturation provide justification for the present studies.

MATERIALS AND METHODS

Antigens and Injection Procedures

Several litters of newborn rabbits were used in the following studies, in which one-half the litter was injected intraperitoneally with antigen as soon after birth as possible (but no longer than 12 hours post-partum) and the remaining littermates were injected at the same time with an equal volume of saline (controls). Two soluble antigens were prepared as described in Ref. 6a with a specific radioactivity of 10 μCi/mg protein; only one of these was used per a litter, either ^{35}S-sulfanilate-bovine serum albumin (^{35}S-BSA) or ^{35}S-sulfanilate-keyhole limpet hemocyanin (^{35}S-KLH).

Sampling and Assay Procedures

Pairs of littermates, one antigen-injected and the other a control were sacrificed at varying times, 12 hours to 6 weeks after injection. Blood was collected both with and without the addition of acid citrate dextrose (ACD); a hematocrit was determined on the former and serum was collected from the clotted blood. Serums were stored at -20°C and assayed by passive hemagglutination (6b) at one time when the collection of samples had been completed for a litter. Blood and bone marrow smears were prepared and excised tissues (liver, spleen, thymus, and nodes) were sampled for histology. The technique of radioautography was essentially as detailed in Ref. 7; the staining of tissue sections with basic fuchsin and fast green was done prior to coating with liquid emulsion. The blood and bone marrow smears were left unstained or were treated with benzidine reagent prior to the processing as radioautographs, after which they were stained with May-Grünwald-Giemsa stains. In addition to the blood smears prepared at the time animals were killed there were also previous small bleedings made by cardiac puncture in order to follow the hematocrit and cellular observations on the same animal at varying periods of maturation.

In addition to the simultaneous tissue assay of a control littermate with an antigen-injected individual, use was made of an occasional control animal of 3-6 months of age which had not been injected previously with antigen to test for adult handling of antigen that was injected intraperitoneally as a 20 mg. dose.

Urine samples were also collected, beginning at 12 hours after antigen injection, continuing at daily intervals for approximately two weeks, and thereafter at intervals of 2-3 days until the animals were sacrificed. Whole urine was used in passive hemagglutination assays (6b) and passive cutaneous anaphylaxis (PCA)(6c) to test for the presence of antibody and in agar diffusion slide tests (6d) to test for the presence of antigen and specific serum antibody.

RESULTS

Failure to Detect Circulating Antibody

The following evidence of unresponsiveness was noted: Passive hemagglutination tests on serums obtained from animals injected with antigen at birth were negative for the presence of antibody. The animals were in a state of unresponsiveness as indicated by the failure to produce circulating antibody when reinjected as adults of 3-6 months of age with the same antigen; the latter test was not routine as most animals were killed without antigen reinjection in order to study in tissues the persistence of a single antigen injection given at birth.

Cellular Detection of Antigen in Tissues

In spleen, nodes and thymus the little antigen that was observed was on freely circulating erythrocytes in the vascular system of the tissue. The liver presented a remarkably different finding in that veins were seemingly filled with erythrocytes that were coated with the antigen and the tissue gave much evidence of active hematopoiesis. In Fig. 1A, both these features are evident as the erythroid precursor cells are the abundant cells which, because of their staining deeply red with the fuchsin stain, are easily visible. It is only with higher magnification of a microscopic field, Fig. 1B, that the pale nuclei of hepatocytes are seen, the latter seemingly crowded by the erythroid cells, and lacking cellular organization characteristic of the adult, Fig. 2, which was from a control littermate that remained uninjected with antigen until three months of age.

At one week after neonatal injection, the very significant amount of antigen that continued to be present on erythrocytes in the liver vascular system is demonstrated in Fig. 3A; the extravascular presence of antigen on erythroid cells and the cellular changes in the liver are seen in another microscopic field, Fig. 3B.

At four weeks, Fig. 4, the findings are similar except some antigen seems more closely associated with the hepatic cells and a greater degree of maturation is likewise obvious. The illustrations represent ^{35}S-BSA as antigen but the findings were similar for ^{35}S-KLH. Other tissues than the liver continued to show little uptake of antigen although intravascular erythrocytes were frequently observed that were coated with antigen.

Hematological Findings

The finding of erythrocytes coated with antigen in the hepatic venules, led to hematological studies to determine the extent to which these cells circulated. (It had been determined as noted previously that erythrocytes coated with antigen were present in other tissues, although not so abundantly as in the liver.)

Hematocrit readings were not significantly different for control and injected neonates and likewise for the immature animal compared with the adult. Despite similar red cell masses, there was a lower cell count per unit blood volume in the perinatal period than after development to an adult, the cellular differences that are apparent in blood smear radioautographs, Figs. 5 and 6, being regularly observed. In 5A, where antigen is associated at 12 hours after neonatal injection with cells that are fairly mature erythrocytes

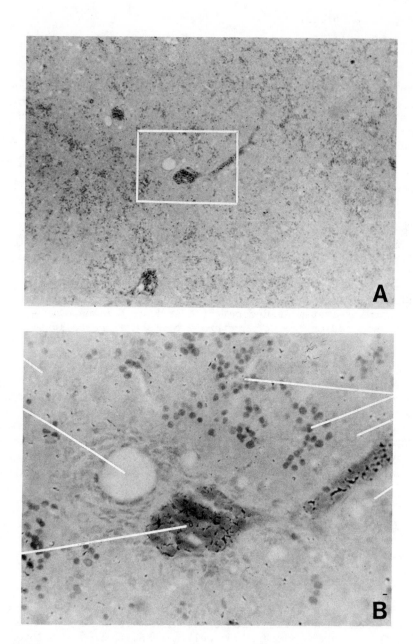

Figure 1. Radioautographs of liver tissue from a rabbit of age 1-2
days, sacrificed one day after injection of ^{35}S-BSA. A. 100 x;
B. 400 x; a-artery, v-vein, h-hepatoblasts, ep-erythroid precursors,
c-capillary. (Magnification factors in this and other figures refer
to optics of microscope.)

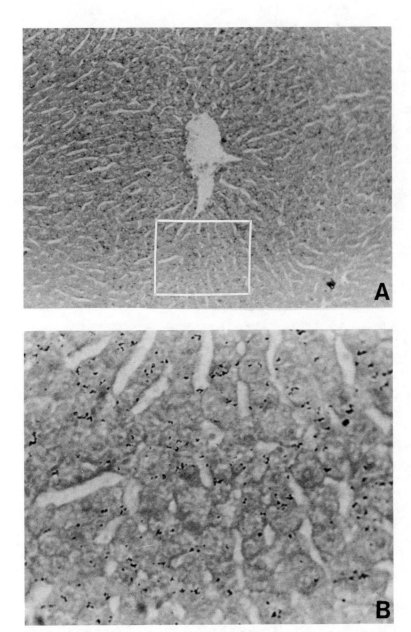

Figure 2. Radioautographs of liver tissue from an adult rabbit, sacrificed 3 weeks after one injection of ^{35}S-BSA. A. 100 x; B. 400 x.

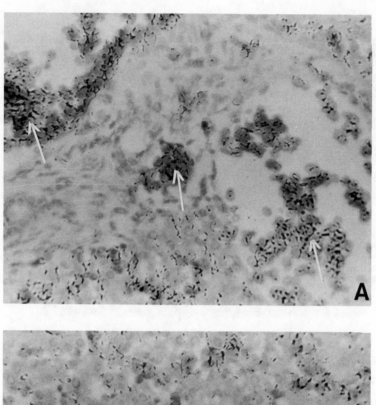

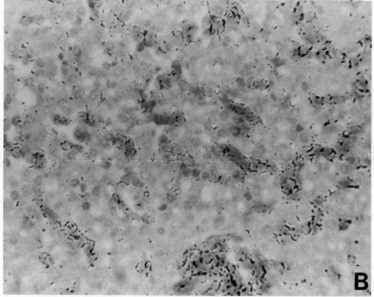

Figure 3. Radioautographs of liver tissue from a rabbit of age about one week that was sacrificed 6 days after injection of ^{35}S-BSA (400 x). A. to show masses of erythrocytes with adherant antigen; B. another field to indicate relative changes in cell types compared to Fig. 1.

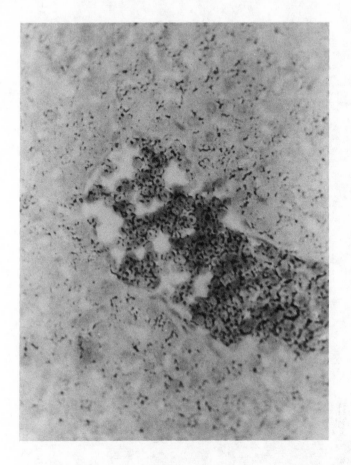

Figure 4. Radioautograph of liver tissue from a rabbit, age and time after injection of ^{35}S-BSA, 4 weeks (400 x).

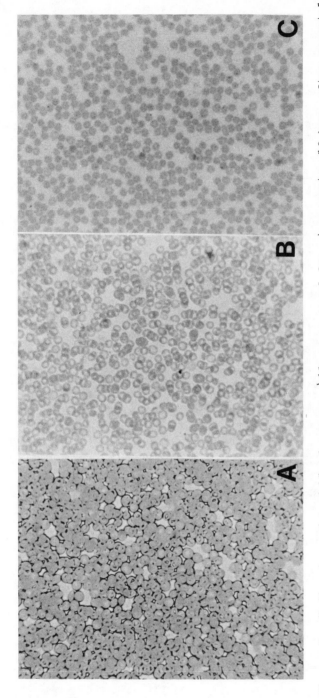

Figure 5. Radioautographs of blood smears, 400 x, prepared from A. neonate, 12 hrs. after neonatal injection; B. control, noninjected littermate of same age, and C. adult, 12 hrs. after initial injection of 35S-BSA at 3 months of age.

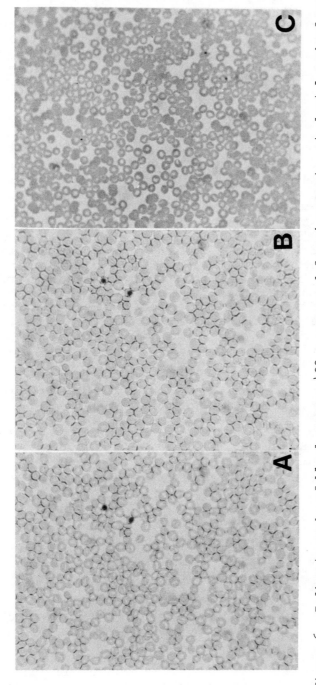

Figure 6. Radioautographs of blood smears, 400 x, prepared from A. neonate, at about 1 week of age, with focus on cells; B. same field as A with focus on grains, and C. control, noninjected littermate of same age.

on the basis of the benzidine test for hemoglobin there are no background grains in the radioautograph and in this respect, there is
similarity to 5B, the control littermate with no antigen injection,
whereas in 5C of an adult, injected 12 hours earlier with ^{35}S-BSA,
the background has a general distribution of grains and a lack of
antigen uptake on cells. Radioautographs A and B in Fig. 6 were
prepared with blood obtained one week after neonatal injection of
^{35}S-BSA, and C in the same Fig. was with blood obtained from a
littermate control of the same age. Although present in fewer
numbers, erythrocytic cells coated with antigen were still apparent
in blood sampled at 4-6 weeks after neonatal injection.

Tests for Antigen and Antibody in Urine and Bile

^{3}H-aniline-azo-bovine serum albumin (^{3}H-BSA) is being compared
currently with ^{35}S-BSA as an antigen for tolerance induction. In
the course of this investigation urine and bile are being collected
routinely for characterization of antigen and detection of antibody.
Since the histological findings of cellular uptake of ^{3}H-BSA appear
similar to ^{35}S-BSA, it may be assumed tentatively that the results
from the more extensive testing of ^{3}H-BSA urines are generally
representative of ^{35}S-BSA. The agar diffusion tests for antibody
in urines were positive for several days following the neonatal
injection, but in the same group of samples, only those collected
during the period of 1-2 days following injection, tested positive
for BSA antigen. These results were supported by PCA tests (6c).
Passive hemagglutination test results were less definitive and
apparently require fractionation (8) prior to testing. Radioactivity,
although not characterized, has been found in the gall bladder whenever sampled in the period 12 hours to 6 weeks after neonatal
injection. The presence of antibody has been investigated in some
bile samples, with the finding of both antigen and antibody for at
least four weeks following neonatal injection of ^{35}S-KLH antigen.
Positive findings by agar diffusion were confirmed by the PCA reaction.

DISCUSSION

An experimental model that gives consistent induction of neonatal tolerance, as generally assayed, has been used to investigate
cellular handling of antigen. The findings indicate an involvement
by erythrocytic cells that is undoubtedly of quantitative, and perhaps
qualitative importance, in the handling of antigen. The liver is the
site of production for these erythrocytic cells, the extravascular
production in rabbit liver having been observed earlier by Sorenson
(9) and McCuskey (10). Characteristic membrane properties may account
for the uptake of antigen by these particular cells and not by erythrocytes at a later stage of development. The erythrocytic cells found
in the liver coated with antigen circulate, and are readily observed

in blood obtained by heart puncture and in the histological preparations of various tissues. Whether such an erythrocyte has merely a
transport function or engages in some antigen processing is not known.

The possibility of antigen undergoing a different metabolic fate
in the neonate compared with the adult as a result of the involvement
with erythrocytic cells in the former has not been approached in
these studies. However, the finding of antibody in the urine and in
the gall bladder is positive evidence for some antibody production,
and together with the finding of antigen on circulating erythrocytic
cells suggests that the latter cells may effectively absorb antibody
thus accounting for the patchy appearance of the antigen-coated cells
in the blood smears (Figures 5A and 6A, 6B), the lack of background
grains in same, and the failure to detect antibody in the serum.

Although radioautographs of liver tissue, example Fig. 4, do
not indicate clearly whether antigen is within the hepatocyte cytoplasm as occurs in the adult tissue (Fig. 2), the presence of radioactivity in the contents of the gall bladder would indicate that
antigen has not only passed through hepatocytes but been processed
en route. The finding of antibody in the gall bladder leads to
consideration of the liver in antibody production. The finding of
antibody in the liver is generally associated with pathological
conditions (11-13), the interpretation being that lymphocyte and
plasma cell infiltration is responsible for the antibody produced.
Since lymphoid cells migrate into liver tissue under "normal" conditions
of antigenic stimulation of adult rabbits and show an increase in such
activity following secondary injections (14), it would seem possible
for an undetectable level of antibody to be produced "normally" in
the liver by lymphoid cells functioning alone or interacting with
cells in the liver. The relative lack of lymphoid cells in the neonatal liver, assuming all the precursor cells observed are erythroid
(9), leads to a consideration of the hepatic cell for the secretion
of either pre- or complete antibody. Whether migrating lymphoid
cells have mainly the function of transporting antibody or producing
it, their absence in the neonate would be a significant factor in
tolerance assayed as a lack of circulating antibody. Support for
these ideas are provided in a recent paper (15) concerned with the
multiple functional units of a liver lobule. One of these, the
sinusoid-central venule functions in erythropoiesis (and was easily
observed in the present investigation because of the presence of
associated antigen, Fig. 1). Another unit is the hepatic cell-
interlobular lymphatic that functions in the secretion of protein.
If the latter is the route of secreted protein rather than into the
central venules, as maintained in Ref. 15, then it seems not surprising
that antibody production like other separate specialized activities
of liver tissue would be observed only under exaggerated conditions
such as development, stress and disease.

CONCLUSION

Evidence has been provided that a fairly mature erythrocytic cell, originating in the extravascular tissue of the liver is involved in the uptake of antigen injected into the neonatal rabbit. The same cell with associated antigen has the capacity of pervading the vascular system of all tissues and of monitoring antigen and antibody on a widespread basis. The presence of antibody in low levels in secretions other than serum was demonstrated in preliminary tests of urine and bile; such antibody would evade detection under the usual experimental conditions that are the criteria for unresponsiveness. If the present findings pertain generally to other states of unresponsiveness, then modification of current concepts of the phenomenon will be required.

ACKNOWLEDGMENTS

The excellent technical assistance of Miss Betty Aalseth and the financial support from United States Public Health Service Research Grant No. AI 01355 from the National Institute of Allergy and Infectious Diseases are gratefully acknowledged.

REFERENCES

1. R. Hanan and J. Oyama, J. Immunol., 73:49, 1954.
2. B. Cinader and J. M. Dubert, Proc. Royal Soc. London, Ser. B Biol. Sc., 146:18, 1956.
3. F. J. Dixon and P. H. Maurer, J. Exptl. Med., 101:245, 1956.
4. R. T. Smith and R. A. Bridges, J. Exptl. Med., 108:227, 1958.
5. P. B. Medawar, in: M. Hašek, A. Lengerová and M. Vojtišková, Eds., Mechanisms of Immunological Tolerance, p. 17. Proc. Symposium, at Prague, Nov. 8-10, 1961. London & New York: Academic Press, 1962.
6a.D. H. Campbell, J. S. Garvey, N. E. Cremer, and D. H. Sussdorf, Methods in Immunology (2nd ed.), New York: W. A. Benjamin Inc., p. 135, 1970.
  b.Ibid. p. 283.
  c.Ibid. p. 360.
  d.Ibid. p. 250.
7. J. S. Garvey and D. H. Campbell, Nature, 209:1201, 1966.
8. J. S. Garvey, D. H. Campbell and M. L. Das, J. Exptl. Med., 125:111, 1967.
9. G. D. Sorenson, Am. J. Anat., 106:27, 1960.
10. R. S. McCuskey, Anat. Rec., 161:267, 1968.
11. J. B. J. Soons and H. G. K. Westenbrink, Bull. Soc. Chim. Biol., 40:1803, 1958.
12. S. Hadziyannis, T. Feizi, P. J. Scheuer and S. Sherlock, Clin. exp. Immunol., 5:499, 1969.

13. F. Paronetto and H. Popper, in: O. Westphal, H. E. Bock and
    E. Grundman, Eds., Current Problems in Immunology, Bayer-
    Symposium I, p. 213, New York: Springer-Verlag, 1969.
14. J. S. Garvey, in: O. J. Plescia and W. Braun, Eds., Nucleic
    Acids in Immunology, p. 487, New York: Springer-Verlag, 1968.
15. E. H. Bloch, Ann. N. Y. Acad. Sc., 170:78, 1970.

CHAIRMAN'S INTRODUCTION TO THE DISCUSSION

INDUCTION AND TERMINATION OF IMMUNOLOGICAL UNRESPONSIVENESS

W. O. Weigle, J. M. Chiller, and C. G. Romball

Department of Experimental Pathology, Scripps Clinic

and Research Foundation, La Jolla, California, U.S.A.

I would like to open the discussion by both commenting on the speaker's data and presenting some data obtained in our laboratory concerning the early events involved in the induction of immunological unresponsiveness. The presentation by de Sousa and Humphrey suggests that an active process is involved in the induction of unresponsiveness to protein antigens in new born mice, resulting in early maturation of the lymphoid tissue. The data presented by Sjöberg and Friedman indicate that this active process may involve the stimulation of antigen reactive cells and/or antibody producing cells. Previous work of others has demonstrated that an induction period is required for the establishment of unresponsiveness. This induction period varies from several hours with in vitro exposure of competent cells to certain bacterial antigens (1, 2) to 24 hours and 5 days with in vivo exposure to bovine serum albumin (BSA) (3) and pneumococcal polysaccharide (4), respectively. Using deaggregated human gamma globulin in mice, approximately 4 days of in vivo exposure was required before establishment of the unresponsive state was complete (5). However, most of the cells in the spleen were unresponsive 6 hours after exposure to the tolerogen (6). The point to be discussed is whether the induction period involved in the establishment of unresponsiveness requires the production of antibody. In addition, the data presented by Nachtigal, concerning the termination and return to the unresponsive state, warrants some comments.

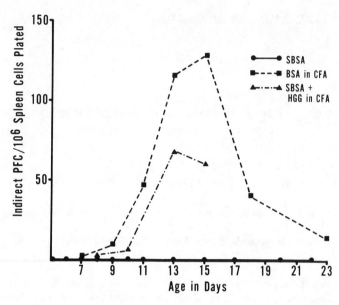

Fig. 1. Cellular response of neonatal rabbits following injections of soluble BSA or BSA in complete Freund's adjuvant (CFA) or soluble BSA and HGG in CFA.

CELLULAR EVENTS INVOLVED IN THE INDUCTION OF
IMMUNOLOGICAL UNRESPONSIVENESS

The injection of rabbits with 500 mg of BSA during the first five days of life results in an unresponsive state that lasts for at least six months. During the first 22 days after the first injection of BSA, given on the day of birth, groups of the rabbits were sacrificed periodically, and their spleens assayed for direct and indirect plaque forming cells (PFC) to BSA (7) using a modification of the Jerne plaque technique (8). At no time during the 22 day period of time were PFC cells to BSA detected (Fig. 1). The failure to find PFC to BSA was specific since the injection of both 500 mg of soluble BSA and human gamma globulin (HGG) incorporated in complete Freund's adjuvant resulted in PFC to HGG but not to BSA. Neonatal rabbits, however, are capable of responding to BSA if injected in certain forms. The injection of rabbits on the day of birth with BSA incroporated in Freund's adjuvant results in the appearance of PFC to BSA in the spleen which peaks on day 15. In addition, rabbits injected on the day of birth with 0.5 mg of heat-aggregated HGG made an excellent cellular response to HGG which also peaked on day 15. The cellular response (PFC) in adult rabbits to aggregated HGG peaked on day 5, but was not significantly greater than the response in neonatal rabbits. It would appear from these results that if an active process is occurring in the lymphoid systems of neonatal rabbits undergoing the induction of unresponsiveness, this process does not involve the synthesis of circulating antibody. The present data do not rule out expansion of populations of antigen reactive cells, a possibility suggested by Dr. Sjöberg's data with Escherichia coli polysaccharide. In view of Dr. Garvey's results showing a difference in the association of antigen with erythrocytes in neonatal and adult rabbits, it is of interest why rabbits respond to either aggregated proteins or proteins incorporated in adjuvant, but become unresponsive following injections of the same proteins in soluble form. It would be important to determine the association of both soluble HGG and heat-aggregated HGG with the hemopoietic tissue of neonatal rabbits. It also has been shown that adult A/J mice rendered unresponsive to HGG by injection of 2.5 mg of deaggregated HGG contain neither direct or indirect PFC to HGG during the first 20 days following injection (9).

Adult rabbits apparently can be made unresponsive to BSA by daily injections of large amounts of soluble BSA (10). In these experiments, it was extremely difficult to verify the existence of a responsive state because of the presence of large amounts of the antigen in the circulation. More recently, the immune response in adult rabbits receiving daily injections of BSA was assessed using the Jerne plaque technique to enumerate PFC to BSA. Adult rabbits were injected daily with one gram of BSA for 36 days. Periodically, groups of the rabbits were sacrificed and their spleens assayed for PFC to BSA. The number of $PFC/10^6$ spleen cells for each individual rabbit is plotted (Fig. 2) and compared with the response detected in normal rabbits injected with 20 mg of aqueous BSA. The response in both situations reaches a peak between the ninth and thirteenth days. In the rabbits receiving daily injections of one gram of BSA, no significant number of PFC were observed after the twentieth day, despite the continuing injections of BSA. Although these results could possibly be explained by "feedback inhibition" as suggested by Friedman for SRBC, the transient appearance of antibody forming cells is most likely the result of recruitment of precursor cells and exhaustive differentiation of memory cells. A similar exhaustion of memory cells to pneumococcal polysaccharide probably occurs in rabbits immunized with intact pneumococci and later injected with pneumococcal polysaccharide (11). It may be of interest to know if antibody producing cells are present in the mice studied by de Sousa and Humphrey and whether appearance of such cells is transient.

TERMINATION OF IMMUNOLOGICAL UNRESPONSIVENESS

The termination of immunological unresponsiveness in rabbits following the injection of cross-reacting antigens is well established (12). This phenomenon is characterized by the ability of

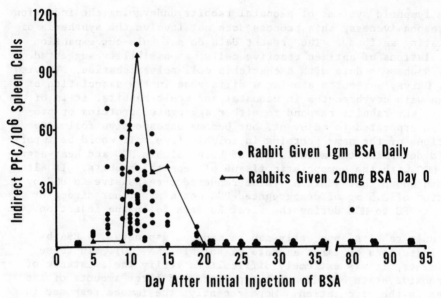

Fig. 2. Cellular response (PFC) of rabbits given daily injections of large amounts of aqueous preparations of BSA.

the rabbits to respond to subsequent injection of the previously tolerated antigen for a limited period of time. The antibody produced following the subsequent injection of the tolerated antigen is directed only to the determinants related to the antigen used to terminate the unresponsive state and can be completely absorbed with this antigen, the rabbits return to the unresponsive state, as evidenced by the results of Dr. Nachtigal. More recently, it has been shown that rabbits rendered unresponsive to BSA by neonatal injections of 500 mg BSA make a normal response to cross-reacting antigens, provided that they receive no additional injections of BSA (13). These rabbits also remain unresponsive to the determinants on BSA not shared with the cross-reacting antigen. Both the amount and quality of antibody to BSA is the same in the unresponsive and normal rabbits. The presence in the unresponsive rabbit of a normal cellular potential to produce antibody to BSA suggests the presence of a normal complement of precursor cells. All the events involved in the termination of unresponsiveness to BSA could be explained if the site of unresponsiveness was at the thymus derived cell and the bone marrow derived cells were unaffected. If both thymus and bone marrow derived cells are required for an immune response to heterlogous serum albumins in rabbits, as has

been shown for BSA in mice (14), unresponsiveness at either population would result in an unresponsive state. In fact, it has been
shown with HGG in mice that if either cell type comes from an unresponsive recipient, it is unable to participate with normal cells of
the other cell type in reconstituting irradiated recipients (15).
However, both thymus and bone marrow cells become unresponsive in
mice injected with deaggregated HGG. Drs. Chiller and Habicht have
recently shown that the unresponsive state in the bone marrow is
unstable and disappears with time, leaving only the thymus cells
unresponsive. Since a three month period of time takes place between the induction of unresponsiveness to BSA in the rabbit and
the injection of cross-reacting antigens, it seems unlikely that
the bone marrow derived cells are still unresponsive. Although the
thymus derived cell population is unresponsive to BSA, there are
present thymus derived cells which can react with determinants on
cross-reacting albumins that are unrelated to BSA and then present
the BSA related determinants to the normal complement of competent
precursor cells specific for these determinants. There is some
evidence that the thymus and bone marrow derived cells interact _via_
different antigenic determinants on the same molecule and that the
antibody is produced to the determinants specific for receptors on
the bone marrow cell (16, 17). The inhibition of the termination
of the unresponsive state to BSA by simultaneous injections of BSA
may be the result of reinducing unresponsiveness in the bone marrow
cells. Dr. Nachtigal's difficulty in terminating the unresponsive
state induced to human serum albumin (HSA) in irradiated rabbits
would be expected if either the unresponsive state in the precursor
cell was not yet lost or the unresponsive state in the precursor
cells was reinforced by the injection of HSA used to test for unresponsiveness. It also has not been possible to terminate the unresponsive state to HGG with cross-reacting antigens in mice which
both the thymus and bone marrow cells are known to be unresponsive
to HGG.

ACKNOWLEDGEMENT

     Publication No. 441 from the Department of Experimental
Pathology, Scripps Clinic and Research Foundation. Supported by
the American Cancer Society Grant T-519, United States Public Health
Service Grant AI 07007 and Atomic Energy Commission Contract AT
(04-3)-410. William O. Weigle is a recipient of United States Pub-
lic Health Services Research Career Award No. 5-K6-GM-693. Jacques
M. Chiller is supported by a Dernham Fellowship (No. J-166) of the
California Division of the American Cancer Society.

REFERENCES

1. S. Britton, J. Exptl. Med., _129_: 469, 1969.

2. E. Diener and W. D. Armstrong, J. Exptl. Med., 129: 591, 1969.

3. N. A. Mitchison, Immunology, 15: 531, 1968.

4. P. Matangkasombut and C. V. Seastone, J. Immunol., 100: 845, 1968.

5. E. S. Golub and W. O. Weigle, J. Immunol., 99L 624, 1967.

6. J. M. Chiller and W. O. Weigle, In preparation.

7. J. M. Chiller, C. G. Romball and W. O. Weigle, In preparation.

8. J. C. Daniels and W. O. Weigle, J. Immunol., 101: 1233, 1968.

9. G. S. Habicht, J. M. Chiller and W. O. Weigle in: I. Richa and J. Sterzl, Eds., Developmental Aspects of Antibody Formation and Structures, New York, Academic Press, 1970.

10. F. J. Dixon and P. H. Maurer, J. Exptl. Med., 101: 245. 1955.

11. B. Benacerraf in: M. Landy and W. Braun, Eds., Immunological Tolerance, p. 6. New York, Academic Press, 1969.

12. W. O. Weigle, Natural and acquired immunological unresponsiveness, Monographs in Microbiology, World Publishing Company, Cleveland, 1967.

13. D. C. Benjamin and W. O. Weigle, J. Exptl. Med., 132: 66, 1970.

14. R. B. Taylor, Nature, 220: 611, 1968.

15. J. M. Chiller, G. S. Habicht and W. O. Weigle, Proc. Nat. Acad. Sci., 65: 551, 1970.

16. K. Rajewsky, V. Schirrmacher, S. Nase and N. F. Jerne, J. Exptl.Med., 129: 1131, 1969.

17. N. A. Mitchison in: M. Landy and W. Braun, Eds., Immunological Tolerance, p. 149, New York, Academic Press, 1969.

DISCUSSION TO SESSION 9
CHAIRMAN, W. O. WEIGLE, CO-CHAIRMAN, N. ODARTCHENKO

F. W. Fitch: The phemonenon of antigenic competition has been mentioned several times at this meeting. I would like to present
briefly some data obtained in my laboratory by Robert Waterston
which indicates that antigenic competition is not due to competition
for cells. Rather, the phenomenon appears to be the result of
regulatory processes operating in the animal, probably to reduce
the number of responding antibody-forming units. At various intervals after intravenous immunization with 5×10^8 pig erythrocytes
(PRBC) DBA/2 mice either received an intravenous injection of 10^8
sheep erythrocytes (SRBC) or spleen cells suspensions were prepared
and cultured *in vitro* with SRBC using the method of Mishell and
Dutton. The number of cells forming antibody to SRBC were enumerated
4 days later using the hemolytic plaque assay.

As other workers have found, prior injection with PRBC depressed
the response of the intact mouse to SRBC (Table I). This depression
was maximal when the interval between injection of the two antigens
was about 4 days. Paradoxically, spleen cells from mice previously

Table I. Spleen anti-sheep erythrocyte plaque-forming cell response
of mice immunized with sheep erythrocytes at various intervals after
immunization with pig erythrocytes.

Interval between pig and sheep erythrocytes	Anti-sheep erythrocyte plaque-forming cells per spleen
1	94,000 ± 23,320
3	58,500 ± 2,110
4	36,750 ± 6,750
7	46,750 ± 9,490
No prior immunization	112,000 ± 12,960

immunized with PRBC had an augmented response to SRBC in culture
(Table II). This augmentation of the response to a second antigen
was maximal when the interval between exposure to the two antigens
was about 4 days. Cell dilution experiments and analysis of the

Table II. Anti-sheep erythrocyte plaque-forming cell response of
mouse spleen cultures prepared at various intervals after immunization with pig erythrocytes.

Interval between immunization of the mouse and initiation of spleen cell culture	Anti-sheep erythrocyte plaque-forming cells per 10^6 cultured cells
2	262 ± 15
4	502 ± 18
6	312 ± 16
8	270 ± 13
No prior immunization	110 ± 7

kinetics of the response indicate that the augmentation of the
response in culture is due to an increase in number of one of the
cell types usually present in limiting numbers. The inhibition of
the response in the animal (antigenic competition) appears to be
due to regulatory processes, probably involving production of small
amounts of antibody, which reduce the number of antibody-forming
units responding to antigen.

        The augmentation of the *in vitro* response to a second antigen
as a result of prior exposure to a "competing" antigen indicates
clearly that antigenic competition observed in the animal is not
due simply to competition for responding cells. It is likely that
the heightened reactivity observed in culture occurs because humoral
and perhaps other regulatory factors operating in the intact animal
are no longer present. Additional studies should yield information
concerning the control mechanisms which regulate the immune response
of the intact animal.

G. Wick: I want to comment briefly on a topic concerned with the
formation of germinal centers after sensitization. The obese strain
of White Leghorn chickens is afflicted with a hereditary, spontaneously occurring, thyroiditis which develops very early in life.
These chickens have circulating auto-antibodies demonstrable by a
variety of methods. Thyroid is severely infiltrated, mainly by
large mononuclear cells, many of which can be identified as plasma
cells. The most prominent finding in the thyroid is, however, a
tremendous number of germinal centers. This high number of germinal

centers, 50 to 100 per cross-section, is by no means an exception in this strain.

Bursectomy on the day of hatching is followed by a significant decrease of incidence and severity of the disease, when checked seven weeks later, as well as of the incidence of thyroglobulin-auto-antibodies. If bursectomy is performed *in ovo*, thyroiditis is even more impressively reduced. On the other hand, neonatal thymectomy has an opposite effect, with a severe infiltration and an increased incidence of auto-antibody formation in 90 to 100% of the thymectomized animals. We feel that it is a fortunate coincidence that such a model occurs in the chickens in which the immune system is functionally and anatomically dissociated into a thymus-dependent and a bursa-dependent part. It might become a very convenient tool to study the pathogenesis of this and perhaps other auto-immune diseases at the cellular level.

O. Mäkelä: Dr. de Sousa, would you consider the possibility that while you paralyze the cells that have reasonable affinity for HSA, you simultaneously immunize cells whose affinity is too low for conventional antibody assays but whose products contribute to the immunoglobulin levels?

M. A. B. de Sousa: Yes, that is precisely what we feel.

N. L. Warner: Could you comment on the quantitative immunoglobulin levels in the tolerant mice?

M. A. B. de Sousa: Yes. There is some increase in the IgM, but it is not as marked as in the IgG.

N. R. Sinclair: Could you take sera from tolerant animals and look for low affinity antibodies by trying to induce rosette-forming cells?

M. A. B. de Sousa: I could not answer that, but that is perhaps something we can consider doing.

R. D. A. Peterson: Dr. Nachtigal, is the disappearance of antibody after the i.v. injection just the consequence of antigen-antibody complex formation?

D. Nachtigal: This is a very durable suppression, but of course the present method does not allow comparison with what happens in animals remaining tolerant throughout their life span. However, formation of antigen-antibody complexes brings about an accelerated elimination rate of antigen from the body. As I mentioned, we found just the opposite phenomenon, which is characteristic of genuine tolerance.

R. D. A. Peterson: So antibody levels did not pop back the next few days?

D. Nachtigal: No.

R. A. Phillips: Dr. Sjöberg, I have two questions. First, how would you call the rosette-forming cells, particularly in normal non-immunized mice? Would you call them T-cells, B-cells, or background antibody-producing cells? Second, Dr. Miller and I have been using cell separation techniques to study the initiation of the immune response to sheep erythrocytes in mice: on the basis of these experiments we would suggest that all B-cells are rosette-forming cells, while functional T-cells cannot form rosettes. Would you comment on this proposal in the light of your experiments on rosette-forming cells in tolerant mice?

O. Sjöberg: We have not tested if there are any thymus-derived rosette-forming cells in non-immunized animals, the background being low. I think that the rosette-forming cells are a mixture of antibody-producing cells and of cells that do not produce antibody.

To your second question, you can show by inhibition with anti-theta serum that T-cells can form rosettes. You must probably have sedimented your cells, by a technique that makes the rosette-forming cells fall down to the bottom. Hans Wigzell has shown that this is possible and it is very difficult to eliminate the helper cells since the affinity of the receptors is very low.

D. Nachtigal: I would be very careful in assigning too much signi-ficance to lymphoid cells bound to antigen-coated surfaces. Dr. Catt in Australia has demonstrated that all plastic surface bind protein solutions at alkaline pH. We have employed this for binding HSA to plastic Petri dishes. Prepared HSA-coated Petri dishes are dried and stored in the cold. Spleen cells are placed on the dishes and rotated. Plates are rinsed after 4 or 5 hours and examined for cells that stick to the protein-coated surfaces. All cells are of lymphoid morphology and this is even most striking with bone marrow. The number of cells that adhere is in the order of 0.5 to 2.5% of the original population. We considered this a non-specific phenomenon, until we observed that the cells that stick can reconstitute irradiated mice specifically to the coating antigen. Our provisional assumption is that the cells that stick consist of two populations, namely, a small minority of specific competent cells and a majority of non-specific binding cells, probably of no immunological relevance.

O. Sjöberg: Yes, it seems likely. I don't know what the connection is between this and the rosette-forming cells that I have tested. In addition you can inhibit binding with an antiimmunoglobulin serum.

M. D. Cooper: About the question of which population of cells, the
T- or the B-cells, form the rosettes, some years ago Peter Dent and
I looked at lymphoid cells from the spleen of agammaglobulinemic
chickens having quite good cellular immune capability. We found no
rosettes even after immunization. Dr. Warner and Dr. Uhr, in an
unpublished study, investigated the same question using *Salmonella
adelaide* and again found no adherent cells in the spleens of agamma-
globulin chickens. I believe that Dr. Peterson and Dr. Alm have
similar findings in such animals. It may not be the complete answer
and I agree that a negative result does not exclude that the receptors, on the thymus cells, whatever they are, can bind antigen.
Nevertheless, it is always fortunate to get away from the hazards
related to cytophilic antibodies.

A. H. Coons: I would like to ask whether any one working with
rosettes has tried to prevent rosette formation by neutralizing
the presumed antibody on the surface with soluble antigen first?

O. Sjöberg: I have done preliminary studies with soluble antigen
and it has proved possible to inhibit the rosette formation to a
certain extent. But others have done more extensive work on it.
Dr. Wigzell, Dr. Howard and Dr. Erna Möller have inhibited rosette
formation too. So it is possible.

K. Merétey: Have you investigated indirect PFC's? We have observed
in rats that *E. coli* 0-induced antibody-forming cells 5 days after
the injection were mostly indirect PFC's.

O. Sjöberg: We have tried to demonstrate indirect PFC's against
this antigen but did not succeed.

H. Lischner: Dr. Garvey, how does the antigen circulate from the
liver to the spleen?

J. S. Garvey: I do not see the antigen on lymphoid cells, but I do
have slides from past investigations showing that there is actual
destruction of hepatic cells upon reinjection of antigen. One sees
the antigen between hepatic cells that are very well degenerated
and the overall appearance is that of an anaphylactic reaction.
We also find antigen-antibody-RNA complexes in the circulation.
Lymphoid cells have sticky surfaces and may take up this material
when it is released from hepatic cells, but in such minute amounts
that it would be below detectable levels. We do see free antigen
between the damaged hepatic cells.

G. J. Thorbecke: I would like to ask Dr. Weigle a question. Have
you already had the time to try if there is a difference in antigen
dose sensitivity for the induction of tolerance between the B- and
the T-cells?

W. O. Weigle: Yes, we have carried out experiments to determine the
dose response in the induction of immunological unresponsiveness
in thymus and bone marrow cells. The concentrations of the
aggregated γ-globulin were 2.5, 0.5 and 0.1 mg and the challenge
injection was given 11 days later. At all doses, the thymus cells
were unresponsive, whereas with 2.5, 0.5 and 0.1 mg only 70, 56
and 9%, respectively, of the bone marrow cells were unresponsive.
It apparently takes a much higher concentration of the tolerogen
to induce unresponsiveness in the bone marrow cells than in the
thymus cells.

IMMUNOLOGICAL REACTIVITY OF MICE INJECTED
WITH LEUKAEMIC CELLS

Ivo Hršak

Department of Biology, Institute Rudjer Bošković

Zagreb, Yugoslavia

INTRODUCTION

Animals infected with leukaemogenic viruses react immunologically less efficiently than non-infected animals, when tested with various antigens (1, 2, 3). Since this defect becomes manifest before the clinical signs of disease (leukocytosis and splenomegaly) appear, hypotheses were advanced that immune depression was an important or even decisive factor in the inception and development of leukaemia (4). Preleukaemic phase of the spontaneously developing leukaemia of AKR mice was also found to involve reduced immunological reactivity (5), although normal reactivity was observed as well (6).

An insight into relation between leukaemic growth and immunological reactivity of the host could also be achieved by investigating the changes induced by transplanting cells of a strain-specific leukaemia. If small number of leukaemic cells is inoculated, a long period of latency will result before leukaemia becomes manifest. This could permit detection of reduced immunological reactivity if such a defect obtains in preleukaemic phase of the disease. With this premise, mice were inoculated with 10^2 cells of a strain-specific lymphoid leukaemia. This dose was 100% lethal, the disease becoming manifest after a lag period of 15-20 days. Reactivity against tissue antigens of sheep erythrocytes and against bacterial antigens of Salmonella typhi murium was tested both in the preleukaemic phase and when the signs of leukaemia became evident.

MATERIALS AND METHODS

Mice of a highly inbred strain A/H were used when 10-14 weeks old. Lymphatic leukaemia, discovered incidentally in an animal of this strain, has been maintained since 1968 by serial intravenous transfers of cells prepared from the enlarged spleens of moribund mice. The leukaemia first invades spleen and liver, than the lymph nodes, but thymus becomes involved only in the terminal phase.

The mice were inoculated intravenously with 10^2 leukaemic cells (which regularly resulted in death 20-40 days later), and at various intervals after inoculation were tested on immunological reactivity against sheep red blood cells (SRBC) and Salmonella typhi murium vaccine (STM). Cells forming haemolytic antibodies against SRBC (plaque-forming cells, PFC) were enumerated in the spleen following the agar plate method of Jerne, Nordin and Henry, and the titre of H-2 agglutinins against STM in the serum was determined by the standard Widal's method.

The extent of leukaemia in each of the animals tested was assessed by counting leukocytes in the peripheral blood, by weighing the spleen, and by macroscopic examination of the spleen, liver, lymph nodes and thymus. Since variations of the spleen weight were less expressed than variations of leukocyte counts, spleen weight was chosen as a measure of the development of leukaemia.

RESULTS

Table 1 shows that the number of cells reacting against SRBC gradually increased in the spleens of A mice inoculated with 10^2 leukaemic cells, so that on days 14 and 19 post-inoculation the number of PFC became more than twice as high as that in the spleens of non-leukaemic animals. In that period, however, spleen weights remained in normal range. When the spleens began to enlarge, after day 25, the number of cells reacting to SRBC started to diminish. The longer the mice lived with leukaemia, the weaker became their reactivity against SRBC . Another correlation was also observed: the larger grew the spleen, the less PFC it contained. Thus, some mice in terminal phases of the disease had their spleens weighing more

Day after inoculation of leukaemia

	4	8	11	14	19	25	29	34
No. of mice	6	4	8	8	6	7	4	6
PFC	21200	25510	34950	60710*	80240*	32280	25660	14470
$\pm$ S. D.	4360	6700	8170	10350	15830	20190	15040	13730
Spleen weight	100	107	91	113	122	172	241	404
$\pm$ S. D.	11	5	8	12	10	38	62	320

Non-leukaemic A mice : PFC 32460$\pm$6880
Spleen weight 102$\pm$15

Table 1: The number of PFC per spleen, and spleen weight in A mice inoculated with 10^2 cells of strain-specific leukaemia.
* The difference from non-leukaemic mice is statistically significant (P < 0.01).

than 500 mg, but possessed no more than 16-600 PFC in them. These data, not included in Table 1, show that animals with final splenomegaly did not react to SRBC whatsoever, or reacted very feebly.

The immunological reactivity of A mice, inoculated with 10^2 leukaemic cells, against <u>Salmonella</u> is presented in Table 2.

Day after inoculation of leukaemia

	6	10	16	21	24	29
No. of mice	4	8	8	4	5	3
$\log_2$ titre	6.7	7.0	7.7	7.2	6.2	5.2
$\pm$ S. D.	0.5	1.0	0.8	0.5	0.6	2.0
Spleen weight	110	105	114	153	198	305
$\pm$ S. D.	13	15	7	26	42	176

Non-leukaemic A mice: $\log_2$ titre 7.0$\pm$0.6
Spleen weight 102$\pm$15

Table 2. The $\log_2$ titre of agglutinins to <u>Salmonella typhi murium</u> in A mice inoculated with 10^2 cells of strain specific leukaemia.

Again, the titre of agglutinins has risen in the phase in which
the disease produced neither leukocytosis nor spleen enlargement, although the rise was not as evident as that in the number of PFC. When splenomegaly did appear, the reactivity
against STM began to decrease, so that mice tested on day 29
after inoculation of leukaemia had the titre of agglutinins
significantly lower than normal mice. In animals tested a few
days before death, the antibody could not be detected at all.

DISCUSSION

After inoculation of a small number of leukaemic cells,
the immunological reactivity against tissue antigens of SRBC
and bacterial antigens of STM was found to be stimulated
rather than depressed in the phase in which the disease has
not yet become manifest. Only in the terminal phase, when the
number of malignant cells started rapidly to grow, did the
immunological reactivity begin to decline (Figure 1). The

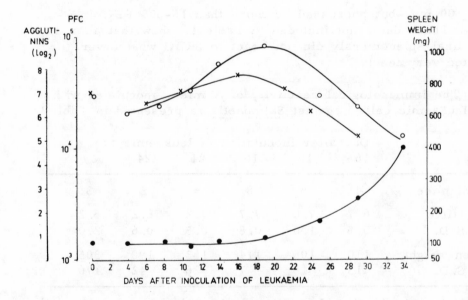

Figure 1. Changes in spleen weight (●), number of PFC per
spleen (o), and $\log_2$ agglutinin titer (x) to <u>Salmonella</u> in A
mice after inoculation of 10^2 leukaemic cells.

turning point occured in the third week after inoculation of leukaemic cells, as if by that time the tumor escaped the control by defence mechanisms of the host and began to proliferate without any restraint.

Increased immunological reactivity in the pre-leukaemic phase is difficult to explain. It could not be attributed to non-specific stimulation, because (as found in another experiment) allogeneic spleen cells failed to boost the reactivity of the host against SRBC although they surely constituted a stronger antigenic stimulus than syngeneic leukaemic cells. Decrease of the immunological reactivity in the terminal phase could be explained by growth of malignant cells that competed with normal cells for space and nutrients. Additional reasons would be that normal, immunologically reactive cells became malignant and lost the ability to recognize or react with antigen, or that viraemia developed and interfered with immunological functions.

Failure to observe decreased immunological reactivity in the preleukaemic phase of mice inoculated with leukaemic cells as compared with mice infected with leukaemogenic viruses, could be explained, in part, as follows. The viruses probably impair function of the thymus (7), as well as the function of antibody-forming cells (8). In animals inoculated with leukaemic cells, however, the amount of viruses liberated was probably small, and the thymus became invaded with malignant cells only in terminal phase of the disease.

I wish to conclude with two remarks. First, the results are consistent with the idea that depression of the immunological capacity need not be always prerequisite for the development of leukaemia, as suggested by Metcalf and Moulds (6). Immune depression is perhaps required for the inception of leukaemias with strong antigenicity, in so far as it will permit growth of aberrant cells, but its role is likely to be accomplished as soon as there emerges a critical number of malignant cells capable of unlimited proliferation. Weakly antigenic leukaemias, including human leukaemias, may perhaps develop without depression of host's immune reactivity. Second, the immune deficit that occurs before leukaemia induced by virus appears, is evidently caused by virus rather than by the presence of malignant cells. The cells depress the immunological function only in terminal phase of the disease.

REFERENCES

1. B.V. Siegel and J.I. Morton, **Proc.** Soc. Exp. Biol. Med.,
    123:467, 1966.
2. M.H. Salaman and N. Wedderbrun, Immunology,
    10:445, 1966.
3. W.S. Ceglowski and H. Friedman, J. Nat. Cancer Inst.
    40:983, 1968.
4. W.S. Ceglowski and H. Friedman, Nature, 224:1318, 1969.
5. J.F. Doré, M. Schneider et G. Mathé, Rev. Franc. Etud.
    Clin. Biol., 14:1003, 1969.
6. D. Metcalf and R. Moulds, Int. J. Cancer, 2:53, 1967.
7. P.B. Dent, R. D.A. Peterson and R.A. Good, Proc. Soc.
    Exp. Biol. Med., 119:869, 1965.
8. M. Bendinelli, Immunology, 14:837, 1968.

IN VITRO IMMUNIZATION FOR IMMUNOTHERAPY [1]

Charles F. McKhann, M.D. and Sreerama M. Jagarlamoody, M.D.

Department of Surgery, University of Minnesota, Minneapolis

Minnesota 55455 USA

The role of the normal immune response in controlling the development of malignant tumors has not yet been defined. However, the increased incidence of malignancy in individuals whose immune response is impaired suggests that this system may be of some importance. Originally demonstrated in experimental animals subjected to thymectomy or irradiation, etc., astonishingly high incidences of malignancy have now been found in patients with congenital or acquired immunologic deficiency diseases or undergoing deliberate immunosuppression for organ transplantation. Regardless of what influence the intact immune response may have on the incidence of new tumors, it is obvious from patients with clinical cancer that it is of little value once a tumor is evident. A rapidly expanding list of human tumors have been found capable of inducing a detectable immune response and the question now underlying any attempt at immunotherapy is whether or not this immune response can be augmented and better adapted to the advantage of the patient.

Optimum Requirements For Immunotherapy: Attempts to immunize the patient against his own tumor should take into consideration the following factors and relationships. (1) The tumor should be of proven antigenicity. (2) When two tumors are used from different patients for cross immunization they should be similar or identical with respect to their tumor antigens. (3) The tumor should be fully antigenic at the time that it is used, avoiding any procedures that may demonstrably lessen its antigenicity. (4) The tumor cells should be

---

[1] Research supported by USPHS Contract NIH-69-2061, USPHS Grant Ca 08832, American Cancer Society Grant T-428.

free of interposed barriers of normal, non-antigenic tissue such as capillary endothelium of host origin. (5) Tumor cells should be free of blocking or enhancing antibody at the time that they are used to stimulate the immune response. (6) Immunologic stimulation should be provided to as many host cells as possible. (7) The injection of viable tumor cells into the patient should be avoided where possible. (8) Production of enhancing antibody should be minimized or eliminated. (9) In vitro methods to evaluate the immune responses should be utilized to monitor alterations in cellular immunity and antibody production.

In Vitro Immunization: Recent studies in our laboratory have employed in vitro immunization as an attempt to meet the outlined criteria for optimal therapy and better delineate the factors and relationships required for successful treatment. As shown diagramatically in Figure 1, cell suspensions are prepared from solid tumors and grown in large numbers in tissue culture where they adhere tightly to the bottom of the vessel. When growth of the tumor is optimal, the tumor cells are overlayed with peripheral lymphocytes obtained from the same patient. The cells are then co-cultivated on a rocking platform for 4 days following which the lymphocytes, which do not adhere to the vessel, are recovered, washed, and reinfused into the patient intraveneously. In order to lessen the danger of implanting viable tumor cells that may have

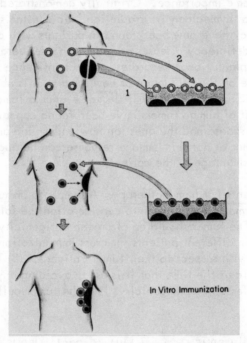

In Vitro Immunization

Legend to Figure 1: In vitro immunization. Lymphocytes exposed for 4 days to patient's own tumor cells growing in vitro, and are then reinfused back into patient.

been released from the surface, the tumor is treated briefly with mitomycin C in culture, prior to addition of lymphocytes. Lymphocytes can be obtained from peripheral blood in numbers up to one billion per 500 ml of blood. The erythrocytes and serum can be returned to the patient after processing. Larger numbers of pure lymphocytes, ranging from 1 to 10 billion per 24 hours can be obtained by thoracic duct cannulation. Once inserted, the cannula must be used continuously, requiring a large number of tumor cells for serial immunization. The potential advantages of this technique are (1) the patient is immunized against his own tumor, (2) the tumor cells are manipulated relatively little and in a form that has been shown to have no detrimental effects on tumor specific antigens, (3) the tumor cells are in a free state with no interposed barriers of capillary endothelium between themselves and immunocompetent cells, (4) cultivation for several days prior to exposure to lymphoid cells should provide adequate elution and dilution of enhancing antibody, (5) lymphoid cells may be exposed to the tumor in far greater numbers in vitro than they may be under normal circumstances in vivo. Moreover, the combination of cell types, including lymphocytes and macrophages, required for optimal immunization can be manipulated. Preliminary studies suggest that macrophages, while not absolutely necessary, greatly potentiate stimulation of lymphocytes in vitro.

Evaluation of In Vitro Immunization: The cellular immune response can be evaluated by determining the capacity of immune lymphoid cells to kill specific target cells in vitro. This is carried out by prelabelling appropriate cultures of target cells with tritiated thymidine and then overlaying the cultures with normal or immune lymphoid cells. Two or three days later the cultures are washed to remove all non-adherent cells and the remaining, viable adherent target cells are digested from the surface and counted for their tritium content. The results are expressed as a percent of controls, these being tumor cells cultivated in the absence of any lymphoid cells or in the presence of non-immune lymphoid cells. Preliminary studies utilized as a model system a human embryonic lung cell, WI38, and allogeneic lymphoid cells from normal donors. Following four days of in vitro immunization against WI38 the lymphoid cells were transferred to fresh cultures of WI38 cells, prelabelled with tritiated thymidine. Control lymphocytes were maintained in culture for a similar period of time. The immunized lymphocytes showed a consistent capacity to kill specific target cells which was related to the number of immune lymphocytes. However, even as many as 20×10^6 lymphocytes added to 50,000 WI38 cells failed to destroy more than 60% of the target cells.

Tumor Neutralization By In Vitro Immunized Cells: Two methylcholanthrene tumors from C3H mice were grown in culture and used to immunize spleen cells recovered from normal mice of the same strain. After 28 and 48 hours of co-cultivation the lymphoid cells were removed, mixed with a predetermined

number of viable tumor cells of each of the two tumors, and assayed for their
ability to inhibit growth of their respectively specific tumors following subcutaneous injection into normal mice. It can be seen from Table 1 that lymphocytes cultivated for 48 hours acquired the capacity to neutralize the
growth of the specific tumor against which they were sensitized. It should be
noted that this is probably the most sensitive but the least stringent of any in
vivo evaluation of tumor immunity. Abortion of the growth of an established
tumor is far more difficult and was not attempted in the present study.

TABLE 1

In vitro immunization of spleen cells against syngeneic MCA–sarcomas:
Tumor neutralization.

Target Tumor	Spleen Cells Immunized Against	Mice Developing Tumors
MC-2	0	5/5
MC-2	MC-41	5/5
MC-2	MC-2	0/5
MC-41	0	5/5
MC-41	MC-2	5/5
MC-41	MC-41	0/5

In Vitro Immunization Against Human Malignant Melanoma: Four patients
with widespread metastatic malignant melanoma were subjected to one or several courses of immunotherapy extending over periods of two weeks to five
months. Only one of the patients, O.Y., showed any stabilization of her
disease. Large tumor masses were seen to regress and disappear but at no time
was she clinically free of disease. The other patients all succumbed to pul-
monary or cerebral metastases which were known to be present before therapy
was initiated. All of these patients had received chemotherapy in the past
and proved to be refractory to it. Studies of one patient are shown in Figure
2. Following an extensive course of immunization, peripheral lymphocytes
from O.Y. were compared with those from a normal donor for their capacity
to destroy tumor cells. It was noted that O.Y.'s lymphoid cells not only inhibited growth of her own tumor in culture but also that of another patient,
R.K. Pre-exposure of both sets of target cells to serum from O.Y. completely
blocked the killing effect of O.Y.'s lymphoid cells. In all four patients a
demonstrable immune response was present prior to immunization but was augmented significantly by the course(s) of immunotherapy. Similarly, in the
three patients where studies for blocking antibody were carried out, such antibody was found to be able to completely inhibit the toxic affect of the

Legend to Figure 2:   Demonstration of direct and cross-reacting cellular immunity and serum "blocking factor" against malignant melanoma. Viable
cells remaining in culture after exposure to lymphocytes and/or serum are expressed as % of control cells (a and f) grown alone. (b) Destruction of autologous tumor cells. (g) Destruction of allogeneic tumor cells. (e and i) Protective effect of blocking factor. (c, d, and h) Controls.

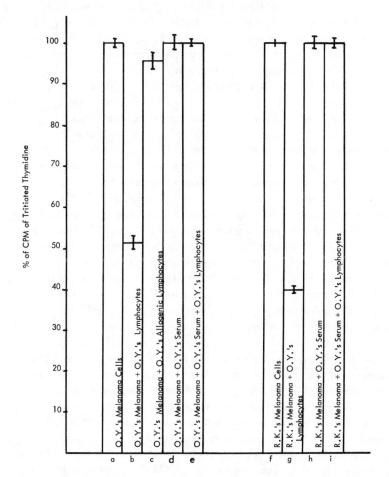

immune lymphoid cells in culture. No attempt was made in these studies to
determine the cytotoxic effect of antibody in the presence of complement.

    Blocking-Enhancing Antibody: A major area for study in the near future
is complete identification of the "blocking" factor in vitro and its relationship to enhancing antibody in vivo. Studies by Hellstrom, including immuno-
electrophoresis and neutralization with immune antiglobulin indicate that the

in vitro blocking factor is probably IgG. It seems unlikely that the administration of large numbers of potentially immune lymphoid cells to a tumor-
bearing patient will have much effect in the presence of even moderate a-
mounts of circulating antibody if the latter is able to protect the tumor. Moreover, it is now clear that the previous concepts of a beneficial cellular immune
response and the detrimental production of blocking or enhancing antibody
must be revised. Immune cells, directly or indirectly by further differentiation, are capable of antibody production. Conversely, cytotoxic antibody of
demonstrable potency in vitro can be prepared against solid tumors. Badly
needed are methods to manipulate the immune response to provide cytotoxic
lymphoid cells and cytotoxic antibody, avoiding production of any blocking
materials. Several methods have been suggested and are being investigated:
(1) Removal of circulating blocking factors in vitro. The passage of serum
through appropriate antigen-bearing columns could remove appreciable
amounts of antibody but would require a great deal of antigen and does nothing to interfere with production of more antibody. (2) Elimination or binding of antibody in vivo by administration of immune globulin would indiscrimi-
nantly decrease the levels of all circulating antibody and would carry considerable risk of damage to kidneys by antigen antibody complexes. (3) Production of antibody has been reported to be inhibited by protein starvation.
(4) "Feed back inhibition" of antibody production might be accomplished with
the administration of specific antibody that was in itself not capable of enhancing tumor growth. (5) Development of drugs that are more specifically
inhibitory to antibody forming cells than they are to those responsible for cellular immunity. (6) The demonstration of antigens specific for plasma cells
and the preparation and administration of antiplasma cell serum (APS) to
selectively depress that aspect of the immune response.

Evaluation of Immune Responses in Cancer Patients: Another area of major
importance is to determine the effects of other forms of therapy in current use,
particularly chemotherapy and irradiation, on the immune responses to antigenic tumors. This may be of particular importance when the patient has
"minimal residual tumor" following conventional therapy, a situation where
the patient's native immune capacity may be of real value to him. Finally,
the importance of in vitro evaluation of the immune responses during any attempt at immunotherapy cannot be over-emphasized. At the present time
most clinical studies are being carried out on patients with advanced disease
in which the likelihood of dramatic regressions or cure are remote. However,
careful documentation of any beneficial alteration in the immune responses
may provide important guidelines to the development of successful therapy
for patients with lesser tumors.

CELLULAR IMMUNITY, ITS SERUM MEDIATED INHIBITION AND

TUMOR-DISTINCTIVE ANERGY TO TUMORS IN MAN

J. Stjernswärd and F. Vànky

Dept. of Tumor Biology, Karolinska Institutet
Radiumhemmet and The Orthopaedic Clinic
Karolinska Sjukhuset, Stockholm 60, Sweden

It is still not known to what extent the cancer patients'
lymphocytes may recognize autochthonous neoplastic cells as foreign.
Increasing clinical evidence indicates that the growth of neoplastic
cells may be subject to limitation by host resistance (1). Among
factors which may limit tumor growth immunological factors may be
relevant. In experimental tumor systems tumor-specific transplantation antigens, capable of inducing immunological rejection reactions
are now well documented (2,3,4).

As summarized earlier (1,3) *in vitro* studies suggest that human
tumor cells may be antigenically alien when compared to the host's
normal non-malignant cells. An important criterion for any postulated
immune surveillance mechanism continuously eliminating malignant cells
as they arise is that the tumor cells are recognized as foreign by
the host's immune responses. The purpose of the present study was
to investigate to what extent cellular immunity against autochthonous
cancer exists in the cancer patient with active disease. However, it
has to be considered that the patient, with an established tumor,
represents a case where immunological surveillance has failed. Possible escape mechanisms (2) such as enhancement, tolerance, antigenic
modulation, escape of tumor cells to immunological privileged sites
and "sneaking through" have also to be considered when evaluating
such results.

Earlier results obtained by a "mixed-lymphocyte-target-interaction-test" (MLTI-test) have demonstrated that the peripheral
lymphocytes of the cancer patient mixed *in vitro* with autochthonous
malignant or non-malignant cells in which DNA synthesis had been
blocked were stimulated to increased DNA synthesis more often and

to a greater extent by neoplastic than by non-neoplastic autochthonous cells (1,5,6,7,8,9,10).

The data presented analyze to what extent various tumors trigger autochthonous lymphocytes to increased DNA-synthesis and represent a search for possible mechanisms of non-reactivity.

MATERIALS AND METHODS

Patients Studied

All patients had active neoplastic disease at the time of testing their lymphocytes against autochthonous cancer cells. Peripheral blood was collected preoperatively.

"Mixed-lymphocyte-target-interaction-test," MLTI-test

This test was described in detail previously (5,7).

Irradiated Tumor Cells, I.T.C.

These were prepared and administered as described in detail elsewhere (10).

Lymph Nodes

Lymph nodes were isolated, weighed and single cell suspension prepared as described in a previous communication (9,10).

RESULTS

Reactivity of Peripheral Lymphocytes Against Autochthonous Tumor

Peripheral lymphocyte stimulation to increased DNA-synthesis after *in vitro* contact with autochthonous tumor cells has been studied in 105 patients. The frequency and degree of reactivity is given in Table I. The results are grouped according to tumor diagnosis and the reactivity indices of lymphocytes against autochthonous tumor cells in the MLTI-test. Tests were run in triplicate whenever possible and the reactivity index has been calculated from each individual test. The reactivity index is the ratio of tritiated thymidine incorporated in test cultures, autochthonous lymphocytes

Table I. Patients with active neoplastic disease whose lymphocytes were stimulated to increased DNA synthesis by autochthonous tumor cells in the "mixed-lymphocyte-target-interaction (MLTI)-test."

Diagnosis	No. reactive / No. tested	Reactivity index against autochthonous tumor		
		1.5<>2	2<>5	5<>10
Burkitt lymphoma	5/18	1/5	2/5	2/5
Renal carcinoma	10/16	2/10	8/10	-
Nasopharyngeal carcinoma	3/4	2/3	1/3	-
Thyroid carcinoma	2/2	-	-	2/2
Breast carcinoma	1/5	-	1/1	-
Testis carcinoma	2/3	1/2	1/2	-
Reticulum cell sarcom	1/1	-	1/1	-
Osteogenic sarcoma	2/4	2/2	-	-
Soft tissue sarcoma	11/36	5/11	6/11	2/11
Malignant melanoma	1/1	-	1/1	-
Brains tumor primary	2/15	-	1/2	1/2
Total:	40/105	13/40	21/40	6/40
	(38%)	(32%)	(52%)	(15%)

Stimulability by autochthonous tumor cells was considered positive where ratio of CPM of autochthonous peripheral lymphocytes, cultured with autochthonlus tumor cells, through CPM of autochthonous peripheral lymphocytes cultured with autochthonous peripheral lymphocytes, was greater than 1.5.

cultured with mitomycin-C treated autochthonous tumor cells, to thymidine incorporation in control cultures, lymphocytes cultured with autochthonous lymphocytes or non-malignant tissue of the same origin as the tumor. In 40 of the 105 patients (38%), the

Table II. Blocking effect of autologous serum in the
           MLTI-test.

Diagnosis	Reactivity-index against autochthonous tumor	
	Tumor cells alone	Tumor cells incubated with serum
Liposarcoma	8.3	2.4
Fibrosarcoma	5.8	1.6
Oligodendroglioma	5.7	2.1
Chondrosarcoma	2.4	2.6
Glioblastoma	1.8	1.9

Tumor cells were after isolation treated with Mitomycin-C. Thereafter 2cc autologous serum was added to $10^7 - 10^8$ tumor cells in
1cc BME. Cells were incubated in serum overnight. After one
washing they were used as target cells.

autochthonous lymphocytes showed DNA-synthesis on contact with
autochthonous tumor cells. Twenty-one of the 40 positive patients
(52%) had indices between 2 and 5, and six (15%) had indices between
5 and 10. Contact with autochthonous tumor cells produced no lymphocyte stimulation in 65 patients (62%). However, these lymphocytes
responded to phytohaemagglutinin and/or allogeneic lymphocytes
indicating that they were viable and capable of responding to a
sufficiently strong stimulus.

Blocking Effect of Sera in the MLTI-test

Autochthonous tumor cells were incubated with sera from patients
with progressively growing tumors prior to cultivation *in vitro* with
the patient's own lymphocytes. The reactivity of peripheral lymphocytes against autochthonous tumor cells was reduced by prior incubation of the tumor cells with the patient's own serum in five out of
nine patients tested (Table II). These results indicate that serum
bound factors may block the cellular immunity of certain patients.

Table III. Reactivity of lymph node cells to
    autochthonous tumor in the MLTI-test.

Lymph node cells	No. positive No. tested	Reactivity index		
Adjacent and draining large tumor	0/5			
Far away from tumor	1/14	2.5		
Far away from tumor - exposed to autochthonous irradiated tumor cells reinjected 10^7, 3-4 times	5/16	9.1	5.6	
		3.4	1.6	1.5

Exposure to relatively small numbers (10^6 - 10^7) of reinjected
irradiated (9000-15000 Rad) tumor cells resulted in tumor-distinctive
stimulation of lymph node cells in 5/16 patients.

Tumor-distinctive Reactivity and Non-reactivity
of Lymphoid Cells from Lymph Nodes

Previous studies showed that the exposure of a lymph node to
reinjected irradiated autochthonous tumor cells leads to an increase
in weight of the exposed lymph node by comparison with the weight
of the contralateral control-exposed lymph node of the same patient.
In 23/28 patients the lymph node exposed to autochthonous tumor cells
was more than 15% heavier than the control lymph node.

Lymphoid cells from lymph nodes draining a large tumor, or from
lymph nodes exposed to small doses of irradiated tumor cells, or from
lymph nodes far away from a tumor and not exposed to irradiated tumor
cells, were compared as what regards ability to be stimulated to
increased DNA-synthesis by autochthonous tumor cells. Table III
summarizes these results. Lymphoid cells from lymph nodes remote
from the tumor were stimulated to increased DNA-synthesis by autochthonous tumor cells in only 1/14 patients. Lymphoid cells from
lymph nodes draining a large tumor and nodes close to the tumor
were non-reactive in the first five patients tested.

DISCUSSION

The results of the MLTI-tests show that primary tumor may induce cellular immune reactions. Peripheral blood lymphocytes from 40 of 105 patients with active disease were stimulated to increased DNA-synthesis after contact *in vitro* with autochthonous tumor cells. Stimulation of lymphocytes by tumor cells, in mixed cultures may represent a method for the detection of antigenic differences between malignant cells and non-malignant cells (5). The present results confirm the first indications from MLTI-tests that lympho-cytes from cancer patients may be stimulated to increased DNA-synthesis by autochthonous malignant cells to a greater extent than by autochthonous non-malignant cells (5,6,7,8,9,10). It is of special interest that also tumor cells of non-lymphomatous origin stimulates in the MLTI-test. We felt it important to always include autochthonous lymphocytes as control target cells as we have found that autochthonous lymphoid cells, by mechanisms yet unknown, may trigger DNA-synthesis in other autochthonous lymphocytes upon *in vitro* contact.

Preincubation of tumor cells with autochthonous serum may abrogate or reduce the tumor cells' ability to stimulate peripheral lymphocytes. This suggests that the stimulating factor is localized at the surface of the tumor cell and indicates that serum-factors, probably antibodies, exist which can block immunolobical recognition of the malignant cells by the lymphocytes. One explanation of the non-stimulability of some patients' lymphocytes by autochthonous tumor cells is that the tumor cells were coated *in vivo* by blocking antibodies. This thesis is open to be tested. *In vito* coating of tumor cells by antibodies has been demonstrated (11,12). The phenomenon of immunological enhancement has been demonstrated *in vivo* (2) and exposure of target cells to humoral antibodies abolished the cytotoxic effect of cellular immunity *in vitro* (13,14,15).

Peripheral lymphocytes were more often stimulated by autochthon-ous tumor cells than were lymphoid cells from lymph nodes. This may reflect a difference in the two lymphocyte populations as well as differences in previous contact with tumor distinctive stimuli.

Tumor distinctive immunological anergy was found in the cells of lymph nodes draining large tumors. Cells from local lymph nodes were not stimulated by autochthonous tumor cells although stimulable by allogeneic cells and P.H.A. The non-reactivity of these cells to tumor cells was not due to lack of tumor cell stimulating capacity since these cells stimulated autochthonous peripheral lymphocytes to increased DNA-synthesis. This may be a demonstration of "local tolerance," and the Mixed-lymphocyte-reactivity test has in fact been shown to be an *in vitro* test for tolerance (16,17,18).

Cells from a lymph node draining the tumor area stimulated autochthonous peripheral lymphocytes to increased DNA-synthesis better than tumor cells. It may be that antigen(s) or tumor cells are trapped in the cells of nodes draining tumor-bearing sites. The lymph node which drains the site of injection of antigen has been demonstrated to trap relatively constant proportions of antigens (19). Antigens associated with macrophages have been shown to be much more immunogenic than native antigens, the difference being greater the smaller the quantities compared (20). Another explanation of the high stimulatory activity of lymph node cells is the fact that antigen activated human lymphocytes release soluble biologically active materials. These include not only migration inhibiting factors (21) and lymphotoxins (22), but also mitogenic factors (23). If draining lymph node cells contain tumor cells or cellular fragments they may be antigen-activated and generate mitogenic factors which could stimulate the DNA-metabolism of peripheral blood lymphocytes exposed to them.

SUMMARY

The extent to which the lymphocytes of a patient with active cancer recognize autochthonous tumor cells immunologically has been investigated. Patients' lymphocytes were mixed *in vitro* with autochthonous malignant and non-malignant cells in which the DNA-synthesis had been blocked by mitomycin-C in a "Mixed-lymphocyte-target-interaction-test," MLTI-test. Peripheral blood lymphocytes from 40 or 105 patients with active cancer were stimulated to increase DNA-synthesis by contact *in vitro* with autochthonous tumor cells. A serum mediated factor which blocked the lymphocytes' immunological recognition of the malignant cells was demonstrated. Indications of tumor distinctive immunological anergy were found in the cells of lymph nodes draining large tumors.

ACKNOWLEDGMENT

The superb technical assistance of Miss Susanne Stenbrink, Dr. Anna-Martha Vånky and Mrs. Yvonne Wiklund is gratefully acknowledged.

This study was supported by grants from King Gustaf V's Jubilee Fund, the Swedish Cancer Society and the Cancer Society in Stockholm.

REFERENCES

1. J. Stjernswärd, Proc. Xth Int. Cancer Congress, Houston, 1970 (in press).

2. G. Klein, Fed. Proc. 28:1739, 1969.

3. K. E. Hellström and I. Hellström, Adv. Cancer Res. 12:167, 1969.

4. L. J. Old and E. A. Boyse, Ann. Rev. Med. 15:167, 1964.

5. J. Stjernswärd, P. Clifford, S. Singh, and E. Svedmyr,
    E. Afr. Med. J. 7:484, 1968.

6. W. A. Fridman and F. M. Kourilsky, Nature 224:277, 1969.

7. J. Stjernswärd, B. Johansson, E. Svedmyr and R. Sundblad,
    Clin. Exp. Immunol. 6:429, 1970.

8. J. Stjernswärd, L. E. Almgård, S. Franzén, T. von Schreeb
    and L. B. Wadstrom, Clin. Exp. Immunol. 6:965, 1970.

9. F. Vànky and J. Stjernswärd, Israel J. Med. Sci. (in press).

10. J. Stjernswärd, P. Clifford and E. Svedmyr, in: Burkitt's
    Lymphona, D. Burkitt and D. Wright, Eds., p. 164. Edinburgh:
    E. S. Livingstone, 1970.

11. E. Klein, G. Klein, J. S. Nadkarni, H. Wigzell and P. Clifford,
    Cancer Res. 28:1300, 1968.

12. I. Witz, G. Klein, and D. Pressman, Proc. Soc. Exp. Biol. Med.
    130:1102, 1969.

13. E. Möller, J. Exp. Med. 122:11, 1965.

14. K. T. Brunner, J. Manuel, J. C. Cerrottini and B. Chapuis,
    Immunol. 14:181, 1968.

15. I. Hellström, K. E. Hellström, C. A. Evans, G. H. Heppner,
    G. E. Pierce and J. P. S. Yang, Proc. Nat. Acad. Sci. 62:362,
    1969.

16. R. W. Dutton, J. Immunol. 93:814, 1964.

17. D. B. Wilson, W. K. Silver and P. C. J. Nowell, J. Exp. Med.
    126:655, 1967.

18. R. M. Schwarz, J. Exp. Med. 127:879, 1968.

19. G. L. Ada, G. J. V. Nossal, J. Pye, Aust. J. Exp. Biol. Med.
    Sci. 42:295, 1964.

20. J. H. Humphrey, Antibiot. et. Chemotherap. 15:7, 1969.

21. B. Bennet and B. R. Bloom, Proc. Nat. Acad. Sci. 59:756, 1968.

22. W. P. Kolb and G. A. Granger, Proc. Nat. Acad. Sci. 61:1250, 1968.

23. R. N. Maini, A. D. M. Bryceson, R. H. Wolstencroft and D. L. Dumond, Nature 224:43, 1969.

TUMOR INDUCTION BY MURINE LEUKEMIA/SARCOMA VIRUSES:

MORPHOLOGICAL AND IMMUNOLOGICAL STUDIES

L. Chieco-Bianchi, N. Pennelli, D. Collavo and G. Tridente

Division of Experimental Oncology, University of

Padova, Italy

Murine sarcoma virus (MSV), injected in immunocompetent adult mice, has the peculiarity of inducing tumors which have a high incidence of complete regression. However, when this virus is injected in newborn mice or in adults, immunosuppressed by various treatments (1,2,3), the induced sarcomas grow progressively and ultimately cause the host's death. Since neoplastic cells release infectious virus and possess a strong antigenicity, it is generally agreed that tumor regression is mediated by an immunological reaction against tumor-specific virus and/or cellular antigens. The operational factors responsible for this regression are controversial. Therefore, we have elected to study the relationship between morphological and biological data on tumor growth and regression in mice injected with MSV. Moreover, preliminary data obtained on the effects of adoptive immunization and pre-infection with murine leukemia virus (MLV) on the oncogenicity of MSV will also be reported.

MATERIAL AND METHODS

MSV(M), (Moloney Isolate) was originally received as lyophilized material (SVRP 104A) through the courtesy of Dr. J. B. Moloney. The virus has been maintained by serial *in vivo* passages in 1-2 week-old BALB/c mice. Tumor cell-free extracts, prepared by homogenization and centrifugation, were diluted weight/volume (w/v) with Hanks Balanced Salt Solution (HBSS). Final concentration ranged from 10^{-1} to 10^{-3}.

Graffi and Passage A Gross strain of MLV have been maintained in this laboratory since 1961 by inoculation of cell-free extracts in newborn C57BL and C3Hf/Gs mice, respectively.

555

BALB/c mice of different ages received 0.05 ml intramuscular (i.m.) injections of the MSV(M) extract in graded dilutions in the thigh region.

One-to-three day old BALB/c mice were injected sub-cutaneously (s.c.) with 0.05 ml of either of the MLV extracts, diluted 20% w/v in HBSS. At 4-6 weeks of age, these mice received 0.05 ml MSV(M) extract i.m.

Adult BALB/c mice, whose primary tumors had regressed, were subsequently injected intra-peritoneally (i.p.) two or three times at week intervals with 0.20 ml of MSV(M) extract diluted 10^{-2}. Ten days after the last injection, spleen cell suspensions were prepared. 10^8 viable cells in HBSS were then injected i.p. in groups of 1 or 10 day old BALB/c mice. Both groups received MSV(M) extract i.m. diluted 10^{-2} at 10 days of age.

Animals were inspected every other day for tumor induction, progression and regression. Survival period was calculated from the date of first detection of local swelling to spontaneous death.

For the morphological study, animals were sacrificed at given time intervals and fragments of tumor, spleen and inguinal lymph nodes were removed and processed for histological examination. Paraffin sections were stained with hematoxylin and eosin and methyl green pyronin. For electron microscopy, small fragments were fixed in 2% gluteraldehyde in phosphate buffer (pH 7.3) at 4°C and then post-fixed in 1% osmic acid in the same buffer. Specimens were embedded in Epon 812. Thick sections (0.5μ) were cut with a Porter-Blum microtome, stained with Giemsa or toluidine blue and examined under the light microscope. Thin sections were cut from the same blocks using an LKB microtome, stained with uranyl acetate followed by lead hydroxide and examined in a Hitachi HV11 electron microscope at 75kV.

                                    RESULTS

Tumor induction. Results concerning development and regression of tumors in BALB/c mice injected at various ages with graded dilutions of MSV(M) extract are reported in Table I. A high incidence of tumors was observed in mice injected at 1-2 weeks of age, which grew rapidly at the injection site causing a high mortality even at the lowest dilution. Animals injected at 4-6 weeks of age had a lower incidence of tumors which decreased in proportion to the extract dilution. Moreover, a very high frequency of spontaneous regression was seen. The mean latent period of tumor appearance (not shown in the Table) was related to the dilution of the virus material: 6, 8 and 15 days in the younger animals, 9, 15 and 21 days

TABLE 1- TUMOR INDUCTION BY MURINE SARCOMA VIRUS (MOLONEY) IN BALB/c MICE.

AGE AT INOCULATION WEEKS	TUMOR EXTRACT DILUTION	TOTAL No. MICE	No. MICE WITH TUMORS	No. MICE WITH REGRESSED TUMORS	No. MICE DEAD WITH TUMORS
1-2	10^{-1}	70	70 (100%)	0	70 (100%)
	10^{-2}	245	239 (97.5%)	5 (2%)	231 (97%)
	10^{-3}	25	21 (84%)	0	21 (100%)
4-6	10^{-1}	12	9 (75%)	6 (67%)	3 (33%)
	10^{-2}	33	16 (48%)	15 (94%)	1 (6%)
	10^{-3}	25	8 (32%)	8 (100%)	0

in adult mice injected respectively with 10^{-1}, 10^{-2} and 10^{-3}. Survival period ranged between 1 and 3 weeks. However, some tumors developed more than 2 months after MSV(M) injection in both age groups. In addition, in some mice whose primary tumors had regressed, there was a reappearance of tumors either at the injection site and/or a different region, i.e., chest muscles, diaphragm, subcutaneous areas of abdomen. Finally, some animals developed leukemia (detailed data on the recovery of MSV(M) from these animals will be reported elsewhere).

Morphology. Early lesions at the site of injection were detectable after 3-4 days and consisted of interstitial edema and focal proliferation of fusiform, rounded or tadpole cells. These cells show abundant pyroninophilic cytoplasm and vesicular nuclei with prominent nucleoli. A few cells exhibited degenerative changes such as cytoplasm vacuolization and enlarged "empty" nuclei. Neutrophilic polymorphs were frequently seen either scattered or in small clusters. In older lesions, pleomorphic tumor cells increased in number. Stellate, spindle, giant straplike or racket-shaped cells with irregular large and often multiple nuclei were seen along the muscle fibers which appeared frequently dissociated, showing signs of atrophy and regeneration. Occasional mitotic figures were observed and degenerative changes similar to those described above were much more evident. Neutrophilic infiltration was quite marked. Vascular proliferation was conspicuous: a rich network of dilated capillaries containing leukocytes and lined by plump hyperplastic endothelial cells was a frequent finding (Fig. 1a). Only rarely, collapsed or obliterated vessels were seen. Cystic spaces containing edematous fluid and small areas of necrosis were also present. Occasionally, bone showed osteolytic changes with clusters

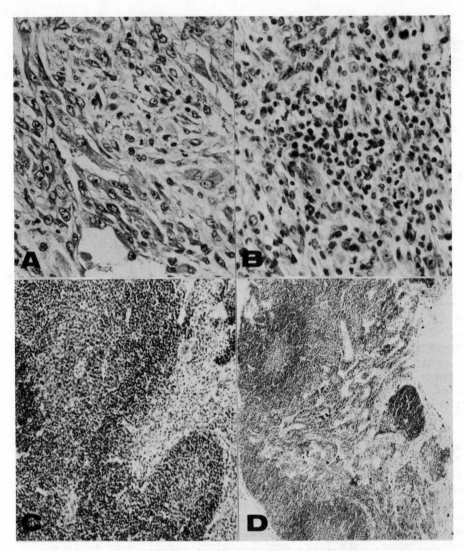

Fig. 1,A. Progressing tumor tissue. Note pleomorphism of neoplastic cells and a newly formed blood vessel lined by plump
endothelial cells. H and E, x 400. (B) Regressing tumor section
showing infiltration consisting mainly of lymphoid cells. H and
E, x 400. (C and D) Spleen and lymph node of a mouse bearing
regressing tumor. Note large lymphatic follicles containing
pronounced germinal centers. H and E, x 160; methyl green
pyronin, x 64.

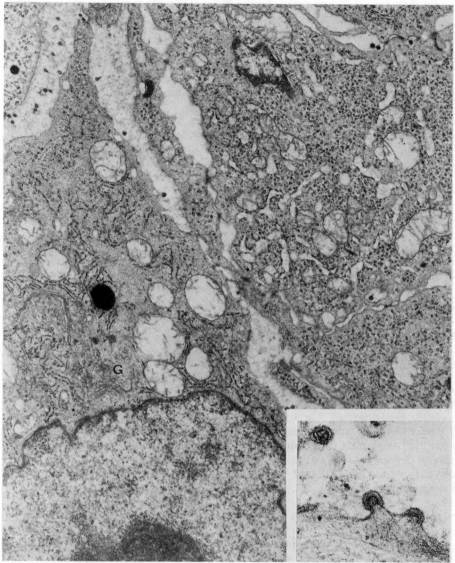

Fig. 2. MSV(M) sarcoma. Poorly differentiated myoblastic tumor cells. Note the characteristic Golgi complex (G) and large number of free ribosomes. The matrix of the mitochondria is relatively electron lucent. Mature and immature particles, indistinguishable from MLV are present on the plasma membrane and in the interstices between tumor cells. In the inset, budding particles and a C-type mature particle. x 15,600; x 49,000.

of osteoclasts mixed together with tumor cells and marked cell
proliferation from the periosteal sheath was frequently observed.
This histologic pattern did not differ during the early or florid
stages of tumor growth in mice receiving MSV(M) as newborns or
adults. However, these latter animals during the regressive phase
showed focal aggregates of lymphocytes among the tumor cells
(Fig. 1b), mixed with pyroninophilic blast-like cells.

On the other hand, striking differences between the two groups
of mice were detected in spleen and lymph nodes. Mice receiving
MSV(M) during the first two weeks of life showed a spleen not significantly enlarged containing small lymphatic follicles with little
or no evidence of pyroninophilic cells within germinal centers and
the periarteriolar area. Occasional erythroid hyperplasia was
observed. Lymph nodes showed a modest increase in pyroninophilic
blast-like cells in the paracortical areas. In mice injected at
adult age and sacrificed during tumor regression, the spleen was
moderately increased in volume and presented follicles with large
germinal centers (Fig. 1c) and plasmocytoid cells in the red pulp.
In the nodes, large germinal centers were frequently seen in the
outer cortex (Fig. 1d). The medullary cords, lining dilated sinuses,
exhibited a high degree of plasmocytosis. Frequently, the paracortical area appeared slightly enlarged and contained scattered pyroninophilic cells.

Electron microscopy. Proliferating tissue consists mainly of
elongated or oval cells which possess an abundance of small free
ribosomes and occasionally cytoplasmic fibrils in varying amounts,
with mitochondria and other cytoplasmic structures located primarily
at the cell periphery. Nuclei were large, oval or elongated, usually
deeply indented and possessing one or more large prominent nucleoli.
Virus particles, indistinguishable from those of MLV, were observed
constantly during the progressive phase of tumor growth in the
intercellular spaces and as buds at the plasma membrane in proliferating sarcoma cells (Fig. 2). Many typical C-type immature particles
were also present within the sarcolemma tubules (T-system) (Fig. 3A)
and in the perinuclear spaces of the individual skeletal muscle
fibers which were frequently isolated by invading sarcoma cells.
In the early stage of tumor proliferation, virus particles were
detected in normal muscle fibers of young mice while they were
extremely rare or absent in the regressive phase of tumor growth in
adult injected animals (Fig. 3B). At this stage, the majority of
neoplastic cells exhibited marked degenerative changes consisting
of vacuolization and appearance of fibrillar and amorphous dense
material in the cytoplasm. Isolated muscle fibers showed an intense
vacuolization of sarcolemma tubules, variable orientation of myofib-
rils and pronounced enlargement of perinuclear spaces. No virus
particles were ever found in the lymph nodes or in the spleen
megakaryocytes.

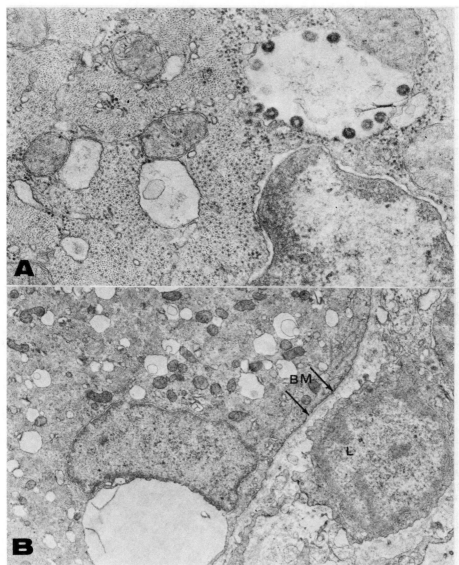

Fig. 3. MSV(M) sarcoma. (A) 13 days after inoculation in 1-2 week old mice. Cross section of an isolated muscle cell with numerous C-type immature particles in a large vacuole of the T-system, x 32,700. (B) 13 days after inoculation in 4-6 week old mice. Cross section of an isolated muscle cell during regression. No virus particles are visible in the sarcoplasmic vacuoles. Note basal membrane (BM) and lymphoid cell (L). x 6,000.

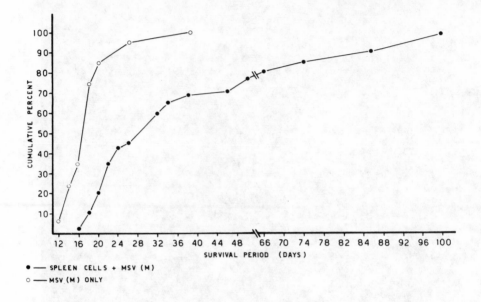

FIG. 4- EFFECT OF SPLEEN CELL TREATMENT ON SURVIVAL PERIOD
OF BALB/c MICE BEARING MSV (M) INDUCED TUMORS.

● — SPLEEN CELLS + MSV (M)
○ — MSV (M) ONLY

TABLE 2 - THE EFFECT OF MURINE LEUKEMIA VIRUSES (MLV) ON ONCOGENICITY OF
MURINE SARCOMA VIRUS, MOLONEY STRAIN (MSV-M) IN BALB/c MICE.

VIRUS INOCULUM		TOTAL No. MICE	No. MICE WITH TUMORS	No. MICE WITH REGRESSED TUMORS	No. MICE DEAD WITH TUMORS
MLV	MSV				
GRAFFI	MSV (M)	35	34	0	34
GROSS	MSV (M)	20	2	0	2
GRAFFI	- -	11	0	0	0
GROSS	- -	10	0	0	0
- -	MSV (M)	25	8	8	0

THE ANIMALS WERE INJECTED AT 1-3 DAYS OF AGE WITH MLV AND AT 4-6 WEEKS OF AGE WITH MSV.
THE MSV TUMOR EXTRACT WAS DILUTED TO 10^{-3}.

Effect of adoptive immunization in MSV(M) injected mice.
Preliminary results concerning the survival period of mice receiving
spleen cells and subsequently injected with MSV(M) are summarized in
Fig. 4. No relevant differences were noted in the two experimental
groups, so data concerning their survival period was plotted together
against the controls. However, as can be seen, their survival period
is longer. Eight out of 12 animals of the newborn-injected group
died with extensive tumor involvement as did all 19 mice of the
group injected at day 10. 25 control mice, receiving MSV(M) only,
showed 100% mortality.

Effect of MLV inoculation on MSV(M) oncogenicity. Data concerning the groups injected at birth with Graffi or Gross virus and then
re-infected with MSV(M) at 4-6 weeks of age are reported in Table 2.
Frequency of tumor deaths in mice dually infected with Graffi virus
and MSV(M) was very high (97%) compared to MSV(M) controls. On the
other hand, inoculation of mice with Passage A Gross virus and MSV(M)
gave only a 10% mortality. In this group, as in that receiving MLV
only, a number of mice developed leukemia. However, since the
survivors at present are 4 to 6 months old, no final data are available on leukemia incidence in the different groups.

                              DISCUSSION

     The results obtained on tumor induction by MSV(M) clearly indi-
cate that, as in other virus-induced systems, development and growth
of tumors are closely related to the dose of infectious virus and
the age-linked immunocompetence of the host. However, the peculiar
and prominent characteristic of MSV(M)-induced sarcomas is represented by the spontaneous regression of established autochthonous
tumors.

     Our morphological study is in agreement with the report of Berman
and Allison (4) which suggests that neoplastic cells may arise from
undifferentiated elements of various sources such as endothelium,
periosteum and muscle sheath. Nonetheless, the constant finding of
virus replication in non-neoplastic muscle cells and a large number
of muscle-derived tumor cells would confirm the recognized affinity
of this virus for muscle tissue. In addition, the observation of
degenerative changes in neoplastic cells, even at early stages of
tumor growth, and a reduction in virus production during the regressive phase further supports the hypothesis that tumor growth is
maintained by continuous recruitment of newly infected and transformed cells. However, while *in vitro* (5) and *in vivo* findings in
the mouse model suggest the non-clonal, "non-stochastic" nature of
MSV-induced sarcomas, there is no experimental evidence to support
the view that tumors of mesenchymal origin represent unsuccessful
host responses (6).

The lymphocytic infiltration seen in regressing tumors and the prolonged survival time noted in tumor bearing mice treated with pre-immunized spleen cells indicate that cell-mediated immune response may operate against tumor proliferation. On the other hand, the very pronounced germinal centers seen in spleen and lymph nodes of animals with regressing tumors suggest that other immune mechanisms come into play as far as regression is concerned. A high virus-neutralizing antibody titer has been found in the serum of animals with regressed tumors but not in animals with progressive tumor growth (1). Furthermore, serum of mice with regressing tumors neutralized both *in vitro* and *in vivo* the oncogenic effect of MSV(M) (1,7). These findings indicate that humoral antibodies with virus-neutralizing activity may also represent a crucial factor in tumor regression.

The enhancement of MSV(M) tumorigenesis by co-infection with MLV has been variably interpreted as the result of an *in vivo* "helper" effect, non-specific immunosuppression and *in vivo* production of more potent MSV-MLV hybrid virions (3,8,9). These interpretations have been recently questioned by the same authors on the basis of the enhancement of MSV(M) exerted by an unrelated arborvirus such as Guaroa virus (10). Furthermore, the possibility that co-infecting viruses may promote the synthesis of "blocking antibody" (11) and consequently potentiate MSV(M) infectivity has been advanced (10).

Our results showing enhancement of MSV(M) oncogenesis by Graffi but not by Passage A Gross leukemia viruses would seem to add further confusion. However, we tend to feel that our findings represent a particular case since Graffi virus and Moloney leukemia virus share a common antigen (12) (which is not true for Gross virus) and consequently a state of specific non-reactivity, i.e., tolerance, can be reasonably expected.

                                SUMMARY

BALB/c mice injected i.m. at various ages with different dilutions of MSV(M) preparations, developed tumors which showed progressive growth as a function of the virus dose and the age of the animal at inoculation. The morphology of these tumors was studied by light and electron microscopy in both the proliferative and the regressive phases which were then correlated to the histological patterns of spleen and lymph nodes.

Mice treated with pre-immunized spleen cells and then injected with MSV(M) showed high tumor incidence but a more prolonged survival period. Mice infected at birth with Graffi or Passage A Gross leukemia virus were subsequently injected with MSV(M). On contrast with controls receiving MSV(M) only, the animals dually infected with Graffi virus and MSV(M) had a high tumor incidence and eventually died from progressive tumor growth. These results are discussed in the light of immunological factors (reactivity vs. non-reactivity) which might influence tumor growth and regression.

ACKNOWLEDGMENTS

We thank Mrs. P. Segato for preparing the manuscript and Miss F. Sanavio and Mr. G. Miotti Scapin for excellent technical assistance.

This research was supported in part by Leukaemia Research Fund, London, Consiglio Nazionale delle Ricerche, Roma, and Associazione Italiana per la Promozione delle Ricerche sul Cancro, Milano.

REFERENCES

1. A. Fefer, J. L. McCoy, K Perk and J. P. Glynn, Cancer Res., 28:1577, 1968.

2. D. A. Shachat, A. Fefer and J. B. Moloney, Cancer Res., 28:517, 1968.

3. W. A. Hook, M. A. Chirigos and S. P. Chan, Cancer Res., 29:1008, 1969.

4. L. D. Berman and A. C. Allison, Int. J. Cancer, 4:820, 1969.

5. R. Bather, A. Leonard and J. Yang, J. Nat Cancer Inst., 40:551, 1968.

6. R. Siegler, in: Int. Conf. on Immunity and Tolerance in Oncogenesis, Perugia, 1969 (in press).

7. J. Bubenik, A. Turano and G. Fadda, Int. J. Cancer, 4:648, 1969.

8. M. A. Chirigos, K. Perk, W. Turner, B. Burka and M. Gomez, Cancer Res. 28:1055, 1968.

9. W. Turner and M. A. Chirigos, Cancer Res., 29:1956, 1969.

10. W. Turner, W. Gibson and M. A. Chirigos, Cancer Res. (in press).

11. I. Hellström and K. E. Hellström, Int. J. Cancer, 4:587, 1969.

12. G. Pasternak, personal communication.

CHAIRMAN'S INTRODUCTION TO THE DISCUSSION

FACTORS CONTRIBUTING TO THE "SUCCESS" OF ANTIGENIC TUMOURS

Peter Alexander

Chester Beatty Research Institute, Institute of Cancer

Research, Belmont, Sutton, Surrey, England

A great deal has been learned in the last decade about the macromolecular constituents which are present in the plasma membrane of tumour cells and absent in all the normal cells of the host. These components are capable of evoking a host reaction which is specifically cytocidal to the tumour cells and are therefore referred to as transplantation-type tumour specific antigens (TTSA). A key problem of tumour immunology is why cells having TTSA succeed in growing into malignant tumours and are not destroyed by the hosts' immune defences. In the early stages of malignant disease - both in man and in experimental animals - the immune mechanism is normal and an impairment in immunity when it occurs is a consequence of the advance of the disease. While immunosuppression facilitates carcinogenesis by oncogenic viruses it is quite clear that it is not an essential component of the aetiology of cancer. The development of specific tolerance to the TTSA has been suggested but there is now convincing evidence that this occurs only rarely if at all and in the majority of tumours studied in man (cf. 1) and in experimental animals (cf. 2) the host has retained the capacity to react against the TTSA of autochthonous tumors. High level tolerance does not operate here!

A hypothesis which is much talked about at present is that the tumour cells are coated by an antibody which is not cytotoxic (e.g., does not bind complement) but which prevents other effector mechanisms from mounting a cytotoxic attack. This hypothetical phenomenon is likened to the well established phenomenon of

immunological enhancement.   This however is a false analogy
since in immunological enhancement antibody is given prior to the
implantation of an allogeneic tumour and the growth of this graft
is facilitated because the antibody combines with the transplantation antigen before these can immunise.   In true enhancement
the antibody acts at either the afferent or central arm of the
immune response.   In spite of much theorising there is no
experimental evidence that <u>in vivo</u> the cells of a progressively
growing tumour are protected by a coating of antibody.   Various
immunotherapeutic procedures have been demonstrated to slow the
growth of tumours in experimental animals (cf. 3) and these
would not work if the tumours were protected by antibody.

It seems much more likely that the success of an antigenic
tumour occurs for the same reasons that permit infectious diseases
to establish themselves and to persist in an immunologically
competent host.   There is no essential difference between the
"success" of tuberculosis or of the bacilli growing on the heart
valve from that of an antigenic tumour and there seems to be no
necessity to involve special phenomena such as tolerance or
blocking antibody for the latter.   The essential point to bear
in mind - and this has been emphasised repeatedly by Gorer (4)
is that there are three independent arms by which the immune
defences exert their action (i.e., circulating antibody,
macrophages and cytotoxic lymphoid cells).   While these different
effector mechanisms supplement one another they suffer from
different limitations.   They are not expressed equally at all
sites and their contributions to the defence of the host as a
whole are limited by anatomical factors which differ for the
different processes.

2. CONTRIBUTION OF CIRCULATING ANTIBODY

TO THE CONTROL OF BLOOD-BORNE METASTASES

Humoral antibodies in conjunction with complement can destroy
tumour cells but their activity is likely to be much greater
against tumour cells in the blood than those at extravascular
sites (e.g., subcutaneously growing tumours) because large macromolecules such as IgM have difficulty in penetrating capillary
endothelium.   There is direct experimental evidence (5) that the
titre of such antibodies in extracellular fluid is much lower than
in blood.   There is also a wealth of clinical experience that
administration of humoral antibody to patients with pneumonia will
sterilise the blood but rarely influences the clinical course of
the disease because the pathogens at extravascular sites cannot
be reached.

In our laboratory we have found that blood-borne metastatic

spread from malignant melanoma in man (6, 1) and autochthonous
chemically-induced sarcomata in rats (7) is controlled by the
presence of circulating antibody, but that this antibody is without effect on the growth of the solid tumours.   Removal of the
antibody in rats with primary sarcomata by draining of lymph
plasma through a thoracic duct fistula results in the appearance
of lung metastases.   Passive administration of serum from a
tumour-bearing animal protects against a subsequent challenge with
the same tumour if given i.v. but not if given s.c.   The finding
that a tumour-bearing rat is unable to resist an autograft of its
tumour when given s.c. but resists autologous tumour cells, when
these are given i.v. is probably due to the fact that the action
of antibody against the TTSA is confined to the blood.   Malignant
melanoma in man remains localised while there is circulating auto- (6)
antibody which seems to be able to destroy blood-borne metastasis
but has no apparent effect on the actual tumour presumably because
of accessibility problems.   When the tumour becomes widely
disseminated no auto-antibodies can be found although the antigenicity of the tumour remains unchanged.   The reasons for the
failure to form antibodies is not known but is not due to a
generalised inability to respond to the antigen because when such
patients are autoimmunized with their own tumour circulating
auto-antibodies to the tumour briefly reappear (1).

3. THE ROLE OF MACROPHAGES IN PROTECTING THE PERITONEAL CAVITY

The phenomenon of concomittant immunity; i.e., the capacity
of an animal to resist an autograft at one site in spite of the
presence of actively growing tumour growth at another site is
shown very clearly in the peritoneal cavity.   We found (8) that
macrophages separated from peritoneal exudate cells of animals,
which had either been immunized against a specific tumour (e.g.,
by pre-treatment with irradiated tumour cells) or have a
progressively growing solid tumour, were capable of specifically
inhibiting the growth of the tumour cells in an in vitro system.
This immunologically specific growth inhibition is associated with
the presence on the macrophages of cytophilic antibody and is
brought about by direct cell-to-cell contact between the immune
macrophage and the target cell.   Phagocytosis is not involved
in the cytotoxic reaction and occurs only after the tumour cells
have sustained lethal damage by an as yet unknown mechanism.
We have been able to demonstrate that a subcutaneous tumour grows
under conditions when there are in the peritoneal cavity sufficient
immune macrophages to destroy all the tumour cells if they could
be brought into contact.   This is a clear situation where the
host defences fail for purely "logistic" reasons, i.e., the
inability of an effector agent present in excess to reach a
critical site.

        The macrophages in the tumour-bearing animal are "armed" by
cytophilic antibody derived from lymphoid (e.g., spleen) cells (8).
We have not been able to arm macrophages with serum from such
animals presumably because the concentration of free cytophilic
antibody is too low.   However when monolayers of non-immune
macrophages are incubated with spleen cells from an animal
immunized with tumour this renders these macrophages specifically
cytotoxic to these particular tumour cells.

        The maximum potential of the macrophage-mediated component
of the immune response may be limited either by the number of
available macrophages or by the amount of cytophilic antibody
present.   Thus a non-specific inflammatory reaction (e.g.,
inoculation of dermal tumours with vaccinia (9)) may lead to an
increased immunologically specific reaction by increasing the
number of available macrophages.

4. CYTOTOXIC LYMPHOCYTES - THE ROLE OF IMMUNOBLASTS

        The third effector mechanism involves immunoblasts and is
ideally suited for the protection of extravascular sites because
these cells possess a remarkable capacity for passing capillary
endothelium and bringing the immune response directly to the cells
of a tumour.   In an earlier paper in this meeting Miss Marilyn
Smith has defined the cells to which we have applied the name
"immunoblast" - originally coined by Damashek.   They are the
large pyroninophilic blast (i.e., DNA synthesising) cells which
appear in the efferent lymph of a node between 50 to 120 hours
following antigenic stimulation.   This cellular response is the
same whether the immune response is of cell-mediated (i.e.,
delayed hypersensitivity type) or involved circulating antibody
(10).   If these cells are removed from the lymph of the draining
node the systemic immune response of the animal is abolished (11).
Some of these cells transform into classical plasma cells (12).
Their most characteristic feature and the one with which
Miss Smith has dealt in detail is that they do not recirculate
between blood and lymph like the blood-borne small lymphocytes
but rapidly extravasate so that within a few hours of injection
they are no longer present in blood or lymph.

        In a variety of in vitro systems studied by us (13, 14)
immunoblasts were shown to be responsible for the cytotoxic action
against specific target cells.   When using lymphoid cells leaving
nodes stimulated with the target cells, highly specific cytotoxic
(i.e., growth inhibiting activity) was only found at those times
when immunoblasts were present in the lymph (i.e., 50-120 hours
after stimulation with the target cells).   The magnitude of the
cytotoxic action was proportional to the fraction of the cells
in the lymph which were immunoblasts.   The cytotoxic action of

the lymphoid cells from lymph was unaffected by 2,000 r of
X-rays (15).   This dose rapidly kills small lymphocytes but does
not appear to affect immunoblasts.   This finding constitutes a
powerful case for the view that it is the immunoblasts and not
small lymphocytes which are the true effector cells of lymphocyte-
mediated cellular immunity.   Ten days or more after immunization
lymphocytes taken from the spleen or lymph nodes of immunized
animals - but not from the lymph - are capable of causing a
specific cytotoxic reaction.   The cells responsible are not
immunoblasts but are sessile and radiosensitive small lymphocytes,
which transform on coming into contact with the target cell into
immunoblasts (15).

Immunoblasts which are specifically cytotoxic to the tumour
cells are formed in response to tumour-specific antigens and have
been recovered from the thoracic duct of rats immunized with
irradiated syngeneic tumour when the only antigenic stimulus is
the tumour-specific antigen (10).   The immunizing tumour was
irradiated so that it should not grow.

Why then are the immunoblasts which, because of their
physiological properties, can gain access to the tumour, not more
effective in arresting the growth of a viable graft or of an
autochthonous tumour?

The reason - at least in the system we have studied (14) -
is that a growing tumour impairs the draining node so that the
immunoblasts are not discharged.   The node draining a growing
tumour is highly stimulated.   It contains many plasma cells and
germinal centres and its cells are cytotoxic to the tumour
in vitro.   However the cytotoxic immunoblasts are not released.
We speculate that this is due to the very large amount of antigen
which is continuously reaching the node from the tumour and which
presumably reacts directly with the immunoblasts.   Whatever the
mechanism, the failure of the immunoblasts to leave the node
effectively severs one very important immunological mechanism
for attacking solid tumours.

Within 24 hours of total excision (partial removal is not
enough) the tumour immunologically specific immunoblasts leave the
node, i.e., the impairment is dependent on the presence of
tumour (14).   This release explains our earlier observation (2)
that an animal is unable to reject a subcutaneous autograft so
long as some of the primary tumour remains, but if the tumour is
totally excised then the rat is able to resist a s.c. autograft.

The impairment produced by a growing tumour is confined to
the draining node and if a piece of the tumour is removed and
transplanted to another site an immunoblast response occurs (14).

This phenomenon has also been observed by G. Currie in our laboratory with human malignant melanoma.

5. IMMUNOTHERAPY INVOLVING IMMUNOBLASTS

The fact that a tumour autograft can cause circulating immunoblasts to appear in a tumour-bearing animal provides an explanation for the growth inhibiting effect of immunizing animals at multiple sites with cells from their own tumour after these had been rendered incapable of growing by exposure to X-rays (16). Like all forms of immunotherapy (cf. 3) treatment with irradiated autologous tumour is only effective if the amount of growing tumour is small.

Immunoblasts obtained from the lymph of allogeneic (17) and heterologous donors (18) immunized with a piece of tumour to be treated have a specific immunotherapeutic effect when injected in large numbers into the tumour-bearing animal. We had postulated that this procedure did not require that the injected lymphoid cells proliferated in the host and referred to it as "passive cellular immunity" in the sense that the injected cells acted directly against the tumour. This procedure seems to have similarities to the administration of antibody in "classical" passive immunity. This hypothesis is strongly supported by a recent experiment (19, 7) in which it was found that the lymphoid cells from thoracic duct of immunized rats retained their full cytotoxic action after irradiation with 1,000 r of X-rays. After this dose the injected cells cannot divide and their anti-tumour action must be attributed to the immunoblasts present in the thoracic duct cells used.

6. CONCLUSION

To understand the host-tumour interaction and to attempt to modify it in a therapeutically useful way it is necessary to consider the full complexity of the diverse effector arms of the immune response and the anatomical factors that limit their expression. Generalisations are likely to be oversimplications and the experience gained from immunity to infectious disease may prove to be very relevant to the problems of the immunological host response to cancer.

7. ACKNOWLEDGMENTS

This work has been supported by grants from the Medical Research Council and the British Empire Cancer Campaign.

REFERENCES

1. R.L. Ikonopisov, M.G. Lewis, I.D. Hunter-Craig,
    D.C. Bodenham, T.M. Phillips, C.I. Cooling, J. Proctor,
    G. Hamilton Fairley, and P. Alexander, British Med. J.
    2:752, 1970.

2. Z.B. Mikulska, C. Smith, and P. Alexander, J. Natl. Cancer
    Inst. 36, 29:35, 1966.

3. P. Alexander, Progr. Exptl. Tumor Res. 10, 22:71, 1968.

4. P.A. Gorer, Advan. Immunol. 1, 345:393, 1961.

5. J.G. Hall, M.E. Smith, P.A. Edwards, and K.V. Shooter,
    Immunology 16, 773:778, 1969.

6. M.G. Lewis, R.L. Ikonopisov, R.C. Nairn, T.M. Phillips,
    G.H. Fairley, D.C. Bodenham, and P. Alexander,
    Brit. Med. J. 3, 547:552, 1969.

7. P. Alexander, and J.G. Hall, Advances in Cancer Research,
    13:1, 1970.   Publ. Academic Press, New York.

8. R. Evans, and P. Alexander, Nature, 1970, in press.

9. I.D. Hunter-Craig, K.A. Newton, G. Westbury, and B.W. Lacey,
    Brit. Med. J. 2:512, 1970.

10. E.J. Delorme, J.G. Hall, J. Hodgett, and P. Alexander,
    Proc. Roy. Soc. (London) B174, 229:236, 1969.

11. J.G. Hall, and B. Morris, J. Exptl. Med. 121, 901:910, 1965a.

12. M.S.C. Birbeck, and J.G. Hall, Nature, 214, 183:185, 1967.

13. S. Denham, J.G. Hall, A. Wolf, and P. Alexander,
    Transplantation, 7, 194:203, 1969.

14. P. Alexander, J. Bensted, E.J. Delorme, J.G. Hall, and
    J. Hodgett, Proc. Roy. Soc. (London) B174, 237:251, 1969.

15. S. Denham, C. Grant, J.G. Hall, and P. Alexander,
    Transplantation, 9, 366:382, 1970.

16. A. Haddow, and P. Alexander, Lancet i, 452:547, 1964.

17. E.J. Delorme, and P. Alexander, Lancet ii, 117:120, 1964.

18. P. Alexander, E.J. Delorme, and J.G. Hall, Lancet $\underline{i}$,
     1186:1189, 1966b.

19. P. Alexander, and E.J. Delorme, Israel Medical Journal,
     1970, in press.

R. Gallily: I have a question regarding macrophages. Dr. Alexander, how do you explain the mechanism of destruction of the tumor cells by sensitized peritoneal macrophages. Why not other macrophages in the vicinity of the tumor or the monocytes in the blood? Will granuloma induction in the vicinity of the tumor in the leg also cause destruction of the tumor?

P. Alexander: Technical difficulties prevent evaluation of the effect of granulomas on the tumor. I think the mechanism of how the macrophage destroys the tumor relates to cytophilic antibodies on the surface of the macrophage and the killing mechanism is a slow one. One does not see it easily by chromium release. This is why to demonstrate it one wants to have cells growing rapidly in culture and lymphoma cells growing in suspension culture are ideal. They are growth inhibitory. The actual destruction of the cells does not occur for 24 to 48 hours. Then the actual lymphoma cells, growing on top of immune macrophages are showing signs of morphological abnormality. Then they begin to be phagocytosed but phagocytosis is not the end effect. The initial destruction is by cell to cell contact via a mechanism which is quite different from the complement dependent antibody lysis because it is a much slower process. We have no idea about the biochemical mechanisms here. Why circulating monocytes should not get to the subcutaneous tumor probably relates to the altered circulation through the tumor and the poor permeation of monocytes into the tumor. We heard from Dr. McKhann that the vasculature of tumors is normal; however, so is the placental barrier, but still lymphocytes cannot pass through it. If we consider that the vasculature of tumors does not allow normal passage of leukocytes this would be an immediate explanation.

I. Witz: I want to emphasize the question of availability of antigens to specific circulating tumor specific antibodies. In a joint paper with Drs. Klein and Pressman we have shown that after injection of radiolabeled specific anti-Moloney sera the antibodies localized only on tumor cells lodging in the spleen and did not localize on tumor cells in the subcutaneous sites. Now the question for Dr. Alexander; you reported that immunoblasts do not pour out of the draining lymph node of the tumor. Stjernswärd before you has reported in some cases anergy of the draining lymph node. I wonder if the draining lymph node was not immunized and no blast transformation occurred from small lymphocytes to immunoblasts, and in fact, that they are not formed at all.

P. Alexander: The facts are unfortunately the exact opposite. These draining nodes, as is well known from clinical observations, are highly stimulated nodes. They are full of plasma cells and contain lots of germinal centers. I once showed Dr. Hanna the local nodes draining one of these tumors, and he commented that it was the most highly stimulated node that he had ever seen. The cells taken from a node draining a tumor, but not from the thoracic duct, are cytotoxic. There are plenty of cytotoxic cells in the node but some defect interferes with their normal physiologic function. This defect, although it may be relatively trivial, is of great importance because if the cells do not get <u>out</u> of the node, then they have no possibility of attacking the tumor. The cells which pour out within 24 hours of surgical removal of the tumor are specifically cytotoxic immunoblasts. There is no essential or necessary difference between Dr. Stjernswärd's and our findings, because he measures the capacity of lymph node cells to transform. I think it is quite reasonable that in highly stimulated nodes there may not be any spare capacity of cells to transform.

R. T. Smith: Do you think then, that the phenomenon of local regression of occurring tumors after injection of BCG, as reported recently by Morton, may be caused by the effect of BCG bringing many active macrophages into the area?

P. Alexander: Yes, I believe one needs two things, the cytophilic antibody and the macrophage. A deficit may be due to deficiencies of either. This is in fact why nonspecific inflammation may effect tumor regression. Nonspecific inflammation may bring in sufficient macrophages and cytophilic antibody. This depends greatly upon the site. Remember that the spectacular regression that Edmund Klein reports is only in dermal tumors. In animals this type of inflammation works terribly well in the skin, or close to the skin. It does very much less to deep tumors.

J. F. A. P. Miller: Dr. Alexander, could you characterize immunoblasts: Are these precursors of antibody-forming cells? Are they involved in delayed hypersensitivity reactions? Are they thymus-derived? Are they generated in thymectomized irradiated rats? Are they inhibited by antilymphocyte serum? Are they a mixed population of T and B cells?

P. Alexander: I really do not feel I should give another lecture. Dr. M. Smith has given a good account of them earlier. Some of them are certainly plasma cell precursors; this is published. If these immunoblasts are labeled with thymidine and reinjected, 24 hours later typical plasma cells carry the label; some of these immunoblasts can therefore transform into plasma cells. We have seen that some of them are the cytotoxic cells. Whether they are related to the thymus, we have no information. They certainly occur in response to all types of antigenic stimuli. This outpouring of immunoblasts occurs after all antigenic stimuli and at that stage of the immune response one cannot tell the difference between a delayed hypersensitivity response or circulating antibody response.

M. G. Hanna, Jr.: Is it possible that the form of the localized antigen (localized possibly in germinal centers) at the time when the immunoblasts stop leaving the draining node is such that it converts the lymph node to humoral antibody production, and therefore the immunoblasts would not need to leave? Have you ever attempted to measure the antibody profile in the fluid that you collect from your draining nodes?

P. Alexander: There are many plasma cells and there is lots of antibody. The explanation you have given is a very reasonable one; that at least some of the immunoblasts, rather than disseminating the immune response throughout the body, may all remain in that node so hence you may get a perfectly good antibody response. This of course is of no use to the subcutaneously growing tumor.

V. Silobrčić: Dr. Alexander, Dr. McKhann has convinced us of the importance of the enhancing antibody with respect to growth of tumors. You, on the other side, have convinced us of the mechanism which you have shown. Now what importance do you put on your mechanism, as opposed to the enhancement in growth of tumors.

P. Alexander: I find it very difficult to believe in the general phenomena of enhancement. If in fact tumors grew because they were protected by some protective antibody, why would one have odd phenomena of concomitant immunity at different sites. Why should tumor cells not disseminate, not go to the peritoneal cavity. Why should they remain confined until the time of breakdown of the immune response. Now, with regard to the test which has been used to argue these points, one can certainly manipulate things in *in vitro*, such as deliberately coating cells with antibody, keep complement away so that they cannot be lysed, and then the immune lymphocytes do not work. These are clear *in vitro* phenomena. However, in the *in vivo* situation we have only one clear set of results. That is if lymphocytes are put against tumor cells they kill, but if the animals' own serum is added it does not kill. This has been called enhancing antibody but it could be circulating tumor antigen. And I would stress that Gold and Friedman have actually demonstrated this in terms of colonic tumors of man. While the tumor is small excess antibody is present, as soon as the tumor gets large excess antigen is the case.

J. Stjernswärd: The earlier remark of Dr. Witz regarding the antigen in the local lymph node is very important. There is no difference between the data of Alexander and our data because we found that local lymph node cells stimulated peripheral lymphocytes more than tumor cells did. The latter finding may be explained by the fact that there is a localization of antigens in the lymph node draining the site of injection. Antigens associated with macrophages in the local lymph nodes have been shown to be much more immunogenic than native antigens

as discussed by Humphrey. Thus, speculatively, it may be possible
that the stronger stimulating effect of local lymph node cells as
compared to that of tumor-cells themselves reflects trapped tumor-
cells or products of them being presented in a much more immunogenic
form.

M. Weiss: Dr. Hršak, the work of Dr. Jerusalem shows that during
prolonged malaria infection the immune response is depressed, as
mice will not reject skin grafts during that time. As the animal
does finally become immune, and the parasite disappears, skin grafts
will be rejected again. So we have a very prolonged period during
which the immune mechanism is depressed. We find that these mice
develop a Burkitt-like tumor later in life. The tumor is often
located in the liver, an area damaged by the infection, so you have
again this correlation of depression of immune response and
conditioning for later cancer.

I. Hršak: Yes, I agree with you, but my point was that depressed
immune response is not a prerequisite for tumor development.

K. Yokoro: I would like to discuss our studies on leukemogenesis in
rats. They indicate the importance of lowered immunological reactivity in initiation and pregression of leukemia. The highly inbred
Wistar/Furth strain rats and a mouse leukemogenic virus of Gross
were employed in our study. All Gross virus-infected rats developed
thymic lymphoma when the virus was given within 48 hours after birth.
However, the susceptibility of the rat to the virus appeared to rapidly
decrease as the age of the rat increased. Thus no leukemia occurred
when the virus was injected at 8 weeks of age. 600 R of total body
irradiation given in 4 split doses at 5 day intervals starting at
4 to 5 weeks of age was also ineffective in inducing leukemia up to
400 days following irradiation. In contrast to these groups, about
60% of rats that received a combined treatment of X-ray and Gross
virus developed leukemia. Also, the immunological reactivity of
these rats given a combined treatment is much lower during the latent
period, as measured by the number of PFCs and serum antibody titers
against SRBC than those of X-ray or Gross-virus infected counterparts.
These results indicate that in leukemogenesis in rats and perhaps in
some other mammals, the direct inducer is virus and radiation merely
promotes an interaction of the virus and its target cells and a
proliferation of antigenically altered lymphoma cells through its
immunosuppressive effect on the host.

C. N. Muller-Berat: I would like to stand on the side of Dr. Yokoro
not only of sympathy, but also because I have the same kind of data.
I think that what both of us would like to say is that if you discard
a viral origin, which after all could fit the human situation, whereby
viral aetiology surely does not fit all the cancer. If you consider
what is relevant to this conference, which is the response of a

lymphopoietic organ which has been disturbed by a proliferative
disorder, what would be the consequence on the immune function? I
have used a model which is far from being satisfactory as far as
extrapolation to man is concerned. It is the L1210 leukaemia. In
8 days we produce a certain disease with a big spleen which is 90%
leukaemic. We use an unrelated antigen as far as the tumor antigen
is concerned, sheep red cells, and we enumerate the plaques forming
cells (PFCs). Therefore we do not measure a cellular response. We
started to ask ourselves a very simple question: if we immunize at
a time when the lymphoid organ is normal, therefore the efferent lymph
of the immune response is kept, what will be the consequence of a
leukaemic proliferation on the number of antibody producing cells?
We have never on any occasion found any decrease of immune response.
On the contrary, as far as direct plaques, indirect plaques, and
rosette-forming cells were concerned, we found a normal response or
an increased one. Moreover, the distribution of these antibodies
should be considered. It has been very well sketched by Dr. Alexander
a few moments ago.

We assayed individual spleens and we looked for the antibody
production. Sometimes we found a normal response at the PFC level
and a decreased humoral antibody response. When we had a big ascites,
there was a trapping of antibody in the ascites fluid giving a wrong
impression of decreased production. I would like to conclude this:
I have never found any immune depression in the L1210 leukaemia when
big spleens are involved. When we have an increased level of PFCs
we think that two possibilities might be put forward. One is very
unlikely, this is that leukaemic cells differentiate to such an
extent that they form antibodies. The second possibility is that
the cellular inoculum has an adjuvant effect.

We would like to emphasize that mechanical trivia, as Dr.
Alexander said, can influence the efficacy of a normally triggered
immune response, whether it is because the tumor has blocked the
lymph nodes or because the humoral antibodies cannot diffuse. Therefore, chemotherapy or surgery should help any nonspecific immunotherapy.

Finally, I would like to explain the difference between Dr.
Yokoro's results and mine. He finds a decreased immune response at
the end of the disease which we never find. This is because you
immunize your animals not only at the time when the spleens are
normal but also when they are invaded; whereas we immunize every
time when the spleen is normal. And, if the notion of the antibody
forming unit not being a cell but an area is right, it may very well
be that the disorganization of a lymphoid organ affects more the
immunization, the afferent lymph more than the efferent lymph of
the immune response.

R. Peterson: Dr. Muller-Berat, I want to add one comment which I think gives a little more dimension. It is possible, as you probably know, to distinguish the suppressive effects of oncogenic viruses on the different types of lymphocytes. Dr. Miller's previous remark was somewhat relevant to this. In the mouse, where many of the oncogenic viruses will impair the thymus or will begin in the thymus, they have a profound effect on the immune response assayed both with cellular immunity and antibody synthesis. In the chicken on the other hand, if you deal with the RPL 12 which has a predilection or a tropism for bursa-dependent lymphocytes, you only see an impairment of the antibody forming system. You see an intact cellular immune mechanism.

L. Chieco-Bianchi: Many leukemia viruses can depress immune reactions, mainly the graft rejection phenomenon and the antibody response to sheep red blood cells. With these two leukemia viruses, namely the Gross and passage A, there is no significant depression in our hands. Thus virus inoculated animals can form cytotoxic anti H2 antibody in a normal way. As far as humoral antibody is concerned there is no significant depression.

M. Weiss: Again going to malaria work performed in collaboration with Dr. Jerusalem, we get enhancement much more often than any type of protection in immunization attempts. We have speculated as to the mechanism by which this enhancement may be brought about just as you did, that a coating of the cells by non-cytotoxic antibody which prevents contact with a cytotoxic lymphocyte is responsible. There is a good suggestion from a number of experiments, that we may be dealing simply with incomplete antibody of very low avidity. First of all, during immunization with attenuated strains, which do not cause disease but will cause complete solid immunity, there is enhancement if the animals are challenged too soon. If you challenge the animals with a virulent strain from 2-4 weeks after immunization you have an enhancement and this seems to be a fancy system of killing the mice even faster. If you wait 6-7 weeks they are solidly protected.

The other line of suggestive evidence comes from the fact that in all of these enhancement experiments there seems to be a dose dependent effect. If you immunize with the small quantities we ordinarily use in the immunization experiments you get enhancement. If you use vast quantities over a long period of time, in terms of 6 to 7 weeks of daily or alternate day injections of antigen prepared in different fashion, you will get protection. Thus with small physiological quantities, which should give you an immunizing effect, you get enhancement. If you use vast quantities you get protection. So we may be dealing with incomplete antibody, or low avidity, which interferes with all kinds of other things. Given enough time, which the animals usually do not give you because they die too fast, then you can get a protective effect with the same dose of antigen that gives enhancement.

R. T. Smith: For the record, a question should be asked of Dr.
McKhann, of Dr. Hellström and also of Dr. Stjernswärd. Have indeed
any of you got any solid unequivocal evidence that the blocking
material in human serum of cancer patients is indeed antibody of
the type we would all accept.

C. F. McKhann: I can only quote the evidence that Hellström provided
last week at a conference in New Hampshire. The blocking material
migrates in the gamma 2 region in the mouse, and, the blocking antibody can be blocked by anti-immune globulin. There is another
possibility (I do not strongly disagree with Dr. Alexander); it may
be an immunoglobulin with antigen fragments on it. We are quite
certain there is an excess of antigen in the animal at that stage.
Furthermore, the Hellströms have found quite a dramatic change over
from the enhancing or blocking antibody (or factor *in vitro*) to a
cytotoxic factor when the tumor has been removed in the experimental
systems. It is a very abrupt change. It would suggest that you are
taking something away quite quickly.

The other thing I might point out is in the *in vitro* studies,
any antibody or any factor that will adhere specifically to the cell
and block the cytotoxic effect of the immune cell will look like
blocking antibody as long as there is no complement there. So that
the definition between blocking antibody as it appears *in vitro*, and
the enhancing antibody or enhancing factor as it might appear *in vivo*
is a distinction that has to be borne in mind still.

J. Stjernswärd: First of all, I must congratulate Dr. McKhann for
his beautiful approach to a new pathway of immunotherapy. Second,
I will raise a warning. As pointed out recently to us by Dr. Trentin,
immunotherapy will be a bandwagon everyone will be hammering on.
However, we know that even in the hyperimmunized host the maximum
kill or elimination of tumor-cells we can get after preimmunization
of the host is 1 or 2 log units above that in an unimmunized host.
We therefore should be very critical when selecting patients for
immunotherapy. I think we should definitely not select patients
with disseminated disease as in your study and most others, with the
exception of Dr. Mathé. There is such an enormous amount of tumor
that even a hyperimmunized host would not be able to affect it. I
think the reputation of immunotherapy may gain if we could agree
upon selecting no patients with manifest dissemination of their
tumors and only patients with no clinical manifest tumor. Then just
a question: Are there not feed-back mechanisms in the body regulating
how many immune competent cells you can commit for one single antigen?
Will this not limit your approach? How many cells can you make
efficiently reactive against one antigen *in vivo*? What do you think
would be your maximum effect, say of tumor-cells killed by the *in
vitro* sensitized lymphocytes?

C. F. McKhann: Are you assuming a patient who has never had a
tumor or where it has been removed and you don't know if there
has been any residual?

J. Stjernswärd: I think the reputation of immunotherapy may gain if
we could agree upon selecting no patients with manifest dissemination
of their tumor.

C. F. McKhann: I think that if the patient has had the tumor, the
dissemination of the immune response could be quite wide. I don't
think for a second that in a person who has had a tumor and, whether
he still has the tumor or not, one tries to further increase his
immune response *in vitro* that this constitutes a primary immune
response. We are almost undoubtedly dealing with a secondary
response, and with presumably substantially more cells than the
patient originally had.

LYMPHOFOLLICULAR HYPERPLASTIC RESPONSES IN ECTOPIC LOCATIONS:

TRACHOMA AS A PARADIGM

A. M. Silverstein and R. A. Prendergast

Wilmer Institute, Johns Hopkins University

School of Medicine, Baltimore, Maryland 21205

Like the ubiquitous butler in many a trite murder mystery, the germinal center of organized lymphoid tissue has long been suspected of playing a central role in the mystery of the immune response to antigenic stimulus. In this situation also, extensive detective work by numerous investigators has produced an almost compelling body of circumstantial evidence to implicate the germinal center, if not as one of the principals, then at least as an important accomplice. As its name implies, the germinal center was long considered to be a hyperactive focus of general lymphopoiesis, and more recently it has been implicated as a center for antigen localization and retention (1,2) or alternatively as the seat of immunologic memory (3,4).

In weighing the evidence presented in favor of one or other role for the germinal center, it may be important to recall that such studies are invariably performed on the organized lymphoid tissue of the lymph node and spleen, where special anatomic relationships may govern or modulate the responses observed. Few studies have been performed on the germinal centers of that other group of organized lymphoid tissues, those occurring at more-or-less discrete locations in the wall of the gastrointestinal tract, and which (with the possible exception of the avian Bursa of Fabricius) appear to respond to stimulus as typical peripheral lymphoid organs. Most neglected of all, however, are those lymphofollicular proliferative responses with typical germinal center formation which may be found associated with a wide variety of different disease processes, and in almost any ectopic site (i.e., a region where organized lymphoid tissue is not normally found). The purpose of this paper is to draw attention to some aspects of the general pathology of the ectopic germinal center, and to make some generalizations from its location and from the nature of the disease processes responsible for its development that may be pertinent to the germinal center of organized lymphoid tissue.

THE GERMINAL CENTER IN THE INFLAMMATORY RESPONSE

The lymphoid germinal center occupies a truly curious position
in the general pathology of inflammation. On the one hand, it is
so conspicuous and prevalent a component of the lymphadenitis
produced by exogenous stimulus that one is encouraged to conclude
that it represents an integral component of this inflammatory
response of organized lymphoid tissues. This conclusion is
reinforced by observations on the diminution or absence of these
structures in germ-free animals (5) or in fetuses prior to
experimental immunization (6) or natural infection (7) (although
the correlation between active immune response and germinal center
formation in the infected fetus [7] or immunized animal is not
absolute). On the other hand, despite the surprising frequency
with which germinal centers may be seen associated with chronic
inflammatory responses in ectopic locations, these structures have
been completely neglected in the discussions of the general
pathology of inflammation, and their potential significance
unmentioned (8,9). Where they are mentioned at all, it is usually
in the context of the differential diagnosis of lymphomas (10,11).

This lack of special interest has probably had three classical
bases. First, where they occur as benign inflammatory lymphoid
masses, they have often been treated as though they were in fact
ordinary organized lymphoid tissue. Thus, Castleman et al (12)
interpreted a group of lymphoid masses of the mediastinum as
being hyperplastic lymph nodes, while other authors have treated
analogous inflammatory masses of muscle (13) or of the soft tissues
of the orbit of the eye (14) as choristomas or hamartomas (although
one does find an occasional expression of surprise at the
occurrence of germinal centers in a site ordinarily devoid of
lymphoid tissue [14]).

Secondly, the pathologist who repeatedly encounters ectopic
germinal centers in association with the lymphocytic-plasmacytic
proliferative responses characteristic of certain disease processes
has often come to consider these cell types and structural
organizations as part of the disease per se, quite unaware of the
mystique with which his immunologic colleagues have surrounded the
germinal center of organized lymphoid tissue.

Finally, those investigators initiated into the arcane
mysteries of the germinal center have generally discussed their
appearance in ectopic locations in a somewhat narrow context,
usually that of the autoimmune diseases. Thus the germinal center
of the thyroid in Hashimoto's disease, of the thymus in myasthenia
gravis, or of the skin in dermatomyositis, has been referred to more

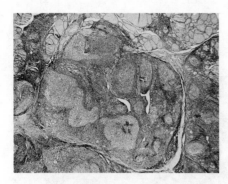
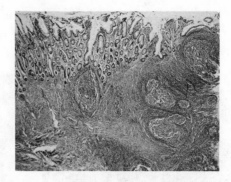

Fig. 1. Thyroid in Hashimoto's disease. Lymphoid hyperplasia with prominent germinal centers has almost completely replaced normal tissue in some areas. H&E, 33X.

Fig. 2. Cecum in Krone's disease. Germinal centers are present at all levels in the intestinal wall. H&E, 33X.

in support of a concept of pathogenesis of these diseases than as an example of general lymphoid function and capabilities in these ectopic locations (15).

Ectopic germinal centers may in fact be seen in diseases of accepted autoimmune pathogenesis such as Hashimoto's thyroiditis (Fig. 1), often in impressive profusion. They may also be seen as part of the chronic inflammatory process in diseases suspected of being related to an autoallergic process. Thus, for example, one may see extensive germinal center formation in the wall of the intestine in regional enteritis, in areas in which these structures are not normally found (Fig. 2). But germinal centers in ectopic locations may also be found in a wide variety of other chronic inflammatory conditions presumably unrelated to any autoimmune process, in some of which the etiologic agent has been well characterized. Although the wall of the stomach does not ordinarily contain lymphofollicular aggregates, the presence of a gastric ulcer may permit these formations to develop (Fig. 3). That this stimulus is not entirely local, but rather may overflow into surrounding areas is shown in Figure 4, where the epigastric lymph node immediately adjacent to the site of the ulcer is seen to be sharing in the lymphofollicular proliferative response. Again, in bacterial infections leading to ascending pyelonephritis, germinal center formation may be seen not uncommonly beneath the epithelium of the ureter (Fig. 5), further up in the pelvis of the kidney (Fig. 6), or even in the kidney parenchyma itself. In a similar manner, bacterial infection of the bladder may lead to a chronic cystitis

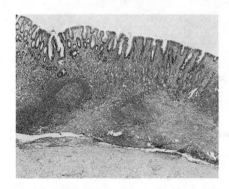
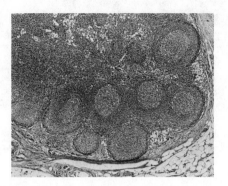

Fig. 3.   Stomach wall adjacent to a gastric ulcer.   H&E, 84X.

Fig. 4.   Epigastric lymph node draining stomach ulcer.   Same case
as Fig. 3.   Note extensive follicular hyperplasia.   H&E, 67X.

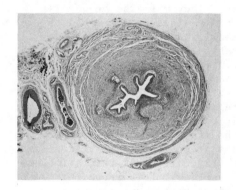
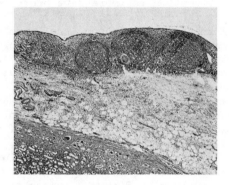

Fig. 5.   Ureter from a case of chronic pyelonephritis.   H&E, 33X.

Fig. 6.   Pelvis of kidney with chronic pyelonephritis.   H&E, 53X.

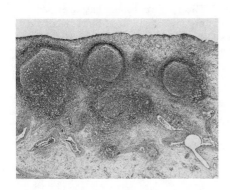
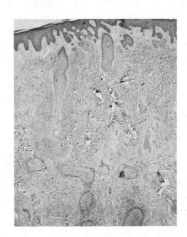

Fig. 7.   Bladder wall in chronic cystitis.   Germinal centers may be found deeper to the epithelium than those pictured.   H&E, 33X.

Fig. 8.   Chronic inflammation of skin at site of tick bite.   H&E, 33X.

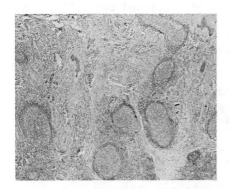
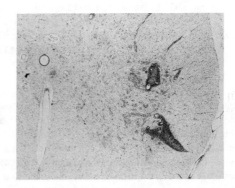

Fig. 9.   Higher power of same case as Fig. 8.   In addition to lympho-follicular response, a deep focus of epithelioid and giant cells was found.   H&E, 50X.

Fig. 10.   Spinal cord of monkey in experimental polio infection. Perivascular lymphoid infiltrates have organized, with many characteristics of germinal center.   Bodian, 33X.

with impressive germinal center formation in the bladder wall (Fig. 7).

It is obvious, however, that chronic inflammation with extensive germinal center formation is not limited to the transfer of stimuli across a mucosal epithelium. Thus, for example, certain insect bites, wherein a portion of the insect itself is left within the dermis or subdermal tissue, may result in the formation of benign lymphofollicular inflammatory masses (Figs. 8,9). Of perhaps greater interest is the occurrence of analogous inflammatory responses in organs which are not only normally devoid of organized lymphoid tissue, but which even lack a lymphatic apparatus. Thus, germinal center formation has been described within the eye in the iris and choroid in cases of chronic uveitis (16), and one can occasionally see structures with many of the attributes of the lymphoid germinal center in association with chronic inflammatory diseases of the central nervous system (Fig. 10).

TRACHOMA AND FOLLICULAR CONJUNCTIVITIS

We have singled out the conjunctiva of the eye for special mention in the context of ectopic germinal center formation for several reasons. First, although it is not widely appreciated, the conjunctiva is perhaps more frequently involved in lymphofollicular proliferative inflammations than any other tissue in the body with the possible exception of the wall of the intestinal tract (17). Second, the nature of many of the external eye diseases associated with germinal center formation has been very well and carefully worked out in etiologic and epidemiologic terms, and some of these diseases are extremely widespread (18). Finally, nowhere in the body is the germinal center more easily visualized or more accessible for biopsy than in the conjunctiva.

The conjunctiva consists of a mucosal epithelium overlying a loose connective tissue stroma. In most species it is normally devoid of any organized lymphoid tissue, although not long after birth diffuse infiltrates of lymphoid cells may develop and persist, presumably a reflection of the accessibility of this highly permeable tissue to air- and finger-borne contaminants. By the same token, however, chronic conjunctivitis may be produced by a wide variety of agents, frequently involving dense infiltrates of lymphocytes, histiocytes, and plasma cells. While many such inflammatory reactions of the conjunctiva do not progress further, it is of some interest that certain agents also elicit the formation and hypertrophy of lymphoid follicles with typical germinal centers, often in great profusion. Typical of such agents are the adeno-3 virus responsible for swimming pool conjunctivitis, a few drugs such as eserine and, most widely known, agents of the psittacosis-lymphogranuloma-trachoma (Chlamydia) family. Among these the most commonly recognized to cause follicular conjunctivitis are trachoma

itself and a group of agents responsible for follicular inclusion
conjunctivitis (including one organism responsible for both
follicular conjunctivitis and cervicitis, a constellation which has
gained local reknown in San Francisco under the name "hippy disease").

In connection with the development of germinal centers, it is
worth emphasizing again that some chronic conjunctivitides may
persist for very long periods of time without resulting in any
organization of the massive lymphoid infiltrates, or in germinal
center formation. Other agents induce a chronic inflammatory
infiltrate with only a slow development of germinal centers, while
some of the adeno viruses produce an acute follicular conjunctivitis
in which germinal center formation may occur in as brief a period
as 4-5 days. In some of these conjunctivides, there is an associated
preauricular lymphadenitis, while in others no spillover of stimulus
to the draining lymph node is evident.

Trachoma is perhaps the most interesting example of this type
of conjunctivitis, in part because it is probably the world's leading
cause of blindness (it has been estimated that some 400 million
persons in the world show signs of this disease), but also because it
presents by far the most interesting pathobiologic story of the entire
group. First, the agent has been isolated, cultivated, and fairly
well characterized (19). Second, the agent infects the epithelial
cells of the conjunctiva, where it forms typical inclusions, but is
not known to leave the epithelium during its sojourn in the host.
Third, the chronicity of this disease is such that the infection

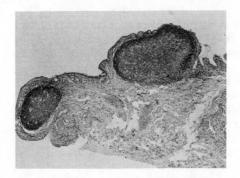 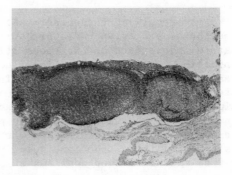

Fig. 11. Conjunctiva, Stage II trachoma. Subepithelial germinal
centers are found, occasionally with little interfollicular
inflammatory cell infiltrate. H&E, 58X.

Fig. 12. Trachoma from same case as Fig. 11. In some areas
massive germinal centers occupy almost the full thickness of the
conjunctiva. H&E, 58X.

and consequent subepithelial inflammatory response may persist for
decades within the conjunctiva. Fourth, the earliest lymphoid cell
infiltrates soon organize into typical germinal centers (20) which
may either be scattered (Fig. 11), or sometimes even appear to
occupy almost the entire depth of the conjunctiva (Fig. 12). There
is usually, in the interfollicular spaces of the conjunctiva in this
disease, an infiltrate of lymphocytes and plasma cells, the
concentrations of the latter cell type sometimes achieving such
proportions as to call to the observer's mind the picture of a
plasmacytoma. Finally, the inflammatory lesion ultimately resolves,
with a fall-off of mitotic activity in the germinal center and an
increase in cellular debris and laden macrophages, suggesting the
picture of what has classically been called the lymphoid reaction
center. The blindness which so often accompanies this disease,
however, results from co-involvement of the cornea in the
inflammatory process as well as extensive fibrosis and scarring of
the conjunctiva.

DISCUSSION

It has been the purpose of this review to remind the reader of
the numerous well-known instances in which germinal center formation
may accompany chronic inflammation in almost any ectopic (extra-
lymphoid) location, and to call his attention to other analogous
conditions which have received less extensive recognition. It is
hoped, from a consideration of the locations and circumstances
under which germinal center formation is seen, that certain
generalizations may be made which are referable back to those tissues
in which lymphoid organization is usually seen.

We may recall at the outset that with the apparent exception
of the thymus and avian Bursa of Fabricius, both of which appear
to mature independent of exogenous stimulus, all other lymphoid
organization in whatever location finds its full expression only
in response to exogenous stimulus. This is attested to by the
immature status of the lymphoid tissues of the fetus prior to
receipt of neonatal stimuli (7) (although infection or experimental
immunization of the fetus results in precocious proliferation,
differentiation, and organization within the lymphoid organs of the
fetus). In addition, the continued lymphoid immaturity of the
germ-free animal further confirms this rule (5).

Where, then, do we find lymphofollicular hyperplastic responses?
Initially, of course, we find them in the lymph nodes and spleen,
organs admirably developed in evolution and located to filter out
exogenous and even autochthonous undesirable substances. Next, we
find these manifestations of host response to exogenous stimulus
immediately beneath those permeable epithelial surfaces exposed to
the outside world, such as the conjunctiva, the bladder, the ureter,

the cervix, or the gut, as a number of the examples of ectopic
germinal center formation described above illustrate. But these
locations are precisely those classified by Aschoff (21) and
Ehrich (22) in their anatomical subdivision of lymphoid tissues:
the subepithelial lymphatic tissue of the respiratory, digestive,
and urogenital tracts possessing no afferent but only efferent
lymphatics. Where better to develop organized lymphoid tissue than
directly at the principal sites of entry into the body of offending
agents?

        Two points, however, are made clear by a consideration of the
follicular conjunctivides and certain of the gastrointestinal
disorders. The first is that the subepithelial lymphoid accumulations
are not "normal", in the sense that an anlage pre-exists with the
intrinsic capacity to respond on call. Rather, we may consider most
if not all of these lymphoid organizations as pathological responses,
not in the sense that all of them cause noticeable disease, but
rather in the sense that they all seem to constitute inflammatory
responses to certain types of exogenous stimuli at presumably specific
threshold levels. Secondly, the distribution of these subepithelial
lymphoid tissues deserves some mention. Access of foreign agents to
the epithelium in question must certainly be of prime importance, so
that it is not surprising to find subepithelial lymphoid tissue in
the digestive or upper respiratory tract, and to find it far less
frequently in the urogenital tract. Beyond this, however, a variety
of local factors must come into play, such as the role of the
permeability of the epithelium in question in governing the type
and distribution of stimuli received and therefore of lymphoid tissue
engendered. Thus, curiously, certain portions of the conjunctiva are
more significantly involved than others in follicle formation in
trachoma. Analogous considerations may govern the local lymphoid
accumulations found in the intestinal tract in the tonsil, Peyer's
patches, and appendix, and the scarcity of similar inflammatory sites
in the lamina propria of the stomach, jejunum, and cecum. It is
perhaps only when the anatomic or physiologic integrity of the
epithelium is disturbed that lymphofollicular proliferation takes
place in response to newly introduced stimuli, as in the cases of
gastric ulcer and regional enteritis described above.

        Ectopic lymphofollicular inflammation is not, however,
restricted to the vicinity of epithelial surfaces to yield what have
been called lymphoepithelial formations. The examples presented
above of these responses in thyroid, in the deep dermis, in muscle,
and in the orbit of the eye suffice to indicate that such
developments may proceed anywhere within the body. Presumably
germinal centers in these locations form much as they do in the
malpighian bodies of the spleen, involving the action of some
further stimulus for organization on a preceding perivascular
accumulation of lymphoid inflammatory cells. This analogy may even
be more clear-cut in the case of germinal center formation within

the eye itself or in the central nervous system, which like the
spleen fit into Aschoff's and Ehrich's third type of lymphoid
tissue: those accumulations along blood vessels possessing neither
afferent nor efferent lymphatics.

Somewhat perplexing is a consideration of the nature of the
stimulus required to induce germinal center formation. We might
conclude from the above discussion that a certain critical mass of
lymphoid cells may be required before structural organization will
occur. This factor, however, cannot be decisive, since certain
agents such as the trachoma organism or some of the adeno viruses
induce germinal center formation with great ease, while other agents
fail to do so despite their elicitation of intensive and long-
standing lymphoid cell inflammatory reactions. It may be that
germinal center formation is encouraged by the presence of certain
chemical constituents present in some of these organisms but lacking
in others, just as the epithelioid and giant cell formations of
granulomas are dependent upon certain types of stimulus. But even
bland proteins and other simple immunogenic molecules are capable
of inducing the formation of germinal centers in lymph nodes and
spleen in association with the general immune response, although in
ectopic locations they seem in the main only able to induce intense
lymphocytic-plasmacytic inflammations without germinal center
formation. The lymph node and spleen thus seem to provide a more
fertile ground for the formation of germinal centers, perhaps
because they are richer in those more primitive cellular elements
upon which germinal center formation may be based. If this were
true, then we might ascribe to those agents able to induce ectopic
germinal center formation the possession of substances capable of
attracting to the local site these special cell types.

It is unnecessary to review the abundant evidence demonstrating
that any tissue in the body may support lymphocytic infiltration,
proliferation, differentiation, and local (ectopic) antibody
formation. The discussion above also makes it clear that under
appropriate circumstances further organization of this lymphoid
tissue into follicles and germinal centers may occur, presumably
employing cells of purely hematogenous origin. We must thus
conclude that there is no function of organized lymphoid tissue
which cannot be reproduced in an ectopic location. Apparently the
only special attribute of organized lymphoid tissues is that they
carry on these same functions with presumably greater ease and
efficiency, a sufficient and even satisfying basis for their evolution.

SUMMARY

The germinal center, as a component of general lymphofollicular
proliferative inflammation, may be seen associated with a variety
of different disease processes in almost any tissue in the body.

Prominent among the diseases which involve the formation of ectopic germinal centers are trachoma and other types of follicular conjunctivitis. Some aspects of the histogenesis and function of this ectopic lymphoid tissue are discussed, as is its relationship to the origin and functions of other lymphoid tissues of the body.

ACKNOWLEDGMENTS

These studies were supported in part by an unrestricted gift from the Alcon Laboratories, Inc., and an Independent Order of Odd Fellows Research Professorship.

REFERENCES

1. G. J. V. Nossal, G. L. Ada, and C. M. Austin, Aust. J. Exp. Biol. Med. Sci., 42:311, 1964.

2. M. G. Hanna, Jr., A. K. Szakal, and H. E. Walburg, Jr., in: L. Fiore-Donati and M. G. Hanna, Jr., Eds., Lymphatic Tissue and Germinal Centers in Immune Response, p. 149. New York: Plenum Press, 1969.

3. G. J. Thorbecke, E. B. Jacobson, and R. Asofsky, J. Immunol., 92:734, 1964.

4. M. G. Hanna, Jr., M. W. Francis, and L. C. Peters, Immunology, 15:75, 1968.

5. G. J. Thorbecke, H. A. Gordon, B. Wostman, M. Wagner, and J. A. Reyniers, J. Inf. Dis., 101:237, 1957.

6. A. M. Silverstein, R. A. Prendergast, and C. J. Parshall, Jr., in: H. A. Waismann and G. R. Kerr, Eds., Fetal Growth and Development, p. 195. New York: McGraw Hill, 1970.

7. A. M. Silverstein and R. J. Lukes, Lab. Invest., 11:918, 1962.

8. H. Florey, Ed., General Pathology, 3rd ed. Philadelphia: W. B. Saunders, 1962.

9. G. Payling Wright, An Introduction to Pathology, 3rd. ed. London: Longmans, 1958.

10. A. H. E. Marshall, An Outline of the Cytology and Pathology of Reticular Tissue. London: Oliver and Boyd, 1956.

11. H. Rappaport, Tumors of the Hematopoietic System. Washington: Armed Forces Institute of Pathology, 1966.

12. B. Castleman, L. Iverson, and V. Pardo-Menendez, Cancer,
     9: 822, 1956.

13. R. Lattes and M. R. Pachter, Cancer, 15: 197, 1962.

14. F. C. Blodi and J. P. M. Gass, Trans. Am. Acad. Ophth. Otol.,
     71: 303, 1967.

15. I. R. Mackay and F. M. Burnet, Autoimmune Diseases.
     Springfield, Ill.:   Charles C. Thomas, 1963.

16. L. E. Zimmerman, personal communication.

17. P. Thygeson, Bull. W.H.O., 16: 995, 1957.

18. Conference on Trachoma and Allied Diseases. Am. J. Ophth.
     63: No. 5, part II, 1967.

19. The Biology of the Trachoma Agent. Ann. N. Y. Acad. Sci.,
     98: 1, 1962.

20. P. Dhermy, G. Coscas, R. Nataf, and J. Levaditi, Rev. Int.
     Trachome, 44: 295, 1967.

21. L. Aschoff, Die lymphatischen Organe. Berlin: Urban and
     Schwarzenberg, 1926.

22. W. E. Ehrich, Am. J. Anat., 43: 347, 1929.

THE BONE MARROW ORIGIN OF LYMPHOID PRIMARY FOLLICLE SMALL LYMPHOCYTES

G. Gutman and I.L. Weissman

Department of Pathology, Stanford University Medical Sch.

Stanford, California USA

Only recently has the morphology of lymphoid tissue been clarified in terms of cell population dynamics and migration streams. Gowans and Knight (1) described in the rat a population of small lymphocytes which recirculate between the blood stream and lymphatics, passing into lymph nodes through the walls of specialized blood vessels, the postcapillary venules (2). This population of cells is represented histologically by the diffuse cortex of the lymph nodes and the periarteriolar white sheath of the spleen; these areas contain the major portion of labelled immigrant thoracic duct lymphocytes and are specifically depleted upon chronic drainage of thoracic duct lymph (3). These have been termed "thymus-dependent areas", since the same pattern of depletion is seen in animals thymectomized early in life (4,5,6). The migration of cells from the thymus has also been shown to be restricted to these areas (7).

At least two areas other than the diffuse cortex are distinguishable in lymph nodes. The medulla consists of a sessile population rich in plasma cells and macrophages, and is also the presumed emigrant pathway of recirculating lymphocytes and, following local immunization, of basophilic and antibody-forming cells to the efferent lymph (1,8). In the outer cortex of lymph nodes (and adjacent to the periarteriolar white sheath of the spleen) lie agglomerations of densely packed small lymphocytes, the primary follicles. The origin of the cells in the primary follicles is not known, although these structures are not depleted in neonatally thymectomized hosts (4-6,9). Experiments suggesting they are bone marrow derived either lacked clear cytological markers (9) or were terminated before the appearance of histologically recognizable follicles (10). We have studied the origin of cells in the primary follicles using fluorescent markers.

MATERIALS AND METHODS: Mice used were C57BL/6Ka (=BL), BALB/cJ (=C)
and the F_1 hybrid between these two strains (=CBF$_1$). Irradiation:
All irradiated mice were given a whole-body dose of 900R (250 Kvp X-
rays, 0.5 mm Cu + 1.0 mm Al added filtration, HVL 1.10 mm Cu, dose
rate 80R/minute). (Abbreviations used: Thymus, Thy; Lymph node, L.N.;
Rabbit, R.; anti-,∝.) Cell Suspensions: Preparations of cell suspensions and injections of newborn liver cells (NBL) were performed
by standard techniques described elsewhere (9). Cytotoxicity was
measured by ^{51}Cr release. ^{51}Cr-labelled cells were incubated for 1
hour in serial dilution of antiserum, plus guinea-pig complement.
Cytotoxicity was calculated by release of ^{51}Cr according to the formula:

$$\frac{(\text{experimental}) - (\text{complement control})}{(\text{freeze-thaw}) - (\text{complement control})} \quad \times 100$$

Antisera used were of two types: BL∝ C (to detect strain-specific
antigen differences, most likely those determined by the H-2 locus;
BL=H-$2^{b/b}$, C=H-$2^{d/d}$), and R∝C Thy (to detect thymus-specific
antigens). The BL∝C antiserum was prepared by 6 weekly injections
of C spleen cells (1/10 spleen equivalent, in 0.1 ml physiological
saline, diluted 1:1 in complete Freunds adjuvant) intraperitoneally
into BL mice, following which ascites was drained, defibrinated with
glass beads, clarified by centrifugation at 20,000 x g for 30', and
stored at -20°C. The R ∝ C thy and R∝ C L.N. antisera were prepared by injecting either 1 thymus or the collected lymph nodes from
from one donor (in cell suspension) i.v. into a rabbit 1x weekly for
4 weeks, followed by exsanguination a week later, and treated as above.
Absorptions were all carried out at 4°C.

     Figure I shows the cytotoxicity titers of the antisera used.
The BL∝ C ascites fluid is specific for cells bearing C antigens.
The R ∝ CThy is toxic to both thymus and bone marrow ; absorption
with newborn liver cells greatly decreases its toxicity for marrow,
while not affecting that for thymus cells.

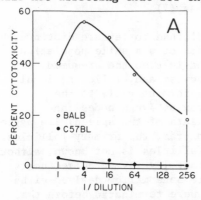 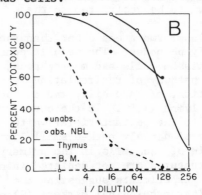

A. Cytotoxicity of BL anti-C lymphoid tissue, against BL and C
thymus cells. The serum is specifically toxic to C cells. B. Cytotoxicity to CBF$_1$ mouse cells, as measured by ^{51}Cr release, of Rabbit
anti-C Thy before and after absorption with NBL. Absorption removes

toxicity to bone marrow while not affecting that to thymus.
Immunofluoresence: Histocompatibility markers were detected by indirect immunofluorescence on frozen sections. Sections were briefly
fixed in acetone before use. Fluorescence staining was carried out
as follows: 15 min. incubation with specific antiserum (BL α C, hyperimmune ascites fluid, used 1:2; or R α C Thy, absorbed with NBL, used
1:6), 6 min. wash in saline, then 15 min. incubation with fluoresceinated
anti-globulin serum (Goat anti-mouse globulin, Cappel Laboratories,
Downington, Pa., used 1:2; or sheep anti-rabbit globulin, Institut
Pasteur, Paris, used 1:40). The sections were then washed, mounted
in buffered glycerine, and examined under far blue illumination.
Control serial sections with various combinations of normal rabbit
or mouse sera and fluorescent sera were routinely examined for non-
specific fluorescence.

Results

I. <u>Bone marrow origin of follicular lymphocytes in a thymusless host</u>:
Adult thymectomized BL mice were lethally irradiated and then injected
i.v. with 3×10^6 CBF_1 newborn liver cells. At varying times thereafter, these hosts were sacrificed and their tissues prepared for
immunofluorescent analysis. The specificity of the BL α C serum is
shown by immunofluorescence in Fig. IIa; the CBF_1 lymph node shows
marked fluorescence, as compared to the adjacent sections of BL node.

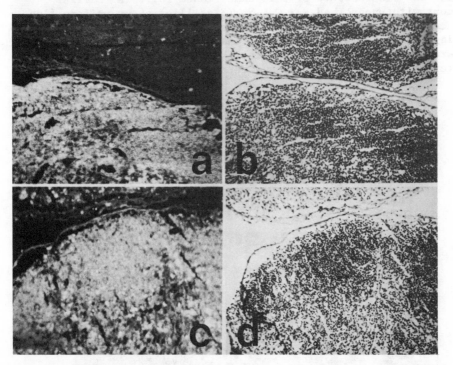

Figure II: a) normal mouse lymph nodes, BL (top) and CBF_1 (bottom),

treated with BL α C serum, followed by fluoresceinated Rα mouse immunoglobulin. c) primary follicle in the lymph node of an irradiated
thymectomized BL mouse, sacrificed 19 days after liver cell injection;
this section was treated in the same manner as in a; the cells in
the follicle are brightly fluorescent, showing they originated from
the injected CBF_1 cells. b,d) hematoxylin-eosin stained preparations
of the same (d) or serial sections (b) to the sections on their left.

Figure IIc shows a lymph node in an adult thymectomized, lethally
irradiated BL mouse, rescued with $3x10^6$ newborn CBF_1 liver cells, and
sacrificed 19 days after the liver cell injection. The cells in the
follicle are uniformly brightly fluorescent with the antiserum directed against the H-2 antigens represented on the inoculated liver
cells. The extra-follicular fluorescence is also specific for the
cells of donor origin; these areas are depleted in lymphocytes and
rich in histiocytes.

II: Distribution of cells bearing thymic antigens in lymph nodes:
Figure IIIe shows a lymph node of a normal CBF_1 mouse. The tissue
sections has been treated with R α C Thy (abs. NBL), followed by
fluorescein-labelled anti-rabbit globulin. The fluorescence of the
primary follicle is markedly less than that of the extra-follicular
cortex. The fluorescence of this same tissue following similar
treatment with unabsorbed R α C L.N. (Fig. IIIg) shows uniform fluorescence over the tissue. This indicates that the lack of follicular
staining in Fig. IIIe is not due to anatomical exclusion of the rabbit
antiserum from the follicle, and is likely to be due to antigenic
differences between follicular and extrafollicular cells.

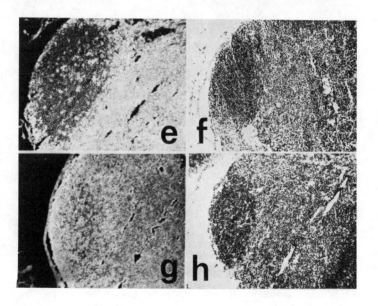

Figure III: e) normal CBF₁ lymph node, treated with RⱰ C thy (absorbed
with NBL) followed by fluoresceinated goat Ɒ R immunoglobulin; the
cortex is brightly fluorescent, except for the dark primary follicle.
g) same as e, but treated with RⱰC L.N.; the tissue is uniformly
fluorescent showing that primary follicles do not exclude rabbit
immunoglobulins. f,h) H+E preparations of sections serial to e,g.

    Figure IV shows a 2° follicle from a normal CBF₁ lymph node. The
follicular lymphocytes show background fluorescence, whereas the
interfollicular lymphocytes and most germinal center cells are
brightly fluorescent.

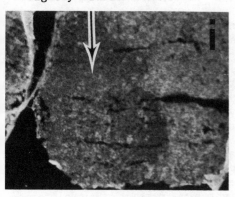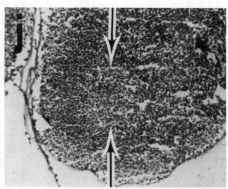

Figure IV   i: Normal lymph node, R Ɒ C Thy, absorbed with NBL
             j: H+E of serial section to L. Arrows outline germinal
                 centers.
                          DISCUSSION

    These results established three points. First, in these ex-
perimental animals, primary follicles can develop from a hemopoietic
cell population (="bone marrow") in the absence of thymic influence.
Second, most follicular lymphocytes in an intact animal quantitatively
lack certain antigens present on thymic lymphocytes and extra-follicular (thymus dependent?) cortical lymphocytes. Third, germinal centers
contain many thymus-antigen positive cells, surrounded by a mantle of
follicular lymphocytes which lack these antigens.

    The work of Claman et al (11) and of Mitchell and Miller (12)
have established that two cell types are involved in the humoral
immune response of mice to sheep red blood cells. The "thymus-
derived cell" is present in the recirculating pool (12,13), may bear
the thymus-specific antigen theta (14-16), may be necessary for expression of some in vitro cellular immune responses (17), and does
not give rise to plaque-forming cells in the response of mice to
sheep red cells (12). The "bone marrow derived cell" is apparently
the precursor of cells synthesizing circulating antibody (12).

    Mitchell and Miller have shown that a two-week "incubation"

period in the irradiated host is necessary for bone marrow cells to cooperate to an appreciable extent with thymus-derived cells (12). Although the nature of this "maturation" has not been clarified, it is during this period that primary follicles appear in the lymphoid tissue.

The role of the primary follicle in the immune response is not known. A key may be provided by findings of several workers showing the localization of injected antigen on the surface of reticular cells within the primary follicle (18,19,20). This localization appears to be related to the hosts' own immunological competence (20,21).

If the bone marrow derived cells in the primary follicle were the precursors of antibody-forming cells, a rationale would be clear for the follicular localization of antigens; the penultimate step of the thymus-bone marrow interaction might take place in the follicle, with the exposure of the bone marrow derived cells to the antigen present locally in high concentration. This interaction may occur on a direct cellular level (thymus-derived cell↔bone marrow-derived cell) or may work through the intermediate of some thymus-derived cell product which would bring about reticular cell antigen binding. In either case, the presence of thymus-antigen positive cells in germinal centers might be significant for the genesis of such inter-actions. The formation of a germinal center, which appears to be an antigen-dependent process (18,22), might also reflect the prolifer-ation of early antibody-forming cells (23,24).

If the primary follicle lymphocytes are to be considered ARC's of nonthymic origin, what is the probability that a single follicle contains a specific ARC for any antigen? A simple calculation reveals that a spherical primary follicle forty cells in diameter contains approximately 30,000 small lymphocytes. Antigen-reactive cells, as measured by cellular antigen-binding in non-immunized animals (25, 26,27), have a frequency on the order of one in 5,000 cells. It is thus apparent that a single primary follicle could contain precursors for virtually every antibody an individual is capable of synthesizing.

Many questions remain to be answered: 1) Is follicular localiza-tion of antigen related to antibody-formation? In the case of a humoral response to thymus dependent antigens, follicular localization of antigen might be dependent on some thymus-derived cell function, and might be a necessary step in the triggering of bone-marrow derived cells into the immune response. In the case of other immune responses, follicular localization might not be thymus dependent. 2) Are cells contained in the primary follicle the immediate precursors of anti-body-forming cells? 3) Is the formation of primary follicles and/or the "maturation" of bone marrow cells to antibody-forming cell precur-sors dependent on some extrafollicular but non-thymic influence (such as gut-associated lymphoid tissue (7,28). 4) To what extent does migra-tion into and out of primary follicles contribute to their steady state (29)? These questions shall be the subject of subsequent studies.

SUMMARY: Lymph node primary follicles develop in adult thymectomized, lethally irradiated mice rescued with F_1 hybrid newborn liver cells; the follicular lymphocytes bear the H-2 antigens of the injected hemopoietic cells. Most follicular lymphocytes in an intact animal quantitatively lack antigens present on thymus cells and on most extra-follicular lymphocytes. In contrast, many germinal center cells bear these antigens.

This work was supported by USPHS grant #AI-09072. GAG is an NSF predoctoral fellow and did this work in partial fulfillment of the requirements for the Ph.D. degree. ILW is a Senior Dernham Fellow of the California Division of the American Cancer Society. We thank Libuska Jerabkova for excellent technical assistance, and Don Lannin and John Santa for performing the cytotoxicity assays.

REFERENCES

1.   J.L. Gowans and E.J. Knight, Proc. Roy. Soc. B. 159:257 (1964).
2.   V.T. Marchesi and J.L. Gowans, ibid., p. 283.
3.   J.L. Gowans and D.D. McGregor, Progr. Allergy 9:1 (65).
4.   D. Metcalf, Brit. J. Haematol. 6:324 (1960).
5.   D.M.V. Parrott, M.A.B. de Sousa, and J. East, J. Exp. Med. 123:191 (1966).
6.   B.H. Waksman, B.G. Arnason and B.D. Jankovic, J. Exp. Med. 116:187 (1962).
7.   I. Weissman, J. Exp. Med. 126:291 (1967).
8.   J.G. Hall and B. Morris, J. Exp. Med. 121:901 (1965).
9.   I. Weissman, in press, in "Developmental Aspects of Antibody Formation and Structure," ed. J. Sterzl and M. Holub, Academic Press, 1969.
10. H. Balner and H. Dersjant, Nature 204:941 (1964).
11. H.N. Claman, E.A. Chaperon and R.F. Triplett, Proc. Soc. Exp. Biol. Med. 122:1167 (1966).
12. G.F. Mitchell and J.F.A.P. Miller, J. Exp. Med. 128:821 (1968).
13. I. Weissman, G.F. Mitchell and L. Jerabkova, in preparation.
14. A.E. Rief and J.M. Allen, J. Exp. Med. 120:413 (1964).
15. M. Schlesinger and I. Yron, J. Imm. 104:798 (1970).
16. E.L. Chan, R.I. Mishell and G.F. Mitchell, Science, in press.
17. D. Lannin and I. Weissman, in preparation.
18. G.J.V. Nossal, G.L. Ada and C.M. Austin, Aust. J. Exp. Biol. Med. Sci. 42:311 (1964).
19. H.O. McDevitt, B.A. Askonas, J.H. Humphrey, I. Schechter, and M. Sela, Immunol. 11:337 (1966).

20. B.M. Balfour and J.H. Humphrey, in "Germinal Centers in Immune
     Responses," ed. Cottier, Springer-Verlag, N.Y., 1967, p. 80.
21. G.L. Ada, G.J.V. Nossal and C.M. Austin, Aust. J. Exp. Biol.
     Med. Sci. 42:331 (1964).
22. M.W. Cohen and G.J. Thorbecke, J. Immunol. 93:629 (1964).
23. R.G. White, V.I. French and J.M. Stark, ibid., p. 131.
24. B. Sordat, M. Sordat, M.W. Hess, R.D. Stoner, and H. Cottier,
     J. Exp. Med. 131:77 (1970).
25. D. Naor, D. Sulitzeanu, Nature 214:687 (1967).
26. G.L. Ada and P. Byrt, Nature 222:1291 (1969).
27. J.H. Humphrey, in press in "Developmental Aspects of Antibody
     Formation and Structure," ed. J. Sterzl and M. Holub, Academic
     Press, 1969.
28. D.Y.E. Perey, M.D. Cooper and R.A. Good, Science 161:265 (1968).
29. C.M. Austin, Aust. J. Exp. Biol. Med. Sci. 46:581 (1968).

EFFECT OF PARTIAL HEPATECTOMY ON IMMUNE RESPONSES

II. ENHANCING EFFECT ON ANTIGEN PRIMED LYMPHOCYTES

Akiyoshi Sakai, M.D. Crevon, M. Sonsino, J. Dormont
A.T.K. Cockett

Division of Urology: University of Rochester
Rochester, New York; Hopital Necker, University of Paris

It is generally known that a major resection of the liver triggers nucleic acid synthesis, not only in the regenerating liver cells (1), but also in lymphoid tissues (2). Partial hepatectomy also stimulates function of the reticulo-endothelial cells. These cells serve as phagocytes which process particulate antigens (3). As previously reported; the number of antibody forming cells detected as hemolytic plaque forming cells (PFC), or immune rosette forming cells (RFC), in the spleen of rats immunized with sheep red cells (SRC), is significantly increased (10 times) after partial hepatectomy (4). The same results have been noted when lymph node cells were employed. Our experiments were designed to elucidate the mechanisms resulting in an increased production of PFC and RFC.

Female Wistar rats, 100-150 gr B.W. were immunized with a single i.v. injection of 1.4×10^9 SRC. Partial hepatectomy was carried out at various time intervals, before and after immunization. Removal of the left and median lobes, which comprises a subtotal hepatectomy (70%), was performed according to Higgins and Anderson (5). PFC's were studied with lymphoid cell suspensions according to Jerne's technique (6). For the determination of mean cell cycle time of PFC, the assay was made every 3 hours after immunization and hepatectomy. Neonatal thymectomy for specific study was made on 60 new born rats within 24 hours after birth. The study of DNA kinetics was accomplished after partial hepatectomy. ^{3}H-Thymidine 0.5/μc/gm B.W. was given intravenously and ^{3}H DNA specific activity was counted in cell suspensions prepared from spleen, thymus and lymph nodes. In vitro incorporation of ^{3}H-Thymidine into lymphoid cell preparations was also determined at varying time intervals, before and after immunization and partial hepatectomy. The cell suspensions (4ml with 7500 cells/mm^3) were incubated during 4 hours

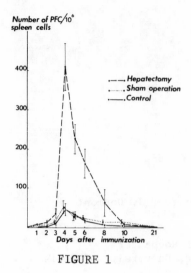

FIGURE 1

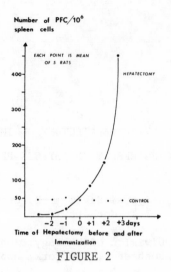

FIGURE 2

with 0.6 μC of ^{3}H-Thymidine. The viability of these cell preparations, as measured with the trypan blue exclusion test, varied from 75% to 94%. For the study of cytological change, the spleen was fixed in Maximow's solution. The sections were stained by hematoxylin-orange G and methyl green pyronin.

When partial hepatectomy was performed after immunization with SRC, the number of PFC was markedly increased in the spleen. An enhancing effect was best seen when assays were completed 24 hours after hepatectomy; the number of PFC in experimental rats in day 4 was 10 times higher than in control or sham-operated animals. The results are shown in Fig. 1, as expressed with mean ± S.D. from 186 rats. Hepatectomy also increased markedly the PFC counts in lymph nodes (8.5 ± 5.2/10^6 cells in control vs 49.0 ± 9.2 in hepatecto-mized 4 days after immunization), slightly in peripheral blood (4.3 vs 7.5) but no increase in either thymus (2.0 vs 2.3) or bone marrow (0).

Time relationship between immunization and hepatectomy is im-portant in showing the effect, however. As shown in Fig. 2, where PFC assay was made 4 days after immunization, partial hepatectomy had no effect on the PFC count when performed before immunization, although in vivo ^{3}H-Thymidine uptake in hepatectomized animals vs controls or sham-operated rats without immunization was markedly enhanced 3 days after partial hepatectomy, either in the spleen (3020 ± 1080 cpm per mg DNA vs 1460 ± 360 cpm), thymus (1650 ± 350 cpm per mg DNA vs 270 ± 90 cpm) or lymph nodes (2260 ± 560 cpm per mg DNA vs 1060 ± 210 cpm). In vitro incorporation of ^{3}H-Thymidine into various lymphoid cells in immunized animals, in contrast to the in vivo data from non-immunized rats, has shown the uptake of the

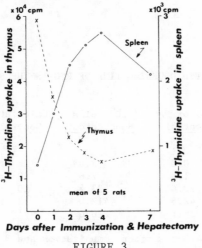

FIGURE 3

DNA precursors to be markedly decreased in thymocytes and increased in splenic cells, but no change in bone-marrow cells, after partial hepatectomy (Fig. 3).

To estimate the PFC doubling-time, the assay was made every 3 hours after immunization and the details of the exponential curve was analyzed. As shown in Table 1, the induction period of antibody synthesis and the mean cell-cycle time was shortened by hepatectomy. Neonatal thymectomy by itself resulted in a marked decrease in the PFC counts ($53.3/10^6$ spleen cells in controls vs $5.5 \pm 2.1/10^6$ assayed at 4th day). The number of PFC remained unchanged after the impact of partial hepatectomy in the thymectomized animals (2.5 ± 1.2 PFC/10^6 cells). Partial hepatectomy constantly stimulated PFC production in animals which had been primed with a sub-optimal dose of the antigen. The result was an increase in number of active antibody forming cells (PFC). SRC (10^6) did not provoke the primary immune response. However, as clearly shown in Table 2, a substantial increase of PFC was readily observed when combined with partial hepatectomy.

Spleen Cytology: Dissociation of the marginal zone with great cell density -- large pyroninophilic cells, lymphoid cells and plasma cells showing many mitosis -- was observed in hepatectomized, immunized animals only (Fig. 4). In normal rat spleen the structure of the arteriole-follicle marginal zone and the red pulp was preserved. Immunization with SRC (4 days) produced some large cells in the follicle with mitosis. Partial hepatectomy alone, either 1 day or 3 days later, increased the number of small lymphocytes and plasma cells to some extent. However, when partial hepatectomy was performed, after immunization, a great hyperplasia was found in

TABLE 1   CALCULATED DOUBLING TIME OF PFC IN THE SPLEEN

Time After Immunization	No. of PFC / 10^6 Cells		Calculated	Doubling Time
	Control	Hepatectomy	Control	Hepatectomy
0	0.1			
24 hrs.	0.3	3.0*	16 hrs.	5.0 hrs.*
48 hrs.	1.8	7.6	10 hrs.	5.3 hrs.
72 hrs.	10.6	33.4	10 hrs.	5.7 hrs.
96 hrs.	42.5	412.0	12 hrs.	4.6 hrs.
120 hrs.	28.1	216.0		10 hrs.

*Assay was made 24 hours after immunization and 8 hours after hepatectomy.

TABLE 2   PFC COUNTS WITH VARIOUS ANTIGEN DOSES

Immunization	Control	Sham	Hepatectomy
10^9	425	492	2982
10^8	132	160	344
10^7	8.2	17.0	61.5
10^6	0	0	9.5

PFC: Assayed four days after priming and expressed per 10^7 spleen cells. Each number: mean of 3 rats.

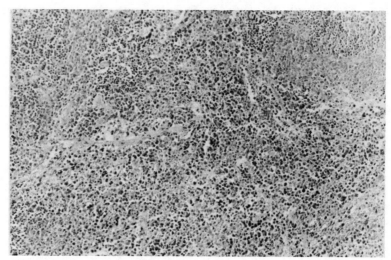

Legend to Figure 4: Rat spleen 4 days after immunization and 1
day after partial hepatectomy (Methyl Green Pyronin Stain). It is
difficult to recognize the structure of the spleen; dissociation of
germinal center (upper right and left corner), a few layers of
cells in marginal zone. Red pulp occupies the most part of the
picture, containing many pyronin positive cells, large and small,
with frequent mitosis.

germinal centers which contained many pyronin stained cells, cros-
sing the follicle and reaching the red pulp where mitosis were frequently observed (Fig. 4).

     The major effect of partial hepatectomy is to stimulate the
production of an increased number of antibody forming cells, notably
of PFC, in the spleen without a significant increase in humoral
antibody titers (4). Although the nature of this phenomenon needs
to be further clarified, one of the contributions of these experiments is that it provides insight into the role of cellular proliferation in the early phase of the immune response.

     The effect in the number of PFC and RFC was most noticeable
when hepatectomy was performed 3 days after immunization and the
organs were assayed on the following day. However, when surgery was
delayed for 10 to 45 days after immunization, no effect in the immune process was observed. It would appear that separate mechanisms
operate on the memory cells and the active antibody forming cells
in terms of synthesizing the m-RNA template.

     Partial hepatectomy stimulates PFC and RFC production in the
spleen and in the lymph nodes. However, similar cells in the thymus

or bone marrow, are not stimulated despite the fact that hepatectomy virtually enhances the ^{3}H-Thymidine uptake of all lymphoid organs tested in non-immunized animals. However, once the animals are immunized, the enhancing effect of hepatectomy is observed only in the spleen on the ^{3}H-Thymidine uptake, but not in the thymus where an actual decrease is observed.

Together with the fact that the number of PFC in neonatally thymectomized rats is no longer increased following partial hepatectomy, we assume that hepatectomy mediates its effect mainly upon thymus dependent lymphocytes. After partial hepatectomy the PFC population is increased and the induction period is shortened. The fact that a marked number of mitosis in the spleen is only observed after immunization and hepatectomy strongly suggests that partial hepatectomy may increase the recruitment of antigen-sensitive cells and/or shorten the mean cell cycle time by acting directly on the proliferation of the antibody forming cells. The latter view is supported by the finding that partial hepatectomy never increased the number of naturally occurring antibody forming cells in the normal animal (4) and that it could initiate the immune response in rats primed with a sub-optimal dose of antigen.

These results suggest that the liver may act in some way on antigen-primed cells. After hepatectomy a factor capable of stimulating cell proliferation could be released. Hepatectomy could also interfere with an inhibitory mechanism controlled by the intact liver. The concept of a "humoral factor" acting upon either virgin-lymphocytes or primed-lymphocytes in partially hepatectomized rats is an extention of our view reported previously (7,8), and the data presented here adds further evidence to this concept.

References:
1. Bucher, N.L.R., Internat. Rev. Cytal., 15:245, 1963.
2. Craddock, C.G., Nakai, G.S., Fukuta, H. and Vanslager, L.M., J. Exp. Med., 120:389, 1964.
3. Fishman, M., J.Exp. Med., 114:837, 1961.
4. Sakai, A., Muller-Berat, N., and Crevon, M.C., Acta Path. Microbiol., Scand. 1970 (in press).
5. Higgins, G.M. and Anderson, R.M., Arch. Pathol., 12:186, 1931.
6. Jerne, N.K., Nordin, A.A., and Henry, C., p.190 Wistar Inst., Press, 1963.
7. Sakai, A., Nature, 1970 (in press).
8. Sakai, A., Transplantation, 9:333, 1970.

REGULATION OF THE IMMUNE RESPONSE. IV. THE ROLE OF THE Fc-

FRAGMENT IN FEEDBACK INHIBITION BY ANTIBODY

N. R. StC. Sinclair and P. L. Chan

Cancer Research Laboratory, The University of Western

Ontario, London, Ontario, Canada

Antigen-antibody complexes affect various types of cells by mechanisms which require the activity of the Fc portion of the antibody. As examples, one can cite systems involving reaginic antibodies, or complement-fixing antibodies in immune complex re-actions. With immunosuppression by specific antibody, there is strong but circumstantial evidence that antibody combines with antigen, forming an antigen-antibody complex (1). Antibody may act by the simple masking of antigen and not through a negative feed-back system in which the Fc portion would play an important role (as with other biological activities of antigen-antibody complexes). Favouring the simple masking of antigen are reports (2-6) that re-moval of the Fc portion by controlled hydrolysis with pepsin pro-duced little, if any, effect on the immunosuppressive activity of specific antibody. Our experience has been the reverse; that is, removal of the Fc portion reduced the ability of specific antibody to inhibit the specific immune response by factors of greater than 10 and sometimes as great as a 1000-fold (7-9). We have been able to rule out the more rapid excretion of $F(ab')_2$ as the sole reason for its low effectiveness in suppressing immune responses by re-placing the excreted antibody on a daily or thrice daily basis (9), and by relating the degree of immunosuppression to the level of cir-culating, passively administered antibody as well as to the amount of antibody injected. With in vitro experiments where excretion cannot be a factor, we have demonstrated a 10 to 30-fold difference between the immunosuppressive activities of $F(ab')_2$ and 7S anti-bodies (10).

Our demonstration of the importance of the Fc portion in immunosuppression by antibody allows one to consider that antigen-antibody complexes may not only be unrecognized by the immune

609

system (simple masking of antigen), but that these complexes also
alter the various cells involved in the immune response through
signals transmitted through the Fc portion. Two possibilities
present themselves: 1) alteration in macrophage functions, and 2)
inactivation (reversible or irreversible) of the immunocompetent
cell or cells. Alteration in macrophage functions induced by antigen-antibody complexes have been reported, but increased destructive phagocytosis of the whole antigen as a whole does not appear to
explain all the immunosuppressive activity of specific antibody
since the immunosuppression has been reported to be determinant
specific rather than molecule specific (1). Data concerning the
inactivation of cells involved in the immune response by antibody
are conflicting (3,11). Inactivation of immunologically competent
cells may imply any effect from a transitory inability to respond
to antigenic stimulation to an irreversible loss of immunological
function or even death of the cells. More recent experiments (12,
13) illustrating more marked inhibition of immune responses when
treatment with antibody was combined with antigen suggest that
antigen, antibody and some part of the immunologically responding
system may interact to cause immunosuppression and even inactivation (3,14,15) of the immunologically responding cells.

When considering an inactivation model for antibody regulation
of the immune response, the problem that faced us was how to correlate the importance of the Fc portion, which is not antigen-specific,
with the obvious specificity encountered in the regulation of the
immune response by antibody. To account for specificity of immunosuppression which requires the non-specific Fc portion, we propose
the following series of events (Fig. 1): 1) attachment of passively
administered antibody to some antigenic determinants on the immunogen, 2) conformational changes involving the Fc portion, 3)
attachment of the antigen-receptor on the immunologically competent
(antigen-sensitive) cell to other antigenic determinants on the
immunogen which are not covered by antibody, 4) transmission of a
negative or inactivation signal from the attached antibody to the
immunologically competent cell via the Fc portion (consequent to
the conformational change and possibly involving complement), and
5) reversible or irreversible inactivation of the immunologically
competent (antigen-sensitive) cell. This tripartite inactivation
model takes what is already known concerning the biological activity of antigen-antibody complexes (that much of the biological
activity is mediated through an Fc ligand), and adds an element of
immunological specificity in that a second (antigen-antibody) ligand
is necessary for the interaction of the complex with an immunologically competent cell. There is likely to be more than one of each
type of ligand and interactions between different antigenic groups
on the same immunogenic molecule would be expected (16).

Such a scheme leads to one obvious prediction. It should be
possible to cover available antigenic determinants with large

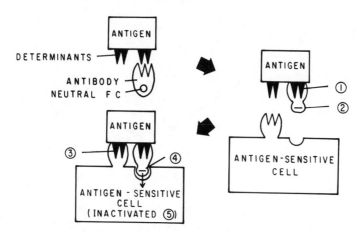

Figure 1:   TRIPARTITE INACTIVATION MODEL.   The numbers refer to the
events (see text) which lead to immunosuppression by antibody.

amounts of antibody so that antigen-receptors on immunologically
competent cells cannot interact with these antigenic determinants.
Under such circumstances, no inactivation should be possible because
the interaction of antigen, inactivating antibody and the immunologically competent cell cannot take place. To study the immunosuppression by antibody under these conditions, the immune response
was initiated with antigen, and then antibody was given in varying
doses one day later. If our model is correct, it should be possible
to demonstrate the inhibition of an on-going immune response by
certain doses of antibody. However, if too much antibody is given,
the immune response should be inhibited to a lesser degree because
antibody would combine with all available antigenic determinants
and no interaction between the immunologically competent cells and
the antigen-antibody complex could take place.

     Inbred male and female Swiss mice, originally obtained from
Carworth Farms, New City, U.S.A., were used for all experiments.
Antibody was obtained from mice given at least two injections of
0.1 ml. of a 10% suspension of sheep erythrocytes. The antibody
sedimented in the ultracentrifuge in the 7S region. Preparation
of F(ab')$_2$ has been described previously (7-9). Serum haemolysin
levels were assessed by the Microtiter method (8). Determination
of 19S and 7S antibody was carried out following ultracentrifugation in sucrose gradients (17). Antibody-forming cells were detected by the local haemolysis in gel technique (18). Irradiation
of mice in a Gammacell 20 (Atomic Energy of Canada Ltd., Ottawa,
Ontario, Canada) were carried out at the absorbed dose rate of 126
rad/minute emmitted from two 1000 curie sources of Cs^{137} (19).

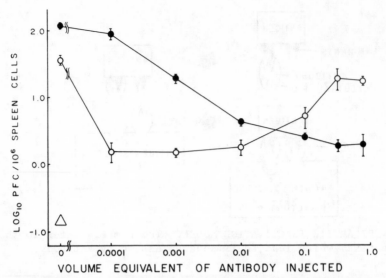

Figure 2: Effect of antibody, given 1 day after initiation of an immune response with low (2 X 10^6 - ◯) and high (5 X 10^8 - ●) numbers of sheep erythrocytes, on the number of plaque-forming cells in the spleen, measured 5 days after the injection of antigen. The triangle represents the background control. Vertical bars indicate one standard error of the reported mean. Number of mice at each point ranged from 5 to 18 (average - 8) and the PFC's were determined in quadruplicate.

        To assess the effect of varying doses of passively administered antibody, 7S haemolysin (titre of 12 $\log_2$ units) was injected intravenously one day after initiation of the immune response by the intravenous administration of either 5×10^8 or 2×10^6 sheep erythrocytes. The dose of antibody administered is expressed as the volume (ml) of the original serum which contained the amount of antibody injected (volume equivalent). The immune response (number of antibody-forming or plaque-forming cells - PFC) was measured 5 days after the injection of antigen. The smaller doses of antibody, given 1 day after 2×10^6 sheep erythrocytes, induced a 20-fold decrease in the number of PFC in the spleen, but larger doses of antibody induced only a 2-fold decrease in the immune response (Fig. 2). With 5×10^8 sheep erythrocytes (Fig. 2), the decrease in PFC response occurred when approximately 500-times the amount of antibody was given (compared to initiation of immune responses by 2×10^6 sheep erythrocytes). Therefore, the range in which inactivation occurred appears to depend on the ratio of antibody to antigen.

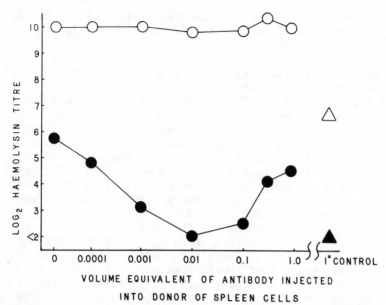

Figure 3: Effect of antibody-treatment of donor on ability of
transferred cells to show 19S (O) and 7S (●) priming. Cells were
transferred to irradiated recipients with 2 X 10^8 sheep erythrocytes 5 days after injection of donor with 2 X 10^6 sheep erythrocytes and 4 days after injection of varying doses of antibody. The
19S (△) and 7S (▲) antibody formation in non-primed cells is indicated and both 19S and 7S memory are demonstrated. Antibody
titres were estimated 7 days after cell transfer.

        As a further measure of the immune response, spleen cells from
animals receiving $2x10^6$ sheep erythrocytes and varying amounts of
antibody were washed 4 times in Medium 199, and 10^7 spleen cells
were transferred with $2x10^8$ sheep erythrocytes into lethally irradiated (900 rad) syngeneic recipients. Cells from animals receiving
$2x10^6$ sheep erythrocytes 5 days previously demonstrated both 19S
and 7S priming (Fig. 3). The 19S priming was not affected by antibody. The 7S priming was inhibited by intermediate doses of antibody but not by high or low doses.

        Our results demonstrate that certain amounts of antibody,
given 1 day after antigen, suppressed both 19S antibody-forming
cells and 7S priming. If too much antibody was given, only minimal
depression of immunological reactivity occurred. In terms of our
model, so much antibody was given that most of the antigenic determinants were masked by antibody so that no interaction took place
between antigenic determinants and antigen-receptors on immunologically competent (antigen-sensitive) cells. This tripartite inter-

action of antigen, antibody and the immunologically competent cell
is essential, in our model, for the inactivation of the immunologically competent cell by antibody.

   In all probability, feedback inhibition operates under two
distinct conditions: 1) when antibody of the suppressive type is
produced initially. Endogenously produced, suppressive antibody
will inactivate the cell producing it after the antibody has
reacted with antigen. The difficulty experienced in initiating 7S
antibody formation in vitro (10) may be due to rapid inactivation
of the suppressive antibody-forming cells as soon as small amounts
of suppressive antibody are formed. 2) when upper limit of antibody concentration in circulation is reached. Circulating (exogenous and suppressive)antibody will bind antigen and prevent the
immunologically competent cells from reacting to exposed antigenic
determinants. By binding antibody via the Fc portion (21), germinal centres may function to control these two types of feedback
inhibition. In the first case, inhibition by endogenous antibody,
the germinal centres may direct the Fc portions of suppressive
antibody away from the cell producing this suppressive antibody,
thus preventing attachment of the Fc portion to the antibody-forming
cell even if the antibody binds to antigen. The correlation between production of large amounts of 7S antibody and germinal centre
function has been commented on previously (22). In the second case,
inhibition by circulating (exogenous) antibody, the germinal centres
may remove adherent antibody from antigen and/or orientate attached
antibody so that the Fc portions are directed away from the incoming immunologically competent cells. We have noted (20) that,
with very high doses of $F(ab')_2$ or 7S antibody, $F(ab')_2$ may show the
better suppression; this may be due to the fact that $F(ab')_2$ cannot
be removed from the surface of the antigen. We envisage that the
removal of adherent antibody from antigen occurs within the germinal centre (or cells with analogous function) in which the Fc portion
acts as a handle for the removal of antibody.

   In summary, $F(ab')_2$ and 7S antibody inhibit immune responses in
markedly different ways, and this difference we attribute to the
loss of the Fc portion of the antibody molecule which functions in
the following ways: 1) prevention of loss of antibody by excretion,
2) facilitation of phagocytosis and degradation of antigen by macrophages by cytophilic and immune adherence mechanisms, and 3) mediation of a negative ('feedback') signal to the immunologically
competent cell. Our present view is that all these mechanisms are
operative in producing the difference in suppressive activity between $F(ab')_2$ and 7S antibody, and that the germinal centres operate to control the third function, that we attribute to the Fc
portion by removing of antibody from antigen. Inactivation via the
Fc portion at certain antigen-antibody ratios may explain high and
low zone tolerance, may be of help in understanding tumour enhancement and lead to effective tumour immunotherapy by blocking Fc-

inactivation, and may explain the curious occurrence of a predominantly anti-Fc IgM antibody (rheumatoid factor) in a number of autoimmune states where lack of feedback inhibition may be significant.

REFERENCES

1. J. Uhr and G. Moller, Adv. Immunol., 8:81, 1968.
2. T.W. Tao and J.W. Uhr, Nature, 212:208, 1966.
3. D.A. Rowley and F.W. Fitch, in: Regulation of the Antibody Response, B. Cinader, Ed., p. 127. Illinois: Thomas, 1968.
4. C.L. Greenbury and D.H. Moore, Nature, 219:526, 1968.
5. J.C. Cerottini, P.J. McConahey and F.J. Dixon, J. Immunol., 102:1008, 1969.
6. H. Chang, S. Schneck, N.I. Brody, A. Deutsch and G.W. Siskind, J. Immunol., 102:37, 1969.
7. N.R.StC. Sinclair, R.K. Lees and E.V. Elliott, Nature, 220:1048, 1968.
8. N.R.StC. Sinclair, J. Exp. Med., 129:1183, 1969.
9. N.R.StC. Sinclair, R.K. Lees, P.L. Chan and R.H. Khan, Immunology, 19:105, 1970.
10. R.K. Lees and N.R.StC. Sinclair, in preparation
11. E. Moller, S. Britten and G. Moller, in: Regulation of the Antibody Response, B. Cinader, Ed., p. 141. Illinois: Thomas, 1968.
12. M. Axelrad and D.A. Rowley, Science, 160:1465, 1968.
13. F.P. Stuart, T. Saitoh and F.W. Fitch, Science, 160:1463, 1968.
14. M. Feldman and E. Diener, J. Exp. Med., 131:247, 1970.
15. E. Diener and M. Feldman, J. Exp. Med., 132:31, 1970.
16. N.I. Brody, J.G. Walker and G.W. Siskind, J. Exp. Med., 126:81, 1967.
17. N.R.StC. Sinclair and E.V. Elliott, Immunology, 15:325, 1968.
18. N.K. Jerne, A.A. Nordin and C. Henry, in: Cell Bound Antibodies, B. Amos and H. Koprowski, Eds., p.109, Philadelphia, Wistar Institute Press, 1963.
19. J.R. Cunningham, W.R. Bruce and H.P. Webb, Phys. Med. Biol., 10:381, 1965.
20. P.L. Chan and N.R.StC. Sinclair, in preparation.
21. C.R. Parish and G.L. Ada, this conference.
22. J.D. Wakefield and G.J. Thorbecke, J. Exp. Med., 128:171, 1968.

Supported by the Medical Research Council of Canada and the National Cancer Institute of Canada. N.R.StC.S. is a Scholar of the Medical Research Council of Canada and P.L.C. is a Fellow of the National Cancer Institute of Canada.

THE ROLE OF THE BURSA OF FABRICIUS IN THE RECOVERY FROM IMMUNOLOGIC TOLERANCE TO BOVINE SERUM ALBUMIN [1]

Raymond D.A. Peterson, Gunnar V. Alm and Suzanne Michalek
The Variety Club Research Center of the La Rabida-University of Chicago Institute, and the Department of Pediatrics, University of Chicago, Chicago, Ill., U.S.A.

It is well known that thymectomy in rodents impairs the recovery from immunologic tolerance (1 - 3). The exact mechanism whereby the thymectomy impairs the recovery process is not fully known. It may be through the removal of the site of differentiation of new immunocompetent, thymus-dependent cells. These cells appear to lack the ability to synthesize and secrete conventional antibody (4).

In contrast the role of the other well established central lymphoid organ, the bursa of Fabricius in the chicken, in the recovery from immunologic tolerance has not heretofore been assessed. The bursa of Fabricius appears to be the site of a critical phase in the differentiation of the actual antibody forming cells (5, 6).

If these cells are involved in tolerance it would be anticipated that the bursa of Fabricius might also, like the thymus, be important in the recovery from tolerance. To test this the following experiment was performed.

MATERIAL AND METHODS

White leghorn chickens were irradiated with 600 R x-ray on the day of hatch as previously described (7). The animals were divided into two groups. One group, controls (C), received intraperitoneal (i.p.) injections of saline twice weekly over the next 5 weeks. The other group, tolerant (T), received i.p. injections

[1] Supported by USPHS Grants Al-08771-02 and AM-05589-03.

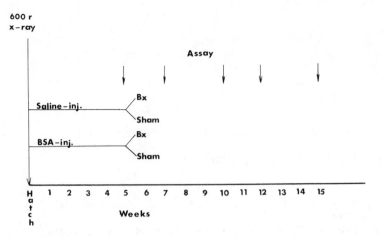

of bovine serum albumin (BSA) twice weekly over the same time
period. The first dose of BSA was 1325 mg/kg body weight. The
subsequent doses were 663 mg/kg body weight. At 5 weeks of age
one half of the chickens were surgically bursectomized (Bx or b),
the other half were sham operated (s). The four experimental
groups were designated C_b, C_s, T_b and T_s. There were 6 chickens
per group per assay time.

Spleen cells forming antibody to BSA were demonstrated by
Jerne's local hemolysis in gel assay, using BSA coupled to sheep
erythrocytes by carbodiimide as the indicator (8). The plaque
forming cells (PFC) were developed with rabbit antiserum to
chicken gammaglobulin, plus guinea pig complement. Seven days
prior to each assay of PFC the chickens were injected i.v. with
40 mg/kg body weight of BSA. Appropriate specificity controls of
the tolerance, using sheep erythrocyte antigen, were run.

The experimental design is shown in figure 1.

RESULTS

As shown in figure 2 the C_s and C_b groups of chickens did
not differ significantly in the antibody response (number of PFC
per spleen) to BSA. Therefore the bursectomy at 5 weeks of age
had no effect on the subsequent immune responsiveness to this
antigen.

The BSA injected chickens (T) were initially significantly
less able to develop PFC to BSA, indicating they were tolerant.

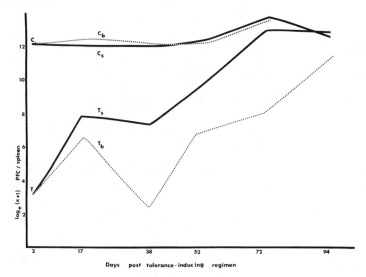

Days post tolerance-inducing regimen

The C and T groups responded equally well to sheep erythrocytes,
showing that the tolerance was specific for BSA.

Further, as can be seen from figure 2, the sham operated
tolerant chickens (T_s) recovered to control levels by 72 days
after cessation of the tolerance inducing regimen. However, the
bursectomized tolerant chickens (T_s) showed an impaired recovery.
The T_s and T_b groups were significantly different at the day 72
(P 0.05) and day 94 (P 0.001) assay times. Furthermore, during
the whole assay period, 9/28 T_b and only 1/28 T_s chickens were
completely unresponsive to BSA. The difference between these
proportions is significant (P 0.025).

DISCUSSION AND CONCLUSIONS

The results of this investigation show clearly that the
bursa of Fabricius, even at 5 weeks of age, has a definite role
in the recovery from immunologic tolerance. They further suggest
that the (potential) antibody forming cells may be made specifically tolerant to BSA. This observation agrees with the recent
report by Chiller et al. (9) that the bone-marrow derived antibody forming cells in the mouse can be made tolerant. It is
suggested that the bursa of Fabricius is the source necessary for
the replenishment of the bursa-dependent antibody forming cells
during the recovery from tolerance. If tolerant peripheral bursa-
dependent cells do exist, they do not recover from the tolerant
state without the bursa.

REFERENCES

1. H.N. Claman and D.W. Talmage, Science 141:1193, 1963.

2. R.B. Taylor, Immunology 7:595, 1964.

3. A.C. Aisenberg and C. Davis, J. Exp. Med. 128:35, 1968.

4. A.J.S. Davies, E. Leuchars, V. Wallis, R. Marchant and E.V. Elliott, Transplantation 5:222, 1967.

5. G.J. Thorbecke, N.L. Warner, G.M. Hochwald and S.H. Ohanian, Immunology 15:123, 1968.

6. P.W. Kincade and M.D. Cooper, Fed. Proc. 29:503, 1970.

7. G.V. Alm and R.D.A. Peterson, J. Exp. Med. 129:1247, 1969.

8. E.S. Golub, R.I. Mishell, W.O. Weigle and R.W. Dutton, J. Immunol. 100:133, 1968.

9. J.M. Chiller, G.S. Habicht and W.O. Weigle, Proc. Nat. Acad. Sci. 65:551, 1970.

CELL DESTRUCTIVE ACTION OF PHYTOHAEMAGGLUTININ (PHA)-STIMULATED HUMAN LYMPHOCYTES;STUDIES ON THE MECHANISM OF THIS CYTOAGGRESSIVE EFFECT IN VITRO [+]

H.Oerkermann,W.D.Hirschmann,K.Schumacher,
G.Uhlenbruck,G.Alzer,G.Wintzer and R.Gross
Medizinische Universitätsklinik Köln,W.-Germany

Under the influence of PHA lymphocytes are transformed into blast-like cells and develop cytoaggres-
siveness against target cells in vitro,i.e.they destroy cultures of various cell types in a very special
manner of action.The cytoaggressive effect has been
described already by several authors (1-4) but the
mechanism of this rather unusual way of cell destruction is still unknown.It has been found that the PHA-
treated lymphocytes enter into a close contact with
the target cells,and this seems to play an important
role in the cytoaggressive reaction.

When we performed time lapse cinematography of HeLa
cell cultures to which human lymphocytes had been added together with PHA we observed that the lymphocytes
were not only passively attached to the target cells
but became very mobile and developed a great activity
almost immediately after they had been added to the
HeLa cell cultures and had come into contact with PHA.
They moved quickly around underneath and upon the cells
of the monolayer and touched the target cells with
fine pseudopodia.They even pushed the nuclei and the
cytoplasm of the target cells to and fro.Only those
target cells which had been "attacked" for a while
died,and this always happened as a sudden and complete
breakdown of single cells,remarkably,without previous
morphological alterations of the cells.The lymphocytes

[+] This study was supported by the DEUTSCHE FORSCHUNGS-
GEMEINSCHAFT.

under the influence of PHA were transformed into blast-
like cells during their cytoaggressive action and exhibited mitotic cell divisions.Similar observations
were performed by AX and coworkers (5).Non-stimulated
lymphocytes in the controls were comparatively immobile,
they did not destroy the HeLa cells and were not transformed into blast-like cells.

To get further information about the mechanism of
the cytoaggressive effect we investigated whether or
not E.coli L-asparaginase (EC-2 A-se) might influence
the cell destructive action of the lymphocytes,too,
since it was found that this enzyme preparation inhibited the PHA-induced transformation of the lymphocytes
into blast-like cells completely (6-8).

In our experiments we used human lymphocytes which
were isolated from the peripheral blood of healthy
donors by means of a glass bead column.They were added
to HeLa cell cultures together with PHA and EC-2 A-se
(3 i.U./ml culture medium).Controls were prepared
simultaneously (see Fig.).To avoid any inhibitory effect
of EC-2 A-se upon the target cells we used a subline of
HeLa cells which had become resistant to EC-2 A-se by
culturing the HeLa cells for several months with increasing doses of this enzyme preparation.The HeLa cells
were labelled with 14C-thymidine previous to each experiment,and the release of 14C-thymidine from the
damaged HeLa cells was measured to determine the extent
of the cytoaggressive effect according to the method
of HOLM and PERLMANN (9).This method was slightly modi-
fied.After 48 hours of incubation each experiment was
stopped and the release of 14C-thymidine determined.

It was shown by the experiments that the release of
14C-thymidine was markedly reduced in those cultures
which had been treated with EC-2 A-se.(Fig).

Time lapse cinematography of those cultures treated
with EC-2 A-se revealed that,indeed,the cytoaggressive
effect of the stimulated lymphocytes was inhibited.How-
ever,and this was an unexpected finding,the typical
action of the lymphocytes was not influenced by EC-2
A-se.As usual they were moving quickly around and acted
in the same way as described above.But the HeLa cells
were not injured any more by their"attack".After 48
hours the monolayer was still intact,and the proliferation of the HeLa cells was undisturbed.The lymphocytes,though highly active,were not transformed into

blast-like cells and did not exhibit mitotic cell divisions.

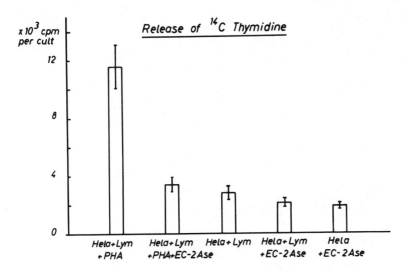

Fig.:: Mean values of three experiments of the same
kind.In all of the tests four cultures were
used for each of the five groups.

From the results it is shown that EC-2 A-se inhibits
not only the blastogenesis of PHA-stimulated lymphocytes
but also their cytoaggressive effect.The PHA-induced
increased motility of the lymphocytes and their typical manner of action which seems to be a sort of "attack"
against the target cells are not influenced by EC-2
A-se.With regard to the mechanism of the cytoaggressive
effect these results lead to the assumption that the
typical "attack" of the lymphocytes alone is not sufficient to bring the cytoaggressive effect about.Ad-
ditional factors must be supposed to play a role in
this special way of cell destruction,factors which
are inhibited by EC-2 A-se but which we do not know
until now.

As EC-2 A-se influences the metabolism of certain
cell types by depriving them of L-asparagine and/or
L-glutamine it seems to be possible that EC-2 A-se stops
the PHA-stimulated lymphocytes to synthesize certain
substances which are additionally necessary to bring
the cytoaggressive effect about.How far the synthesis
of those substances is connected with the blastic trans-

formation of the stimulated lymphocytes remains to be seen.Since the blastic transformation and the cyto-aggressive effect are both suppressed by EC-2 A-se such a connection is anyway conceivable.Finally it must be considered whether or not the blastic transformation itself represents the additional factor for the cyto-aggressive effect: The stimulated lymphocytes entering into the blastic transformation and preparing cell division have an increased nutritional requirement and this might induce them to develop a sort of "parasitic properties" towards the target cells.By withdrawing essential components from the target cells they might cause the cell destruction in vitro.

REFERENCES:

1.   Rosenau W.,Moon H.D.
     J.Nat.Cancer Inst.,1961,27,471

2.   Wilson D.B.
     J.Cell Comp.Physiol.1963,62,273

3.   Holm G.,Perlmann P.,Werner B.
     Nature 1964,203,841

4.   Möller E.
     Science 1965,147,873

5.   Ax W.,Malchow H.,Zeiss J.,Fischer H.
     Exper.Cell Res.1968,53,108

6.   Astaldi G.,Burgio G.R.,Krc J.,Genova R.,Astaldi,A.A.
     Lancet 1969,1,423

7.   Ohno R.,Anderson M.D.
     Proc.Amer.Ass.Cancer Res.1969,10,66

8.   Oerkermann H.,Hirschmann W.D.
     Proc.6th Internat.Congr.Chemother.,Tokyo,1969,in
     press

9.   Holm G.Perlmann P.
     Nature 1965,207,818

ON THE MECHANISM OF GERMINAL CENTER FORMATION[1]

T. Mariani, T.J. Linna[2], and R.A. Good

Pediatric Research Laboratories, University of

Minnesota Hospital, Minneapolis, Minnesota, USA

The purpose of this communication is to present evidence for a new model of germinal center formation. Extensive investigations have been conducted in our laboratory at Minnesota concerning syngenic skin graft rejection, so-called heterogenization or antigenic alteration of normal tissue in mice with Gross passage A virus-induced lymphoma (1,2,3). Concurrently, light microscopic examinations of germinal center formation during leukemogenesis were undertaken. As early as 12 hours following intraperitoneal transfer of Gross passage A (GPA) lymphoma (ascites form) in the $(C_3H/Bi$ x $DBA/2)F_1$ hybrid mice, germinal centers were observed in the mesenteric nodes of these injected animals, whereas, they were absent in the untreated animals. We also observed germinal center formation in the spleen of the injected animals. However, they were not as prominent as those found in the mesenteric nodes.

To clarify the mechanism of germinal center formation in this experimental model, mice were injected with cell-free peritoneal fluid from tumor-bearing animals. The same kinetics of

1. Aided by grants from The National Foundation March of Dimes, and the American Cancer Society, Inc., Public Health Service grants NB 02042 from the National Institute of Neurological Diseases and Blindness and AI 00292 and AI 08677 from the National Institute of Allergy and Infections Diseases; and the Minnesota Division of the American Cancer Society, Inc.

2. Present address: Department of Histology, Institute of Human Anatomy, University of Uppsala, Uppsala, Sweden.

germinal center formation with their very early appearance could
be found. The frequency of these centers in the mesenteric nodes
was approximately the same as when the ascites was used. Because
of these findings, i.e., this frequency of germinal center formation with or without tumor cells, attempts were made to minimize the chance of injecting live GPA virus. Thus, the next stage
of experimentation sought to determine the effect of the following preparations on germinal center formation. Four groups of
animals received heat-killed or repeatedly freeze-thawed virus
from either cell-free filtrates from leukemic tissues or from
cell-free peritoneal fluid. A fifth group was injected with
supernatants from ultracentrifuged cell-free peritoneal fluid;
these supernatants were obtained by centrifuging the cell-free
peritoneal fluid at 125,000 g for as long as 3 hours. The sixth
group of mice received live purified GPA virus which was prepared from leukemic tissues according to procedures initially
described by Gross (3). In all these groups, we could still observe germinal center formation as frequently as before and as
early as 12 hours after injection of these preparations. These
data indicate that germinal center formation with this model is
not primarily caused by either tumor cells or live GPA virus.

We were, of course, puzzled by these findings, and we
wanted to relate them to more conventional antigens. Thus, in
other groups of animals, we injected intraperitoneally, for
example, Brucella antigen and BSA. There was also included a
third group of animals which was treated with purified endotoxin prepared and supplied to us by Dr. Y.B. Kim, Department
of Microbiology, University of Minnesota. With all these preparations, we observed germinal center formation as early as
3 hours after injection of the agents (Fig. 1); this has been
the earliest time thus far that we have examined the tissues.

Because we have obtained early appearance of germinal
centers even with endotoxin, our data indicate that germinal
center formation may not require immunologic specificity. Approximately 30 years ago, Hellman (5) described formation of secondary lymphoid follicles as a result of various noxious agents including antigens. He introduced the term "reaction nodule" for
these structures. Our findings support strongly his interpretation. The extraordinarily early appearance of germinal centers
in our studies, we believe, can be more easily explained in
terms of transformation of cells in situ into germinal center
cells rather than cell traffic from other organs, or proliferation of preexisting cells.

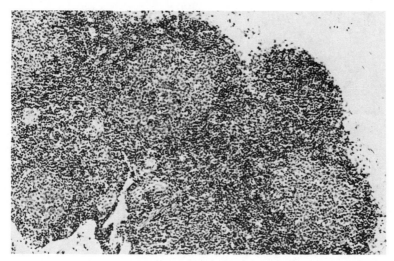

Text for Figure 1: Germinal centers in a mesenteric lymph node
3 hours after endotoxin administration (x100).

REFERENCES

1. T. Mariani, Fed.Proc., 27:715, 1968.

2. T. Mariani, P.B. Dent, and R.A. Good, J. Nat. Cancer Inst.,
   44:319, 1970.

3. T. Mariani, Y. Maruyama, Fed. Proc., 29:560, 1970.

4. L. Gross, Proc. Soc. Exptl. Biol.Med., 94:767, 1957.

5. T. Hellman, in: W.v. Möllendorff, Ed., Handbuch Der Mikro-
   skopischen Anatomie Des Menschen, Vol VI/4, p. 200. Berlin:
   Springer-Verlag, 1943.

APPENDIX AND BONE MARROW CELL SYNERGISM IN EARLY ANTIBODY

RESPONSE TO SHEEP ERYTHROCYTES[1]

H. Ozer[2] and B.H. Waksman

Department of Microbiology, Yale University, New Haven,

Conn. 06510

With regard to the problem of whether the rabbit appendix is a central or peripheral lymphoid organ, the evidence from our laboratory indicates that the first possibility is the more likely. Our recent experiments have shown that the early response of rabbits to sheep red blood cells (SRBC) requires the presence of both appendix and bone marrow cells.

MATERIAL AND METHODS

New Zealand albino rabbits received 2×10^9 SRBC i.v., and their spleen cells were assayed 5 days later for direct plaque-forming cells (PFC) by a modification of the technique of Jerne et al. (1). Appendectomy, 900 rads whole body irradiation (central axis dose), and shielding of femoral bone marrow (after excision of both popliteal lymph nodes) were carried out by techniques already described (2, 3). Some animals were reinjected, immediately after irradiation and 3-4 hours prior to immunization, with $1-5 \times 10^9$ autologous appendix cells i.v., while others received a similar number of allogeneic spleen cells. Control animals were reinjected with appendix cells disrupted by hypotonic lysis (in 20 ml distilled water) and two cycles of freeze-thawing; microscopic examination showed that no viable cells remained following this treatment.

[1] Supported by USPHS grants AI-06112 and AI-06455.
[2] Predoctoral Fellow, USPHS Medical Scientist Training Program GM 02044-01.

Table I

Group	No. of rabbits	PFC/10^6 spleen cells Average (range)	PFC x 10^3/spleen Average (range)
Normal	5	201 (183-213)	174 (150-210)
Appendectomy + 900 r			
(BM)	5	8.6 (7-19)	2.3 (1.8-2.5)
(App)	5	16 (9-28)	4.5 (0.4-10)
(BM + App)	5	91 (47-118)	33 (18-43)
(BM + App$^+$)	4	5.3 (3-7)	1.2 (0.7-1.7)
(Spleen)	4	132 (84-178)	90 (33-143)

BM: Shielding of femoral marrow

App: 1-5 x 10^9 autologous appendix cells

Spleen: 1-5 x 10^9 xenogeneic spleen cells

$^+$: Hypotonic lysis and freeze-thawing

RESULTS

The direct 5-day PFC response in the spleen was almost completely abolished by the combination of appendectomy and lethal whole body irradiation. Shielding of the bone marrow or re-injection of living autologous appendix cells restored the response to a slight extent (Table I). The two cell types in combination gave between 5-10 times more PFC than either alone or than the sum of the two. This degree of restoration was, however, slightly less than that achieved by injecting a similar number of living allogeneic spleen cells. The response observed did not depend on an adjuvant effect of endotoxin present in the appendix cell preparation, since killed appendix cells failed to restore the PFC response. With the number of cells employed, the maximal response attained was less than the minimum seen in normal animals.

DISCUSSION

The data presented here show that the early splenic antibody response to SRBC in the rabbit requires the presence of two cell types provided, respectively, by the bone marrow and the appendix. We thus confirm in a direct manner the results of extirpation experiments (4, 5) which suggest that the appendix, sacculus rotundus, and Peyer's patches act as the source of a cell essential to M-antibody formation in this species. Our finding also supports the hypothesis (3) that this cell is not immunocompetent in itself but must normally migrate to peripheral lymphoid organs such as the spleen, where it can interact with antigen in cooperation with a marrow-derived cell. Since spleen cells respond in high degree to the SRBC stimulus, it is clear that antigen can act directly on progeny of the marrow and appendix (or similar organs) which have already entered the peripheral lymphocyte pool. However, in animals whose bone marrow and appendix are shielded during irradiation, antigen injected directly into the appendiceal artery immunizes very effectively (2). This implies, in agreement with the present results, that appendix cells possess specific reactivity for antigen before they leave to enter the peripheral pool.

These findings and those of others who have recently studied ɣM responses in the rabbit (2-8) provide an interesting contrast to the findings in rats and mice (see reviews in 9). In these species the response to SRBC is in large part thymus-dependent and there is good evidence to show that thymus-derived and bone marrow-derived lymphocytes must co-operate, the antibody-forming cell originating directly from the marrow-derived partner. The function of the lymphoepithelial organs in the rabbit bowel is apparently not affected by thymectomy and irradiation (4, 5). There is therefore a strong presumption that in this species these organs may carry out part of the function usually ascribed to the thymus, that related to ɣM responses.

REFERENCES

1. N.K. Jerne, A.A. Nordin and C. Henry, in Cell Bound Antibodies (B. Amos and H. Koprowski, Eds.). Wistar Inst. Press, 1963, p. 109.

2. M. Hanaoka, K. Nomoto and B.H. Waksman, J. Immunol., 104:616, 1970.

3. M. Hanaoka and B.H. Waksman, Cellular Immunol., submitted.

4. S. Konda and T.N. Harris, J. Immunol., 97:805, 1966.

5. R.A. Good, W.A. Cain, D.Y. Percy, P.B. Dent, H.J. Meuwissen, G.E. Rodey and M.D. Cooper, in Lymphatic Tissue and Germinal Centers in Immune Response (L. Fiore-Donati and M.G. Hanna, Jr., eds.). Plenum, New York, 1969, p. 33.

6. C. Henry, W.D. Faulk, L. Kuhn, J.M. Yoffey and H.H. Fudenberg, J. Exp. Med. 131:1200, 1970.

7. M. Richter, B. Rose and N.I. Abdou, Int. Arch. Allergy, 38:269, 1970.

8. N.I. Abdou and M. Richter, J. Immunol., 104:1087, 1970.

9. Antigen-sensitive cells (G. Möller, Ed.). Transpl. Rev., 1:1, 1969.

THYMUS-MARROW CELL INTERACTION IN VITRO

Enhancing Effect of Different Bone Marrow Constituents on PHA
Response of Thymocytes

G.Tridente, G.Biasi, L.Chieco-Bianchi, L.Fiore-Donati

Division of Experimental Oncology, University of

Padova, Italy

In the series of complex events which characterize the immune response the role of cell cooperation between different cell
types has recently received much attention. In particular it has
been shown that different classes of lymphocytes may cooperate
togheter and/or with other cells, such as macrophages, in producing an immunological response (I-3). Moreover, cell interaction
can occurr between lymphoid precursors and produce immunocompetent cells (4-6). On this basis we have been studying possible
interactions in vitro between thymocytes and bone marrow cells
by using Phytohemagglutinin (PHA) stimulation, in order to establish wether cell cooperation can also occurr entirely in vitro
and produce PHA-responsive cells, known to be related to the
thymus-dependent population of lymphocytes responsible for cell
mediated immune reactions(7-9). We report here evidence that
such interactions can be determined in this in vitro system and
attempts to individuate the cell types involved.

MATERIALS AND METHODS

CBA mice of both sexes were used as thymus and bone marrow
donors. Bone marrow cell suspensions were obtained from femurs
and tibiae of normal 4-6 months old animals by forcing 0.3 ml of
fresh medium (Hanks-Eagle Minimal Essential Medium - MEM - Gibco,
N.Y., USA) into the bone cavity. Cells were washed once and resuspended in MEM additioned with 20 percent heat-inactivated Fetal Calf Serum (FCS, Gibco, N.Y., USA). Part of this suspension
was brought to 2×10^6 viable cells/ml in the same medium to be

cultured; part was brought approximately to 30 x 10^6 viable cells/ml and transferred to a nylon column to be separated in two cell populations on the basis of their property to adhere or not to nylon fibers. Columns were prepared by packing nylon (Filtralon, ARA, Amsterdam) into 20 ml syringes or in water jacketed glass columns (I.5 cm diam. x 20 cm high). Nylon was cleaned in hot 7X (Linbro Chem. Co., New Haven, Conn.,USA) rinsed overnight in tap water, then in several changes of distilled water. Columns were sterilized, washed with MEM $\pm$ IO percent FCS and brought to 37 °C just before use. 25-65 x 10^7 nucleated cells in approximately 8 ml medium were incubated for 40 min at 37 °C. Non adhering cells were then washed out with 30-40 ml pre-warmed medium, pooled and centrifuged. Final cell concentration was adjusted at 2 x 10^6 viable cells/ml as for the unfractionated bone marrow. The collected cell fraction (Fr) contained approximately 90% mononucleated cells mostly resembling small lymphocytes and late erythroblasts and represented 20 $\pm$ 5 percent of total cell population of the respective unfractionated bone marrow. When higher yields of this fraction were obtained, due to contamination with larger proportions of other cell types, the collected suspension was refractionated by incubation for 20 min in another nylon column. In the water jacketed column a constant flow of the cell suspension to be fractionated was achieved by connecting the cell suspension container to the column by a blood transfusion set and adjusting the flow at I-2 ml/min. The results obtained with the two systems were superimposable and therefore the syringe system was more frequently used for practical reasons. The adhering cell population was removed from nylon by adding 0.02 percent EDTA in Ca^{++} and Mg^{++} free Hanks solution + IO percent FCS, for 5-IO min then washing with 20 ml of the same solution.

Thymus lobes from 2-3 days old mice were removed without damaging the capsule and carefully cleaned to avoid mediastinal lymph node or blood contamination. The intact lobes were then washed twice in MEM + 20 percent FCS and gently forced trough a multilayer nylon sieve. Final cell suspension was adjusted at 2 x 10^6 viable cells/ml. Viability ranged between 85-95 percent in all cell suspensions and was determined by the Eosin Y exclusion test.

Triplicate cultures with and without 0.025 ml PHA (Wellcome, Beckenam, England, diluted as reccomended by the manufacturer) containing 2-6 x 10^6 cells in a standard volume of 3 ml medium were prepared from thymus and bone marrow cell suspensions.

Mixtures of both cell types in varying ratios were also set up. In another group of cell mixtures thymus or bone marrow cells were alternatively treated with Mitomycin C (30 ug/ml - A. Christiaens, Bruxelles) according to a modified technique for one-way directional cultures (IO) in order to establish which of the two cell populations is responding to PHA after the interaction. Similar experiments have been performed by using the lymphoid marrow fraction (Fr), or the adhering cell fraction in the place of unfractionated bone marrow with the aim of individuating the cell type involved. Control cultures consisted of both mitomycin treated and untreated single cell suspensions employed in the relative cell mixtures. Finally fibroblasts and peritoneal macrophages were cultured in the place of bone marrow cells in isogenic combinations with thymocytes in order to establish the specificity of the marrow constituent(s) involved in the interaction.

PHA response was evaluated as increment in DNA synthesis in stimulated cultures of all the experimental groups compared to the spontaneous incorporation of 3H-thymidine (3H-TdR) of the respective controls. I.5 uC/ml 3H-TdR (Thymidine-methyl-H3, spec. activity 2.0 C/mM, NEN, Boston) per culture was added six hours before harvesting and processing the cultures for liquid scintillation counting.

In addition, to better establish the cell types present in the (Fr) fraction,different amounts of unfractionated bone marrow and the respective (Fr) cell fractions were injected in iso genic adult mice lethally irradiated (850 rads) and the number of Colony Forming Units (CFU) was determined after 9 days in the spleen according to the technique of Till and McCulloch. The same cell suspensions were also assayed for the presence of PHA responsive cells and for the interacting capacity with thymocytes.

RESULTS

Previous work developed in this laboratory has shown that mouse lymphocytes from different sources respond to PHA with different degrees of cell transformation and DNA synthesis (I2-I4). More recently we have studied the PHA response of thymus cell cultures and shown that these cells, in our system, react poorly to PHA, especially thymocytes obtained from normal adult animals (7-9).Bone marrow cell cultures showed a slight increase in 3H-TdR uptake after PHA stimulation with a moderate peak at 96 hours of incubation.

However, when newborn thymus cells were mixed with isogenic

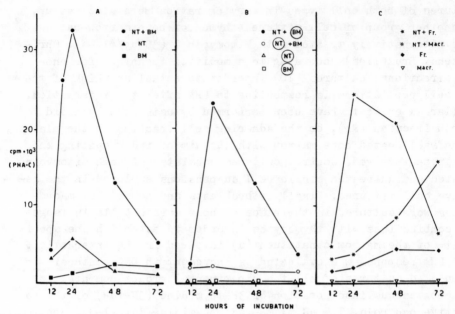

Fig. I - 3H-TdR incorporation induced by PHA in thymus-marrow cel-
l mixtures. A: unblocked cell cultures. B: one-way directional
cultures. C: interacting effect of different marrow cell fractions.(see text)
NT: newborn thymus; BM: bone marrow; Fr: marrow lymphoid cell fraction; Macr: macrophage rich fraction; ◯:mitomycin-treated.

marrow cells a remarkable increase of isotope uptake in PHA stimulated mixtures was observed, compared to the response of the
respective single cell suspensions (Fig. I,A). This response was
strictly dependent on the number of thymocytes in the mixture
and the total cell concentration per culture. Optimal thymus-marrow cell concentration was found to be $4+2 \times 10^{6}$ cells/culture
and the typical PHA peak response was detected after 24 hours
of incubation. Under similar culture conditions thymocytes obtained from adult animals proved to be slightly effective in increasing the PHA response of the mixtures.

  Data obtained from one-way directional cultures clearly
showed that intact thymocytes mixed with mitomycin-blocked marrow cells give a PHA response strikingly similar to that observed in unblocked cell mixtures (Fig. I,B). On the other hand,
no significant PHA response was registered when blocked thymo-

Table I - Presence of CFUs and PHA responsive cells in unfractionated and nylon-fractionated mouse bone marrow.

	CFU assay[1]		PHA assay[2]	
	No./10^4 cells	CF	PHA-C ($cpm \times 10^3$)	CF
Bone Marrow	3.6 ± 1	1.0	3.9 ± 2	1.0
Marrow Lymphoid Fraction (Fr)	14.4 ± 2	4.0	11.3 ± 1	2.9

(1)- spleen colonies according to Till and McCulloch(11).
(2)- net PHA-induced incorporation of 2×10^6 cells at 96 hours.
CF - concentration factor
Fr - nylon non-adhering mononuclear cell fraction, representing
     20 percent of total bone marrow.

cytes were cultured with intact marrow cells. Moreover, an increase in the number of blocked marrow cells over 2×10^6 cells/
culture did not enhance the response of a constant number of thymocytes. Similarly, by increasing the number of blocked thymocytes no effect was observed on the PHA response of intact bone
marrow cells.

Particularly interesting were the results obtained from nylon-fractionated bone marrow cell cultures. The non-adhering
cell population (Fr) proved to be as effective as unfractionated
bone marrow in enhancing the PHA response of newborn thymocytes
(Fig. 1,C). However, the adhering fraction as well as peritoneal
macrophages (Macr), although ineffective in producing the typical 24 hour peak modified the PHA response of thymocytes in that
a progressive increase of isotope uptake was found after the first day of culture, with peak values at 72 hours.

No enhancing effect was registered when fibroblasts were
added to thymus cell cultures in the place of bone marrow cells.

Finally, the (Fr) cell fraction, which contained the early-
interacting cell population, appeared also to yield a higher number of CFUs and of PHA responsive cells compared to unfractionated bone marrow (Table I). The relative concentration factor(CF)

demonstrated in fact, a four fold increase of stem cells and approximately three fold increment of the PHA-sensitive cells in the fractionated cell population.

DISCUSSION

Considerable evidence suggests that the cell type which is stimulated in vitro by PHA is related to the immunocompetent cell population responsible for typical cell-mediated immune reactions such as graft rejection, delayed type ipersensitivity, graft-vs-host (I5-I8). Moreover, in many experimental models the PHA test parallels the in vivo conventional tests for cellular immunity, i.e. skin graft rejection, the Simonsen assay, the appearance of acute secondary disease (I4,I9).

Murine thymus and bone marrow are known to contain a low number of immunocompetent cells able to elicit cell-mediated reactions. On the other hand they contain immature precursors which may cooperate in raising an immune response in the anti-sheep erythrocyte system (4-8) as well as in others (20).

In this study we have obtained evidence that the PHA response can also be enhanced in vitro by using proper mixtures of newborn thymus and bone marrow cells. Moreover, data from one-way directional cultures,which allow only one cell population to respond to PHA, clearly show that the potential PHA-responsive cell is in the thymus and is triggered by a bone marrow constituent(s). It is noteworthy that the marrow component is still effective when its DNA synthesis is blocked. The trigger cell(s) which produce the early and more pronounced peak of incorporation are present in the nylon non-adhering cell fraction which morphologically appears lymphoid in type and represents approximately IO-I5 percent of total bone marrow population. In addition,this component seems to be specific for bone marrow or bone marrow-derived cells since we have also obtained evidence that spleen cells from newborn-thymectomized animals are equally effective as bone marrow cells(9). This specificity is further substantiated by the finding that substituting fibroblasts for marrow cells does not increase the thymic response to PHA.

On the other hand, peritoneal macrophages and the nylon-adhering marrow cell fraction also seem to enhance the thymic response to a certain extent and with a different kinetics, which would indicate that different mechanisms and/or cells come into play in this in vitro interaction.

Particularly interesting was the finding that the marrow lymphoid fraction (Fr) contained a higher number of stem cells (CFU) and PHA responsive cells then unfractionated bone marrow, thus showing the efficacy of the nylon columns in concentrating these cell types. It is noteworthy that a stem cell CF factor of 4.0 was similarly obtained by others using glass bead columns (2I) which confirms the possibility of employing bone marrow fractionation on the basis of cell adherence in order to concentrate stem cells. This fraction also contained the interacting cell population responsible for the early increase of PHA response of thymocytes. However, since this effect proved not to be strictly dependent on the dose of (Fr) component in the mixture no evidence could be obtained wether the fractionation procedure was also effective in concentrating this cell type.Possible relations between all these cell types present in (Fr) fraction remain to be ascertained.

We consider all these observations as supporting the hypothesis that more then one cell type is involved in the production of an immune response in typical cell-mediated, thymus dependent systems. Moreover, they confirm that PHA responding cells pertain to this compartment and are thymus-derived cells.

ACKNOWLEDGMENT

The capable technical assistance of Mr. A. Leorin and Mr. S. Mezzalira is acknowledged. Mrs. P. Segato kindly revised the manuscript.

Supported in part by Consiglio Nazionale delle Ricerche, Roma and by the Leukemia Research Fund, London.

REFERENCES

I. D.E. Mosier, Science, I58:I573, I967.

2. C.W. Pierce, and B. Benacerraf, Science, I66:I002,I969.

3. R.C. Seeger, and J.J. Oppenheim, J. Exp. Med.,   :44, I970.

4. H.N. Claman, and E.A. Chaperon, Transl. Rev., I:92, I969.

5. J.F.A.P. Miller and G.F. Mitchell, Transpl. Rev., I:3, I969.

6. G.M. Shearer, and G. Cudkowicz, J. Exp. Med., I29:935, I969.

7. G. Tridente, D. Collavo, L. Chieco-Bianchi, and L. Fiore-Donati, Exp. Hematol., 19:53, 1969.

8. G. Tridente, D. Collavo, L. Chieco-Bianchi, and L. Fiore-Donati, Exp. Hematol., 20:56, 1970.

9. G. Tridente, and G. Biasi, in preparation.

10. F.H. Bach, and N.K. Voynow, Science, 153:545, 1966.

11. J.E. Till, and E.A. McCulloch, Rad. Res., 14;213, 1961.

12. G. Tridente, G.M. Cappuzzo, and L. Fiore-Donati, Tumori, 53:
    565, 1967.

13. G. Tridente, G.M. Cappuzzo, Rec. Progr. Med., 46:1, 1969.

14. G. Tridente, and D.W. van Bekkum, in: Lymphatic Tissue and
    Germinal Centers in Immune Response, L. Fiore-Donati and M.
    G. Hanna, Jr., Eds., Plenum Press, New York, 1969, p.371.

15. M.F. Greaves, I.M. Roitt, and M.E. Rose, Nature 220:293,1968.

16. F. Daguillard, and M. Richter, J. Exp. Med., 130:1187, 1969.

17. E.M. Hersh, and J.J. Oppenheim, Cancer Res., 27:98, 1967.

18. W.O. Rieke, Science, 152:535, 1966.

19. K. Dicke, G. Tridente, and D.W. van Bekkum, Transpl. 8:422
    1969.

20. R.B. Taylor, Transpl. Rev., 1:114, 1969.

21. K. Shortman, personal comunication.

MIGRATION, RECIRCULATION AND TRANSFORMATION OF LARGE DIVIDING LYMPH NODE CELLS IN SYNGENEIC RECIPIENT RATS FOLLOWING INTRAVENOUS INJECTION

D. Guy-Grand, C. Griscelli, P. Vassalli and R.T. McCluskey
C.H.U. Necker - Enfants Malades, Paris (15e), and Depts. of Pathology, University of Geneva, Switzerland, and State University of New York at Buffalo, New York, U.S.A.

Lymph node cells were obtained from Lewis rats, either from "peripheral" lymph nodes (popliteal, axillary, lumbo-aortic and cervical nodes) 4 days after a foot-pad injection of B. Pertussis, or from mesenteric nodes. Cell suspensions were incubated for 60' to 120' in medium 199 containing 15% rat serum and 1 μC/ml of H_3-thymidine. Autoradiography of cell smears showed that at the end of the incubation 3 to 3.5% of the cells were labelled, most of the labelled cells being classified as large lymphocyte (LL) or large pyroninophilic cells (LPC); labelled small lymphocytes were not observed (1). 200-500 millions incubated cells were injected intravenously into Lewis recipient rats, which were killed at various intervals between 30' and 15 days after transfer. The fate of the large labelled cells in the recipient rats was followed by autoradiography of tissue sections and cell smears obtained from lymphoid organs.

Migration of the labelled cells in lymphoid organs.
Numerous labelled LL and LPC were found in the spleen red pulp as soon as 30' after transfer. In the lymph nodes, labelled cells appeared in significant numbers only 2-3 hours after transfer: they accumulated in the deep cortex, probably by traversing postcapillary venules, since some labelled cells were observed within the wall of a postcapillary venule.

Recirculation of LL and LPC.
Labelled LL and LPC are found in the thoracic duct lymph collected during the first 12 hours following transfer (Fig. 1). That LL and LPC are capable of leaving lymph nodes to enter thoracic duct lymph was also observed in experiments in which rats were cannulated 3 and 4 days after immunization in the foot-pads, and lymph collected

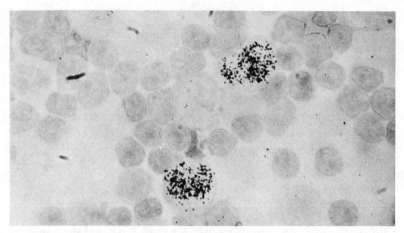

Fig. 1. Smears of thoracic duct lymph cells collected during the first twelve hours following transfer of lymph node cells labelled in vitro with H_3-thymidine. (x 800).

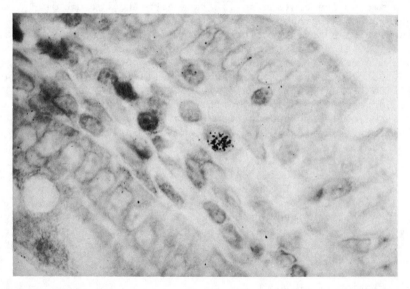

Fig. 2. Intestinal mucosa containing a labelled plasma cell, 20 hours after transfer of mesenteric lymph node cells labelled in vitro with H_3-thymidine. (x 800).

after in vivo injection of H_3-thymidine to label rapidly dividing cells; the number of large labelled cells found in the lymph was about 4 times larger in immunized rats than in normal animals. These findings correlate with those of Hall et al. (2) in the sheep, and show that recirculation and migration through the walls of post-capillary venules is a property not only of small lymphocytes, but of LL and LPC as well.

Transformation of labelled LL and LPC after transfer. Among the labelled cells observed on section and smears of the recipient at various times after transfer, LL and LPC disappear progressively while small lymphocytes and plasmocytes appear in increasing number. 1) Small lymphocytes are present in all the organs examined as soon as 24 hours after transfer, and represent after this time the majority of the labelled cells. With a few exceptions, they become progressively less highly labelled and their number appears to decrease progressively after 4 days. In lymphoid organs, they are present throughout the lymph node cortex as well as in the spleen red and white pulp, but are observed only exceptionally in the lymphoid follicles or germinal centers. 2) Plasma cells: labelled plasma cells are conspicuous in the spleen red pulp (as well as in the liver sinusoids and lung capillaries) 24 hours after transfer. They are highly labelled and are still observed with high labelling in the spleen red pulp after 15 days indicating little or no cell division. In contrast, labelled plasma cells are practically never observed in the lymph nodes: this is interpreted as indicating that young plasmablasts can stop in the spleen sinusoids and home within the red pulp, but cannot cross the postcapillary venules to home within lymph nodes. Plasma cells precursors of mesenteric nodes origin, however, appear to behave differently than precursors obtained from peripheral nodes: 24 hours after the transfer of large, labelled mesenteric node cells, large numbers of labelled plasma cells begin to appear in the intestinal mucosa (Fig. 2).

REFERENCES

1. C. Griscelli, P. Vassalli and R.T. McCluskey, J.Exp.Med., 130: 1427, 1969.

2. J.G. Hall, B. Morris, G.D. Moreno and M.C. Bessis, J.Exp.Med., 125:91, 1967.

IMMUNOSUPPRESSION BY L-ASPARAGINASE[*]

H. Friedman

Department of Microbiology, Albert Einstein Medical

Center, Philadelphia, Pennsylvania

During the last year there have been several reports from a
number of laboratories showing that L-asparaginase has profound
immunosuppressive effects in animals (1-15). Until recently, this
enzyme was generally considered to have specific anti-leukemic
effects (16-18). However, it is now evident that asparaginase may
be a useful immunosuppressive agent, inhibiting antibody formation
(6,7,9-11,13,14), lymphocyte transformation (1-3), the graft-vs.-
host reaction (8) and graft rejection (4,12,13,15). We have studied
the effects of L-asparaginase derived from Escherichia coli on the
antibody plaque response of mice to sheep erythrocytes and E. coli,
as well as its effects on the allograft rejection phenomenon.

For the study on the immune response, mice were injected with
varying doses of L-asparaginase either before, simultaneously with,
or after challenge immunization with sheep erythrocytes. For the
allograft study, mice were treated with the enzyme during the first
week after transplantation of a full thickness skin graft from a
donor mouse strain differing at the H2 locus.

Mice injected at the time of immunization and during the following 2 to 3 days with varying doses of asparaginase, such as 10 to
100 international units (I.U.), had a marked depression in the
number of antibody plaque forming cells (PFC) to sheep red blood
cells throughout an observation period of 10 to 30 days. Whereas
normal control mice had a vigorous response to the sheep erythrocytes, with 50,000 or more PFCs in their spleen 4 days after immunization, enzyme-treated mice generally responded with fewer than 1000

[*] Supported in part by grants from U.S. National Science Foundation.

Table 1. Effect of L-asparaginase on appearance of antibody plaque
forming cells to sheep erythrocytes in spleens of treated mice.

Asparaginase treatment (I.U.)[a]	Day after immunization							Mean peak titer ($\log_2$)
	2	4	6	8	10	12	20	
None	4,310	54,650	21,200	9,300	6,220	4,100	956	7.3
100	654	960	875	641	320	159	100	< 2.0
50	730	865	910	510	430	210	159	< 2.0
10	2,310	5,100	4,760	4,110	3,260	2,950	1,860	< 2.0
5	5,200	18,750	1,430	9,350	7,310	6,900	2,100	4.3
1	4,980	59,650	25,310	14,600	12,650	5,310	1,300	6.5

[a] Groups of mice injected i.p. with indicated dose of asparaginase
on day of immunization and on following 2 days.

PFCs at the same time (Table 1). Furthermore, suppression of the
PFC response was noted throughout the time of the expected immune
response, with very few PFCs at 2, 4, 6, 8, 10 or 12 days after
immunization (Table 1).

The suppressive effect was dose dependent in that a smaller
concentration of enzyme resulted in less suppression. Furthermore,
the suppressive effect was also dependent upon the time of administration of the enzyme relative to the day of immunization. For
example, when asparaginase was injected into a test mouse before
antigen challenge, there was only a slight and probably insignificant suppression of the immune response. These results, plus other
experiments, suggest that L-asparaginase affects the immune response
by interfering with cells stimulated by antigen. The most generally
accepted mechanism at present is that the enzyme depletes the blood
and tissue level of an important amino acid, asparagine, so that
stimulated lymphoid cells lack a required nutrient during the time
when they would normally react and proliferate into antibody-forming
cells after antigenic stimulation.

The effects on the graft rejection response were as marked as
that observed for the PFC response. Treatment of recipient C57BL/6J
mice with L-asparaginase during the first week after grafting with
BALB/c skin resulted in a prolonged graft survival time (Table 2).
Whereas control mice rejected a test skin graft with a mean survival time (m.s.t.) of approximately 9 to 10 days, mice treated
with 20 I.U. enzyme, from day 0 to +8 after grafting, had an m.s.t.
of approximately 16 to 17 days. Larger doses of enzyme resulted
in a greater graft prolongation time.

Table 2. Effect of L-asparaginase on survival of BALB/c skin grafts on C57B1 recipient mice.

Asparaginase treatment (I.U.)[a]		No. of recipient mice	m.s.t.	Range
None		18	9.4	8-12
L-asparaginase	100	12	19.6	15-23
	50	14	17.9	12-25
	10	10	14.8	8-17

[a] Mice treated with indicated dose of asparaginase on day of skin grafting and subsequent 7 days.

It seems apparent from these results, as well as those presented by others, that L-asparaginase derived from E. coli may effectively depress the immune response to antigenic stimuli, as examplified by the cellular antibody plaque response to sheep erythrocytes and the allograft rejection response to allogeneic skin grafts.

REFERENCES

1. G. Astaldi, G.R. Burgio, J. Krc, R. Genova and A.A. Astaldi Jr., Lancet I:423, 1969.

2. T.J. MacElvain and S.K. Hayward, Lancet I:527, 1969.

3. H.K. Schulten, G. Giraldo, E.A. Boyse and H.F. Oettgen, Lancet II:644, 1969.

4. J.J. Dartnall and A.L. Barkie, Lancet I:1098, 1969.

5. R.S. Schwartz, Nature 224:275, 1969.

6. G.N. Muller-Berat, Acta Path. Microbiol. Scand. 17:750, 1969.

7. H.P. Hobik, Naturwiss. 56:247, 1966.

8. M.C. Berenbaum, Nature 225:580, 1970.

9. M.C. Berenbaum, H. Ginsburg and D.M. Gilbert, Nature 227:1188, 1970.

10. A.K. Chakrabarty and H. Friedman, Science 167:869, 1970.

11. S.D. Nelsen, M.B. Lee and J.M. Bridges, Transpl. 9:566, 1970.

12. A. Shons, T. Jetzer and J.S. Najarian, Transpl. 10:280, 1970.

13. M.E. Weksler and B.B. Weksler, these proceedings. p. 429.

14. H. Friedman and A.K. Chakrabarty, Transpl. Proc., in press, 1970.

15. J.E. Broome, J. Exp. Med. 118:1217, 1963.

16. E.A. Boyse, L.J. Old, H. Campbell and L.T. Mashburn, J. Exp. Med. 125:17, 1967.

17. J.E. Broome, J. Exp. Med. 127:1055, 1968.

IMMUNOSUPPRESSIVE PROPERTIES AND SIDE EFFECTS OF E. COLI

L-ASPARAGINASE *

K. Schumacher, G. Alzer, H. Oerkermann, and W.D.
Hirschmann
Medical University Clinic, Cologne, Germany

The immunosuppressive properties of L-Asparaginase (L-Ase) were studied by different test systems. First we tested the inhibition of the cellular immun-reaction after immunization of mice with sheep red blood cells by means of counting the "rosettes" forming cells in the spleen.

As shown in fig. 1, at least 2000 units of L-Ase per kg mouse had to be applicated to obtain an immunosuppressive effect. The best results were obtained after application of 5000 and 10000 μ/kg.

Compared with Cyclophosphamide, Imurel and rabbit antimouse-lymphocyte serum the effect of L-Ase was less impressive.

A significant reduction of the hemagglutination titres after L-Ase treatment could not be observed (1).

In a second test system we studied the inhibitory effect of L-Ase on the blast cell transformation of human lymphocytes after stimulation with Phytohemagglutinin (PHA), cultivating the lymphocytes in Millipore chambers in the peritoneal cavity of rats (2).

We found (fig. 2) a dose dependent immunosuppressive effect of L-Ase, if the time between the last L-Ase application and the implantation of the chamber, i.e. the start of the stimulation did not exceed 24 hours.

---

* Supported by Deutsche Forschungsgemeinschaft.

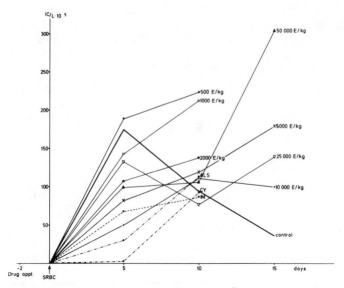

Fig. 1. "Rosettes" forming cells per 10^5 spleen cells. Drug
application two days before immunization with 10^0 sheep red blood
cells. Thin solid lines indicate the cell counts after different
doses of L-Ase. The broken lines show the cell counts after
application of other immunosuppressive substances: CY = cyclophosphamide (40 mg/kg), IM = Imurel (10 mg/kg), ALS = rabbit antimouse-lymphocyte serum (0.2 ml/animal). Each point indicates an
average of 10 animals.

These findings are extended by our investigations on the
inhibitory effect of L-Ase on the cytoaggressive activity of PHA-
stimulated lymphocytes against target cells, which were pointed
out by the film demonstrated at this conference.

Further, we studied some side effects of L-Ase. In the serum
of patients with acute leukemia treated with L-Ase in a dose range
of 5000-25000 µ/kg totally, we found a significant decrease of the
coagulation factors and of albumin (fig. 3) (3).

In the same patients the immunoglobulins showed at the same
time a significant increase (tab. 1).

The histologic examination of three of the ten patients
showed a severe fatty degeneration of the liver cells.

From these results we conclude:
1. L-Ase has a suppressive effect on cellular immunreactions but
   little or no inhibitory effect on antibody synthesis. In relation to other immunosuppressive agents such as cyclophospham-

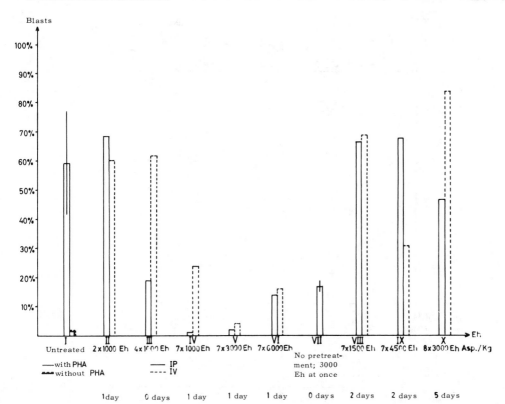

Fig. 2. Percentage of blast like cells (10^3 cells counted) in the chamber after stimulation with PHA and pretreatment with L-Ase. Drug application either intraperitoneally (solid columns) or intravenously (dotted columns). The last line indicates the time in days between the last drug application and the implantation of the chamber (from 2).

ide or Imurel, no complete suppression of the immunreactions could be observed, even with extreme doses.

2. The best immunosuppressive effect of L-Ase could be obtained by permanent treatment before stimulation by antigen or PHA. 24 hours after the last application of L-Ase the immunosuppressive effect decreases rapidly.

3. The main problem of the immunosuppressive treatment with L-Ase is the fact that immunosuppressive doses of L-Ase cause dose and time dependent severe side effects. These are the inhibition of the protein synthesis in the liver (coagulation factors and albumin) and a toxic fatty degeneration of the liver cells with a reactive increase of the immunoglobulins, similar to other toxic influences (4).

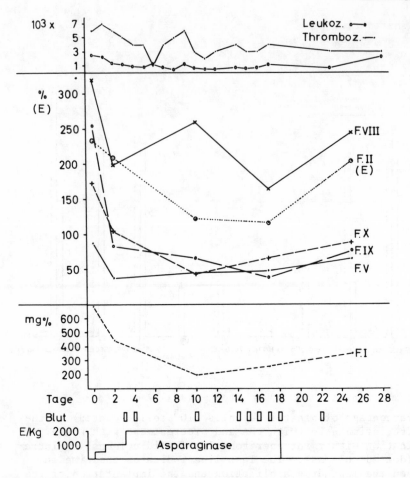

Fig. 3. Behaviour of some coagulation factors under treatment with L-Ase of a patient with acute leukemia (from 3).

4. The necessity of using high doses of L-Ase supports our previous results (5) which suggest that the active principle of E. coli L-Ase may be the glutaminase activity rather than the asparaginase activity.

Table 1. Quantitative determination of the immunoglobulins IgG, IgA, IgM before and under treatment with L-Ase of patients with acute leukemia.

Case No.	IgG mg/ml				IgA mg/ml				IgM mg/ml			
	bef. treatment	under	%	days treated	bef. treatment	under	%	days trented	bef. treatment	under	%	days treated
1	10.0	26.6	266	10	2.16	4.12	190	25	1.12	3.60	323	25
2	24.0	29.6	123	10	1.20	2.40	200	10	0.27	0.50	135	10
3	18.8	21.2	113	13	1.28	2.24	175	13	0.97	3.18	328	13
4	21.6	41.5	192	11	2.80	3.84	137	18	0.82	1.62	197	18
5	13.2	22.6	171	15	2.40	6.20	258	15	0.97	1.95	201	15
6	28.0	35.0	125	55	4.64	5.50	118	5	1.12	3.62	323	9
7	16.6	20.0	121	13	1.16	1.00	86	13	1.17	1.82	155	13
8	10.2	13.4	131	5	1.52	1.72	113	5	1.50	1.50	100	5
9	25.4	16.6	65	5	1.36	2.04	150	5	1.00	1.00	100	5
10	13.4	15.2	113	6	1.00	1.04	100	6	0.37	0.67	181	6
$\bar{x}$		142.0				152.7				205.3		

REFERENCES

1. K. Schumacher, G. Sichert, and H. Sichert, Unpublished results.

2. A. Pappas, W.D. Hirschmann, P.G. Scheurlen, and W. Esser, Med. Welt 21:1288, 1970.

3. E. Lechler, K. Schumacher, and W.D. Hirschmann, Med. Welt, 1970 (in press).

4. K. Schumacher, and R. Gross, Klin. Wschr. 47:123, 1969.

5. H. Oerkermann, and W.D. Hirschmann, Proc. 6th Internat. Congr. Chemother., Tokyo, 1969 (in press).

CHRONIC HISTOINCOMPATIBILITY AND LYMPHOMAGENESIS IN MICE[1]

Leonard J. Cole

Immunobiology Program, Life Sciences Division, Stanford

Research Institute, Menlo Park, California USA

There is a growing body of knowledge suggesting that immunological factors may play a critical role in the induction of neoplasms. Apart from the evidence that immunosuppression *per se* may permit the growth and development of autochthonous tumor cells bearing neoantigens, it is possible that lymphoproliferative diseases such as malignant lymphomas may be the consequence of chronic, persistent histoincompatibility reactions involving immunocompetent cells, in a host animal which for one of several causes may, in effect, be an isoantigenic mosaic or chimera. Such a possibility derives not only from certain theoretical formulations by Burnet (1), Tyler (2), Dameshek and Schwartz (3), and Kaplan and Smithers (4), but also from earlier observations in two different types of experiments: the incidence of lymphomas in mouse radiation bone marrow chimeras from our laboratory (5), and the work of Schwartz and Beldotti (6) and of Walford and Hildeman (7), on the occurrence in populations of mice subjected to graft-versus-host reactions.

From our previous studies (5), we know that syngeneic radiation chimeras, i.e., lethally X-irradiated (C57L x A/HeJ)F$_1$ hybrid mice (H-2a,b) receiving an injection of normal syngeneic bone marrow or neonatal spleen cells show a very low lymphoma incidence (approaching zero) for their total natural life span; whereas, in contrast, allogeneic BM chimeras, i.e., irradiated LAF$_1$ mice transfused with C3H (H-2b) marrow cells exhibit a definite incidence of malignant lymphomas—9% in our series and an additional 9% with atypical proliferations in the spleen.

---

[1]Supported in part by funds from the Office of Naval Research.

Table I.   Lymphomas in X-irradiated F_1 hybrid mice
surviving graft-versus-host disease*

Cells injected into irradiated (500 R) LAF$_1$ mice	Time of sacrifice (month)	Lymphoma no./total (%)	Lymphoid hyperplasia no./total
Fresh A-lymph node	25	0/12 (0)	5/12
Incubated A-lymph node	25	10/17 (59)	1/17
A-lymph node incubated with prednisone	25	4/9 (44)	3/9
None (irradiation controls)	20-24	17/132 (13)	—

*15×10^6 cells injected iv, or 30×10^6 injected ip.   The cells were
incubated at $37°$ for 2 hr in buffered saline, with or without added
prednisone (100 μg/ml) prior to injection.

In view of these considerations, we have carried out experiments
on parental-strain F_1 hybrid bone marrow and lymphoid chimeras as
model systems in the attempt to determine whether (1) overt graft-
versus-host reactions are necessary preconditions for increased
lymphomagenesis in allogeneic chimeras and (2) the lymphomas are of
donor or of host origin.

RESULTS

In our experiments (8), adult (10-12 week-old) male (C57L x A/He)F$_1$
hybrid mice (so-called LAF$_1$) received a whole-body sublethal exposure
of 500 R of 250 KVP X-rays, followed in a few hours by a single intravenous injection of 15×10^6 fresh parental strain lymph node cells
or an intraperitoneal injection of 30×10^6 lymph node cells from
adult A/He donors (H-2a).   In some cases the lymph node cells were
incubated *in vitro* at $37°C$ for 2 hours, with or without added prednisone, prior to their injection--this procedure designed to reduce
the severity of the graft-versus-host reactions.

Lymphoma Incidence

A definite increase in lymphoma incidence occurred in the recipient mice injected with incubated parental strain lymph node cells, as
compared with radiation controls (Table I): a total of 14 among the

26 animals (combined) which received the incubated lymph node cells
exhibited lymphomas, compared to a 13% incidence among radiation
controls (p < .01). Histologically, the lymphomas did not differ
significantly from those previously observed in either irradiated or
nonirradiated LAF$_1$ mice. The majority were lymphosarcomas composed
of sheets of medium and large lymphocytes, usually extra-thymic in
origin and involving the spleen, various lymph nodes, kidney, and
liver. The most common variant consisted of more undifferentiated
and pleomorphic cells shading into a reticulum-cell pattern. Tumors
resembling follicular lymphoma, Hodgkin's disease, and plasmacytoma
were observed once or twice each.

Another set of experiments were carried out in which parental
bone marrow cells were injected instead of lymphocytes. A group of
500 R irradiated LAF$_1$ mice received a single intravenous injection of
4 X 10^6 fresh bone marrow cells from normal, adult A-strain donors.
In addition, a group of A-strain mice were first subjected to 900 R
of X-radiation, with one limb of each mouse enclosed in an external
lead shield during the irradiation. Such marrow shielding is known
to permit the migration of viable bone marrow stem cells into the
circulation and into the peripheral tissues, and brings about the
subsequent functional cellular repopulation of the radiation-depleted
hemopoietic and lymphoid systems (cf. 9). Seven days after this procedure, the spleen and liver from these donors were removed and
injected intraperitoneally as separate cell suspensions in TC-199
medium into LAF$_1$ mice which had just received 500 R of X-radiation.
Each recipient LAF$_1$ mouse received either the equivalent of 50 mg wet
weight of A-liver cells from these donors, or the equivalent of one
A-spleen. A control group of 16 sublethally X-irradiated LAF$_1$ mice
received liver cells from whole-body lethally X-irradiated (900 R)
A-strain donors.

When the marrow-injected mice were sacrificed 23 months later,
76% of the group of 17 exhibited malignant lymphomas (Table II).
Similarly, in the F$_1$ hybrid mice receiving liver or spleen cells from
900 R X-irradiated A-strain mice (with one limb lead-shielded during
irradiation) about 80% of a group of 18 showed lymphomas 23 months
later. As a control, liver cells (equivalent to 50 mg liver) from
900 R whole-body irradiated A-strain mice were injected into LAF$_1$
mice; under these conditions, no lymphomas were seen at 25 months
among 16 mice thus treated. However, in a small group of 500 R
irradiated LAF$_1$ mice each receiving a single intravenous injection
of a suspension of normal A-strain liver cells, derived from 50 mg
wet weight liver, 50% developed lymphomas.

Thus, the transplantation of adult parental strain bone marrow
cells directly, or of cells in the irradiated spleen and liver recently
migrated from the shielded femoral bone marrow leads to a significant
augmentation of lymphoma frequency in the F$_1$ hybrid recipient (p<0.01).

Table II.   Lymphomas in X-irradiated F_1 hybrid mice (500 R)
            receiving parental strain marrow cells*

Irradiated (500 R) LAF$_1$ mice	Time of sacrifice (month)	Lymphoma (no./total)	(%)
4 x 10^6 A-marrow	23½	13/17	76
Liver from 900 R limb-shielded A-mice*	23	8/10	80
Spleen from 900 R limb-shielded A-mice*	23	6/8	75
Liver from 900 R whole-body irradiated A-mice*	25	0/16	0
None (irradiation controls)	20-24	17/132	13

*Tissue removed 7 days postirradiation.

   The lymphomas arising in 6 of the marrow cell-injected mice were
each injected intraperitoneally as a cell suspension (approximately
10^7 cells from the leukemic spleen and lymph nodes) into nonirradiated
adult A-strain and LAF$_1$ hybrid recipient mice (3 each) in order to
determine whether these cells would exhibit malignant growth and show
specificity as regards their donor or host origin. Among lymphomas
thus examined, all grew and infiltrated in the A-strain recipients
sacrificed 9 weeks after injection of the lymphoma cells; in all these
cases the spleens, as well as the mesenteric lymph nodes, were greatly
enlarged and lymphomatous; thymic and liver involvement was grossly
evident in 2 cases. At the same time, no evidence for lymphoma takes
was seen in the LAF$_1$ recipients. The lymphomas from 3 of these
A-strain recipient mice were each retransplanted in turn into 5 nonirradiated adult LAF$_1$ mice and 5 A-strain mice. In all cases, the
tumors again grew in the A-strain recipients but not in the LAF$_1$
mice. We conclude from these observations that many, if not all of
the lymphomas arising in parental-strain F_1 hybrid bone marrow chimeras
were of donor, i.e., parental strain, bone marrow cell origin.

   We are presumably dealing here with a condition of persistent
chronic histoincompatibility, associated with the parental-strain F_1
hybrid reticuloendothelial cell chimerism. Albert Tyler's hypothesis
(proposed in 1960) suggested analogies between tumor etiology and
pathology and graft-versus-host reactions (what he called transplantation disease). It is evident that the state of chimerism such as
described here would lead to the stimulation of the immunologically
competent parental strain cells by the host isoantigens, resulting

in blastogenesis, new RNA synthesis and proliferation of these cells. We suggest that such repeated and prolonged proliferative activity increases the probability of the occurrence of a carcinogenic alter-ation in the immunologically stimulated parental strain lymphocytic cells. However, the occurrence of such carcinogenic changes depends importantly on the genotype of the cells. This follows particularly from recent observations by Huebner *et al.* (10) which reveal marked differences among various mouse strains in the susceptibility to be activated or "turned on" with respect to vertically transmitted oncogenic virus. These workers (11) also postulate, from cell culture evidence and sero-epidemiological studies, that cells of vertebrates contain information in the genome (the virogene), for producing C-type RNA viruses. However, in some strains of Swiss mice the information for the expression of oncogenic virus is completely repressed. Thus, expression of oncogenic potential is controlled by the genetic makeup of the host, but is also influenced by extrinsic environmental factors, such as chemical carcinogens and ionizing radiation.

In the present context, we propose that chronic histoincompati-bility reactions, blastogenesis, and lymphocytic proliferation consti-tute another additional mode of activation of such endogenous oncogenic viruses.

DNA Synthesis in Lymphoid Tissues

From the data so far presented, we do not know the magnitude of, nor the duration or "chronicity" of the proliferative stimulus to the cells under discussion, in the chimeras. In order to obtain infor-mation on this point, and in addition--incidentally--to be able to measure graft-versus-host reactions quantitatively, we have developed a procedure based on measuring the incorporation of injected H^3-thymidine into the spleen DNA fraction of lethally irradiated mice which receive a single intravenous injection of allogeneic lymphocytes. The transplanted immunocompetent cells are stimulated by the host isoantigens and mount a graft-versus-host reaction, reflected in the increased DNA synthesis, typically measured at 3 and 6 days by scintillation counting. Figure 1 presents some typical data. Graft-versus-host response ratios as high as 17-fold over radiation controls is seen 6 days after injection of parental A-strain lymph node cells, thymus cells, and peripheral leukocytes; note the lack of response with 10^7 syngeneic lymph node cells. The data of Figure 2 illustrate another aspect of the genetic specificity of the method. A-strain irradiated recipients give no proliferative response following the injection of syngeneic lymph node cells and also of F_1 hybrid cells. Therefore the graft-versus-host reaction in this case is undirectional, i.e., parental cells reacting against F_1 hybrid isoantigens. Figures 3 and 4 show the effect of number of injected parental and allogenic cells on H^3-thymidine incorporation.

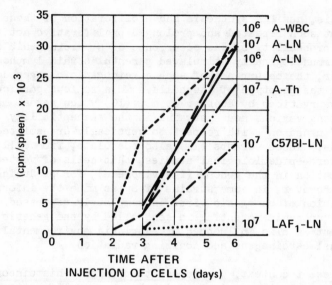

Fig. 1. Quantitative assay of graft-versus-host reactions. Incorporation of H^3-thymidine into spleen DNA fraction of 900 R X-irradiated LAF_1 mice.

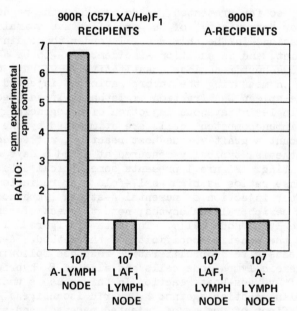

Fig. 2. Genetic specificity of quantitative graft-versus-host reaction assay.

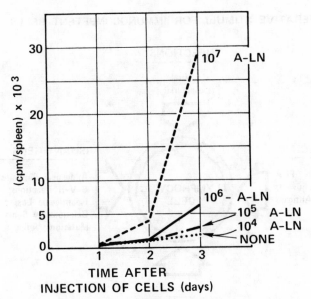

Fig. 3. Injection of parental strain (A) lymph node cells into X-irradiated LAF₁ recipients. Effect of cell number on graft-versus-host reactions.

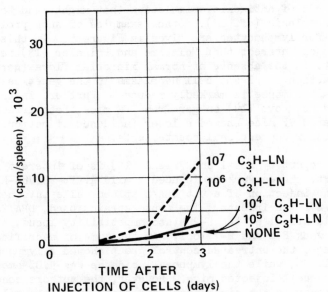

Fig. 4. Injection of allogeneic (C3H) lymph node cells. Effect of cell number of graft-versus-host reactions.

PROLIFERATIVE STIMULI FOR IMMUNOCOMPETENT CELLS

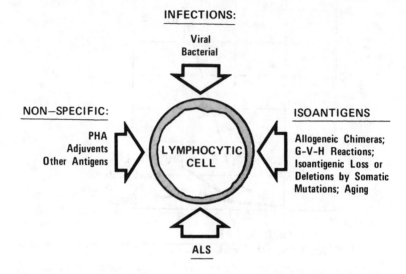

Fig. 5. Possible modes of proliferative stimuli for lymphocyte cells.

Isoantigenic stimulation of immunocompetent cells is, of course, not the only mode of antigenic stimulation that might lead to the induction of neoplasia (cf. 12). Other examples of such proliferative stimuli for lymphocytes are given in Figure 5. In this connection, it is of interest that McIntire and Princler (13) reported last year that, in the absence of normal microbial flora (germ-free mice) the induction of plasma cell neoplasms in the genetically susceptible BALB/c mouse is markedly reduced. Further, in the studies of Walburg and Cosgrove (14) on germfree RFM mice, both irradiated and nonirradiated GF mice showed a lower incidence of reticulum cell sarcoma than their conventional counterparts.

A recent report by Rossi and Friend (15) is of interest in the present context. These workers induced a mild graft-versus-host reaction by the injection of adult DBA/2 spleen cells into newborn (BALB/c X DBA/2)F_1 recipients. The mouse strains used, DBA/2J and BALB/cJ, are identical at the H-2 histocompatibility locus, but differ at the weak H-1 and H-7 loci. At the time of sacrifice, at 18 months of age, the untreated control group showed a lymphoma incidence of 1.67%, while the lymphoma incidence was 9.0% among the parental spleen cell-injected mice. However, the authors consider that this increase is not significant and state that "the relation of immunologic phenomena to neoplastic proliferation remains to be clarified."

Using this procedure, we have measured the H^3-thymidine (4-hour pulse labeling with 10 μc H^3-thymidine) incorporation in the spleen and lymph node cells of 500 R X-irradiated LAF_1 mice which had been injected with 4 X 10^6 parental strain marrow cells 5 months before. The preliminary data thus far obtained show a 250% increase in mean H^3-thymidine incorporation per spleen in these animals, compared with irradiated controls which had received no cell injection. A corresponding increase in H^3-thymidine incorporation into the cervical lymph node DNA, expressed in terms of incorporation counts per 10^6 lymph node cells was also observed.

These data indicate that a significantly increased proliferative activity occurs in the spleen and lymph nodes of the F_1 hybrid mice which had received sublethal X-irradiation plus parental strain lympho-hemopoietic cell injection 5 months earlier--the same treatment which gave rise in other groups of similarly treated mice to increased lymphomagenesis.

In addition, the injection of 4 X 10^6 A-strain marrow cells into 500 R X-rayed LAF_1 mice gives a 2-day response ratio (H^3-thymidine incorporation) as high as 4.4 with respect to saline controls, whereas syngeneic marrow injected controls gave a response ratio of only 1.4. These data suggest that some cells in the injected parental strain bone marrow cell population were undergoing new DNA synthesis, presumably due to immunological stimulation. We are now making continuing determinations of this type on groups of chimeric mice being maintained for lymphoma incidence studies, over their entire life span.

DISCUSSION

On the basis of the data presented and of the proposed hypothesis, at least two types of additional experiments suggest themselves as being worthy of pursuit:

1. Investigations on lymphomagenesis in parental-strain F_1 hybrid chimeras using immunologically nonreactive fetal liver cells as the donor cells in place of adult marrow. Fetal liver contains potential immunoreactive cells, i.e., stem cells, which are known to develop tolerance in appropriate F_1 hybrid hosts (16). Therefore, the interesting question could be posed as to whether early induction of specific tolerance on the part of parental strain precursor cells to host isoantigens precludes lymphomagenesis under these conditions.

2. Since the expression of oncogenic virus is so importantly a function of mouse genotype, it would be valuable to study lymphomagenesis in parental marrow-F_1 hybrid chimeras among strain combinations showing high and low susceptibility to derepression of the oncogenic virus, for example, A versus BALB/c.

We conclude on the basis of the presently available experimental evidence that the relationship of immunological factors to lymphomagenesis in mice is a multifactorial one. More studies will be required to resolve the question as to the relative importance of, and the interrelationships among, the following factors in lymphomagenesis:

1. Immunosuppression *per se* resulting from graft-versus-host reactions.

2. The degree and duration of chronic proliferative stimulation of the reacting cell population.

3. The strength of histocompatibility differences between the cell populations involved--whether as a result of chimerism, mutations, etc.

4. The mouse genotype, i.e., the relative susceptibility of the host to expression, activation or derepression of endogenous oncogenic virus.

REFERENCES

1. M. G. Burnet, Brit. Med. Bull., 20:154, 1964.

2. A. Tyler, J. Nat. Cancer Inst., 25:1197, 1960.

3. W. Dameshek and R. S. Schwartz, Blood, 14:1151, 1959.

4. H. S. Kaplan and D. W. Smithers, Lancet, 2:1, 1959.

5. L. J. Cole, P. C. Nowell, and M. E. Ellis, J. Nat. Cancer Inst., 17:435, 1956; W. E. Davis, Jr., L. J. Cole, W. A. Foley, and V. J. Rosen, Jr., Radiation Res., 20:43, 1963; L. J. Cole, Proc. Int. Sympos. R. E. S. 4th, Kyoto, Japan, p. 364, 1964.

6. R. S. Schwartz and L. Beldotti, Science, 149:551, 1965.

7. R. L. Walford and W. H. Hildemann, Amer. J. Pathol. 47:713, 1965; R. L. Walford, Science, 152:78, 1966.

8. L. J. Cole and P. C. Nowell, Proc. Soc. Exptl. Biol. Med., 134:653, 1970.

9. P. C. Nowell and L. J. Cole, J. Cell Physiol., 201:37, 1967.

10. J. W. Hartley, W. P. Rowe, W. I. Capps, and R. J. Huebner, J. Virol., 3:126, 1969.

11. R. J. Huebner and G. J. Todaro, Proc. Nat. Acad. Sci., U.S.A.,
     64:1087, 1969.

12. D. Metcalf, Brit. J. Cancer, 15:769, 1961.

13. K. R. McIntire and G. L. Princler, Immunol., 17:481, 1969.

14. H. E. Walburg, Jr., and G. E. Cosgrove, in: Germ Free Biology,
     p. 135. Plenum Press, 1969.

IMMUNOLOGICAL EFFECTS OF CORTISONE CAUSED BY INTERFERENCE WITH LYMPHOID CELL TRAFFIC

A.A. van den Broek

Department of Histology, State University of Groningen

Groningen, Holland

Dietrich and Dukor (1) have shown that a regimen of 5 daily injections of cortisone-acetate may severely affect the antibody response against sheep erythrocytes in mice. Suppression was most pronounced when the cortisone treatment was given just prior to the antigen. Similarly Elliott and Sinclair (2), using a single, large dose of cortisone-acetate, found maximal suppression of both IgM- and IgG-response when the cortisone was given before antigen. Recovery from this cortisone-induced immunological depression was shown to be independent of the thymus but correlated with increase of blood lymphocyte numbers. Everett and Tyler (3) demonstrated that hydrocortisone preferentially affected the short-lived category of lymphocytes in blood and peripheral lymphoid tissue. According to Esteban (4) especially those in the thymus and bone marrow were highly susceptible to cortisone. Together these results suggest that cortisone might affect lymphoid cells - possibly including antibody-forming-cell-precursors - prior to their stimulation by antigen.

The experiments to be presented here were conceived to investigate the possibility of cortisone affecting the antibody response by interfering with the *cell traffic* of these lymphoid elements. The effects of 7 daily i.m. injections of cortisone-acetate (20 mg/kg) on the H-agglutinin response against Salmonella paratyphi Java vaccine (0.1 ml. containing 6×10^8 formol killed organisms/i.v.) were studied in normal rabbits and in rabbits subjected to local irradiation of the spleen (700 rads) and - 24 hrs. later - whole body irradiation (450 rads) with the spleen shielded.

Local irradiation of the spleen or a lymph node has been shown by Keuning and Bos (5), Bos (6) and Simic (7) to give rise to immediate repletion of the irradiated organ with blood-borne small lymphocytes. Two types of lymphocyte traffic were distinghuised (6):

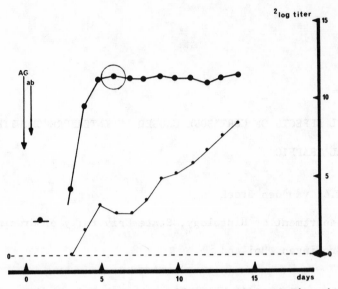

Fig. 1. Mean H-agglutinin titers of control rabbits (see
table 1).

(i) a relatively slow repletion of thymus-dependent areas, absent
in thymectomized animals (8), and (ii) a rapid and massive repletion of the follicles, leading to typical marginal zone cell formation within a few days. When the local irradiation was followed -
24 hrs. later - by a total body irradiation with the previously irradiated node (or spleen) shielded, the immune potential of the im-
migrated cells could be assessed. The thymus dependent first type
of lymphocyte influx led to restoration of cell-mediated immune potential; the non-thymus dependent follicular type of lymphocyte repletion to repair of antibody and follicular center responsiveness
(Veldman (8)).

RESULTS

The mean course of H-agglutinin titers in a group of 6 control rabbits is shown in fig. 1. In all instances a small amount of
anti-H hyperimmune serum was given (up to a passive titer of 2 to
3) 6 hrs. after vaccine administration to restrict the period of effective antigenic stimulation and more or less synchronize the antibody response. In this model the endpoint of IgM accumulation,
which is reached about 6 days after antigen administration, can be
used as a parameter of antibody forming potential, representing under certain conditions a measure of the number of antibody-forming-
cell-precursors stimulated by the antigen (Keuning et al (9) and unpublished data). The individual 6th day (peak) titers are given in
table 1.

Table 1

Treatment	6th day (peak) titer
Ag-controls	14. 13. 12. 11. 11. 10
Cortisone (-6 through 0d.) + Ag	12. 10. 9. 8. 7.
Spleen irrad.(-3d.) and shielded (-2d.) + Ag	9. 9. 2. 2.

Cortisone (-6 through 0d.) +
    spleen irrad.(-3d.) and
    shielded (-2d.) + Ag
	<3. <2. <1. <1. 0.

Cortisone given on days -6 through 0, i.e. prior to antigenic
stimulation (day 0), clearly depressed the antibody response as
measured by the 6th day (peak) titers (table 1). It may be added
that cortisone treatment from day -3 through +3, or from day 0
through +6 did not affect the antibody response.

Histologically a moderate atrophy of lymph node and splenic
lymphoid tissue was already found 24 hrs. after the first cortisone
injection. Signs of lymphocyte destruction were few in these organs.
The histological changes remained nearly constant over the entire
period of cortisone treatment. Foto nr. 1 shows the splenic white
pulp of an untreated control rabbit. Foto nr. 2 representing a corresponding area 24 hrs. after the last of six cortisone injections,
shows as the most prominent feature: a complete absence of follicular (coronal) lymphocytes, unmasking an intact or even over-deve-
loped (?) marginal zone cell system. A similar change was found in
the lymph node outer cortex. In the thymus dependent periarteriolar
lymphocyte sheaths (spleen) and paracortical areas (lymph node) a
slight to moderate reduction of lymphocyte numbers was observed.
This was in agreement with the observation of perfectly normal skin-
allograft rejection times (10-12 d.) in 4 rabbits, and the occurrence
of vigorous immunoblast reactions in the paracortical areas of the
allograft draining lymph nodes. In contrast to spleen and lymph nodes
the thymuses within a few days of cortisone treatment exhibited a
nearly complete cortical lymphocyte depletion with early signs of
large scale lymphocyte destruction.

Local irradiation of the spleen on day -3, followed by total
irradiation with spleen shielding on day -2 and antigen administered
like before on day 0 gave good responses in two animals (table 1);
the poor responses in two others are unexpected in view of other
data (a.o. lymph node experiments) and may not be representative.
Histologically the lymphocyte repletion 24 hrs. after local irradiation of the spleen (from one of the high titer animals) is shown
in foto nr. 3. The two types of lymphocyte-influx, periarteriolar
and follicular, are easily distinghuised.

A group of 6 rabbits, similarly treated but in addition given

cortisone-acetate from day −6 through 0, completely to produce
measurable amounts of antibody (table 1). Foto nr. 4 clearly demonstrates the complete and nearly complete absence respectively of
follicular and periarteriolar lymphocyte repletion in one of these
cortisone treated animals. Similar observations were done on lymph
nodes with experimental conditions adapted.

CONCLUSIONS AND DISCUSSION

From the observations described it is concluded that cortisone
severely affects lymphoid cell traffic towards spleen and lymph
nodes under the conditions of these experiments. The lymphocyte repletion of both follicles and periarteriolar lymphocyte sheaths
(resp. paracortical areas) was blocked by cortisone. There can be
little doubt that the blockade of follicle-bound lymphocyte traffic
was responsible for the suppression of antibody forming potential
in these experiments (cf. 10). It should be mentioned, however, that
with longer periods between local irradiation of the spleen and total irradiation with the spleen shielded, a number of cells escaped
this blockade; weak to moderate antibody responses were observed in
these cells.

Evidence is accumulating which suggests that the follicular
lymphocytes of primary lymphoid follicles and at least part of the
coronal lymphocytes of secondary follicles represent non-thymus
derived blood-borne lymphocytes that are continuously being supplied
under normal conditions; they probably contain the "mobile" antibody-forming-cell-precursors (11). Maintenance of antibody responsiveness would in that case depend on a continuous supply of these
cells. Our experiments suggest that the known effects of cortisone
on the antibody response might, at least in part, be due to blockade
of this particular type of lymphoid cell traffic.

It remains to be decided whether this blockade mainly affects
bone marrow output, as with mononuclear phagocyte precursors (12),
or peripheral cell traffic as well.

Lastly further experiments are needed to establish a possible
role of a blockade of lymphoid stem cell supply in cortisone induced

---

Fotomicrographs: White pulp of rabbit spleen.
1. Normal control: periarteriolar lymphocyte sheath and follicle
   with marginal zone.
2. 24 Hours after the last of six cortisone injections: absence of
   follicular lymphocytes unmasking marginal zone cell system.
3. 24 Hours after local irradiation: repletion of follicles and
   periarteriolar lymphocyte sheaths.
4. 24 Hours after local irradiation of cortisone treated animal:
   blockade (complete) of follicular repletion and (partly) of periarteriolar lymphocyte sheath repletion.

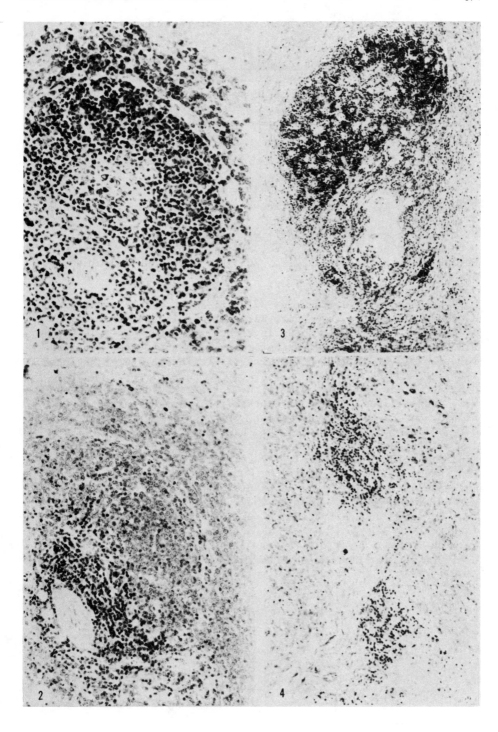

thymic atrophy, in addition to lymphocyte destruction.

ACKNOWLEDGEMENTS

This investigation was supported by a grant of the Foundation for Basic Medical Research (FunGO).

The skilful help of Miss H.M.J. Kramer, Miss A.S. Wubbena and Mr. M. van der Zee is gratefully acknowledged.

REFERENCES

1. P. Dukor and F.M. Dietrich, Inter. Arch. Allergy Appl. Immunol. 34: 32, 1968.
2. E.V. Elliott and N.S. St.Sinclair, Immunology 15: 643, 1968.
3. N.B. Everett and Ruth W. Tyler (Caffrey), in: International Review of Cytology, vol. 22, p. 205. New York and London: Academic Press, 1967.
4. Jose N. Esteban, Anat. Rec. 162: 349, 1968.
5. F.J. Keuning and W.H. Bos, in: H. Cottier, N. Odartchenko, R. Schindler and C.C. Congdon, Eds., Germinal Centers in Immune Response, p. 86. New York: Springer Verlag, 1967.
6. W.H. Bos, Recirculatie en Transformatie van Lymfocyten (doctoral thesis). Groningen: University of Groningen (The Netherlands), 1967.
7. M.M. Simić and M.Z. Pétrović in: H. Cottier, N. Odartchenko and C.C. Congdon, Eds., Germinal Centers in Immune Responses, p. 419. New York: Springer Verlag, 1967.
8. J.E. Veldman, Histophysiology and Electron Microscopy of the Immune Response (doctoral thesis). Groningen: University of Groningen (The Netherlands), 1970.
9. F.J. Keuning, P. Nieuwenhuis, N. Mulder and G. Hoekstra, in: International Symposium on Adjuvants of Immunity, Utrecht 1966, p. 183. Basel/New York: Karger 1967.
10. F.J. Keuning and A.A. van den Broek, Exp. Haematol. 17: 4, 1968 (abstract).
11. P. Nieuwenhuis, these proceedings, p. 25.
12. J. Thompson, in: Mononuclear Phagocytes, Oxford (G.B.) Blackwell 1970.

IMMUNOLOGICAL UNRESPONSIVENESS TO SOLUBLE ANTIGENS IN ADULT MICE

Vesna Tomažič and B. Vitale

Laboratory for Tumor and Transplantation Immunology

"Rudjer Bošković" Institute, Zagreb, Yugoslavia

Specific immunological unresponsiveness has been induced in a variety of animal species, and its effectiveness and duration varied with different regimens of injections and dosages of antigens. In adult mice, specific immunological unresponsiveness can be provoked after repeated inoculations of large doses /high-level paralysis/ and after repeated injections of minute doses of the same antigen /low-level paralysis/(1). According to the hypotesis of Mitchison and Dresser (2), excess of antigen acts directly upon immunologically competent cells, causing their blocade or death. However, this hypotesis can not explain the effects of minute doses of antigen in provoking the specific immunological unresponsiveness. Reapproaching this problem, the aim of our investigations was to find out whether the mechanism of induction of the specific immunological unresponsiveness caused by multiple injections of large or minute doses of antigen is the same, or two different processes resulting in similar effects.

MATERIALS AND METHODS

CBA mice of both sexes, 12 to 14 weeks old, weighing 20 to 22 grams were used. They were divided into 3 large groups and injected intraperitoneally with saline solution of crystalline bovine serum albumin (BSA) /Albumin Bovine Plasma cryst., A grade, Calbiochem, Los Angeles, California, batch No. 901689/, three times per week over the period of 50 days. The dosages for different groups of mice were: 0.01, 1.0 and 20.0 mg per injection. Three mice from each of the experimental groups mentioned above were sacrificed every second day. Mice were bled from jugular vessels, and serum from each animal was tested for the presence

673

of antibodies. These were detected by means of passive haemagglutination technique with Takátsy microtitratior. Spleen and lymph nodes of bled animals were taken for preparing smears and for histological analysis. The smears were fixed in methanol, and the tissues embedded in paraffin were cut in 4μ sections. Both the smears and the sections were stained with methyl-green pyronine. In each smear, 2,000 cells were counted, recording the percentage of large pyroninophilic cells and plasma cells. In a parallel experiment, mice received antigen according to the same schedules, and then half of them were challenged with BSA /7 mg of BSA incorporated in Freund's adjuvant/ after 16 days, and another half after 30 days of treatment. Three mice from each of these experimental groups were sacrificed every second day and analysed in the manner described previously.

RESULTS

In the group of mice receiving immunizing doses of BSA /1.0 mg per injection/, antigen provoked cyclic changes in the number of spleen blast cells (Figure 1) with maximums on days 2, 9 and 16 after the beginning of multiple injections. The number of blast cells observed on days 2 and 9 were significantly higher /P < 0.01/ that the values in nontreated mice. Inspite of the fact that the regimen of BSA injection continued, after the 16th day no further changes did occur in the number of blast cells. Significant increase in the number of plasma cells was observed on days 3 and 7 after the initiation of the treatment, and their number was permanently increased from the 25th day onward /P<0.01/. In the sera of these mice, antibodies never appeared before the 14th day after the beginning of the injection protocol, and were present in the sera up to the 40th day. Their titer varied, with maximums on days 16, 25 and 35.

In the groups of mice which were multiply injected with large or small doses of BSA, the number of blast and plasma cells in the spleen did not differ from the values in control animals. Antibodies were formed only in the sera of mice receiving large doses of BSA, but were present in very low titer. They appeared in the same time as in the group of mice injected with the immunizing doses of BSA . In this group of animals, antibodies were produced although the number of blast and plasma cells in the spleen did not increase above control values. Histological analysis, however, revealed changes in the structure of the spleen which were compatible with a weak immunological reaction. In the white pulp of the spleen of these mice scattered large pyroninophilic cells could be often detected. Thus, the weakened antibody production in the group of mice which were multiply injected with large doses of BSA could be attributed to the activity of a small number of immunologically competent cells, which were still active.

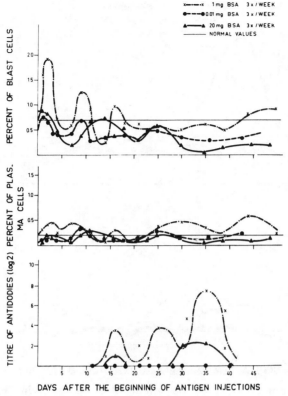

Figure 1. Cytological changes in the spleen and production of antibodies in mice multiply injected with various doses of BSA.

In order to test the effectiveness of multiple injections of large and small doses of BSA in provoking specific immunological unresponsiveness, mice in all three experimental groups were tested with a challenging dose of BSA incorporated in Freund's adjuvant. The challenge was given on day 16 and 30 after the initiation of multiple injections of BSA. When tested on day 16, mice in all three experimental groups reacted equally. In the spleen of these mice, the number of blast and plasma cells was significantly increased. When tested on day 30 after the initiation of multiple injection /Figure 2/, mice treated with immunizing doses of BSA reacted with proliferation of blast and plasma cells in the spleen, and 16 days later with appearance of antibodies in their sera. The kinetics of the appearance of antibodies followed the pattern of the kinetics observed in non-treated mice which only received a single injection of BSA incorporated in Freund's adjuvant. However, animals

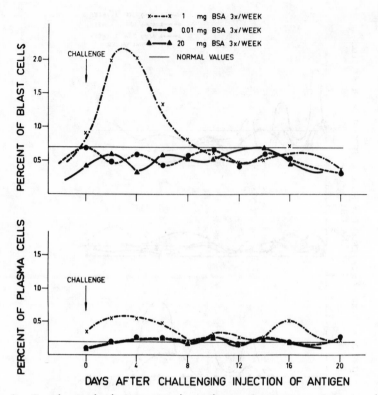

Figure 2. Cytological changes in the spleen of mice receiving multiple injections of various doses of BSA for 30 days, and then the challenging injection of the same antigen.

injected with large and small doses of BSA showed neither proliferation of blast and plasma cells in the spleen, nor production of humoral anti-bodies /Table 1/. In the sera of a small percentage of mice pretreated either with the small or the large doses of BSA , antibodies could be detected. Titer of these antibodies was practically identical with that observed in non-treated mice which only received a single injection of BSA incorporated in Freund's adjuvant. Thus, after the regimen of multiple injections of large or small doses of BSA over the period of 30 days, approximately 75 to 80% of all animals were rendered completely unresponsive to the challenging dose of the same antigen. Those mice which did react inspite of the paralysing treatment, produced antibodies in normal fashion.

Table 1. Antibody production in mice receiving multiple injections of various doses of BSA for 30 days, and then the challenging injection of the same antigen.

DOSE OF BSA PER INJECTION (mg)	PERCENT OF REACTIVE ANIMALS AT DAYS AFTER THE BEGINNING OF MULTIPLE INJECTIONS OF BSA				
	16 – 30	30	31 – 40	41 – 50	51 – 60
0.01	0 (0/25)*		0 (0/18)	11 (1/9)	33 (2/6)
20	24 (6/21)	CHALLENGE	45 (8/18)	45 (4/9)	17 (1/6)
—	—		0 (0/18)	33 (3/9)	100 (6/6)

* IN PARENTHESES INDIVIDUAL SCORES (NUMBER OF REACTIVE ANIMALS / TOTAL NUMBER) ARE INDICATED

DISCUSSION

Analysis of the smears and histological sections of the spleen and lymph nodes of mice multiply injected with small doses of BSA revealed that this treatment did not provoke any visible changes in the lymphoid organs. Also, no antibody production occured. These data suggest that the mechanism responsible for this type of immunological areactivity is probably blocade of differentiation and proliferation of immunologically competent cells. Those animals in which this mechanism, by some reason, did not operate, reacted after the challenging dose with normal production of antibodies.

Mice multiply injected with large doses of BSA also did not show significant changes in lymphoid organs. However, histological analysis of the spleens and the analysis of the sera revealed the existence of an immunological reaction. Between days 31 and 40, when antibodies were produced in all mice receiving the immunizing schedule of BSA injections, low titer of antibodies was detected only in 45% of animals treated with large doses of BSA . These findings suggest that large doses of BSA first induced an immunological reaction, which was then suppressed by subsequent injections of antigen (3). At the time of testing, only 45% of mice had antibodies in their sera, but in very low titer. These antibodies evidently appeared due to the treatment with multiple injections of BSA and not due to the challenging injection, because in mice which only received a single injection of BSA in Freund's adjuvant, antibodies do not appear before day 14 after imunization. As a consequence of pretreatment with large doses, the challenging dose of the same antigen was ineffective in triggering the production of antibodies in 83% of animals. Again, mice which did react, produced antibodies in the same amount as control animals which only received a single injection of BSA in Freund's adjuvant.

In conclusion, our data suggest 1. that mice pretreated with multiple injections of BSA in doses which induce specific immunological unresponsiveness, react after the challenging dose of the antigen in an all-or-none fashion. In other words, if the paralysing treatment operated, it rendered animals completely unresponsive, 2. that there are probably two different mechanisms by which the specific immunological unrespon-siveness may be induced. One by multiple injections of minute amounts of antigen which inhibit differentiation and proliferation of immunologically competent cells, and the second, by multiple injections of large doses of antigen which gradually suppress the already provoked immunological reaction.

REFERENCES

1.   N.A. Mitchison, Proc. Roy. Soc. B., 161 : 275, 1964.

2.   D.V. Dresser, and N.A. Mitchison, Adv. Immunol., 8 : 129, 1968.

3.   J. Šterzl, Nature, 209 : 416, 1966.

THE IMMOBILIZATION OF LYMPHOID CELLS IN THE DEVELOPING PALATINE

TONSIL OF THE RABBIT

W. Leene

Laboratorium v. Elektronen-Mikroscopie

Amsterdam, The Netherlands

During the embryonic development of the rabbit, the palatine tonsils are the first lympho-epithelial organs in which lymphoid cells appear.

It seems relevant to the problem of the ontogenetic precursors of plasma cells in mammals to investigate the nature of the first appearing lymphoid cells in the palatine tonsil.

On the 22nd day of gestation lymphoid cells appear underneath the bottom of the primary crypt. On the 23rd day, junctions are formed between lymphoid cells and cells of the condensed mesenchyme. In the same stage the first lymphoid cells are seen to migrate into the epithelium of the bottom of the crypt.

The ultrastructure of the lymphoid cells in the different localizations will be demonstrated by the following electron micrographs:

a) lymphoid cell from the outside of the tonsillar area having the features of a mobile lymphoid cell;

b) junctions between lymphoid cells and mesenchymal cells in the area of condensed mesenchyme (the two cell types are easy to distinguish);

c) the junctions are "close junctions" (according to Trelstad, the formation of this type of junctions may result in the cell motility being inhibited);

d) changed morphology of lymphoid cells contacting mesenchymal cells after 24 hrs; cells and nuclei are round, the pseudo-pods have disappeared, the cytoplasm no longer contains fibrils, the cell density increases, but the junctions are of the same type as in earlier stages.

From these observations it may be concluded that: 1) in the palatine tonsil of the rabbit there are no transformations from epithelial or mesenchymal cells into lymphoid cells; 2) the lymphoid cells are therefore of extrinsic origin; they migrate into the area of condensed mesenchyme, and subsequently into the epithelium; 3) in the area of condensed mesenchyme the lymphoid cells are immobilized by the formation of "close junctions" with mesenchymal cells, which may point to a possible mechanism for the "homing" of lymphoid cells in this lymphatic primordium.

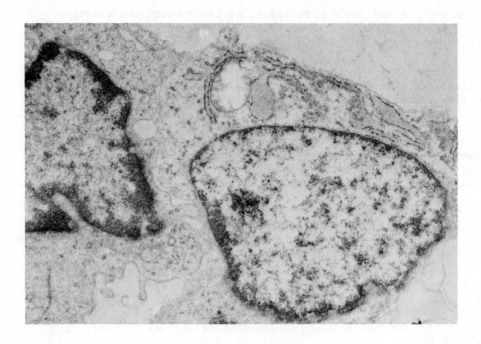

Fig. 1. Lymphoid cell contacting mesenchymal cell in a 23 days' embryonic rabbit palatine tonsil.

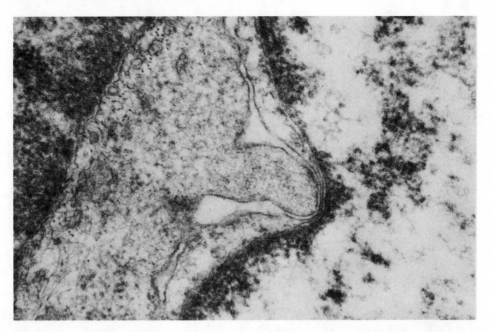

Fig. 2. A newly formed "close junction" between a lymphoid cell and a mesenchymal cell in a 23 days' embryonic rabbit palatine tonsil.